Pharmacology and Medicines Management for Nurses

For Churchill Livingstone:

Senior Commissioning Editor: Ninette Premdas
Project Development Manager: Mairi McCubbin
Project Manager: Derek Robertson
Designer: Judith Wright

Pharmacology and Medicines Management for Nurses

George Downie MSc FRPharmS
Medicines Unit Manager/Trust Chief Pharmacist, Grampian Primary Care NHS Trust, Aberdeen, UK

Jean Mackenzie BA(Open) RGN SCM DipN(Lond) RCT RNT
Lecturer, School of Nursing and Midwifery, The Robert Gordon University, Aberdeen, UK

Arthur Williams OBE FRPharmS
Formerly Chief Administrative Pharmaceutical Officer, Grampian, Orkney, Shetland and Tayside Health Boards

THIRD EDITION

ELSEVIER
CHURCHILL LIVINGSTONE

Edinburgh London New York Oxford Philadelphia St Louis Sydney Toronto 2003

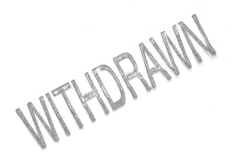

CHURCHILL LIVINGSTONE
An imprint of Elsevier Limited

First edition 1995
Second edition 1999
Third edition 2003
Reprinted 2004, 2005

ISBN 0 443 07176 4

British Library Cataloguing in Publication Data
A catalogue record for this book is available from the British Library

Library of Congress Cataloguing in Publication Data
A catalogue record for this book is available from the Library of Congress

Notice
Medical knowledge is constantly changing. Standard safety precautions must be followed, but as new research and clinical experience broaden our knowledge, changes in treatment and drug therapy may become necessary or appropriate. Readers are advised to check the most current product information provided by the manufacturer of each drug to be administered to verify the recommended dose, the method and duration of administration, and contraindications. It is the responsibility of the practitioner, relying onexperience and knowledge of the patient, to determine dosages and the best treatment for each individual patient. Neither the publisher nor the authors assume any liability for any injury and/or damage to persons or property arising from this publication.
The Publisher

The publisher's policy is to use **paper manufactured from sustainable forests**

Printed in China

Contents

Preface

For this third edition we have taken into account the many helpful suggestions made by both readers and reviewers. The chapters in the new Section 1 have been enhanced and the order has been changed to reflect the vital importance of the nurse in achieving the safe and effective management of medicines. The administration of oral, parenteral and transdermal medicines is covered in Chapter 9. Other methods of administration are included in association with the relevant drug treatment chapter. New appendices, and a glossary have been introduced, and it is hoped that these will be useful to nurses, midwives and students.

It should be noted that the text is intended for nurses involved in the care of adult patients. However, where it is felt to be appropriate, some consideration is given to particular aspects that affect the drug treatment of infants and children. The guidance given in the BNF regarding the name changes of medicinal substances has been followed. Rapid developments in both new drugs and new treatment methods have been included as far as this is possible in an era of great scientific progress.

We are conscious of the pressures being experienced by all healthcare professionals in meeting the high standards rightly expected of them. Our sincere hope is that this book will make a positive contribution in one very important aspect of the nurse's care of patients.

Aberdeen 2003

George Downie
Jean Mackenzie
Arthur Williams

Acknowledgements

Grateful acknowledgement is made for the help and support received from colleagues working within the NHS in Grampian. We recognise the value of being able to draw on the expertise of colleagues practising in a number of specialities. In particular, Mrs Jill Kettle has given invaluable advice on the chapter on drugs acting on the CNS. Mrs Thora Baeyens has expertly advised on the role of the nurse in the community; Mrs Fiona Crowther on the role of the practice nurse; and Miss Carol Edgar on the role of the community midwife. Our sincere thanks go to Dr D. M. Levy (Queen's Medical Centre, Nottingham) for the chapter on anaesthetic agents. Mrs Lesley Anderson has once again risen to the challenge of completing the mammoth task within a tight timeframe. Lesley is an invaluable member of the team who has made an outstanding contribution to this publication.

SECTION 1

Medicines management

SECTION CONTENTS

CHAPTER CONTENTS

1

Medicines today

INTRODUCTION

Mankind has always been subject to injury and disease. Our ancestors perhaps faced less self-inflicted illness than is seen today (due to unhealthy lifestyles) but then, as now, medicines were needed to alleviate pain and suffering. Our expectations of medicines have increased, just as they have in other technological aspects of our lives. Today, those who prescribe, administer and use medicines rightly demand safety, efficacy, economy and convenience from their medicines. Even after decades of very significant progress these demands cannot always be fully met. Great progress has been made on the safety of medicines, but events of recent years demonstrate that there is no room for complacency. Efficacy has also improved but we still have very few cures; indeed, effective treatment for a number of conditions still appears to be many years away. Nevertheless, we do have some cures and a range of products which help to control symptoms and improve the quality of life for many people. However, the very real advances of recent years have not been achieved without the expenditure of vast sums of money. The development of new drugs is a very high-risk business, and the costs of new treatments reflect this. An individual course of treatment can now cost several thousand pounds and, even then, benefits to the patient may not be seen and cannot be guaranteed. Just as the drugs have been improved so have the means of delivery, thus increasing convenience to the user as well as reducing adverse effects and improving targeting.

On the establishment of the National Health Service in 1948, the range of safe and effective medicines available to the prescriber was very limited indeed. Most of the drugs that are now taken for granted were not even a gleam in the eye of the molecular chemist in 1948. Safe and effective cardiovascular drugs, anticancer agents, oral diuretics and psychoactive drugs did not exist. In the 1950s, simple, though not always harmless,

Table 1.1 Progress in drug development in the last 80 years

Decade	Drugs developed
1920s	Insulin
1940s	Penicillin and streptomycin
1950s	Chlorpromazine, corticosteroids and thiazide diuretics
1960s	Benzodiazepines, ampicillin, vinblastine, melphalan, propranolol and cytarabine
1970s	Cefalexin, enflurane, doxorubicin, clotrimazole, naproxen, streptokinase and cimetidine
1980s	Clozapine, salmeterol, lisinopril, goserelin, erythropoietin and ranitidine
1990s	Monoclonal antibodies, colfosceril and lamotrigine, third-generation cephalosporins, anticancer agents, and products such as insulin lispro produced by recombinant techniques using sophisticated biological methods
2000s	Gene therapy, more drugs from natural sources, more emphasis on chemoprevention, cell/organ transplantation. Safer drugs

inorganic and organic chemicals and products of very dubious composition derived from naturally occurring products such as roots, leaves and barks were widely prescribed. Natural products remain a very important source of valuable medicines but today we have sophisticated methods of extraction, purification and standardisation which, in the case of licensed medicines, guarantees consistency of quality. Methods of drug delivery were also very basic indeed, with oral solid dosage forms adequate but crude by today's standards. Simple oral liquid preparations were often poorly formulated, foul-tasting and inconvenient to use. Although some quality assurance procedures were in place, these were aimed at testing the final product rather than controlling the whole manufacturing process. The Medicines Act of 1968 marked a new beginning in the control of all aspects of the production, testing and marketing of medicines. Some idea of the progress made in the last 80 years can be gained from the summary shown in Table 1.1.

There is no doubt that the efforts of the pharmaceutical industry will continue to be directed towards producing medicines that meet the needs of both patients and health professionals caring for them. Standards of production and quality assurance are very high indeed. Before a product can be given a product licence and marketed, safety and efficacy must be established, although proof of a therapeutic advance over existing products is not required in the UK, nor is evidence of cost-effectiveness.

Figure 1.1 gives an outline of the stages involved in bringing a new medicine into use in the UK. Only

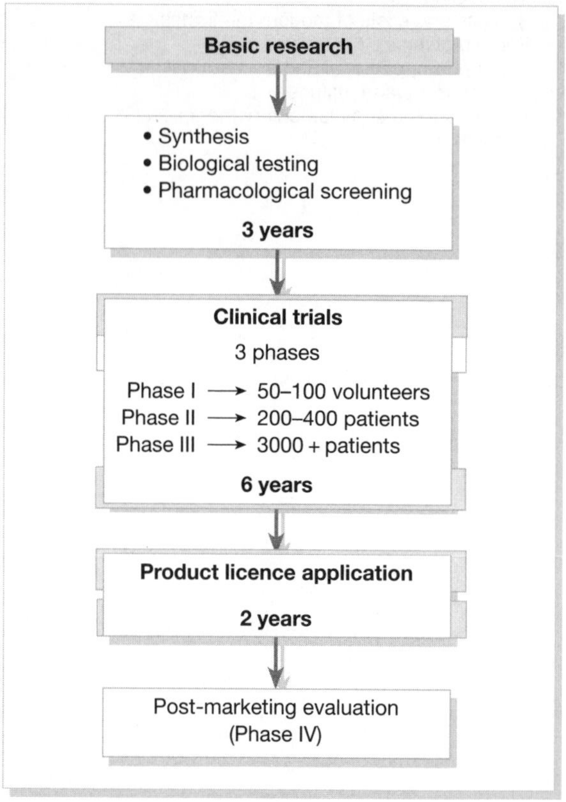

Figure 1.1 Stages in the development of a new medicine.

international companies with vast resources can hope to remain competitive in the global market. The whole process may cost several hundred million pounds. In view of the high cost of drug development, it is not surprising that the large drug companies use very sophisticated marketing techniques in order to maximise their returns. A strict code of practice covers the pharmaceutical industry's promotion of medicines to members of the health professions.

BENEFITS AND COSTS OF MODERN MEDICINES

Today, many patients are enjoying both a longer and better quality of life as a result of drug treatment. Perhaps the most dramatic example of this is the control of certain infections which, 50 years ago, would almost certainly have had a fatal outcome. Drugs acting on the cardiovascular system, the newer insulins, oncolytic agents and psychotropic drugs have prolonged and improved life for many patients. Safer anaesthetic agents have played a major part in the surgical advances of recent years. At a time when the resources available for healthcare are under great pressure, health service managers are required to examine carefully all competing demands. The drug bill is no exception to this process. Unfortunately, techniques for economic evaluation of drug treatments have not been fully developed and, as a result, the debate on cost benefits of drug treatments may be based on consideration of drug costs only. There is a need for an informed public debate on this aspect of healthcare, especially when issues of rationing care and inequalities of provision are involved. The pharmaceutical industry has an excellent record of innovation, and the new drugs produced must be sold in order to recover costs and make profits for further investment. Sales promotion may cause tensions and pressures within the NHS but improved understandings are developing, especially in the context of the development of joint working between hospitals and community-based services. In order to avoid 'postcode prescribing' (variation in the availability of medicines between different points of the country (UK)), national mechanisms are now in place to evaluate new drug treatments and make recommendations on prescribing. The National Institute for Clinical Excellence (NICE) covers England and Wales, and the Health Technology Board fulfils the same functions to the NHS in Scotland. The British National Formulary (BNF) reproduces NICE guidance on a number of drugs, e.g. on the taxanes and other oncolytic drugs. Choices do have to be made between various forms of treatment. Local drug formularies help the process of choice so that prescribing costs are contained without compromising treatment, safety and efficacy. The public debate on inequalities of provision of healthcare in different locations in the UK will intensify as pressure on resources increases.

SOME PROBLEMS

Although many patients derive great benefit from their medicines, the search for the 'magic bullet' goes on, especially in oncology. All medicines have the potential to cause harm to the patient, even when used in standard doses. Many patients, especially older patients, suffer from more than one condition, resulting in multiple drug therapy. The risk of drug interactions thus increases but the risk of actual harm to the patient is low in well-managed situations since the professionals involved in the management of medicines take steps to protect the patient from such eventualities. Chapter 4 describes the vital contribution made by the nurse in helping to ensure that the patient derives benefit from the prescribed treatment.

The emergence of bacterial resistance to even the newer drugs is of great concern, and improved methods of preventing and treating blood-borne viral diseases will be required.

Abuse of chemicals is of growing concern throughout the world, a particular concern being the use of so-called 'recreational' drugs. Much drug abuse is based on the use of illegal substances but medicines can be abused with equally devastating outcomes for the abusers and their families. Dependency on drugs may arise as the result of bona fide medical treatment but this is rare. There is increasing concern about the extent to which patients may become dependent on benzodiazepines and other anxiolytic drugs. Legislation is in place designed to reduce the likelihood of drugs being diverted for abuse but there can be no substitute for vigilance by all members of the healthcare team when involved in the management of medicines with the potential for abuse. Even in the best-regulated organisation there will always be a need to dispose of time-expired, surplus and obsolete drugs. Legal and environmental considerations require that such drugs be disposed of in a way that does not damage the environment. Incineration under controlled conditions may be needed to meet the legal requirements.

SOME PUBLIC, PERSONAL AND PROFESSIONAL PERCEPTIONS AND ATTITUDES

Health promotion resources are targeted at prevention strategies, such as a healthy lifestyle, but the belief that health can be achieved or maintained by the use of medicines is still widely held. All health professionals must seek to ensure that patients have realistic expectations of their drug therapy, and know when and why drug therapy is needed.

Economic and other pressures have led to campaigns designed to encourage people to take more responsibility for their own health and to form health alliances. One outcome of this is the increasing sales of proprietary medicines both of the traditional type and less orthodox remedies. There can be no doubt of the importance of self-medication in healthcare. The NHS would collapse if all the demands for medicines had to be met from NHS resources alone. There are dangers in assuming that proprietary over-the-counter (OTC) medicines are completely safe and can be treated as placebos. As more medicines are made available for supervised sales by pharmacists, the likelihood of drug interactions or other complications will increase.

One key objective of the NHS is to provide patients with comprehensive information about all aspects of their treatment. Linked with this is the need to ensure that patients and their carers have all the necessary information to enable courses of drug treatment to be completed successfully. A coordinated approach between professionals is called for on the provision of relevant non-conflicting information. The recognition of the need for a wider range of information on treatment is a product of both consumer pressures and changing attitudes within the professions. Care is needed to ensure that the information needs and views of ethnic minorities are recognised and responded to.

As yet, prescription medicines cannot be advertised to the public in the UK. In the USA such advertisements are allowed, and free telephone numbers offer callers a detailed information service. Even money-off coupons have been used to promote the use of certain products. Web site addresses are given where detailed information can be accessed. Patients, especially those involved in an 'interest group', may, on occasion, be better informed on the details of a particular treatment than some health professionals.

Personal factors

The realisation that patients and their families hold, and are entitled to hold, their own beliefs about treatment is recognised by the Patient's Charter (Scottish Office Home and Health Department 1991). Patients (and their families) can formulate views on a proposed treatment only if they are in possession of relevant information about the condition, the nature and effects of the treatment, the alternatives available and the consequences of not accepting treatment. The right of the patient or client follows the principle of informed consent which is based on the individual having the necessary knowledge to make a decision (NMC 2002). There may be situations, however, where it is in patients' best interests not to provide full information on their drug therapy.

From time to time it may be necessary to change a patient's drug therapy. The reasons for any changes must be clearly explained to the patient by the prescriber, particularly where changes are made for economic reasons. A medicine which has proved to be highly successful in treating a particular condition plays an important part in the patient's life. There may be an understandable reluctance, on the part of the patient, to accept the change. Nurses and pharmacists can play an important part in providing the patient with any necessary reassurance when drug treatment is changed for whatever reason. It should be remembered, too, that the patient has the right to refuse to take the medication. Were this to happen, details of the refusal must be documented. Major problems could arise if insulin or high-dose steroids, for example, were refused.

Social factors

The ethical issues relating to medicines with which society is confronted raise questions rather than provide answers. For example, should the pharmaceutical industry be making profits out of illness? Some would argue that profits are the result of innovation and great capital investment which must be rewarded. Should animals be used for testing new drugs? Clearly, animal rights campaigners think not, whereas others regard such practice as acceptable if humanely carried out. What then of clinical drug trials on humans? In the advanced stages of testing there is no practicable alternative. Wider issues about pollution of the environment, with chemical waste arising from the manufacturing processes involved in drug production, may also be a concern. Very strict legislation does provide a high degree of protection, but concerns will always exist. Dependence, addiction and over-reliance on drugs raise doubts in the minds of many health professionals. Nurses are required to enter into the debate on the ethical aspects of the use of medicines as part of their professional role. Local ethics committees provide guidance on specific matters, particularly on ethical aspects of clinical trials. There may be situations where, on religious grounds, a nurse cannot be involved in a particular form of treatment. This stance has to be respected and accepted by colleagues without any form of sanction being applied. Nurses in such situations will receive the support they need but, as always, the best interests of the patient must be served.

Professional factors

Doctors want to be able to help their patients get better. However, there are factors which doctors must consider before deciding which is the best treatment (or indeed whether or not to treat the patient at all). For example, the decision may be influenced by the likely side-effects, the risk of dependence on the drug, the age of the patient and the patient's prognosis. Difficulties may arise when there are conflicting professional views on prescribing. Medical misadventures can also have a profound effect on a doctor's prescribing behaviour many years after the event. Downward pressure on prescribing costs must not be allowed to compromise patient care. Well-researched prescribing policies and protocols must take into account cost factors, but all healthcare professionals have a duty to provide the best for their patients in the light of the current state of knowledge. When to withhold treatment may be a more difficult decision than when to initiate treatment.

ALTERNATIVE AND COMPLEMENTARY THERAPIES

Interest in alternative and complementary medicine is increasing. Patients seek relief from a range of problems such as pain, allergies, gastrointestinal and psychological conditions. In a study by Moore et al (1985) it was found that patients interviewed were not 'cranks' and had not lost confidence in conventional medicine. A high percentage of patients often felt better after the treatment.

The range of alternative therapies is very wide but only those involving the use of medicines are briefly discussed here. Homeopathy has been a source of help for many patients over the years, and homeopathic treatment is available via the NHS. Herbal remedies are used by many people in the belief that they are natural and completely safe. A number of studies have shown that this belief may be seriously flawed (MacGregor et al 1989). Side-effects arising from herbal treatments are well documented. Hepatotoxicity, pulmonary and veno-occlusive disease have been shown to be caused by herbal remedies. However, it should not be forgotten that many valuable and effective drugs are derived from natural sources. There appears to be no doubt that patients will continue to seek relief from alternative and complementary medicines. In many instances patients have access to complementary therapies in addition to conventional therapy, a holistic approach being adopted by the responsible health professionals.

THE FUTURE

Based on experience since the establishment of the NHS, it can be confidently predicted that the search for new and more effective drug treatments, using technologies as yet unknown, will continue and that the search will be successful. Efforts will be made to ensure that drugs are more specific in their actions and can be delivered to the site of action. Gene therapy may provide a more fundamental approach to the control of certain diseases. Research on the use of embryonic stem cells, although controversial, appears to offer great promise for the future.

Patients and their carers will become even better informed, and the legislation controlling all aspects of the marketing and use of medicines may be reviewed in the light of changes in the provision of healthcare. In the USA, a drug company arranged to meet patient groups to discuss plans for clinical trials and clinical research. AIDS patients lobbied doctors and politicians and this led to fast-track approval for certain innovative treatments (Fricker 1997).

It seems certain that information technology will become increasingly important in supporting the safer use of medicines by such developments as electronic prescribing and telemedicine. Drug costs have always been a major cause for concern in the NHS. It appears certain that this and other concerns will continue to test the mettle of those who provide and manage health services.

As with all developments in healthcare, nurses in both community and hospital practice will continue to play a key role. Increased provision of care in the community will place additional demands on nurses. The development of nurse prescribing will further expand that role, which it is hoped will continue to develop in line with the needs of our patients.

REFERENCES

Fricker J 1997 The AIDS effect. Rx The Sunday Telegraph, 30 November 16–17

MacGregor F B, Abernethy V E, Dahabra S et al 1989 Hepatotoxicity of herbal remedies. British Medical Journal 299:1156–1157

Moore J, Phipps K, Mareer D et al 1985 Why do people seek treatment by alternative medicine? British Medical Journal 290:28–29

Nursing and Midwifery Council (NMC) 2002 Code of professional conduct. NMC, London

Scottish Office Home and Health Department 1991 The patient's charter: a charter for health. SOHDD, Edinburgh

FURTHER READING

Association of British Pharmaceutical Industries (ABPI) 2001 Code of Practice for the Pharmaceutical Industry. ABPI, London

Brown M E 2001 What is a drug? Pharmaceutical Journal 267:301–302

Edworthy S M 2001 Editorial: Telemedicine in Developing Countries 323:524–525

McCarthy A 2001 Pharmacogenetics. British Medical Journal 322:1007–1008

Mintzes B, Barer M L 2002 Influence of direct to consumer pharmaceutical advertising and patients' requests on prescribing decisions: two site cross sectional survey. British Medical Journal 324:278–279
Moynihan R, Heath I, Henry D 2002 Selling sickness: the pharmaceutical industry and disease mongering. British Medical Journal 324:886–890
Sculpher M, Drummond M, O'Brien B 2001 Effectiveness, efficiency and NICE. British Medical Journal 322:943–944
Vincent C 2001 The safety of acupuncture. British Medical Journal 323:467–468
Westbrook J I, Duggan A E 2001 Prescriptions for antiulcer drugs in Australia: volume, trends and costs. British Medical Journal 323:1338–1339

CHAPTER CONTENTS

2

Control of medicines in hospital and community

INTRODUCTION

Medicines are subject to a range of control in terms of legislation as well as local policies and procedures. This is necessary to ensure that:

- medicines are manufactured to the highest standards
- medicines are tested and evaluated before being licensed
- the potential for abuse is minimised
- medicines are stored securely under appropriate conditions
- medicines are used in such a way as to minimise risk to both patient and donor
- medicines are administered appropriately to enable the best possible therapeutic outcome to be achieved.

The manufacture, packaging and distribution of medicines depend on the expertise of the pharmaceutical industry. At local level the pharmaceutical service provides a comprehensive service designed to meet the needs of patients and those providing medical and nursing care. The objectives of achieving successful patient care depend on the integrity and security of all stages of the supply chain from manufacturer to patient. All those involved in using medicines for diagnosis, treatment or palliation must be aware of the need to ensure compliance with their legal and professional responsibilities.

LEGAL CLASSIFICATION OF MEDICINAL PRODUCTS

The supply, storage and use of all medicinal products are controlled by the Medicines Act 1968. Three classes of products are defined in the Act; these are shown in Box 2.1. Additional legislation for Controlled Drugs is provided by the Misuse of Drugs Act 1971. The

Box 2.1 Classes of products defined by the Medicines Act 1968

General Sale List (GSL)
Medicines which can be sold in a general store. (Some GSL medicines may only be sold in a pharmacy but direct pharmaceutical supervision is not required.)

Pharmacy medicines (P)
Medicines which may be sold only under the personal control of a pharmacist. There is no statutory list of pharmacy medicines.

Prescription-only medicines (PoMs)
Medicines that can be sold or supplied on prescription only.

Medicines Act is concerned primarily with regulating the legitimate use of medicines; the Misuse of Drugs Act is concerned with the prevention of the abuse of Controlled Drugs.

Certain legal requirements apply to the sale, supply, dispensing and labelling of each class of medicinal product. These requirements are applicable mainly in the community, e.g. sale/supply of medicines by community pharmacists and others. In hospital practice, all medicines are treated in the same way, no distinction being made between the different classes listed in Box 2.1. However, Controlled Drugs are subject to additional security and recording requirements. The key elements of the legislation that affect nursing practice are described below.

Prescription-only medicines

There are three classes of PoM:

- medicinal products containing listed substances
- medicinal products containing a drug controlled under the Misuse of Drugs Act 1971
- medicinal products for parenteral use (there are some specific exemptions).

The Medicines Act provides that no one may administer a PoM otherwise than to himself, unless he is a practitioner (registered doctor, dentist or nurse) or is acting in accordance with the directions of a practitioner. Certain exemptions to this rule are made in the case of life-saving drugs, e.g. adrenaline (epinephrine), certain antihistamines, antidotes, etc.; normally this exemption would not apply in hospitals.

The administration of medicines is normally covered by a health authority policy statement which permits administration of medicines *only* in accordance with the written prescription of a medical, dental or nurse practitioner. The only exception to this rule is where a Patient Group Direction has been set up (see p. 44).

Prescribing of PoMs

In hospital practice the inpatient prescription includes directions to the nurse for administration of the medicine. If a prescription is written for an outpatient, more details of the patient are required than would be the case for an inpatient, e.g. address of patient and quantity of medicine to be supplied. In the community, a prescription from the patient's general practitioner is required. These are mostly computer generated.

Emergency supply of PoMs

In hospital practice, situations under which medicines can be supplied without a prescription will be defined in the local code of practice for medicine management. A community pharmacist can, under specified conditions, supply PoMs in an emergency without a prescription, on the request of a doctor or an individual patient.

Exemptions from controls

Special arrangements apply to particular classes of persons, e.g. midwives, chiropodists, ophthalmic opticians, ambulance paramedics and Masters of ships (consult specialist literature for details).

Labelling of medicinal products

Standard labelling requirements are described in the Act. This is a matter for the manufacturer or pharmacist to comply with (Figs 2.1 and 2.2). The main particulars included on a label of a medicinal product are listed below – it is important to note that the information on the label must be clear, legible, comprehensible and in English:

- the name of the product – this may be an approved name and/or a proprietary name
- the pharmaceutical form, e.g. tablets, capsules, etc.
- the strength of the product, distinguishing between active and non-active ingredients
- the quantity in the container expressed in appropriate terms, e.g. in the case of tablets the number of dosage units, in the case of an ointment the weight contained in the pack
- list of excipients known to have a recognisable action
- any special storage instructions including a warning to keep out of the reach of children
- method/route of administration

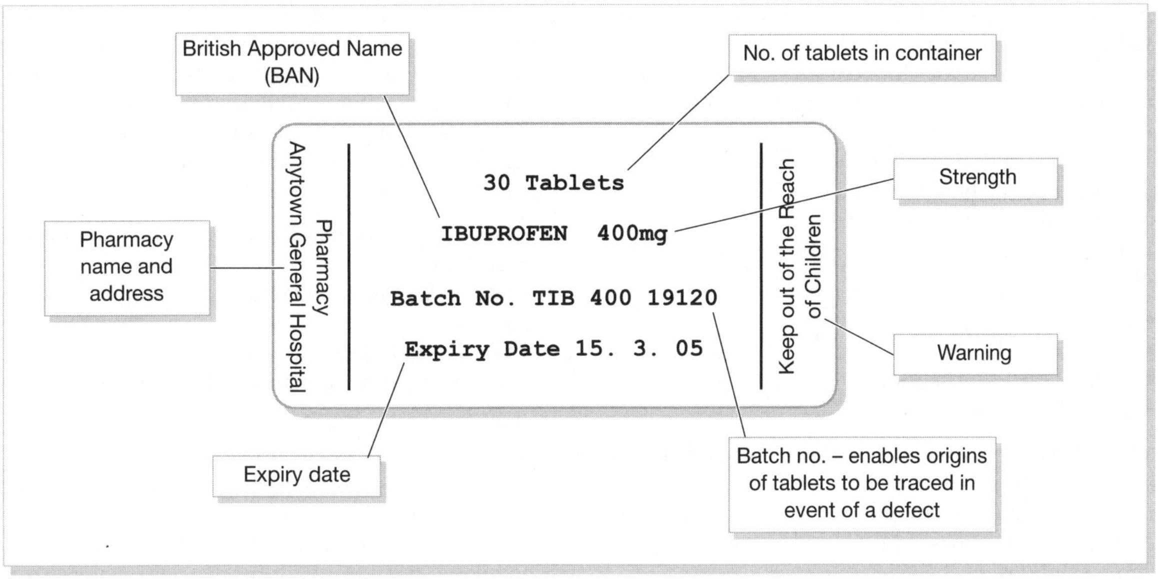

Figure 2.1 Example of a pharmacy-generated label.

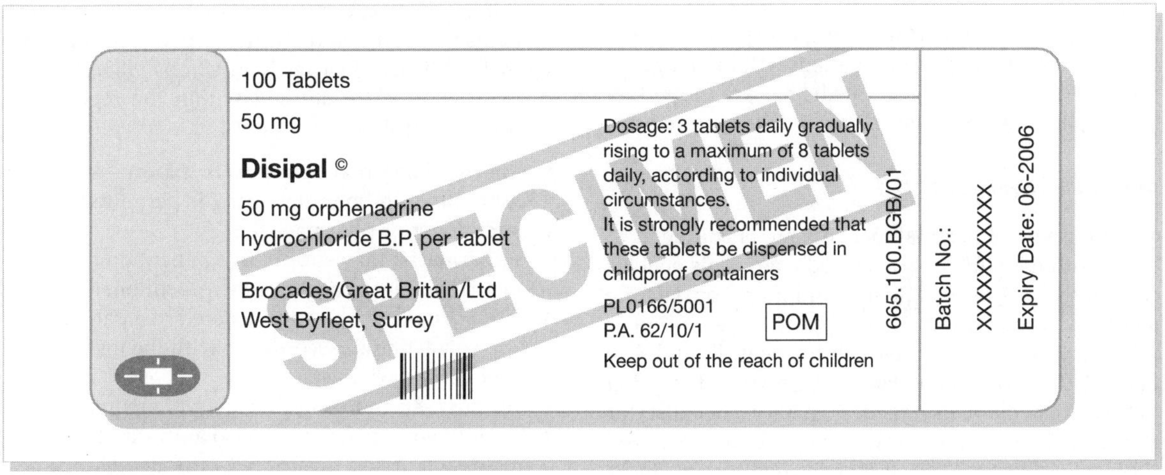

Figure 2.2 Example of information on manufacturer's original pack.

- a date after which the product should not be used (expiry date)
- any special warnings required by the marketing authorisation for the product
- name and address of the holder of the marketing authorisation and number of this authorisation
- batch reference number
- instructions for use if for self-medication
- special precautions for disposal.

Particulars of special labelling requirements are given in the literature, e.g. if a product contains hexachlorophene the label should carry a warning 'not to be used for babies'.

Additional labelling requirements apply to dispensed medicines. It is common in hospital practice for the pharmacist to add further information to labels in response to local need such as colour change of tablet.

Storage of medicinal products in hospital

Although different classes of drugs are recognised under the Medicines Act, in hospital practice *all* medicinal products are treated in the same way, i.e. secure storage in locked cupboards. In many instances, the controls applied to the different types of medicine in hospitals exceed the basic legal requirements. This is necessary to ensure the protection and safety of both patients and staff. Health authorities have a duty to ensure that regulations are drawn up and applied to all aspects of the use of medicines.

Separate locked cupboards are required for the following:

- internal medicines
- external medicines
- disinfectants/antiseptics
- clinical reagents.

A lockable drug refrigerator is also required. Separate sections will be required within a cupboard or refrigerator, e.g. to segregate oral preparations from injections. Other storage facilities are provided for larger-volume sterile solutions.

Self-administration systems

Where it is considered appropriate (e.g. during the week before discharge) for a patient within an agreed protocol to self-administer medicine, an individual locked patient medication cabinet will be required.

Patients' own drugs (PODs)

On admission to hospital, patients are encouraged to bring with them their current medicines. This enables current therapy to be validated and if appropriate the medicines can be used. There appear to be a number of advantages in using PODs in hospital (Fradgley & Pryce 2002). However, risks may be involved in using PODs. To avoid these risks a quality checklist for assessment of patients' own drugs should be used (Fradgley & Pryce 2002). If it is decided to use PODs, suitable arrangements must be made for safe storage of the drugs. Separate storage in a locked individual patient medication cabinet may be appropriate, especially if the patient is to self-administer medicines. It should be remembered that the medicines brought in by patients are the patients' property and permission should be sought either to use them or dispose of them.

CONTROLLED DRUGS

Drugs of addiction which produce dependence (see Ch. 18) such as diamorphine and pethidine require special controls. The Misuse of Drugs Act 1971 and the Misuse of Drugs Regulations 1985 regulate the importation, export, supply and use of such drugs. The misuse of drugs is a very serious offence. Offences are dealt with taking into account all circumstances including the harmful nature of the drug that is misused.

Controlled Drugs are classified according to their potential to cause harm if abused. Drugs in Class A are the most harmful.

- Class A, e.g. cocaine, diamorphine, methadone and morphine
- Class B, e.g. oral amfetamines, barbiturates and codeine
- Class C, e.g. buprenorphine, most benzodiazepines, cannabis and clenbuterol.

Within the regulations, five schedules are defined. The details in the schedules are not of great practical interest to nurses but aspects of supply, possession, prescribing and record keeping are important. Most drugs used in clinical practice are subject to Schedule 2 requirements. Schedule 3 includes barbiturates and temazepam. Strictly according to the law, records are not required to be kept of temazepam, but in view of the great potential for abuse, Controlled Drug records are made.

The use of Controlled Drugs in medicine is permitted by the Misuse of Drugs Regulations 1985. Different levels of control are applied within the regulations. The main controls are as follows:

- A licence is needed to import or export.
- Compounding/manufacturing is permitted by a practitioner or pharmacist.
- A pharmacist may supply to a patient on the prescription of an appropriate practitioner.
- These drugs may be administered to a patient by a person acting in accordance with the instructions of a doctor or dentist.
- Safe custody and record keeping are required.
- The following persons are also authorised to be in possession of and to supply Controlled Drugs:
  - medical or dental practitioner
  - matron or acting matron of a hospital or nursing home
  - the sister or acting sister for the time being in charge of a ward, theatre or other department.

The authority is limited to obtaining ward stocks from no other source than the pharmacist responsible for the dispensing of medicines in the particular hospital. In some situations, where there is no on-site pharmacy, the hospital pharmacy normally providing the pharmaceutical service is regarded as being within this provision. Limitations are applied to the authorisations, in that they apply only so far as is necessary for the practice or exercise of their profession. A sister or acting sister in charge of a ward, theatre or department may not supply any Controlled Drug other than for administration to a patient in accordance with the prescription of a doctor (or dentist). It should be noted that, apart from healthcare personnel, other groups of workers are permitted to possess/supply Controlled Drugs, e.g. the Master of a ship, person in charge of a recognised laboratory, manager of an offshore installation.

Certain barbiturates and appetite suppressants (e.g. diethylpropion) are also classed as Controlled Drugs. All the requirements for prescription writing, ordering, recording and storing Controlled Drugs apply to the following drugs:

- amobarbital
- butobarbital
- phenobarbital
- secobarbital.

Because of its use in the treatment of epilepsy, the regulations covering phenobarbital are not so comprehensive in that neither the handwriting requirements (see below) nor the storage and recording requirements for Controlled Drugs apply.

Supply of Controlled Drugs to addicts

Special regulations are applicable to the supply of Controlled Drugs to persons who are dependent on such drugs. For example, only a doctor who holds a licence issued by the Secretary of State may prescribe certain Controlled Drugs (e.g. diamorphine, dipipanone) for a dependent person. (Any doctor may prescribe Controlled Drugs to an opioid-dependent person for the treatment of pain.) A special prescription form is used to enable people dependent on opioids to receive daily supplies of methadone for consumption under supervision. This procedure is designed to limit the diversion of methadone for illegal purposes. Prescribers in drug treatment centres may be given exemption to 'own handwriting' requirements. This allows the use of rubber stamps for prescribing.

Controlled Drugs in hospital

Certain of the legal requirements concerning drug control do not apply in hospitals. However, health authorities are required to institute safe procedures in accordance with official circulars, reports, etc. Failure to institute or comply with these procedures would leave the health authorities or individuals liable to legal action. In practice, a positive attitude to all aspects of safe use of medicines will benefit patients and safeguard healthcare workers.

Legislation and responsibility of staff

Procedures involved in the handling of Controlled Drugs are drawn up by health authorities against the background of the legal and professional responsibilities defined in the documents listed below and may be supplemented where necessary in accordance with local requirements:

- The Misuse of Drugs Act 1971
- Misuse of Drugs Regulations 1985
- The Aitken Report – Control of Dangerous Drugs and Poisons in Hospitals 1958
- The Roxburgh Report – Control of Medicines in Hospital Wards and Departments 1972
- The Duthie Report – Guidelines for the Safe and Secure Handling of Medicines 1988.

Prescribing

Preparations which are subject to the prescription requirements of the Misuse of Drugs Regulations 1985 are distinguished throughout the British National Formulary by the symbol CD (Controlled Drug).

A Controlled Drug may only be prescribed by a doctor or dentist who is registered or provisionally registered. Controlled Drugs must never be prescribed by telephone. In community hospitals where there is no doctor on site, a prescription for a Controlled Drug may be faxed to the ward. The original prescription must be sent to the ward within 24 hours of it being faxed. The fax must be retained in the patient's notes.

Inpatient prescriptions are normally written on a standard prescription sheet.

For outpatients (or patients on discharge from hospital) detailed information is required. It is not lawful for a practitioner to issue a prescription for a Controlled Drug (included in Schedule 2 or 3), or for a pharmacist to dispense it, unless it complies with the following requirements. The prescription must:

- be in writing and signed by the person issuing it with his usual signature and be dated by him
- be in ink or otherwise so as to be indelible
- except in the case of an NHS or local health authority prescription, specify the address of the person issuing it
- have written on it, if issued by a dentist, the words 'for dental treatment only'
- specify (in the handwriting of the person issuing the prescription) the name and address of the person for whose treatment it is issued
- specify (again in the prescriber's own handwriting) the dose to be taken, the form of the medicine and, where appropriate, the strength of

the preparation, and either the total quantity (in both words and figures) of the preparation, or the number (in both words and figures) of dosage units to be supplied
- in the case of a prescription for a total quantity intended to be dispensed by instalments, contain a direction specifying the amount of the instalments which may be dispensed and the intervals to be observed when dispensing.

Ordering

Controlled Drug supplies for hospital wards and departments may be ordered only by a sister or acting sister. Although the Misuse of Drugs Act/Regulations use this precise terminology, today this would be interpreted as the nurse-in-charge of the ward or his/her deputy. Using the order book (Ref No 90–500) provided for the purpose, the following details must be provided for each product:

- the name of the preparation (in block letters); modified-release preparations should normally be entered using the brand name, although where there is no doubt regarding bio-equivalence between brands, a generic description may be used
- the formulation
- the strength (in figures and words), and
- the total quantity (in figures and words).

A separate page should be used for each product (Fig. 2.3). The nurse signs and dates the order, adding his/her designation. Unless the order has all the necessary detail written in the correct manner, the pharmacist cannot supply the drug.

The whole order book is sent to the pharmacy department where the pharmacist prepares the order and signs the requisition. The person acting as messenger for the return of drugs to the ward or department also signs the requisition. The original requisition is then retained in the pharmaceutical department. In situations where supply of a Controlled Drug is required outwith normal working hours and there is no pharmacy on site, the order may be faxed to the central pharmacy department followed by confirmation by telephone. In rural hospitals it may be necessary to have two Controlled Drugs order books since one may be in transit between the hospital and the pharmacy department.

If an order which has been written is incorrect or no longer requires to be supplied to the ward or department, it must be clearly cancelled by writing cancelled diagonally across the order between two parallel lines and the cancellation must be signed by the nurse. The cancellation must appear on both the white original and pink copy of the order book. At no time should any entry be obliterated. Cancelled orders should not be torn out.

Order books should be stored in the Controlled Drugs cupboard whenever possible. Replacement order books are obtained from pharmacy departments.

Delivery and receipt

Delivery of Controlled Drugs may be made in a locked box or by a designated messenger. If Controlled Drugs are collected from the pharmacy, the appropriate

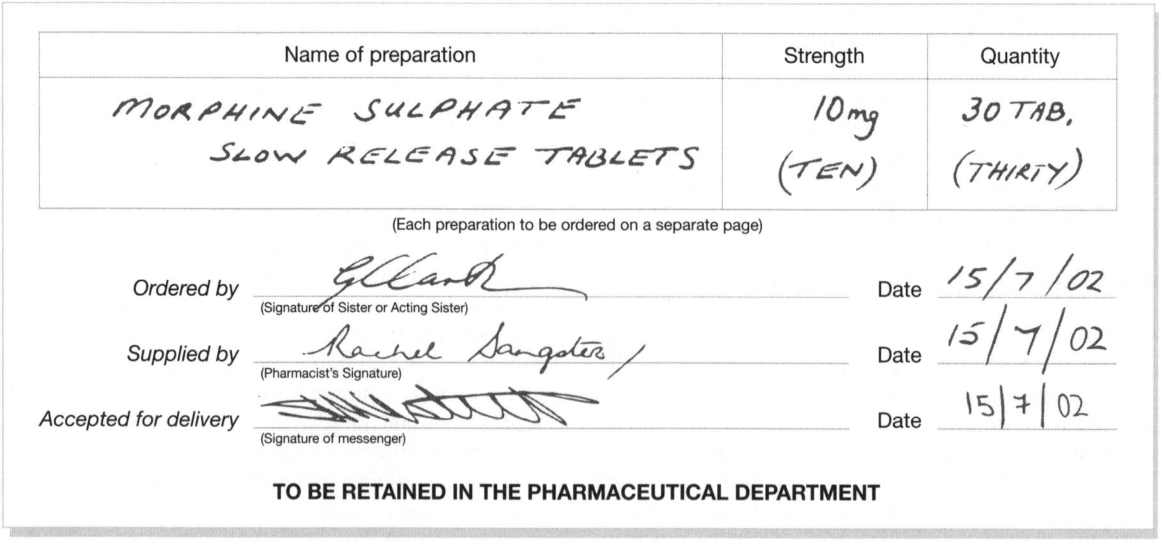

Name of preparation	Strength	Quantity
MORPHINE SULPHATE SLOW RELEASE TABLETS	10mg (TEN)	30 TAB. (THIRTY)

(Each preparation to be ordered on a separate page)

Ordered by (Signature of Sister or Acting Sister) Date 15/7/02

Supplied by (Pharmacist's Signature) Date 15/7/02

Accepted for delivery (Signature of messenger) Date 15/7/02

TO BE RETAINED IN THE PHARMACEUTICAL DEPARTMENT

Figure 2.3 Order form for Controlled Drugs.

section should be completed by the messenger. Careful consideration should be given as to persons suitable to act as messengers carrying Controlled Drugs.

On receipt of supplies of a Controlled Drug and the order book by a ward or department, two nurses one of whom is a registered nurse should check the drugs against the copy requisition. If all is found to be correct, the copy requisition is signed (Fig. 2.4) and the order book retained in the ward or department. If there is any discrepancy, the pharmacy should be notified at once.

An entry is then made in the ward Controlled Drugs record book (Ref No 90–501) with details of the new supply, keeping records of the different forms and strengths of each preparation in separate sections or pages (Fig. 2.5A). The page is headed with the name of the preparation (in block letters), its form and strength. The columns are filled appropriately to include the number of tablets or vials, or the volume of liquid received, the date and the serial number of the requisition. Where there is continuity of use of a page or section, the existing stock balance is added to the new supply. When it is necessary to start a new section or page, the index is amended accordingly.

Storage

Controlled Drugs are required to be stored in a *separate* locked cupboard constructed to prevent unauthorised access to the drugs. It is customary for this cupboard to be within another locked cupboard. Preferably, the cupboard should be sited where it is visible to nursing staff on duty. With this recommendation, however, there is the disadvantage that 'visible' cupboards are also often in the busiest parts of a ward – for example, at the nurses' station or within the patient area of a Nightingale-type ward. These locations are not conducive to a clear, uninterrupted environment in which to concentrate on checking drugs, and so extra care is essential. A warning light indicating when the cupboard is open is normally provided. The locked compartment in the cupboard must not be used for the storage of any other items.

The key to the Controlled Drugs cupboard must be kept *separate* from other keys and held in the possession of the designated nurse-in-charge of the ward.

Spare keys for Controlled Drugs cupboards are generally kept in the hospital pharmacy. If there is no pharmacy on site, local arrangements are usually made for spare keys to be held in the safe-keeping of the senior nurse manager concerned. In departments where Controlled Drugs are stored but which do not have 24-hour supervisory cover – such as outpatient clinics – arrangements must be made for the safe-keeping of the key(s) to the Controlled Drugs cupboard out of working hours.

Loss or suspected loss of keys should be reported in the first instance to the senior nurse manager on duty

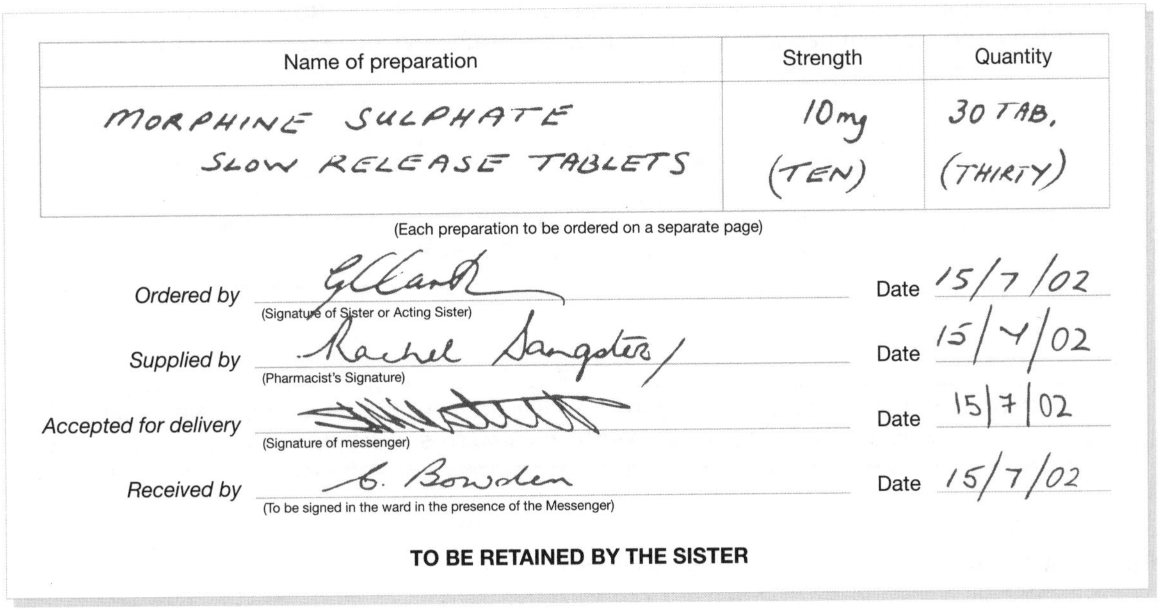

Name of preparation	Strength	Quantity
MORPHINE SULPHATE SLOW RELEASE TABLETS	10mg (TEN)	30 TAB. (THIRTY)

(Each preparation to be ordered on a separate page)

Ordered by (Signature of Sister or Acting Sister) Date 15/7/02

Supplied by (Pharmacist's Signature) Date 15/7/02

Accepted for delivery (Signature of messenger) Date 15/7/02

Received by (To be signed in the ward in the presence of the Messenger) Date 15/7/02

TO BE RETAINED BY THE SISTER

Figure 2.4 Copy order for Controlled Drugs.

NAME, FORM OF PREPARATION AND STRENGTH DIAMORPHINE INJECTION 10 mg

AMOUNT(S) OBTAINED			AMOUNTS ADMINISTERED						
Amount	Date received	Serial no. of requisition	Date	Time	Patient's name	Amount given	Given by (signature)	Witnessed by (signature)	STOCK BALANCE
20 AMP	7/9/02	07							20 AMP
			9/9/02	7.10am	A. PATIENT	10 mg	J. Milne	G. Bennett	19 AMP
			9/9/02	11.35am	A. PATIENT	20 mg	J. Milne	M Edgar	17 AMP
			10/9/02	-	STOCK CHECKED AND	FOUND CORRECT	S. Smith	SISTER	17 AMP
10 AMP	16/9/02	08							

(A)

NAME, FORM OF PREPARATION AND STRENGTH MORPHINE IN CHLOROFORM WATER 20 mg in 5 ml

AMOUNT(S) OBTAINED			AMOUNTS ADMINISTERED						
Amount	Date received	Serial no. of requisition	Date	Time	Patient's name	Amount given	Given by (signature)	Witnessed by (signature)	STOCK BALANCE
200 ml	16/8/02	06							200 ml
			18/8/02	3.20pm	A. PATIENT	10 ml	J. Milne	M Duncan	190 ml
			18/8/02	6.40pm	B. PATIENT	5 ml	I. Cowie	M Stewart	185 ml
			↓	↓	↓	↓	↓	↓	
									*60 ml
200 ml	23/8/02	11	———	———	———	———	———	———	260 ml
			25/8/02	5.20am	A. Patient	10 ml	Lorna Sutherland	J. Riddell	250 ml

THE ABOVE PROCEDURE TO BE ADOPTED IF THERE IS CONTINUITY OF USE AND AN ACCURATE BALANCE ALTERNATIVE PROCEDURES WHERE THEORETICAL BALANCE DOES NOT EQUAL ACTUAL BALANCE

Amount	Date received	Serial no. of requisition	Date	Time	Patient's name	Amount given	Given by (signature)	Witnessed by (signature)	STOCK BALANCE
									170 ml
			19/9/02	9am	F. BROWN	10 ml	L. Armstrong	C Cameron	160 ml
				↓	↓	↓	↓	↓	40 ml
			23/9/02	STOCK CHECKED	J. Murray	SISTER	LOSSES ON	MEASURING	30 ml
			23/9/02		BALANCE RETURNED	TO PHARMACY	J. Murray		NIL
200 ml	23/9/02	14	23/9/02	———	———	———	———	———	200 ml

OR

IF THERE IS CONTINUITY OF USE THE <u>CORRECTED BALANCE</u> SHOULD BE ADDED TO NEW SUPPLY WHERE LOSSES APPEAR EXCESSIVE PHARMACY SHOULD BE NOTIFIED

(B)

Figure 2.5A, B Extract from ward Controlled Drugs record book.

whose duty it is to inform a senior member of the pharmacy staff and, if necessary, the security officer for the hospital.

As with all other drugs, Controlled Drugs should not be transferred to other containers but must be retained in the original container, which should not be defaced in any way.

Administration

The basic procedure for giving any medication applies also to the giving of a Controlled Drug. Instructions relating specifically to Controlled Drugs are as follows:

- Two persons must be involved in the administration of a Controlled Drug, one of whom must be a registered nurse or a registered doctor.
- The keys to the Controlled Drugs cupboard are obtained from the nurse-in-charge.
- The stock amount of the drug to be used is checked against the last entry in the Controlled Drugs record book.
- After the dose is selected, the remaining stock is returned to the cupboard which is then locked.
- The date, the name of the patient, the amount of the drug to be given and the stock balance are entered in the record book (Fig. 2.5B).
- Both persons involved take the prepared drug to the patient, one to administer the drug, the other to act as witness.
- The time of administration and the signatures of the two persons are entered in the record book.
- The keys of the Controlled Drugs cupboard are returned to the nurse-in-charge.

Keeping ward or department Controlled Drugs record books

Strictly according to the regulations, the sister or acting sister is not required to keep a drug register. However, in practice, the keeping of a drug register at ward or department level is always required by the health authority. The record book must be kept in accordance with the guidance given on page 16. At no time should any entry be obliterated. Replacement ward Controlled Drugs record books are available from the pharmacy department.

When Controlled Drugs are dispensed by the pharmacy for a named individual inpatient, each supply should be recorded in a separate section of the ward Controlled Drugs record book.

When arriving at a stock balance of liquid oral medicines, it may not always be possible to obtain exactly the theoretical number of doses from each container. Accordingly, records may be made as illustrated in Figure 2.5B.

Checking stock balances

By nurses. This is undertaken in accordance with locally agreed procedures. Regular checks are part of ward drug management. The intervals vary from on a shift basis, daily, to weekly.

By pharmacists. These checks are made at least at 3-monthly intervals but may be required more frequently. A written record of the check is made in the ward Controlled Drugs record book by the pharmacist carrying out the check.

Procedure to be adopted if (a) the Controlled Drugs order book and/or ward Controlled Drugs record book and/or (b) Controlled Drugs are missing

In the event of loss or suspected loss of these items, the nurse-in-charge of the ward or department should contact the senior nurse manager on duty who will inform the senior pharmacy manager if this becomes necessary.

Disposal of Controlled Drugs

An individual dose of a Controlled Drug which is prepared and is unsuitable for taking back into stock should be disposed of in the ward or department and a record made in the ward Controlled Drugs record book. The destruction must be witnessed by a registered nurse. The same procedure should be adopted where only part of the contents of an ampoule is required for administration. Any accidental breakage should be dealt with in the same way.

In all cases of disposal or loss of small amounts of a Controlled Drug, the amount should be recorded beside the entry in the Controlled Drugs record book. Similarly, if after a dose is removed from its original container the patient refuses the medicine, it should be flushed down the sink with running water. An entry recording refusal by the patient should be made and signed by two nurses one of whom is a registered nurse. If the contents of a syringe used in a syringe driver are only partly used, a similar procedure is followed. Spills and breakages should be similarly accounted for and the pharmacist should be contacted to correct any imbalance in stock. Used fentanyl patches may contain a small amount of fentanyl and so should be disposed of by folding in half and placing in a special medicines waste collection. No record of the disposal is required.

Destruction of Controlled Drugs

It is illegal to destroy Controlled Drugs (and other medicinal products) by means of the public sewerage system. Although it is acceptable to dispose of part of an ampoule or unit dose vial or unused dose at ward level by flushing down a sink with running water, quantities in excess of this should be returned to the pharmacy for destruction. The pharmacist will arrange for safe destruction within the professional and legal requirements.

Controlled Drugs brought in by patients on admission

Some problems can arise at ward level with Controlled Drugs brought in by patients on admission. These will have been obtained by the patient on prescription. Technically it is illegal for the ward sister to receive these drugs from the patient. However, in such situations the pharmacist may lawfully accept such drugs for destruction. On rare occasions a patient may be in possession of illicit Controlled Drugs. This is obviously a very delicate matter and is dealt with having regard to all clinical and legal considerations. At the present time it is illegal for the pharmacist to receive such drugs and it may be necessary to call in the police to deal with the matter. In such situations medical confidentiality will be observed unless there are compelling reasons to the contrary.

Unwanted or time-expired Controlled Drugs held at ward/departmental level

These should be returned to the pharmacy, having made suitable records in the ward Controlled Drugs record book.

Retention of records

All Controlled Drugs order books and record books must be retained for 2 years after the date of the last entry. After this time, such documents should be destroyed by burning or shredding.

OTHER ASPECTS OF THE CONTROL OF MEDICINES

While legal aspects of the control of medicines remain central to all hospital medicine policies, it is important to recognise the changes that are occurring which make an impact on the way medicines are controlled. Computerised medicine management systems provide the opportunity to follow the movement of medicines from the manufacturer through to the administration of a dose to the patient.

Although security must be maintained throughout all transactions involving medicines, it is also vitally important to provide information to the users of medicines as to costs, compliance with formulary, etc. (see p. 39). The Duthie Report (DoH 1988) defines the 'Medicine Trail', which is the path taken by medicines from manufacturers (or other supplier) via the hospital pharmacy to the ward. At each point on the trail appropriate safeguards and procedures are recommended to ensure that there are defined responsibilities, appropriate record keeping and reconciliation (checks on receipts/issues/balances). Many of the responsibilities etc. defined in the Duthie Report will be undertaken by the hospital pharmacist.

Some specific points from the Duthie Report which relate to the duties and responsibilities of the nurse (and are not dealt with elsewhere) are summarised below.

Controlled stationery

The term 'controlled stationery' refers to any stationery which, in the wrong hands, could be used to obtain medicines fraudulently (DoH 1988). All medicine order books and stationery of this kind must be kept in a secure place so as to reduce the likelihood of misuse.

Samples and clinical trial materials

It is essential to ensure that all such materials are received from the pharmaceutical department and not directly from a manufacturer.

Medicines liable to diversion

The security of all medicines is vitally important, as is the security of medicines that may be especially attractive to the drug user (e.g. temazepam). Such drugs should be subject to checks as agreed with senior nurse and pharmacy managers.

Borrowing of medicines

Legislation to remove Crown Immunity (Medicines Control Agency 1992) means that the practice of borrowing medicines between wards is no longer acceptable.

Community clinics, family planning clinics

Just as with wards and departments in hospitals, clear guidance is needed for all staff working in clinic settings. Responsibilities must be defined at all stages from ordering to use of the medicine.

Management of medicines in day hospitals

The day hospital aims to provide facilities for assessment, diagnosis and rehabilitation of patients who do not require hospital admission as well as to maintain the level of rehabilitation achieved by patients discharged from inpatient care. Such departments are an accepted component of healthcare for elderly people and also for psychiatric patients. Day hospitals operate during daylight hours and cater for the needs of appropriately selected patients, allowing them to remain in the community.

The management of medicines in a day hospital is many-sided as elderly patients present a wide range of conditions which require to be assessed and treated. On the first visit to the day hospital, patients should be asked to bring all their medicines with them. The medicines should be examined by the doctor, and patients asked in detail what each is being taken for, the number to be taken, the frequency and so on. At this time, patients should also be asked if they are able to gain access to the medicines or if they are experiencing any other difficulties with them. If there is any doubt about a patient's ability to cope with the medicines at home, appropriate action should be taken. This may involve contacting a relative of the patient, the general practitioner, the district nurse or the community pharmacist. The use of a suitable compliance aid should be considered. If necessary, the liaison health visitor will be asked to visit the patient at home to try to assist with the problem. Since patients attending a day hospital are outpatients under the care of their GP, the geriatrician does not normally prescribe medicines for them. The geriatrician may, however, withdraw medication immediately from a patient for a suspected adverse reaction; suggest to the GP the need for a medicine or a change in prescription; and, in response to laboratory results or the severity of symptoms, prescribe a course of antibiotics – for example – when otherwise there might be an unacceptable delay in written advice reaching the patient's own doctor.

On subsequent visits, the patient is normally required to bring only those medicines which have to be taken during the period of the visit. It is tempting for the patient to transfer to smaller containers only those medicines which will be required but this practice is to be discouraged.

Some of the patients attending the day hospital may be capable of remembering to take their medicines as well as undertaking the procedure involved. Others, who normally are supervised or assisted in taking their medicines by relatives or a neighbour, will need this support maintained by the day hospital staff. The nurse is in an ideal position to supervise patients taking their medicines. It is important to be alert to the possibility of unwanted side-effects which can have serious consequences, especially in older people.

Small amounts of medicines for the relief of unexpected discomfort in patients may be held in the day hospital; these include simple analgesics and antacids. Supplies of certain medicines which must never be omitted should also be kept. These may include antibiotics, oral antidiabetic drugs and antihypertensives.

Apart from medicines, other nursing procedures involving pharmaceutical products may have to be carried out. These may include urine testing, catheter irrigation, stoma care and surgical dressings. Resuscitative measures may have to be instigated if a patient collapses, and so the nurse must ensure that relevant and updated emergency medicines are available. The importance of keeping accurate records of medicines which patients attending the day hospital are taking, and of maintaining good lines of communication between all personnel involved, cannot be overemphasised. The principles and practice of medicine management apply to day hospitals as much as in other situations. The notable feature of the day hospital in this context, however, is that the patients form a mobile and ever-changing group – making patient identification and staff stability of the utmost importance.

Disposal of time-expired and unwanted medicines

Under the Environmental Protection Act 1990 a 'duty of care' requirement was introduced. The effect of this legislation was to place very clear responsibilities on healthcare staff to ensure that time-expired and unwanted medicines (and in some cases containers) are safely disposed of. Both community and hospital pharmacists must provide the necessary disposal services within the legal framework, ensuring avoidance of environmental hazard. Nurses need to be aware of the provisions of the legislation so that in their own practice, and in giving advice to patients and carers, they can be confident of working within the law. The duty of care requirements also apply to the disposal of other clinical waste such as used syringes and needles.

Control of substances hazardous to health

The Control of Substances Hazardous to Health Regulations (1988) are designed to provide a framework of control within which all substances hazardous to health can be used safely. Many substances used in healthcare and healthcare settings are hazardous to health. The administration of cytotoxic drugs presents particular hazards to staff. These are discussed in more detail elsewhere (see p. 351). Key elements of the COSHH regulations are listed below:

- Responsibility for ensuring compliance with the regulations lies with the employer.
- In practice, responsibility is delegated to the manager of a department or safety officer.
- Known health hazards must be given high priority.
- Microbiological hazards are included.
- Having determined that a substance is hazardous the following action must be taken:
  - assess the risk in the particular setting where the product is used
  - control the risk
  - produce data sheets (on procedures to be followed) for guidance of staff
  - introduce and monitor compliance with data sheet requirements
  - carry out review of procedures and health surveillance of staff involved.

The assessment of risk should take the form of a written statement and should be carried out in a systematic way. All the controls introduced are designed to either avoid exposure to the hazardous substance or limit the exposure to an accepted safe level. Control methods range from the use of protective clothing to the use of mechanical ventilation systems. An outline of the contents of a COSHH data sheet is given in Box 2.2.

As with all procedures, it is essential to monitor compliance with the controls and ensure that any equipment used to contain the risk is maintained in good order. All staff share the responsibility of achieving and maintaining safe working practices within the COSHH regulations. In seeking to improve the health of patients, every effort must be made to avoid damaging the health of those caring for them. Risks to patients from administered medicines are outside the scope of the COSHH regulations.

Box 2.2 Contents of COSHH data sheet

Name of substance
Chemical formula
Occupational exposure limit
Form of product
Uses of product
Specific health hazards
Sensitisation
Other harmful effects
Specific hazards
Dealing with spillages
Disposal of surplus material
First aid

Hazard warnings and drug withdrawals

Every precaution is taken by manufacturers and distributors of medicines to ensure that all medicines comply with the relevant standards and are safe for their intended use. However, mistakes do occasionally occur in either the manufacturing, packaging or labelling. In order to avoid any risk to patients or staff, it is the responsibility of the Health Departments to issue any hazard notification without delay. This is normally done through health service channels on a 24 hours/day basis. Nurses would be provided with written information on the particular hazard by the pharmacist. It may be necessary to check ward stocks and withdraw the affected product from use. On occasion, where there is a risk to public health, warnings regarding a particular product will be communicated via the news media.

Following the receipt and evaluation of clinical data regarding hitherto unknown clinical hazards, the Medicines Control Agency (MCA) may withdraw a product licence. The effect of this is to remove the product from use.

Product licences

All products marketed for human use in the UK must have a product licence. Normally, licensed products are used for the indications defined in the licence. On occasion, doctors may need to prescribe a drug for a non-licensed indication or may prescribe a non-licensed drug on a 'named-patient' basis. Pharmacists will advise their professional colleagues on the implications of prescribing outwith the product licence arrangements. Some drugs are restricted to prescribing by hospital specialists owing to potentially dangerous side-effects, e.g. phenylbutazone.

REFERENCES

Control of Substances Hazardous to Health Regulations 1988 Statutory Instrument No. 1657. HMSO, London
Department of Health (DoH) 1988 Guidelines for the safe and secure handling of medicines (Duthie Report). DoH, London
Environmental Protection Act 1990 HMSO, London
Fradgley S, Pryce A 2002 An investigation into the clinical risks in the use of patients' own drugs on surgical wards. Pharmaceutical Journal 268:63–67
Medicines Act 1968 HMSO, London
Medicines Control Agency (MCA) 1992 Guidance to the NHS on the licensing requirements of the Medicines Act 1968. MCA, London
Misuse of Drugs Act 1971 HMSO, London
Misuse of Drugs Regulations 1985 Statutory Instrument No. 2066. HMSO, London

FURTHER READING

Atwell C 1990 Control of substances hazardous to health. Surgical Nurse 3(6):10–13
Department of Health/Welsh Office/Scottish Office Home and Health Department 1989 Guide to the Misuse of Drugs Act 1971 and the Misuse of Drugs Regulations
Prescription Only Medicines (Human Use) Order 1997 Statutory Instrument No. 1830. HMSO, London
Royal Pharmaceutical Society of Great Britain 1997 Medicines, ethics and practice: a guide for pharmacists. RPS, London

CHAPTER CONTENTS

3

Pharmaceutical services

THE PHARMACIST'S ROLE

Safe and effective management of drug therapy depends on many factors, not least of which is the availability of a comprehensive pharmaceutical service.

The pharmacist has an important role in advising on the prescribing of medication as part of the multidisciplinary team providing patient care. Safety, efficacy and cost-effectiveness are key elements. The role includes the provision of advice on the choice of therapy to the prescriber and information to the patient. This information is provided verbally and reinforced in the form of a patient information sheet. Technical services designed to contribute to the achievement of optimal drug therapy include dispensing, the compounding of sterile preparations for parenteral administration and the provision of a radiopharmaceutical service. These specialist services are generally provided by highly trained technicians working under the direction of a pharmacist. With the development of clinical pharmacy, the role of the pharmacist continues to expand as the focus is increasingly on issues that relate directly to patient care rather than the medical product. However, suitability of the product for its intended purpose remains a vital responsibility.

CLINICAL PHARMACY

The use of highly structured documentation for recording the prescribing and administration of medicines has made it possible for pharmacists to discharge their professional responsibilities at ward level. By visiting the ward, they are able to obtain detailed information on the medicines prescribed for each patient. They are able to contribute their professional skills on all facets of the use of medicines. Ideally, the pharmacist will be present as part of the ward team and advise on medications to be prescribed. However, this is not always possible. As a member of the team, the pharmacist is

Box 3.1 Key elements of a clinical pharmacy service

- Review of prescriptions:
  - dosage
  - route of administration
  - adverse drug reactions
  - drug interactions
- Rapid response to changing needs for medicines
- Advice on formulation/presentation of medicines to meet the needs of individual patients
- Formulary management systems – development and monitoring
- Advice on aids to patient compliance

well placed to advise professional colleagues on a wide range of topics related to drug therapy. Interpretation of prescriptions, checking dosage levels and monitoring prescriptions for possible drug interactions are a vital part of the pharmacist's role but, working at ward level, the pharmacist has access to more information on the patient's clinical condition, special problems, etc. than would be the case if working solely within the pharmaceutical department. As electronic links between clinical areas and the pharmaceutical department are developed the pharmacist's role will be enhanced. Decentralisation of pharmaceutical services will also contribute to improved pharmaceutical care.

Clinical pharmacists with specialist skills are integral members of directorate teams. They undertake such roles as medication review, drug history-taking, discharge planning, education and training, and formulary management (see Box 3.1). Pharmacist-led clinics (anticoagulant and pain control) are becoming well established.

PHARMACEUTICAL CARE

The concept of pharmaceutical care developed in the USA continues to receive attention in the UK. It refers to the pharmaceutical contribution to direct patient care resulting from the practice of clinical pharmacy. In effect, it involves helping patients to get the most benefit from their medicines. In practical terms, the provision of pharmaceutical care follows a problem-solving approach with several key elements which are familiar to nurses:

- assessment of the patient's drug-related needs
- determination of the patient's actual or potential problems
- development with other health professionals of a pharmaceutical care plan designed to deal with problems identified
- implementation and monitoring of the plan.

The rate and extent to which pharmaceutical care will be further developed in the UK depends on many factors, in particular the availability of resources. Nevertheless, with increasing emphasis on care in the community, plans are needed for patients receiving complex therapy in their own homes. Cooperative working between pharmacists and community healthcare staff (especially nurses) is essential if effective pharmaceutical care is to be implemented successfully.

Significant benefits can be achieved for individual patients in introducing a system whereby the pharmacist prepares a pharmaceutical care plan. As with clinical pharmacy services, the overall objective is to utilise the skills of the pharmacist so that the benefits of drug treatment are fully realised for the patient. Table 3.1 outlines the process by which a pharmaceutical care plan can be established.

MEDICINES MANAGEMENT

In an attempt to prevent avoidable ill-health from the use of medicines, reduce NHS waste and help patients get the most from their treatment, a government initiative known as medicines management is being implemented in both primary and secondary care organisations throughout the UK. Medicines management is a system of processes and behaviours that determines how medicines are used by patients and by the NHS. Medicines management services provide patient-focused care based on need and include all aspects of supply and use of medicines from the level of an individual patient to that of the organisation. The services include:

- reviewing prescriptions
- monitoring medication
- managing repeat prescribing
- providing services for nursing and residential homes
- educating patients about their medicines.

Improving working relationships across the primary–secondary care interface is seen as important to the success of this initiative. A uniform approach to prescribing using an agreed formulary must be encouraged.

The greatest impact on nursing staff will be the utilisation of patients' own drugs while in hospital. Newly prescribed medicines and medicines issued on discharge will be supplied increasingly in patient packs. It is anticipated that original pack dispensing will lead to greater efficiency overall through a reduction not only in waste but also in the need for hospital dispensing and the delays associated with the discharge process. A further benefit of the system includes facilitation of the self-administration of medicines (see Box 3.2).

Table 3.1 Development of a pharmaceutical care plan

Stage	Action by pharmacist	Notes
I	Establish contact with the patient	The need for a good professional working relationship cannot be overstated
II	Collect and interpret information on patient's condition and drug history (including use of non-prescription medicines)	Aspects that will require particular attention include: • non-compliance of the patient • practical problems with medicine use • drug interactions • incidence of side-effects • poor medicine hygiene/storage
III	List patient's problems in priority order	It will be important to establish the degree of risk involved in order to prioritise the problems
IV	Establish whenever possible the desired *outcome* of each problem identified	In some situations the outcome may be very easy to define, e.g. improve the storage of medicines. Thereafter, outcomes may be less easy to define but every effort must be made to do so
V	Examine alternatives available and choose the best in particular circumstances	As with all stages, the needs of the *individual patient* will be the paramount consideration
VI	Design and implement a monitoring plan based on patient's needs	The plan should focus on outcomes which can be measured
VII	Implement plan	Effective communication within the healthcare team is vital, especially between community nursing staff and the pharmacist
VIII	Follow-up to determine overall success of the plan	It is emphasised that pharmaceutical care plans have an overall requirement of a long-term commitment to the patient

Box 3.2 Advantages of original pack dispensing

Patient aspects
- Greater acceptability
- Improved convenience
- More focused on patient's need
- Improved information about the medicine
- Fewer changes to the medication
- Increased opportunity to take responsibility for own medicines and their administration
- Reduction in delays at time of discharge from hospital
- Improved compliance

Safety aspects
- Increased security
- Child resistance
- More hygienic
- Better labelling
- Reduction in medication and dispensing errors
- Reduction in prescription fraud

Economic aspects
- Reduction in wastage of medications
- Stock control
- Reduction in dispensing time

PRESCRIBING BY PHARMACISTS

Schemes are currently being undertaken by suitably trained community pharmacists to prescribe within agreed clinical management plans for individual patients. The schemes are intended to enhance patient care by providing quicker and more efficient access to healthcare through an increased and flexible use of pharmacists' skills. This form of prescribing is classed as supplementary prescribing, i.e. the responsibility for clinical management of a specified patient will be passed to the pharmacist *once a diagnosis has been established or a treatment plan has been prepared* (DoH 1999). The management plan will specify in detail the dose, frequency and formulation of the medicine. In hospital practice, pharmacists are often involved in managing prescribing for patients on discharge into the community.

DISTRIBUTION OF MEDICINES AND PHARMACEUTICAL PRODUCTS

Distribution to hospital wards

Several different methods are used to supply medicines to wards. Depending on circumstances, the system of medicine distribution used is a product of many factors including availability of resources, clinical need, local geography and overall strategy of the trust being served.

The overall aim of any medicine distribution system is to ensure that the necessary medicines of the appropriate quality are available when required in quantities that reflect both current and to some extent future usage. Increasingly automated/computer-controlled systems of medicine distribution are being developed, with the joint aims of reducing labour costs and increasing patient safety.

Significant quantities of medicines and related products which are not routinely prescribed are supplied for use in wards. These can be considered broadly as:

Resuscitation packs. These are supplied by the pharmacy in accordance with local policy. The packaging and presentation of drugs will be a matter for the pharmaceutical service. It is vital to ensure that the contents are presented for quick access and replenished immediately following an emergency, and that regular checks are made to ensure the products are not allowed to pass their expiry date.

Nursing care products. In order to avoid multiplicity of products in use for nursing care procedures such as catheter care, skin care and eye bathing, a formulary of nursing care products is an effective approach (see p. 45). Such a formulary contains monographs on the products which are available for use by nurses without medical prescription. The items contained in the formulary are often supplied on a routine 'top-up' basis.

Diagnostic agents. Clinical reagents are normally supplied on a routine stock basis. Other more specialised agents are supplied on request.

Disinfectants, antiseptics, skin cleansers, etc. It is now standard practice for wards (and departments) to use a range of products as agreed by the control of infection committee. The disinfection policy will contain information on the use of products together with supporting technical information. The products are supplied on a routine indenting or topping-up basis. A brief discussion of the properties and uses of disinfectants appears in Chapter 28. In view of the limitations of chemical agents, physical means of disinfection are preferred.

Distribution to hospital departments

The distribution of medicines and related products to departments (e.g. to operating theatres) often involves considerable bulk, but the product range is less extensive than is supplied to wards. However, it is still important to achieve standardisation since duplication of products is costly and may cause confusion. Pre-printed drug indents facilitate the introduction and maintenance of a standard range of products. Specialised clinical pharmacy services are also required in hospital departments.

Special arrangements are often required in accident and emergency departments, such as the provision of 'patient-ready' packs of analgesics and antibiotics which can be issued to patients without nurses having to undertake 'dispensing'. Such packs issued to patients should be accompanied by patient information leaflets.

TECHNICAL SUPPORT SERVICES

The drug distribution arrangements previously described are supplemented by specialist technical support services. These are dispensing services which require pharmaceutical expertise and special environmental conditions such as those provided in an aseptic suite. These central, pharmacy-based services have been developed in response to the growing complexity of drug therapy and the need to provide the highest possible standards of patient care.

Central intravenous additive services (CIVAS). The addition of drugs to intravenous fluids is best performed in an aseptic dispensing suite rather than a clinical area where full aseptic standards may be impossible to achieve. By providing these services centrally, nurses are relieved of time-consuming manipulative tasks and are able to concentrate on clinical care. On occasion it will be necessary to make an addition to an intravenous fluid at ward or departmental level but this should be undertaken only where there is no alternative.

Parenteral nutrition services (see also p. 385). The administration of nutrients, vitamins and minerals in combination in a single container presented ready for use represents a far safer method of administration than that provided by using a series of separate containers. Containers of suitable volume are prepared under strict aseptic conditions within the pharmacy. This reduces the risk of infection and helps to ensure accuracy of the therapy.

Cytotoxic reconstitution services (see also p. 352). The risks inherent in reconstituting cytotoxic drugs without due attention to the safety of the doctor or nurse undertaking this task are well recognised. Full protection of operator and product can be achieved only within a specialised unit having all the necessary facilities such as vertical laminar air flow cabinets, air-conditioning and facilities for staff to change into sterile protective clothing. As with the other specialist services, the medicine is provided as an accurately compounded, fully labelled, ready-to-use sterile product. Although this greatly reduces hazards, care is required when administering the medicine so as to avoid aerosol formation or spillage which may contaminate the environment and thus any persons in the immediate vicinity.

Radiopharmaceuticals. Major hospital pharmaceutical departments provide a supply service of sterile radioisotope injections for use in specialised diagnostic procedures. The injections are formulated in order to accumulate in a particular organ or part of the body, e.g. phosphate injection becomes concentrated in bone;

thiosulphate in the liver; albumin microspheres are temporarily trapped in the lung capillaries. These chemicals are labelled with a short-acting radionuclide such as ^{99m}Tc (half-life 8 hours), which rapidly decays. A camera which is sensitive to the radioactive particles emitted by the technetium scans the organ or part of the body. This illustrates different concentrations within a particular organ and in this way abnormalities can be located.

MEDICINE INFORMATION SERVICES

The provision of information on many aspects of the use of medicines and properties of drugs is an integral part of pharmaceutical services. The organisation of this service and method of provision will vary considerably, depending on circumstances. In larger acute hospitals, a department under the control of a full-time specialist pharmacist will provide the service on a local, regional or national basis. The pharmacist providing clinical services will also be a source of information on drugs. Medicine information pharmacists work closely with their clinical colleagues when the nature of the query requires highly specialised information that can be obtained only by a literature search. Pharmaceutical manufacturers are an important source of product information, and professional bodies such as the Royal Pharmaceutical Society of Great Britain provide invaluable technical information to practising pharmacists.

All specialist drug information services are available to health professionals but are not normally available directly to members of the public. With the rapid development of information technology (internet), drug information is widely available to health professionals and the general public. Queries received by pharmacists cover a wide range of topics, including dose, route of administration, adverse effects, interactions, contraindications and, increasingly, information on cost/benefits of particular treatments. Information on medicines is provided in response to specific requests and in regular bulletins.

An important part of the practising pharmacist's work is also to provide patients with the necessary information to enable them to use their medicines in the most effective way. This aspect is discussed in more detail in Chapter 11.

COMMUNITY PHARMACY SERVICES

Community pharmacists are responsible for the supply of medicines to patients in the community. In addition, they are responsible for the provision of a wide range of healthcare products, surgical appliances, dressings, etc.

Medicines are supplied on prescription and, where legislation permits, are also sold over the counter. In many instances, an individual will seek the pharmacist's advice and guidance on a particular health problem. This may result in a medicine being recommended and sold to the client, or the pharmacist may suggest self-referral to the general practitioner. There is considerable and increasing use of proprietary medicines by the public and this should always be borne in mind by healthcare staff in both community and hospital practice. Members of the public often regard purchased medicines as being little more than ordinary household commodities. As a result, important information on the patient's full current medications may not be readily ascertained. Community pharmacists will provide information on the use of medicines to community healthcare staff and give invaluable support and guidance to their clients.

For many years community pharmacists have played a vital part in healthcare provision. There is great potential to extend further the contribution that they can make, not only in the treatment of illness but in prevention of ill-health. With the growing emphasis on self-care for the treatment of self-limiting conditions, more people are seeking the professional advice of the pharmacist for the treatment of minor ailments. Such advice is provided within the context of locally agreed protocols.

The use of computer technology enables the pharmacist to exercise a monitoring role (e.g. on repeat prescriptions) by maintaining patient medication records including information on allergies to specific drugs.

The provision of information on the use of medicines is of growing importance. The pharmacist is well placed to provide the necessary information in the most suitable form for patients and their carers. Internet pharmaceutical services may develop in the years ahead.

As more patients are cared for in their own homes and in the community, the community pharmacist's services are becoming more important. In addition to providing services to patients suffering from chronic diseases, the community pharmacist provides a range of services to patients with special needs, such as people who abuse drugs.

Participation in health promotion campaigns is an accepted part of the community pharmacist's role. There is great potential for an expansion of this increasingly important role in areas such as dental health, safer sex, skin care and smoking cessation.

REFERENCES

Department of Health (DoH) 1999 A review of prescribing, supply and administration of medicines (Crown Report 2). DoH, London

FURTHER READING

Bellingham C 2002 Pharmacists who prescribe: the reality. Pharmaceutical Journal 268:238–239

Burton S S, Duffus P R S 1995 An exploration of the role of the clinical pharmacist in general practice medicine. Pharmaceutical Journal 254:91–93

Department of Health (DoH) 2002 Proposals for supplementary prescribing by nurses and pharmacists and proposed amendments to the Prescription Only Medicines (Human Use) Order 1997. DoH, London

Editorial 2002 Consultation starts on supplementary prescribing by pharmacists and nurses. Pharmaceutical Journal 268:521

Hassell K, Whittington Z 2001 Managing demand: transfer of management of self limiting conditions from general practice to community pharmacies. British Medical Journal 323:146–147

CHAPTER CONTENTS

4

The role of the nurse in drug therapy

THE ROLE OF THE NURSE

From the earliest days of their career, nurses are involved to some extent in the management of medicines. Although responsibilities increase and change with time, the safe and effective management of medicines remains a high priority for all practising nurses. The importance of establishing a firm basis of learning during pre-registration training is well recognised, as is the need to progress to wider aspects, as part of professional development. Thus, nurses build upon the knowledge and skills acquired to prepare themselves for the particular responsibilities and duties in their chosen speciality. As with all health professionals, nurses have a responsibility to keep up to date and to make their contribution to professional issues of the day.

Although it is recognised that the emphasis will vary depending on the speciality in which the nurse works, the role of the nurse in drug therapy can be broadly summarised under the following headings:

- to ensure that the correct dosage is given at the correct time and by the correct route, observing any special requirements
- to observe/report any side-effects and consequences of drug interactions
- to take action to alleviate unavoidable side-effects
- to observe and assess the patient so that medical and nursing decisions can be made
- to participate in education and guidance of patients (and in some cases their relatives) with regard to their drug therapy
- to take action to promote patient compliance and the achievement of therapeutic objectives
- to provide nursing care to help reduce, or obviate, the need for drug therapy
- to follow recognised procedures for the control of medicines and pharmaceutical products

- to contribute to the evaluation, research and development of new treatments, and/or the reassessment of existing treatments
- to contribute to the development of medicine management in a changing environment.

It is fully recognised that the discharge of every aspect of the nurse's role in drug therapy is essential for the well-being of the patient.

The nurse's role is much more than a mechanical achievement of objectives. It is a professional role requiring knowledge, skill, judgement and commitment.

The standards expected of each individual registered nurse, midwife and health visitor with respect to medicines are made eplicit by the Nursing and Midwifery Council (NMC 2002a). To meet such standards, the expectation is that nurses are personally accountable for their practice and in so doing act at all times to promote and safeguard the interests and well-being of patients and clients. This requirement applies to all persons on the Council's register, irrespective of the part on which their name appears.

Having outlined the current role of the nurse in drug therapy, it is important to realise that many changes and developments continue to take place within both healthcare and the health professions. A number of changes are having, and will continue to have, an increasing impact on the practising nurse, whether in hospital or community. Some of the areas of significant development are as follows:

- provision of healthcare in the primary care sector
- complexity of drug therapy in both hospitals and the community
- specialisation in the use of drugs
- new drug-delivery systems
- drug presentation, packaging, and drug-distribution systems
- side-effects of drug treatment
- interest in alternative medicine
- the need to use resources effectively
- the need to ensure that whoever is administering the drugs is not harmed by them
- the need to ensure the safe and effective use of medicines by older people
- the use of computers in clinical practice, both in hospitals and the community
- self-care
- access by the general public to technological information about medical conditions and their treatment
- clinical pharmacy services
- professional aspirations of healthcare workers.

The practising nurse cannot fail to be aware of the great benefits as well as the potential dangers of drug therapy. As nurses are accountable for their clinical actions, it is essential that well-founded confidence is acquired in whatever is undertaken. This confidence is achieved through the acquisition of practical skills supported by the necessary theoretical knowledge. No matter how careful and expert the prescribing doctors, or dispensing pharmacists, the consequences for patients may be disastrous if nurses are ill-equipped to discharge their vital role to the full.

Knowledge/information

In order to be safe in the administration of medicines and to be able to advise patients appropriately, the nurse requires a knowledge of basic pharmacology as well as physiology. A knowledge of the medicines in use, and their management, is equally important. It is necessary also to know and understand the policies and procedures which relate to medicines. Along with this background knowledge, nurses require to have basic information on their patients, including any special points about them, which could have a bearing on the successful management of their medication.

Pharmacology and physiology

Basic pharmacology includes:

- drug absorption mechanisms
- the metabolic action of the liver
- the method by which substances are transported in the bloodstream
- cell transport and activity
- the excretory function of the kidneys (see also Ch. 21).

Without an appreciation of the relevant physiology, nurses' understanding of how drugs act in the body is incomplete and their safety and effectiveness in practice is therefore open to question. A lack of specialist knowledge of the physiology of extremes of age may hazard the very young or very old patient who is often more at risk from adverse drug reactions than patients in other age groups.

Legal and professional responsibilities

Nurses, midwives and health visitors are professionally accountable for their practice (NMC 2002b), and work must be conducted according to the standards set by the Council. Each health authority is required to establish policies and procedures which set out in detail instruction and guidance on the administration and storage of medicines. These policies are derived from statutory sources and circulars of guidance issued by the Department of Health (DoH). The nurse must be fully conversant with policies and procedures and adhere to them at all times.

The medicines

A working knowledge of the medicines used includes:

- range of presentation of medicines
- ordering/requisitioning procedures
- storage of medicines and disposal of unwanted medicines
- legislation and health authority policies
- prescribing/recording procedures
- dosage levels
- routes/methods of administration
- rationale for the particular therapy
- safe handling of drugs known to be hazardous
- methods of promoting effectiveness of and/or reducing the need for drug therapy.

The following areas of knowledge are also important:

- mode of action of drugs
- recognition of side-effects and methods of minimising/dealing with unavoidable side-effects
- signs and symptoms of drug toxicity
- methods of dealing with effects of drug toxicity
- drug–drug interactions
- drug–food interactions
- effects of disease states on drug therapy
- potential dangers of self-medication
- use of clinical reagents
- use of drugs in diagnostic tests
- aspects of research into drugs
- achieving/improving patient compliance.

The patient

It is essential that the nurse is aware of the relevant details of the person who is to receive the medication. In hospital, the patient's name, date of birth and unit number are required for correctly identifying the patient. A knowledge of the patient's medical diagnosis, physical capabilities and mental capacity is essential in achieving safe and effective drug treatment. The nurse must be aware also of any special instructions relating to a particular patient's drug therapy. For example, it is important to be aware of hypersensitivity which a patient may have to a particular medicine so that it is never given to that patient. The nurse should be alert to changing circumstances such as the patient who is temporarily to be given nothing by mouth, and be able to respond appropriately in terms of medicine administration.

Knowledge and information are vital. Acquiring and using knowledge contribute to safety in the administration of medicines. By understanding the theory behind the administration of medicines, nurses can act with confidence. In the exercise of professional accountability, however, nurses must be prepared to acknowledge any limitations to their knowledge. It is important, too, to recognise that information about medicines and their management keeps changing, and that practising nurses have a responsibility to keep pace with new developments. Even up-to-date knowledge, of course, is not in itself sufficient to guarantee safe practice.

Skills

As well as knowledge, a number of skills have to be mastered for the successful management of medicines.

Observational skills

By continual observation, a nurse assesses the patient's condition before and after drug treatment, and in so doing helps to establish when treatment is indicated and whether it is being beneficial or otherwise. Nurses routinely measure and record indices such as blood pressure, pulse rate and weight, but it is the ability to note (and report) significant changes in these recordings that is important.

Observable changes in a patient receiving specific forms of drug therapy may include:

- allergic reaction ranging from skin rash to anaphylaxis
- muscular weakness arising from potassium loss in diuretic therapy
- bruising or overt bleeding arising from too high a dose of an anticoagulant
- euphoria associated with corticosteroid therapy
- depression associated with antihypertensive drug therapy
- anorexia in patients receiving digoxin therapy
- breakdown of oral mucosa in patients receiving cytotoxic drugs.

Communication skills

From the moment people become patients, their continued well-being (and eventual restoration to health) depends on effective communication with them, and between healthcare personnel. Nowhere is this more important than with all aspects of drug therapy.

At a very early stage, interviewing skills are needed when eliciting a patient's history. This will involve collecting details of current drug therapy, prescribed or non-prescribed, and any difficulties the patient has in taking medicines. The patient may reveal a belief in alternative medicine or some form of lay medicine and this should never be discounted. Information on a patient's medical condition and/or drug therapy may be obtained from the medical pendant or bracelet worn by some patients.

An equally important part of the communication process is a willingness to listen. Patients are often happy to talk about their illnesses and treatments, and by appropriate questioning and astute follow-up of cues, nurses can assess how much patients understand their disorder and which problems are most real to them. By non-verbal means, such as a gesture, facial expression or mood, patients can convey, respectively, the nature or location of pain, their like or dislike of taking a medicine, and the likelihood of their actually taking the medicines.

Particular opportunities for communication between nurse and patient arise when medicines are being administered. For example, when applying a preparation to an area of broken skin, nurses may help to ease pain by engaging patients in some topic of conversation so as to divert their attention from the procedure. It is not always appropriate, however, to deal with detailed questions at the time of administration as this may cause too much delay or increase the risk of error in the procedure itself. Nevertheless patients are entitled to know the name of the medicine, why it is being given, the dose they are to have, how often it is to be taken, and, if known, the length of the course of treatment. It may also be appropriate to advise patients of any likely side-effects. If questions cannot be dealt with fully at the time, patients should be assured that a more detailed explanation will be given later. Patients may need additional explanation and reassurance when a new treatment is begun or when a medicine is changed or discontinued.

The nurse should also be prepared to learn from the patient (see Ch. 11). Many patients, especially those suffering from chronic conditions, such as dermatological conditions, asthma, myasthenia gravis or Parkinson's disease, will almost certainly have far more practical experience than the nurse in managing their condition. For example, these patients know, by personal experience, the optimum time for administration of their medicine.

Teaching skills

Rodman & Smith (1974) suggest that nurses should aim to teach about drug therapy so that, at the time of discharge from hospital, patients can display a full understanding of their illness and medicines, and can take their medicines in accordance with the prescription. The assumption is that patient teaching promotes independence by facilitating self-administration of the medication, and thus the achievement of therapeutic benefit. By alerting patients to potentially harmful situations (e.g. taking aspirin when receiving warfarin therapy), nurses can contribute significantly to patients' continued well-being. Increased understanding may help patients in deciding to comply with the prescribed therapy.

Teaching is an essential part of the management of patients, and time must be found for it in spite of other pressures. Moreover, as so much of what we learn results from copying others, nurses must display a high level of precision and professionalism in all aspects of the management of medicines and, in so doing, teach by example. Individual factors do, however, influence learning and, consequently, the approach to teaching. These include the patient's level of intelligence and maturity, knowledge, past experience, physical ability and motivation. Where a patient is unable to acquire the necessary skill, the nurse may have to teach a relative or friend.

Some practical points to remember when teaching patients and/or relatives are listed in Table 4.1.

Motor skills

Apart from the situations where patients manage their own drug therapy, medicines are administered by nurses using skills acquired through learning and practice. Improvements in drug presentation (e.g. pre-filled syringes and aseptic dispensing services) continue to improve the safety of drug administration. On the other hand, application of modern technology in clinical areas has placed additional demands on nurses' skills and technical abilities. The use of electronically controlled drug delivery systems, pumps, and other devices requires skills quite different from those traditionally associated with nursing. Against this background, however, it is vitally important that the traditional practical skills of the nurse should not be neglected.

The degree of skill required in the administration of medicines varies considerably, depending on the form of dosage used, the route/method of administration, and the extent to which the patient cooperates or is able to cooperate.

Table 4.1 Teaching patients and/or relatives about medicines*

Action	Discussion
Make sure the time is right for teaching	Teaching should be carried out at a time mutually convenient to patient and nurse. In this way, the patient is less likely to be hurried, and there will still be time left to deal with any difficulties which arise (e.g. the occurrence of an unexpected side-effect)
Consider whether the patient can hear you	The noise created by equipment or others in the vicinity may prevent instructions from being heard. Patients who wear a hearing aid may require assistance in its use
Consider the patient's visual acuity	Many patients need to wear spectacles for reading and at other times. Some patients may use a magnifier. Good lighting is necessary
Avoid creating a mirror image	When demonstrating how to load a syringe, for example, sit or stand alongside patients rather than face them so that they can observe the procedure from the stance in which they will perform it
Adopt a positive approach	For example, 'Hold the syringe this way'
Keep speech and demonstration separate	When learning a skill for the first time, a limited amount of information can be absorbed at one time
Break the teaching into stages	Do this whenever possible, and select important points which require special emphasis
Do not assume that the patient is literate	Obviously, great tact is required to establish the extent of the patient's ability to read and write. People with literacy difficulties often wish to deny them and are skilful at concealing their problems. Conversely, do not 'talk down' to patients. Where English is not understood, the help of an interpreter will be required

* One of the ways considered to be good for improving one's knowledge and understanding of a subject is teaching it to somebody else.

The giving of a tablet to a relatively well, intelligent, and cooperative adult presents few problems. Administering a small volume of a liquid medicine from a dropper to a severely handicapped child presents a greater challenge. To succeed in administering an intramuscular injection to a very agitated and uncooperative patient demands experience, skill and tenacity. The motor skills required include manual dexterity, coordination of hand and eye, coupled with lightness and delicacy of touch. Specialised situations, such as those met with in dermatology and ophthalmology, call for skills which are acquired only through repeated practice.

Numeracy skills

With the increasing potency and specificity of modern drugs it is now more than ever vital to ensure accuracy when administering medicines. It is essential, therefore, that the nurse has a sound working knowledge of SI units of mass and volume and can calculate in these units. Recognition by pharmacists that it is important to supply medicines to wards and departments in a suitable range of strengths has reduced the need for calculations prior to the administration of medicines. Nevertheless, a nurse may be called upon to calculate how to obtain a dose of, say, 50 micrograms from a dosage form that contains 250 micrograms in 2 mL. Attempts to do this have unfortunately resulted in errors of 10-fold or even more. Nurses should also have an understanding of proportions and percentages. It is suggested that these alone represent a minimal level of attainment. Nurses working in intensive care units would be expected to have considerably greater numerical skills and knowledge. Guidance on basic calculations is given in Chapter 8.

Attitudes

The least tangible part of the nursing role is the nurse's overall attitude to patients and the management of their medicines. Relevant skills and knowledge are vital if nurses are to discharge their basic responsibilities. However, without an informed respect for drugs generally, the full benefits of drug therapy will not be achieved and drug therapy may fail.

On a professional level, the nurse should have an awareness of the place of all medicines in the care of the patient. It is vital to recognise the reasons for the need to be systematic in adherence to both national (legal) and local standards. The recognition should be based on a broad understanding of the principles involved, not merely the mechanical following of a set of rules. An overall sense of the need for security in its widest sense is required, coupled with an appreciation of economic factors. An enquiring attitude of mind associated with a knowledgeable, well-informed approach, will give the nurse confidence to play a full part in ensuring safe and effective drug therapy.

It is also important, however, to consider those attitudes which are, to a large extent, linked with personal qualities. These include powers of observation and the ability to keep calm and work under pressure. Being selective in dealing with interruptions during procedures involving medicines calls for judgement, patience and, occasionally, a sense of humour. The nurse must exercise judgement, since a degree of flexibility may be called for on occasion; firmness, linked with tact, is a prerequisite. The balanced assessment of one's own knowledge, or lack of it, is important, as is the willingness to ask and seek advice.

Against this background it should not be forgotten that nurses have a duty to encourage patients to regard all medicines with respect, without at the same time causing anxiety. In exercising the necessary skills and demonstrating the correct attitude, nurses set an example for patients to follow. Special emphasis on certain aspects, such as the need for safe storage of medicines, can be reinforced by the attitude adopted by nurses and the care and concern which they show. A patient may be reluctant to take the medicines and/or unable to see the need for them. This demands patience and perseverance by the nurse. Often the problem arises with those in greatest need of the treatment. With a responsibility to act as a role model in health education, the nurse should respect medicines at all times, both on a professional and a personal level.

THE ROLE OF THE NURSE IN THE COMMUNITY

The community nurse

With the continuation of the trend towards care in the community, the role of the community nurse in relation to drug therapy continues to expand. Early discharge from hospital, an ageing population and as a consequence of modern medicine the increase in the number of people surviving chronic disease and disability have all contributed to this expanded role. Whether urban or rural, community nurses throughout the UK provide a daytime nursing service and an on-call system at night which ensures there is equity of care for all. The nurse plays a key role in the community alongside other health professionals such as general practitioners (GPs) and those in professions allied to medicine. The flow of accurate information interprofessionally as well as intraprofessionally regarding drug therapy is of vital importance. Information technology is of increasing assistance in meeting this requirement.

The vast majority of people taking medicines at home take complete responsibility for this and therefore there is no involvement of the community nurse. Where the community nurse, for whatever reason, is asked to make a home visit, certain key principles with regard to drug therapy must be adhered to. Assessment is a vitally important responsibility. Where there is physical or mental impairment, the nurse's powers of observation must be used constantly to spot clues suggestive of non-compliance. Checks are made to see that the medicines are being taken as prescribed and are being managed safely and effectively in all respects. In the over-75 age group, the use of a checklist may assist this process (see Box 4.1).

Box 4.1 Sample of an over-75s medication review

Is the patient able to read the labels?
Can the patient open all the containers?
Are the medicines being taken as prescribed?
Does the patient understand the reason for taking the medication?
Is the patient managing the medication with regard to constipation, nausea, difficulty swallowing, drowsiness?
Are any OTC medicines being taken on a regular basis? If so, what are they?
Are the medicines suitably stored?
Does the patient have a compliance device? If so, is it being used correctly?
Has the patient acceptable quantities of current medicines?
Have all discontinued medicines been returned to the pharmacy or GP?

In some situations, older people may be found to be having difficulty as the result of stiff, weak or shaky hands, or because their short-term memory is failing. In such cases, assessment may have to extend to establishing whether a family member, home carer or neighbour is able to assist. Home carers are not permitted to administer medicines, although they are allowed to prompt, encourage and facilitate the taking of a medicine.

The community nurse gets to know her patients especially well and, as a result, is in a good position to assist in the monitoring of all drug therapy. The nurse must have a keen awareness at all times of possible side-effects or drug interactions that may arise from the prescribed drug therapy and take appropriate action. If there is any uncertainty whatsoever, reference should be made to the BNF. The occurrence of side-effects should be documented and of course reported to the prescriber so that, if necessary, changes in therapy can be made.

The community nurse must be aware that patients may receive conflicting advice about their medicines from the media and from well-meaning neighbours, relatives and friends. This may cause confusion in the patient's mind which may lead to non-compliance.

Patients should be encouraged and if necessary helped to read the manufacturer's instructions. Community nurses are often able to give the patient suitable guidance with the help of the GP and community pharmacist where necessary.

As part of the assessment process, the nurse should be aware also of the possibility that the patient may be taking OTC medicines. Patients may purchase proprietary medicines some of which could conflict with prescribed medicines. For example, aspirin-containing preparations potentiate the effect of oral anticoagulants and should therefore be avoided by patients receiving this therapy. Normally the GP and community pharmacist will give the patient guidance but the patient may be unaware of the presence of aspirin in a proprietary product. The BNF contains lists of products (in therapeutic groups) which cannot be prescribed on the NHS. However, these products may be purchased from a pharmacy. Whenever possible, it is advisable for patients to obtain their medicines from the same outlet.

Patients may use a 'lay' (unorthodox) remedy or some form of complementary medicine. Unless there are specific difficulties, the patient's wishes in the matter should be respected.

Increasingly, community nurses, provided they have undertaken the relevant training, are involved in prescribing certain medicines in certain situations. This calls for in-depth understanding of pharmacology and the increased responsibilities involved (see Ch. 6).

Essentially the community nurse has the same responsibilities with regard to the administering and recording of medicines as the hospital nurse. Naturally, there is a difference in emphasis but the principles are the same. The patient's consent must always be obtained. The detailed guidelines given in Chapters 7 and 9 apply equally to the community nurse but, of course, a second nurse will not be present to carry out the checking procedure. Where appropriate, relatives may be asked to check drugs – helping them to feel part of the caring team instead of being simply bystanders. Full records of medicines administered by the nurse, normally only parenteral forms, are kept in the patient's home and maintained and signed by the community nurse.

In an emergency, a medicine may be administered on the authority of a verbal message or facsimile but must be confirmed in writing by the medical practitioner within 24 hours. Controlled Drugs will be prescribed by the patient's GP and supplied by the community pharmacist. Community nurses, unlike hospital nurses, do not keep stocks of Controlled Drugs. The drugs are the patient's property and are kept in the patient's home along with formal written authorisation from the GP for the nurse to administer the medicine. The nurse has a responsibility to check that medicines are prescribed in appropriate doses. In palliative care, for example, where the patient's need for pain relief may change, and although the GP has prescribed the medicine, the nurse has a responsibility to know the safe limits of dosage of the particular medicine. The community nurse keeps a record in the home of doses administered together with the balance remaining.

Normally, community nurses do not carry any medicines other than those required for the treatment of anaphylaxis. They are responsible for ensuring that they know the current treatment and dosages of medicines used for anaphylaxis and that expiry dates on the products are not exceeded.

Theft from cars is a major concern for the community nurse. Medicinal products should always be out of sight and the vehicle locked. Once the nurse gets to know clients and their families, it may at times be necessary to weigh up what is the best action – to take the bag when calling on the patient or leave it in the car.

In very exceptional cases, a nurse may collect dispensed medicines for delivery to a patient if in the nurse's professional opinion the patient's safety and/or comfort would otherwise be in jeopardy. The nurse must balance the risk of contravening the law and professional guidance with a duty of care to the patient. In any event, security must be maintained throughout the time the medicines are in the nurse's possession. The safe-keeping and correct storage of medicines in the home are aspects of the role where advice may be sought from the patient or family, or offered by the nurse. Prescribed medicines are the property of the patient and should always be regarded as such by the community nurse. If a nurse has any concerns about leaving medicines (or equipment associated with the use of medicines) in the patient's home, the nurse manager or patient's GP should be consulted. Patients should be advised to store all medicines in a cool, dry and safe (although not necessarily locked) place out of the reach of children. The need for special storage requirements (e.g. refrigeration for insulin and for certain eye drops) should be stressed. The importance of noting and responding to expiry dates (e.g. eye drops must not be used beyond 4 weeks of opening) should also be emphasised.

Since the GP prescribes the vast majority (generally in the region of 80%) of all medicines, it follows that the scope for improving patient compliance in the community is considerable. Many of the strategies for improving compliance by the patient, discussed in Chapter 11, can be used by the community nurse.

Where a monitored dosage system ('tablet box') is to be introduced, the community pharmacist should provide this service. This includes dispensing the medicines into the compliance aid, labelling it and sealing it. Regular assessment of the patient's ability to use the aid safely and of the continued suitability of the aid in use should be made. Where it is not possible to get a compliance aid filled by the pharmacist and nurses choose in the patient's interests to place the dispensed medicines into the compliance aid, they must ensure the same level of accuracy and be aware that they are accountable for their actions (NMC 2002a). Despite strenuous and ingenious efforts by the nurse, family, neighbours and the home care team, the severely confused patient may be beyond immediate help, and alternative arrangements such as admission for long-term care may be required in the patient's best interests.

The scale of unused medicines in the community is now being fully recognised. Wasteful though it may seem, it is too dangerous to recycle even completely unopened packages and containers. Many patients, when a medicine is no longer required, simply do nothing about disposing of it. Others hang on to medicines in the belief that they may find a use for them on some future occasion and, besides, do not want to see them wasted. While doctors are being urged to prescribe realistic quantities of medicines, nurses need to encourage patients, relatives and carers of the need for safe disposal of unwanted medicines via the community pharmacist or GP/chemist. The Environmental Protection Act 1990 demands the safe disposal of pharmaceutical products. It is not acceptable to flush away unwanted medicines. Specialist advice should be sought when necessary from the community pharmacist, especially where larger quantities are to be disposed of.

Sharps containers should be supplied where necessary and advice given regarding safe disposal of sharps, storage of such containers in the home and arrangements for their ultimate removal.

The practice nurse

With the number of procedures previously undertaken in hospital outpatient departments now being carried out in GP practices and health centres, the role of the practice nurse (PN) has taken on increasing importance. As well as having either a community nursing qualification or a practice nurse qualification, PNs are trained to carry out a range of procedures which extend beyond those required of a registered nurse. The majority of PNs work in a treatment room within the practice, although some also do home visits. A variety of clinics (asthma, diabetes, well woman, wart removal, weight reduction, smoking cessation, etc.) are practice-nurse led. Dressings, ear syringing and administration of injections (e.g. hydroxocobalamin for pernicious anaemia; flupentixol for mental health problems; parenteral progestogen-only contraception) are routinely performed. An especially busy time for the PN is from October to December when much time is taken up with the annual administration of influenza vaccine. The vaccine is recommended for everyone over the age of 65 and for those in long-stay facilities. People of any age with a chronic condition of the lungs, heart or kidneys, or who have diabetes or are immunocompromised are also given the vaccine. Immunisation may be recommended for healthcare staff in years when the risk is considered to be higher than usual. With the increase in world travel all the year round and to far-flung regions, the PN has a wide variety of travel immunisations to attend to. The relevant vaccine(s) for the geographical region being visited, the vaccination programme, storage instructions and any particular advice can be accessed by the PN on an internet database. New patient medical checks, blood pressure checks for hypertensive patients and venepunctures required by the GPs are all done by the PN. First aid, treatment of minor injuries and assisting with minor surgery add to the many skills required. Only those PNs who have undergone the nurse prescribing course and gained authorisation to do so are permitted to prescribe. Patient Group Directions are drawn up by some practices. The PN is responsible for the ordering and safe storage of medicines held in the treatment room. Of special importance is ensuring medicines are 'in date', that all medicines including Controlled Drugs are appropriately stored, and that vaccines are stored at the correct temperature in a locked refrigerator.

The community midwife

The general principles of prescribing, administering and recording of medicines apply similarly in relation to community midwifery. All medicines being taken by the mother and any medicines administered to her during labour and to the baby must be recorded. Community midwives who also work in a hospital maternity unit may be permitted, without a medical prescription, to administer certain drugs which are listed on agreed standing orders previously signed by the doctor. The list is likely to include:

(i) for the mother:

- a narcotic analgesic, intramuscularly
- a local anaesthetic (for infiltrating the perineum prior to episiotomy)

- an anti-emetic, intramuscularly
- Syntometrine, intramuscularly (to prevent haemorrhage in third stage of labour)
- a mild analgesic, oral
- an antacid
- a mild laxative
- cream/suppositories (to soothe haemorrhoids).

In addition, a dose of ergometrine and a dose of naloxone may be listed for administration to the mother in the event of haemorrhage and opioid-induced respiratory depression respectively.

(ii) for the baby:

- phytomenadione, intramuscularly (vitamin K_1) (see BNF caution)
- naloxone, intramuscularly (to reverse depressant effect of opioids).

For a planned home confinement, the drugs required may be either obtained (and stored) by the patient from the community pharmacy on production of a GP's prescription, or provided by the GP for use by the community midwife and stored in the community hospital until required by the patient. The drugs required will be similar to those previously mentioned in the standing orders. Requisitions for medical gases can also be made by the community midwife.

The triple duty nurse

In remote areas, special arrangements for the management of medicines need to be made to cover the wide range of duties undertaken by the triple duty nurse.

The health visitor

It is customary for vaccinations to be administered by health visitors in clinics. The administration of immunological agents by nurses can be facilitated by a Patient Group Direction.

Specialised drug therapy in the home

In addition to haemodialysis and peritoneal dialysis, several forms of therapy more usually associated with inpatient care are carried out in the patient's home. The number of patients involved is not large but this trend is steadily increasing. There are many benefits to treatment at home:

- less time in hospital
- less risk of infection
- care at home
- greater autonomy
- ability to return to work
- best option for those living in remote rural areas
- frees up beds
- saves money.

The extent to which the community nurse is involved in the therapy will depend on several factors. In a number of situations patients will be taught to carry out procedures themselves but will need support and guidance from the nurse who will also carry out periodic checks on the patient's technique. Technical support services (e.g. equipment maintenance) will also be required.

Home intravenous therapy

Intravenous therapy may be continued at home using a centrally placed access device which was inserted in hospital when treatment was initiated. Examples of such devices include the Hickman catheter (skin-tunnelled, cuffed catheter inserted via the subclavian vein and with its tip lying in the superior vena cava) and the Port-a-Cath (catheter inserted into the subclavian or internal jugular vein and ending in an implanted subcutaneous disk-covered port). Devices such as these are introduced to save frequent venepunctures. Three main groups of patients may be taught to self-administer intravenous medication by one of these methods.

Patients suffering from cystic fibrosis, advanced bronchiectasis or cytomegalovirus retinitis (in immunocompromised patients) are taught to administer intravenous antibiotics. The specific benefit for these patients is the reduced risk of developing nosocomial infections (Kayley 1996).

Home parenteral nutrition (see also p. 385) is used for patients with severe intestinal failure. In most instances the therapy is required in the short term where the condition is reversible but in some patients therapy must be continued for life. Oncology patients may receive intravenous cytotoxic therapy at home or may be intermittently admitted to hospital for repeat pulses of treatment. In each case, the community nurse may be involved in the maintenance of the line and in providing ongoing support for the patient and carer(s).

Continuous intravenous administration of drugs using a syringe pump is available for use in the patient's home for pain control in terminal care (see Ch. 30) and other specialised forms of therapy such as insulin. A battery-operated syringe pump is also available for the intravenous injection of drugs in boluses at regular but infrequent intervals.

The subcutaneous route using a syringe driver may also be used in the domiciliary setting for the continuous infusion of drugs used in palliative care. It is essential that nurses involved in setting syringe driver rates are adequately trained to avoid a common source of drug error.

Home nebulisers for the treatment of asthma

Nebulisers are occasionally prescribed for asthmatic patients who have been found unresponsive to conventional treatment. Dangers associated with this form of treatment have been identified, particularly when the nebuliser in use has not been prescribed.

The forms of home therapy briefly described above have a number of advantages, the greatest of which is the fact that many patients are able to resume a reasonably normal lifestyle. In addition, home therapy is more economical than hospital-based therapy. Obviously, care in patient selection for any form of sophisticated home therapy is extremely important, as is the need for training and continuing support. In certain situations the community nurse will need special instruction on the techniques involved, which can best be provided in the ward where the treatment is initiated. Community nurses, in responding to this technological revolution, are working to ensure that their patients receive maximum therapeutic benefit.

REFERENCES

Environmental Protection Act 1990 HMSO, London

Kayley J 1996 Use of IV antibiotics at home. Community Nurse 2(7):15–16

Nursing and Midwifery Council (NMC) 2002a Guidelines for the administration of medicines. NMC, London

Nursing and Midwifery Council (NMC) 2002b Code of professional conduct. NMC, London

Rodman M J, Smith D W 1974 Clinical pharmacology in nursing. Lippincott, Philadelphia

FURTHER READING

Beecham L 2000 UK health secretary wants to liberate nurses' talents. News. British Medical Journal 320:1025

Carlisle D 2002 Hidden agenda. Nursing Times 98(21):24–27

Davies C 2000 Getting professionals to work together: there's more to collaboration than simply working side by side. British Medical Journal 320:1021–1022

Doyal L, Cameron A 2000 Reshaping the NHS workforce: necessary changes are constrained by professional structures from the past. British Medical Journal 320:1023–1024

Iliffe S 2000 Nursing and the future of primary care: handmaidens or agents for managed care? British Medical Journal 320:1020–1021

Salvage J, Smith R 2000 Doctors and nurses doing it differently: the time is ripe for a major reconstruction. British Medical Journal 320:1019

Zwarenstein M, Reeves S 2000 What's so great about collaboration?: we need more evidence and less rhetoric. British Medical Journal 320:1022–1023

USEFUL WEB SITES

Nursing and Midwifery Council: http://www.nmc-uk.org

Royal College of Nursing: http://www.rcn.org.uk

CHAPTER CONTENTS

5

Formularies

DEVELOPMENT OF FORMULARIES

Today, it is widely accepted that a drug formulary is an essential element in the drive to achieve safe and rational prescribing while at the same time controlling costs. Box 5.1 outlines the stages in formulary development which would be followed by a Drug and Therapeutics Committee (D&TC) in hospital with a multidisciplinary membership of doctors, pharmacists, nurses and finance officer.

The method of presentation of the formulary varies from a simple listing of products to a compendium giving full details of the formulations, actions and uses of each drug, side-effects, dosage levels and costs. Presentation of the information is increasingly by means of computerised systems which also facilitate monitoring of formulary compliance. The choice of drug for inclusion in the formulary is based on safety, efficacy, cost and advice provided centrally (see p. 5). The classification system used by the British National Formulary (BNF) is generally adopted in local formularies for ease of reference.

Government policy has strongly encouraged the development of drug formularies throughout the NHS. Drug formularies have significant advantages for

Box 5.1 Stages in formulary development in the hospital setting

Stage I	Request for inclusion of product by consultant(s)
Stage II	Consideration by D&TC
Stage III	Inclusion in formulary (or rejection or suggestion of alternative)
Stage IV	Publication of information on product to prescribers
Stage V	Monitoring of impact/cost/benefits
Stage VI	Depending on outcome, use of drug extended, curtailed or discontinued

patient care, especially when linked electronically with prescribing systems. Some of the advantages and disadvantages postulated are summarised in Box 5.2.

Although opponents of drug formularies may still be heard, there can be little doubt that, as the range of drugs available to the prescriber continues to expand and costs continue to escalate, formularies will become even more important.

Effective multidisciplinary working methods and consultation can do much to reduce the difficulties outlined above. Collaborative effort leading to ownership is a key element of formulary development. On the advice of government departments, health authorities have been given the responsibility to develop joint formularies where agreement is reached between primary and secondary care regarding which drugs should be prescribed.

The nurse plays an increasingly important role in both formulary development (as a member of the D&TC) and formulary management. Devolved drug budgets are an incentive to nurses in achieving and monitoring formulary compliance. To carry out this important task, the need for accurate, up-to-date information on the usage of medicines is vital. Pharmaceutical services are provided in such a way that staff who are responsible for the use of medicines receive regular feedback on levels of use of both formulary and non-formulary drugs. The introduction of a formulary system may create problems for nurses when patients receiving a non-formulary medicine are admitted for inpatient care. The approach to this problem will vary depending on local arrangements. For example, patients may continue to be given the medicine(s) using supplies they have brought in on admission. This approach needs the support and advice of the clinical pharmacist (and/or prescriber) to ensure that the medicine(s) are suitable for use. When the prescriber considers it to be appropriate, another medicine may be substituted. In such situations, nurses can help to explain to patients the reasons for any change in therapy. On the other hand, the nurse may become the patient's advocate and ask that the patient be maintained on the original therapy where, in the nurse's professional view, it would be disadvantageous to change the patient's therapy. In addition to formularies designed to meet the prescribing needs of doctors, formularies of nursing care products have been developed (see p. 45).

Box 5.2 Advantages and disadvantages of drug formularies

Advantages
- Lower prescribing costs
- Encourage generic prescribing
- Improve drug safety
- Improve patient care (by linking with prescribing systems)
- Reduce range of products to be stored
- Facilitate drug purchasing in hospitals
- Educational value
- Provide opportunity for multidisciplinary working
- Improve continuity of care, especially where a joint hospital/community formulary is in place

Disadvantages
- Restrict clinical freedom
- Inhibit introduction of new products:
  - reduce research efforts
  - stifle innovation by pharmaceutical industry
- Restrict the patient's choice
- Reduce treatment options

PATIENT PROTOCOLS

Shared-care protocols

Doctors in general practice and hospitals are developing shared-care protocols for the care of patients suffering from chronic illnesses such as asthma, diabetes and hypertension. Patient protocols have strong links with drug formularies, since protocols contain details of drug treatment regimens. Shared-care protocols represent an agreement between consultant, GP and patient on the approach to diagnosis and treatment of a particular illness. The purpose of the protocol is to standardise treatment and to help ensure continuity of care and involvement of the patient. An outline of a shared-care protocol is given in Box 5.3.

Computerisation of the management of patient care greatly assists in the introduction, monitoring and audit of the benefits (or otherwise) achieved by use of the protocol. Shared-care protocols also provide a framework

Box 5.3 Outline of a shared-care protocol

Brief introduction to condition dealt with in protocol
Objectives of protocol
Responsibilities of consultant, e.g.:

- communication between consultant ↔ patient ↔ GP
- source of supply of medicines
- treatment regimen drug/dose/route/etc.

Responsibilities of GP, e.g. prescribing (and administration) of the drug(s)
Responsibilities of patient, e.g. attendance at clinic(s)
Contact telephone numbers, etc.

within which the patient can become fully involved in the treatment plan.

Nurses will normally be involved in drawing up shared-care protocols, especially those nurses working in close liaison with their colleagues in the community.

In addition to shared-care protocols, GPs are adopting protocols for use within their own practices on the treatment of such conditions as urinary tract infection (UTI), intractable pain and chronic bronchitis.

Protocols may be seen by some doctors as limiting clinical freedom and as a potential threat to innovation. There are also legal implications and concerns that patient protocols may be unduly influenced by cost factors. Advantages claimed for patient protocols include improved patient care, elimination of the wide variation in diagnosis and treatment, and opportunities for the introduction of clinical audit. A protocol for the treatment of UTI in general practice contained the following elements:

- organisation of care, e.g.
  - aims of treatment
  - organisation of diagnostic services
- assessment and treatment of the patient
- problem solving and follow-up
- patient checklist
- practice audit.

As protocols are developed, there will be many opportunities for nurses to contribute to their development.

Local policies

In small hospitals with no resident doctor, in specialist units and in some community settings, the strict criteria laid down by the NMC (2002) with respect to the administration of medicines either cannot be applied or, if applied, could introduce dangerous delay with consequent risks to patients. In these situations, an agreed local policy may be drawn up for use by nurses. Where a policy of this kind applies it must clearly state:

- the circumstances in which particular 'prescription-only medicines' may be administered in advance of examination by a doctor
- the form, route and dosage range of the medicines so authorised
- which nurse(s) are allowed to be involved in the administration of these medicines.

THE FUTURE OF FORMULARIES

There can be no doubt that the financial pressures arising from the introduction of new drugs will continue to mount. The general public and patient support groups will press health authorities to find the necessary resources to fund all forms of new technology. New drugs are part of the technological revolution. NICE and the Health Technology Board for Scotland provide central guidance on drugs which have been approved for prescribing within the NHS. Nurses and their colleagues have great opportunities to contribute to the achievement of safe and cost-effective drug treatment through the development of formularies.

One approach that may provide a framework for future development is the management of medicines in patient-focused care. This concept, developed in the USA, seeks to address the fragmentation that so often is seen in the provision of patient care. Key aspects of patient focused care are:

- improving continuity of care
- decentralisation of services within the hospital
- introduction of total quality management
- establishing critical care pathways/protocols.

The excellent cooperative working between nurses and clinical pharmacists augurs well for the future.

REFERENCES

Nursing and Midwifery Council (NMC) 2002 Guidelines on the administration of medicines. NMC, London

FURTHER READING

Audit Commission 2001 A spoonful of sugar. Medicines management in NHS hospitals. Audit Commission, London

CHAPTER CONTENTS

6

Nurse prescribing

BACKGROUND

The prescribing of medicines by nurses is a significant development of their professional role. First recommended by the Royal College of Nursing in 1980 (Blatt 1997) and addressed in more detail in the Cumberlege Report (DHSS 1986), nurse prescribing evolved with the growing realisation that much of patients' and community nurses' time was being wasted in waiting to get prescriptions signed by a doctor when in many cases it was the nurse who had recommended the dressing or appliance in the first place. It was also apparent that community nurses were becoming increasingly skilled in managing pain relief for terminally ill patients (Humphries & Green 1999). Clarification of professional responsibilities was long overdue. The Crown Report (DoH 1989) took the matter further with the recommendation that suitably qualified nurses working in the community should be authorised to prescribe in defined circumstances from a limited list, i.e. a nurse prescribers' formulary. A further recommendation was that nurses should be able to supply medicines within group protocols. The legislation permitting nurse prescribing within the NHS received the Royal Assent in March 1992. This primary legislation was introduced to permit appropriately qualified nurses working in community practice who had had the recognised additional training to prescribe (within the NHS) medicines and appliances (surgical dressings, etc.) needed for the nursing care of their patients.

In 2000, further proposals to extend the range of prescription-only medicines which may be prescribed by independent nurse prescribers were issued for consideration. These wider prescribing powers were granted in 2001 (Scottish Executive 2001a). Similar powers have been granted in other parts of the UK.

LEVELS OF AUTHORISATION

For many years, nurses had access to a range of medicinal and nursing care products which were used without medical prescription. With the interests of patient need and the effectiveness and safety profile of the products in mind, written protocols were subsequently developed. Such protocols took the form of, for example, a formulary of nursing care products. Guidance included in the protocols was determined jointly by clinical staff.

A number of levels of authorisation are now in place which, depending on the training and accreditation the individual has received, allows nurses to utilise their knowledge of patients and make informed judgements of a patient's requirements.

SYMPTOMATIC RELIEF POLICY

A symptomatic relief policy provides a framework which allows the nurse to use a limited number of simple medications used in the treatment of minor ailments. The drugs on the limited list are generally agreed between nursing, medical and pharmacy staff and may include for example simple analgesia, aperients and demulcents. *Doctors initiate* symptomatic relief for *individual* patients by entering the words SYMPTOMATIC RELIEF on the prescription along with their signature and the date. Nurses use their professional judgement in selecting the appropriate preparation and dose from the agreed limited list and then administer and record it. Provided the guidelines which accompany the symptomatic relief policy are adhered to by the nurse administering the medicine(s), it is the *doctor who is accountable* for the effects of the medicine(s). The policy is designed to benefit patients, doctors and nurses by speeding up the process of relieving the patient's symptoms, reducing the number of times doctors are interrupted and allowing nurses to exercise their professional role in order to meet the needs of patients.

Nurses are well placed to both adjust dosages/frequency of administration and prescribe certain medicines without the need for medical intervention. It is emphasised that dosage adjustment and prescribing must be in accordance with agreed written guidelines. Relief of symptoms will generally include the relief of pain, constipation, sore throat and mild upper respiratory tract problems. Nurses can often prescribe for the relief of gastrointestinal symptoms. They may also prescribe and use local instillations to the bladder, especially where indwelling catheters have to be maintained. While the policies on prescribing for symptom relief are applicable widely, a doctor may wish to make certain exceptions in the case of a particular patient. For example, 'symptom relief except laxatives' may be entered on the patient's case notes/prescription sheet. Nursing staff permitted to administer medicines in this category must be registered with the Nursing and Midwifery Council and be able to demonstrate competence following appropriate additional training.

PATIENT GROUP DIRECTIONS

Following concerns about the legality of group protocols highlighted in the Crown Report (1999), changes were made to the Medicines Act 1968 which allow the legal supply and administration of medicines under Patient Group Directions (PGDs) replacing the term group protocol. Patient Group Directions are *written* instructions for *groups of patients* in *specific situations* who have not necessarily been individually identified (DoH 1999). They allow prescription-only medicines to be administered on the 'direction' of a doctor.

PGDs have been introduced in both hospital and community practice to reduce the time patients have to wait for treatment. Increased use of the nurse's professional skills, it is believed, will result in more effective utilisation of resources. Those authorised to supply or administer medicines under PGDs include individually named registered nurses, midwives, health visitors, pharmacists and a range of professionals allied to medicine who have undergone training and accreditation relevant to the clinical condition(s) to be treated and medicine(s) to be used. Each PGD is formally established by local professional advisory groups in wide consultation with senior representatives of the appropriate professional group. In line with the legislation, the Direction must provide among other things details relating to the specific clinical condition, medicine(s), healthcare professional involved and health organisation to which it applies. All authorisations must be signed and dated. A senior doctor, senior pharmacist and senior nurse must sign the PGD and authorisation must be granted by the appropriate health authority/trust.

Staff participating in PGDs must have the approval of their professional manager and be provided with written authorisation to provide care within the specified Direction. Examples of PGDs include:

- the administration of individual vaccines (a separate Direction will be compiled for each: for example, administration of polio vaccine; administration of diphtheria, tetanus and pertussis vaccine; administration of hepatitis B vaccination)
- the administration of travel vaccinations

- the administration of sodium chloride 0.9% injection for flushing intravenous catheters/ cannulae
- the administration of adrenaline (epinephrine) in cases of suspected hypersensitivity and/or anaphylactic reactions
- the administration of products contained in the formulary of nursing care products
- treatments for minor injuries
- administration of emergency hormonal contraception
- test doses of salbutamol.

Many more, no doubt, will be developed.

All nurses supplying and/or administering medicines under a PGD must sign to confirm they understand its contents and have received the appropriate training. A register of those nurses who have been authorised to supply/administer medicines under PGDs must be maintained by the senior nurse manager, and continuing education provided for those whose names are on it.

Summary

The majority of patients receiving clinical care will continue to receive medicines which have been prescribed on an individual basis. In contrast, PGDs provide a system for authorising appropriately trained nurses and other healthcare professionals to supply and administer named medicines in identified clinical situations without the need for a separate, signed prescription for each individual patient. The benefits of PGDs are significant and include the production of an evidence-based quality standard with improved response to anaphylaxis, earlier treatment and less administrative work (Jones 2001).

Responsibility rests with senior medical, pharmacy and nurse managers to ensure that Patient Group Directions are suitably prepared and that training is provided for those participating. Individual nurses, having been instructed on the bounds of professional responsibility, must not act beyond their professional competence. To do so would be in breach of the law.

NURSE PRESCRIBING

District nurses, health visitors and those practice nurses with a district nurse or health visitor qualification who have successfully completed a training programme in nurse prescribing are permitted to prescribe from the limited list set out in the Nurse Prescribers' Formulary, based on their own judgement and without consulting a doctor. They are legally accountable for their actions.

Prescribing is restricted to a limited range of medicines and appliances. Community pharmacists are not able to dispense any prescriptions written by nurses for products outwith the approved list. Products available for prescribing by nurses include laxatives, stoma care products, analgesics associated with minor trauma, bladder instillations, preparations for the treatment of simple skin and ear conditions, surgical dressings, and treatments for head lice. It should be pointed out that treatments initiated by nurses should always be fully recorded and communicated to the patient's doctor as soon as possible.

Nurses are expected to have a suitable level of background knowledge of clinical pharmacology and therapeutics in order to be able to benefit fully from the training. Training programmes focus on the need for the nurse to be able to prescribe effectively from the Nurse Prescribers' Formulary. In addition to knowledge of clinical pharmacology and therapeutics, the nurse is required to demonstrate a knowledge of the relevant legislation and to be fully aware of issues of accountability and professional responsibility. The overall training requirements of nurse prescribers are as follows:

- basic clinical pharmacology and therapeutics
- legislation
- professional role/accountability
- role of the professions (doctor, nurse, pharmacist)
- principles, practices and procedures of nurse prescribing
- knowledge of actions/uses/hazards of products included in the Nurse Prescribers' Formulary
- economic aspects.

Good prescribing is based on a number of fundamental principles. A seven-step model represented as a prescribing pyramid is advocated (Fig. 6.1) (National Prescribing Centre 1999). A thorough, holistic assessment of the patient's needs should always be carried out before any other action is taken. All treatment options should be considered including not to treat at all. Where there is a genuine need to prescribe, care should be taken to select a product that is effective, appropriate for the patient, safe and cost-effective. As far as possible, the patient should be encouraged to participate in the process of deciding on the most suitable product. A regular review of the patient is essential to ensure that the prescribed treatment is effective, safe and acceptable. It is a professional requirement for nurses to keep records that are both accurate and up to date (NMC 2002).

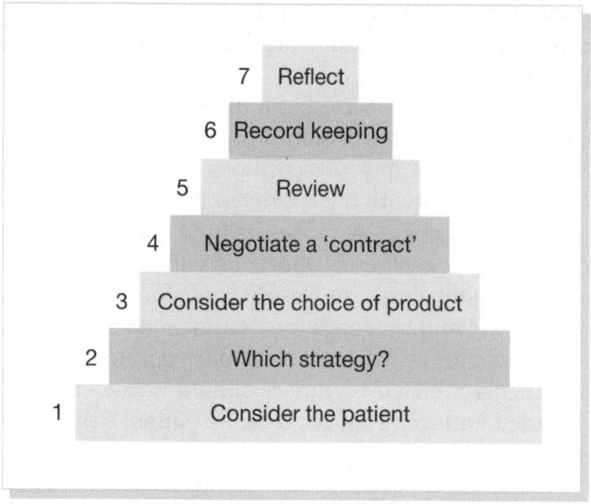

Figure 6.1 The prescribing pyramid. Each step should be considered carefully before the next is approached. (From National Prescribing Centre 1999, with permission.)

Finally, much can be learned from reviewing prescribing practice.

EXTENDED NURSE PRESCRIBING

The extended prescribing of prescription-only medicines (PoMs) by independent nurse prescribers is intended to enhance patient care by:

- providing quicker and more efficient access to healthcare
- making better use of nurses' skills
- allowing doctors more time to deal with more serious cases (Scottish Executive 2001b).

Suitably trained nurses will be permitted to prescribe all General Sale List medicines and all Pharmacy medicines that are prescribable by GPs under the NHS with the exception of Controlled Drugs and antibiotics. In addition, they may prescribe a range of PoMs linked to specific medical conditions/situations arising in the following areas

- minor ailments, e.g. haemorrhoids, upper respiratory tract infections
- minor injuries, e.g. burns, lacerations
- health promotion, e.g. smoking cessation, emergency contraception
- palliative care, e.g. symptomatic relief of dry mouth, hiccup, nausea.

The amended Prescription Only Medicines (Human Use) Order 1997 gives independent nurse prescribers, who have had additional training to the required level, powers to prescribe any medicinal product containing one or more of the POM substances listed under the recommendation of the Committee on the Safety of Medicines. No other POM substance may be prescribed. Nurses permitted to prescribe from the *extended* list of prescription-only medicines require to be first level registered nurses who have successfully completed an *enhanced* programme of preparation for nurse prescribing and are subsequently recorded in the professional register as having successfully completed that programme. A 3-month programme of preparation at degree level involving approximately 25 taught days (or equivalent) must be undertaken plus additional self-directed learning. An essential element of the training programme is time spent learning in practice with a prescribing mentor. Both theoretical knowledge and competence in practice are assessed on completion of the programme. Approval and monitoring of the programmes is to be undertaken.

Preparations are underway to train large numbers of nurses and midwives to undertake the extended nurse prescribing role. Priority is to be given to:

- community midwives in midwife-led units
- nurses in community hospitals
- specialist nurses in nurse-led clinics.

Provided the criteria for entry to the training programme are met, however, there is no reason to prevent other nurses from applying. Practice nurses and hospital nurses in specialist practice are expected to seek early application.

This latest development is seen as a further opportunity for nurses and midwives to enhance patient care. Its success is dependent on high-quality education provision and multiprofessional support systems.

FUTURE DEVELOPMENTS AND IMPLICATIONS FOR NURSES

In time, it is anticipated that some oral antibiotics may be added to the Nurse Prescribers' Formulary. Eventually, certain Controlled Drugs may also be included.

The advent of nurse prescribing within community practice in the NHS, will, in time, also have an impact on the role of the nurse in hospital practice. Hospital nurses have always had certain prescribing responsibilities and it seems likely that these will develop in the years ahead. Nurse prescribing can be seen as having special relevance as care in the community gathers momentum. Continuity of care between hospital and the community will be greatly facilitated by nurse prescribing.

The introduction of nurse prescribing brings into even stronger focus the principles of medicine management and associated responsibilities already familiar to the professional nurse. Nurses authorised to prescribe are required to utilise to the full their knowledge of the actions and uses of medicines and their skills in observation, communication and recording. Furthermore, prescribing nurses take a greater part in decision-making and thereby have increasing reasons to be accountable for their actions and inactions.

Proposals are currently under discussion (DoH 2002) which would allow prescription-only medicines to be prescribed by healthcare professionals (suitably qualified nurses and pharmacists) following clinical assessment and 'once a diagnosis has been established or a treatment plan prepared' (DoH 1999). Those undertaking this role would be classed as supplementary (dependent) prescribers.

The clinical management plan would be a written document relating to a named patient and to that patient's specific condition. It would be agreed and signed by both the independent and supplementary prescriber. The range of medicines would be specified in the plan along with the circumstances within which the dosage, frequency and formulation of the medicines could be varied.

It may be argued that prescribing medicines is simply another medical task that has been devolved to nurses primarily to relieve hard-pressed doctors of a time-consuming chore. Many nurses and other health professionals, however, consider that the development of nurse prescribing is part of a logical progression which recognises the needs of patients and how these can best be met. Nurses have, for many years, exercised considerable influence on the prescribing process. All the indications are that when nurses assume wider professional responsibilities the outcomes are greatly beneficial to patient care. As always, nurses expect to encounter a new set of challenges and opportunities. Prescribing is not a simple mechanistic act. Relationships between patient and prescriber can be subject to tensions and perhaps unreasonable demands on the part of the patient. It is vitally important to ensure that all parties to the prescribing process have a clear understanding of the remit of the nurse and the constraints of a limited formulary within which the nurse is working. Prescribing, whether by doctors or nurses, should never be seen as a substitute for preventive measures or the use of basic household remedies. Patient education, information and counselling must not be neglected. Community nurses are especially well placed to monitor the patient's total use of medicines, both prescribed and non-prescribed. As more potent medicinal products become available without prescription, this aspect of the nurse's responsibilities will become increasingly important. Nurse prescribing must not, and will not, be allowed to become purely a supply service, important though this is. As with all aspects of nursing care, the clinical needs of patients should be uppermost in the minds of nurses when they decide to prescribe for them.

REFERENCES

Blatt B 1997 Nurse prescribing: are you ready? Practice Nursing 8(12):11–13

Department of Health (DoH) 1999 A review of prescribing, supply and administration of medicines – final report (Crown Report 2). DoH, London

Department of Health (DoH) 2002 Proposals for supplementary prescribing by nurses and pharmacists and proposed amendments to the Prescription Only Medicines (Human Use) Order 1997. DoH, London

Department of Health and Social Security (DHSS) 1986 Neighbourhood nursing: a focus for care (Cumberlege Report). HMSO, London

Department of Health (DoH) 1989 Report of The Advisory Group on Nurse Prescribing (Crown Report). DoH, London

Humphries J L, Green J (eds) 1999 Nurse prescribing. Macmillan, Basingstoke

Jones P G W 2001 How to decide when a patient group direction is needed. Guidelines in Practice 4(9):78–84

Medicines Act 1968 HMSO, London

National Prescribing Centre 1999 Signposts for prescribing nurses – general principles of good prescribing. Prescribing Nurse Bulletin 1(1):1–4

Nursing and Midwifery Council (NMC) 2002 Guidelines for records and record keeping. NMC, London

Prescription Only Medicines (Human Use) Order 1997 Statutory Instrument No. 1830. HMSO, London

Scottish Executive 2001a News release: Deacon – nurses to be given wider prescribing powers. Scottish Executive, Edinburgh

Scottish Executive 2001b Extended prescribing of prescription only medicines by independent nurse prescribers. Scottish Executive, Edinburgh

FURTHER READING

Courtenay M, Butler M 1999 Nurse prescribing: principles and practice. Greenwich Medical Media, London

Jones P G W 2001 How has the patient group directions website contributed to patient care? Pharmaceutical Journal 268:371–373

USEFUL WEB SITES

British National Formulary: http://www.BNF.org

Department of Health nurse prescribing: http://www.doh.gov.uk/nurseprescribing

National Prescribing Centre: http://www.npc.co.uk

Nurse Prescribing Bulletins (published by National Prescribing Centre): http://www.npc.org.uk

Nurse Prescribers' Formulary: http://www.doh.gov.uk/nurseprescribing

Patient Group Directions: http://www.rpsgh.org.uk

CHAPTER CONTENTS

7

The principles of medicine administration

INTRODUCTION

Medicine administration is a multifaceted process. This chapter considers the basics of the administration of medicines in any setting. It should be read in conjunction with other chapters in this section.

A number of basic rules apply to the administration of medicines irrespective of the method of administration used or whether the patient is in hospital, in a clinic or at home.

FOLLOWING THE POLICY

Policies regarding the storage, checking and administration of medicines are established by health authorities from a number of sources. These include:

- legal requirements
- government health circulars
- Nursing and Midwifery Council codes of practice, guidelines, etc.

In addition, local policies which relate to a functional unit, e.g. hospital or ward, may exist within this wider context. Copies of the relevant policies should be readily accessible. It is incumbent on nurses to become fully conversant with these policies and to adhere to them at all times.

ASSESSING PATIENTS AND THEIR MEDICINES

When compiling a profile of any patient, whether newly referred to the district nurse or on admission to hospital, the nurse is ideally placed to identify actual or potential problems the patient may have in relation to his or her medicines. It is important to gather personal data including age, address and available family support as these may have a bearing on the likelihood of patients managing to take their medicines at home. Dietary, cultural and economic influences should also be noted.

Patients should be asked if they are taking medicines of any kind – prescribed or non-prescribed – and whether they are experiencing any difficulty with them. The effect that individual drugs are having, or may be suspected of having, on the activities of living should be considered such as the constipating effect of some analgesics may affect elimination; the nauseating effect of an antibiotic may interfere with eating and drinking; a sedative drug may make communication difficult. An examination of medicines brought into hospital by the patient may reveal patient non-compliance. Through questioning and/or observation, the nurse may be the first to discover that the patient is hypersensitive to a medicine.

The initial assessment of patients' physical capabilities and mental capacity helps in estimating the degree of dependence they are likely to have on others for assistance, including the taking of medicines. Patients' learning needs with respect to their medicines may also be established at this time. Thereafter, assessment of a patient's condition and needs is carried out on a continual basis. Finally, just prior to the administration of any medicine, the nurse must consider whether, according to the condition of the patient at the time, it is appropriate to proceed.

Some of the difficulties (actual or potential) which patients have that can interfere with safe and effective medicine management, and the nursing implications, are given in Table 7.1. The activities of living as categorised by Roper, Logan & Tierney (1996) serve as a suitable checklist.

PLANNING DRUG THERAPY

Medicines are prescribed by the doctor, taking into account the patient's age and other factors including body mass, physical and mental condition, concurrent illness and, in some instances, the patient's specific requests or beliefs. The nurse can assist in suggesting times of administration that will fit in with other activities in which the patient is involved. Where the presentation of the medicine (e.g. a large tablet) is likely to pose a problem, the nurse can draw the doctor's attention to the patient's difficulty. In this situation, the clinical pharmacist can be of particular assistance. When an intravenous infusion is to be begun, it may be possible to take into account the patient's preference of which arm to use. Here the nurse should act as the patient's advocate as necessary.

WRITING THE PRESCRIPTION

Responsibility rests with the prescriber to provide the statutory components of a prescription, clearly and indelibly written or computer generated, authorising the administration of any medicine(s) irrespective of whether the prescriber or another person is going to administer the medicine(s). Unless provided for in a specific protocol, or in very exceptional circumstances, instruction by telephone to administer a previously unprescribed substance is not acceptable (DoH 1988). On occasion, in community hospitals, for example, there may be no alternative to a prescription being ordered by telephone. In such cases, locally agreed procedures should be followed. A registered nurse, in all situations, must take the message, repeating it to the doctor to ensure accuracy. Where possible, a second nurse should also take the message, again repeating it to the doctor to ensure accuracy. An entry should be made by the nurse(s) taking the message on the appropriate prescription sheet. The prescribing doctor should sign the entry at the earliest possible opportunity. Local policy will demand that, in any event, the prescription is signed within a set period of time, for example, within 24 hours. New prescriptions for Controlled Drugs must never be ordered by telephone. An alternative to telephoning prescriptions is using facsimile transmission (fax). Computerised prescribing systems are being developed for use in hospitals. In primary care, many general practitioners use computers for both acute and repeat prescribing. Whatever the method used, where the new prescription replaces an earlier one, the latter must be clearly cancelled and the cancellation signed and dated by a registered medical practitioner.

INTERPRETING THE PRESCRIPTION

All prescriptions must bear:

- the full name of the patient
- the patient's address if at home or, in the case of an inpatient, the hospital and ward
- the patient's age/date of birth and unit number.

Six items must be present as part of the actual prescription before administration can take place. These are:

- The *date* (including day, month and year) of prescribing of each individual medicine which should be coincidental with the date of commencement. As far as possible, medicines should not be prescribed prospectively although it is recognised that, for practical purposes, preoperative medicines and diagnostic agents may have to be prescribed in this way.
- The *name* of the medicine prescribed, written in full in block letters using the approved (generic) name

Table 7.1 Identifying problems that can interfere with medicine management

Activity of living	Patient problems and nursing implications
Maintaining a safe environment	When compliance is likely to pose a problem, it may be necessary to ask a relative or friend to supervise or assist the patient with medicines on discharge from hospital. Extra emphasis on safety with medicines is essential when there are children
	Any drug or medicine sensitivity known to the patient should be clearly entered in nursing and medical records including medicine prescription sheets
	Patients and/or relatives should be warned of potential harm from side-effects, e.g. drowsiness, dizziness. Hypotension may occur when benzodiazepines are in use, leading to falls
	Patients should be discouraged from 'hoarding' unused medicines and instructed about safe disposal
Communicating	Any knowledge deficit should be identified and corrected. Guidance and instruction in the administration of medicines must be matched to the patient's level of understanding. Advice from each member of staff must be consistent. Nurses must help patients to appreciate the importance of taking medicines correctly. Relatives may be asked to provide further support
	Many older patients have difficulty seeing their medicines. Small white tablets against a white background, or clear liquids in a clear medicine glass can be overlooked. Nurses should ensure that good light is provided and that patients are wearing their spectacles
	The successful taking of medicine depends on receiving accurate instruction, most of which is verbal. When patients are weak and depressed, hearing is less acute. Language difficulties may require the help of an interpreter. Compliance aids may be needed where forgetfulness is a problem
Breathing	Where severe breathlessness makes swallowing difficult, an alternative route, such as the rectal route, may be used
Eating and drinking	Inability to swallow will necessitate the use of alternative routes of administration (e.g. via nasogastric tube, per rectum or by injection). Patients with dysphagia may require oral medicines in liquid form
	Nausea and vomiting often prevent successful administration of oral medicines. Patients may indicate ways they have devised to overcome this problem
	Large volumes of fluid should be discouraged where the daily intake is restricted (e.g. in renal failure). Patients taking certain sulphonamides require to take copious amounts of liquid
	The concurrent use of alcohol with prescribed medicines may result in dangerous interactions
Eliminating	Loss of control of the anal sphincter or faecal impaction may make it impossible for the patient to retain rectal medication. Constipation may interfere with the free flow of urine per urinary catheter and may make bladder irrigation difficult
Personal cleansing and dressing	Lack of interest in personal hygiene or embarrassment may make the patient reluctant to accept treatment for such problems as body odours or head lice
	Some topical applications stain clothing, bedding and the bath, which may be the cause of non-compliance
Controlling body temperature	Some drugs may affect the heat-regulating mechanism, e.g. phenothiazines, causing hypothermia in older people. Requirements of clothing and room temperature should be adjusted accordingly
Mobilising	Patients should be in the most upright position possible for taking oral medicines. Great care must be taken to avoid inhalation when giving medicines to patients who have to be nursed in the prone or recumbent position
	Restrictions may be imposed on patients' mobility so that nurses must adapt their approach to the administration of medicines accordingly
	Where there is loss of the use of both hands or where tremor is very severe, considerable assistance will be required with the taking of medicines. Strategies for overcoming the difficulty of mild tremor, stiffness of the hands, or having the use of one hand only, can be taught. The use of an appropriate aid should be considered.
	Lack of mobility may prevent patients from obtaining their medicines when at home
Working and playing	Poorly motivated patients are less likely to take an interest in their medicines. Encouragement should be given to all patients but especially to those who will have to manage their medicines at home. Importance should be attached to drugs which constitute replacement therapy or control of disease
	Those in full-time education or employment may have difficulty maintaining compliance in taking their medicines
Expressing sexuality	Embarrassment may interfere with the satisfactory insertion or application of certain preparations (e.g. pessaries, vaginal creams). Nurses should be tactful in their approach and ensure maximum privacy. Whenever possible, self-administration should be encouraged
Sleeping	Very drowsy patients may be unable to cooperate in the taking of medicines, and other routes may have to be used. Special care must be taken to avoid accidental inhalation of medicines
Dying	In terminal care, injections should be minimised. Where they cannot be avoided, the volume of reconstituting fluid used should be the minimum compatible with the physical and other properties of the drug. A smaller needle may be required for giving an intramuscular injection, e.g. 23G, 1 inch, for an adult
	Control of pain is achieved through thorough assessment of the pain, careful choice of analgesic, appropriate dosage, and administration at regular and suitable intervals. There is no place in terminal illness for 'analgesics as required'

for single-ingredient preparations. If the product is a compound formulation (i.e. contains more than one active component), the name of a proprietary (trade) product may be used. In some instances, the name will include the strength of the medicine to be used (for example, glucose 5%) or in the case of a compound the ratio of strength of the components (for example, co-amilofruse 2.5/20).

- The *dosage* of the medicine to be given each time, prescribed using the metric system. Substitutes for actual dosage (e.g. 1 tab instead of 250 mg; 1 vial instead of 100 mg) must be avoided except in the case of multi-ingredient formulations. Decimal fractions should be avoided (e.g. 250 micrograms and not 0.25 mg). When writing prescriptions the word 'micrograms' (or nanograms) should be written in full and not abbreviated.
- The *route* (method) of administration, which may be abbreviated as follows:

SL	sublingual
PR	per rectum
PV	per vaginam
TOP	topical
INHAL	inhalation
SC	subcutaneous
IM	intramuscular
IV	intravenous
ID	intradermal.

Oral and other forms of administration should be written in full using block letters. 'O' for oral is not a recognised abbreviation and may lead to error if linked to the dose prescribed. Further requirements for giving the medicine may have to be stated specifically. For example:

ORAL after food
TOP to both eyes
INHAL via mask – 24% at 2 litres per minute.

A list of internationally recognised abbreviations and symbols is included inside the front cover of the BNF. Some of these are used in prescription writing such as e/c (enteric-coated) and s/c (sugar-coated) (see also Abbreviations, p. 487). Instructions of any length will obviously require to extend to the next prescription line. When using the documents of the Aberdeen system of prescribing and recording medicines, the code letter opposite the name of the medicine is (as always) the one that is used (Crooks et al 1965).

- The *time(s)* ticked or entered in writing. The prescription must specify the time of administration with the exception of 'as required' prescriptions. In this situation, the prescribing instructions must be written in English stating the symptom(s) to be relieved and the maximum frequency (for example, 'As required for headache every 4 hours'). For once-only prescriptions, the actual time should be indicated. A term such as 'monthly' can lead to inaccuracies or omissions and is better to be written as 'four-weekly' or 'every 28 days'. Where a specific number of doses of, or number of days, a medicine is to be given, instructions to this effect must be clearly written. In an outpatient or community setting, the duration of the course of treatment before review should also be stated on the prescription.
- The full *signature* of a registered (or provisionally registered) practitioner for *each* individual prescription. Initials do not suffice, and an unsigned prescription has no validity.

Additional information may be provided in conjunction with the prescription. For example, if the doctor has agreed to allow the patient to keep a particular medicine within reach, the doctor should enter this on the prescription. The registered nurse may enter a specific preference of the patient in relation to the medicines such as 'takes with a biscuit'. The clinical pharmacist will advise on aspects of the storage of all medicines. The monitoring of prescriptions by the clinical pharmacist working at ward level provides additional safeguards for the patient.

Irrespective of who is the prescriber, the nurse administering the medicine is accountable for his or her actions (and inactions). *If any part of the prescription is unclear, absent or, in the nurse's view, incorrect, the nurse must seek clarification before administering the medicine.* When two nurses are involved in the administration of a medicine, each takes full responsibility for every step of the procedure, i.e. reading the prescription, selecting the medicine and witnessing its administration.

MINIMISING CROSS-INFECTION

Prior to any procedure involving medicines the hands should be at least socially clean. If the procedure involves an aseptic technique then an antiseptic handwash is required.

As far as possible, the hands should not come into contact with the medicine. Tablets and capsules are tipped out into the cap of the medicine container before being placed in a medicine measure or spoon; medicines from a blister pack are pushed through the foil side of the pack. Gloves should be used when applying creams or ointments, although the main reason for this is to protect the nurse from receiving an unwanted dose of the active drug. Medicine trays should be washed after use, and sticky medicine bottles wiped before being returned to the trolley or cupboard. All storage and preparation areas should be kept clean.

CHECKING THE PRODUCT

The label and/or packaging nearest to the product must be checked before administration. It is not sufficient to check the outer box or packet in which a bottle, ampoule or blister pack is contained. If there is any doubt about the legibility of the container information, the medicine must not be used and the container with its contents should be returned to the pharmacy.

Medicines should remain in their original container until required for use. They should not be transferred to another container.

Pharmaceutical products should be used only if they are in date, and their colour, appearance/consistency and smell are unaltered. Unsuitable medicines should be returned to the pharmacy and the advice of the pharmacy technician and/or the clinical pharmacist sought.

IDENTIFYING THE PATIENT

The patient must be identified correctly. In hospital and in clinics, this becomes especially important and a variety of methods are used. The patient may be addressed by name or asked to state his or her name. A check may be made of the name on the bed label or chart kept at the bedside. Factors contributing to ease of identification include knowing the patients in your care, checking medicines with a second nurse and making proper use of identification bracelets/photographs. However, shift work, staff shortages, movement of staff from ward to ward or from team to team and a high turnover of patients can create difficulties in knowing patients well. Moreover, not all staff like patients to be 'labelled' (i.e. using identification bracelets) or to have the patient state his or her name. Encouragement of patients to be more mobile and to socialise away from the bedside in day rooms can add to the problems, while deafness and confusion can compound them.

Not uncommonly, patients with the same name appear in a ward. It is of paramount importance that the nurse-in-charge draws the attention of the patients concerned and all staff to this occurrence. Checking each patient's hospital unit number *and* date of birth is the only safe means of distinguishing patients in this situation.

POSITIONING THE PATIENT

For safety and comfort, patients should be suitably positioned in advance of being given a medicine. For example:

- an upright position will assist the swallowing of a medicine
- for giving an injection, bladder irrigation or rectal medicine, only the area involved should be uncovered
- to facilitate the administration of an injection or a rectal medicine, the nurse should encourage the patient to relax.

SELECTING, CHECKING AND ADMINISTERING THE MEDICINE

Medicines should be administered by permanent staff on the ward who are more likely to be familiar with the patients (and the medicines most often used there), although it is recognised this is not always possible. There are many other tasks which may be assigned to relief staff, which are potentially much less hazardous.

An essential part of the administration of medicines is the carrying out of a series of checks. Checking a medicine is an *active* process. The guiding principles of the checks involved are listed in Box 7.1.

Before any medicine is administered it is essential to check on the recording sheet that it has not already been given. The prescription is then carefully read and the appropriate form of the medicine identified. These two are *compared* and any calculation of dose carried out. The medicine is removed from its container and the label *re-checked* before the container is returned to trolley or cupboard. Where two nurses are involved, *each* nurse must read both the prescription sheet *and* the details on the container. The medicine is finally made ready for administration and the patient identified. There is thus a series of checks to be made on every occasion. In the event of another member of staff or the patient questioning any aspect of the medication, the nurse must be willing to make further checks.

Although medicines require to be administered according to the prescription, they are often linked to other aspects of the patient's care. It falls to the nurse to integrate the administration of a patient's medicines with nursing care, investigations and other treatments without departing from the general instructions contained in the prescription. To achieve an optimal outcome, nurses must base their decisions on a sound knowledge of the purpose of the medication. However, some medicines do not need to be given at a specific time of day but do need to be given in conjunction with

Box 7.1 Guiding principles of checking

Work from the assumption that something may be wrong rather than presuming most things are likely to be right.

Checking involves *comparing* two things, e.g. product against prescription, identification bracelet against prescription:

Read on *prescription*	Read on *product*
• Name of medicine	• Name of medicine
• Strength to be used	• Strength available
• Dose to be given	• Dose available
• Route to be used	• Route medicine intended for
• Additional information not already given	• Any specific instructions
	• Expiry date

Check details on outer wrapper *and* inner container, e.g. ampoule, blister pack:

Read on *prescription*	Read on *identification bracelet*
• Patient's name	• Patient's name
• Date of birth	• Date of birth
• Hospital unit number	• Hospital unit number

If necessary, seek clarification from:

- nurse-in-charge
- medical staff
- ward pharmacist
- BNF, MIMS, Data Sheet Compendium
- Medicines Information department.

If in doubt, STOP/CHECK/ASK/ASK AGAIN.

Stand back; ask yourself 'is this reasonable?'

Never be reluctant to get things checked.

Two persons, at least one of whom is registered, *should* be involved when administering:

- insulin
- heparin
- high doses, e.g. corticosteroids
- cytotoxic chemotherapy (IV)
- any other medication locally stipulated.

Controlled Drugs *must* be checked by two persons at least one of whom is registered.

Where two persons are involved:

- stand side by side
- *both* persons must be able to see both prescription *and* product
- use finger as pointer
- *read out* details one by one first on prescription, then on product, then re-check prescription
- stress each syllable, e.g. flu-o-cin-o-lone
- make calculation of what is to be given, independently and then compare answers
- do not hesitate to use pen and paper to work out dose.

Do NOT proceed without further checking if:

- the number, e.g. of tablets, ampoules, etc., or volume to be given appears excessive
- the dose prescribed is outwith the normal range.

a nursing procedure. For example, topical medicines may need to be applied in association with bathing, a surgical dressing or oral hygiene.

USING PROFESSIONAL JUDGEMENT

The nurse must be alert to those occasions when it would be unsafe to proceed in giving a medicine exactly as prescribed. For example:

- digoxin is not administered unless the pulse rate is 60 beats per minute or above
- depending on the patient's baseline blood pressure and the severity of pain, it may be inappropriate to administer narcotic analgesics in the early postoperative period
- permission to use an alternative route of administration should be sought following an upper endoscopy when the throat has been anaesthetised or when a patient is being fasted.

When a dose has to be omitted or reduced (or the medicine is refused by the patient or not immediately obtainable) a record of the fact must be made, giving the reason and initialled by the member(s) of staff involved.

TEACHING THE PATIENT

Through careful explanation prior to the administration of medicines, and by acting as a good role model in relation to medicines, the nurse gradually builds up the patient's knowledge of, expertise in handling, and respect for his medicines. Every opportunity should be taken to teach hospital patients and/or their relatives about the medicines which will require to be continued following discharge. A period of self-administration of medicines prior to discharge has been shown to be worthwhile (see p. 110). It may be important, for example, for patients to increase their fluid intake while taking a particular medicine. Instruction in the proper technique to use is essential for patients who have to use an inhaler.

Teaching newly diagnosed diabetic patients how to administer insulin to themselves calls on the nurse's ability to demonstrate the procedure, and to provide the necessary encouragement and supervision. It is also the nurse's duty to draw the attention of patients, as appropriate, to patient information leaflets, videos, etc. concerning their condition.

PROMOTING THE EFFECTIVENESS OF MEDICINES

In addition to administering medicines correctly, nurses have a responsibility to do their utmost to promote the medicines' effectiveness. A knowledge of how medicines act, along with thoughtful prescribing, allows the nurse to play a considerable part in improving efficacy of the drugs the patient is receiving. For example:

- The absorption of some antibiotics (e.g. flucloxacillin) taken by mouth is decreased by the presence of food in the gut and so it is advisable to give the medicine at least half an hour before a main meal.
- By restricting salt in the diet of those patients receiving diuretic therapy, there is less sodium to be reabsorbed by the renal tubules. Less water will be absorbed and therefore more urine is produced.
- In the terminal stages of a painful illness where comfort has become the prime concern, careful attention to timing of the giving of analgesics is essential to obtain complete pain relief. If this is done, the medicine can relieve pain just as it is due to break through, the only drawback being that this may mean wakening the patient.

MONITORING THE EFFECT OF MEDICINES

Indices recorded by nurses which reflect the effect of commonly used groups of medicines are referred to in Table 7.2.

Although nurses are greatly assisted in monitoring the effect of medicines by these recordings, there is no substitute for using general powers of observation. Nurses are ideally placed to get to know their patients well and, although they may not always fully understand what process is developing, often know intuitively when even the most minor change in the patient's condition is taking place.

In addition to the indices monitored by nurses, laboratory tests are used as a basis for making adjustments to doses/frequency of administration of certain medicines:

- *Prothrombin times* (reported as international normalised ratio (INR)) indicate the capacity of the blood to clot and are used to monitor the effect of anticoagulant drugs. Daily dosages are calculated according to the prothrombin time. While maximum anticoagulation is the aim in the prevention of thrombus formation, extreme caution is required to prevent over-anticoagulation and subsequent bleeding.
- *The white blood cell count* (WBC) reflects the patient's resistance to infection. Frequent checks of the white blood cell count are carried out on patients receiving immunosuppressant or cytotoxic therapy as these drugs can reduce the count to a dangerously low level and hence lower the patient's resistance to infection.

Table 7.2 The effect of medicines on the patient's vital signs and other indices

Index	Effect
Temperature	Body temperature will be *reduced* when: • an appropriate antibiotic is given for bacterial infection • an antipyretic is used to control disturbance of the heat-regulating centre • an antithyroid drug is used to treat hyperthyroidism
Pulse	The heart rate is *slowed*, steadied and strengthened by: • cardiac glycosides (The radial and apical rates may require to be measured by two nurses simultaneously) The pulse is *increased* by: • antimuscarinic drugs • thyroxine
Respiration	The rate and pattern of breathing are likely to be *improved* by: • diuretics • bronchodilators • antibiotics (The forced expiratory volume (FEV) may require to be estimated using a peak flow meter before and after inhaling bronchodilators) Analgesics, by relieving pain, may make breathing more comfortable, but in high doses may *depress* respiration to a dangerous level
Blood pressure	The blood pressure can be *raised* by: • corticosteroids High blood pressure is treated with: • antihypertensives (They may cause the blood pressure to fall sharply when the patient stands up and therefore close monitoring, including records of lying and standing blood pressure, is essential) The blood pressure can be *lowered* when using: • strong analgesics (Extreme caution is needed in states of shock and following anaesthetic)
Weight	Weight *loss* (or lack of it) may reflect the beneficial (or otherwise) effect of a high-dose diuretic (A careful record of the patient's weight taken at the same time each day in the same clothing should be kept when high doses of diuretic are being given)
Urinary output	Urine formation is *increased* with diuretics Retention of fluid in the tissues with subsequent *oliguria* occurs with corticosteroids (A record of both intake and output of fluid helps monitor fluid balance)
Glycosuria	The blood glucose level and consequent presence of glucose in the urine are *lowered* by: • insulin • sulphonylureas and *raised* by: • corticosteroids • thiazide diuretics (Monitoring of diabetes is now largely done by testing a sample of capillary blood taken from the thumb or ear lobe several times per day. Patients receiving high doses of corticosteroids or thiazide diuretics may have their urine tested for glucose at regular intervals)

• *Therapeutic drug monitoring* (TDM). Laboratory techniques are also used to determine the level of a particular drug in the plasma. Doses are adjusted to achieve or maintain the desired therapeutic level of drug in the patient's blood. Such monitoring is commonly used in the management of epilepsy and certain psychiatric conditions.

As technology advances, analyses can be carried out at ward level, obviating the need for samples to be sent to a central laboratory, e.g. blood gas determination. Not only is time saved by carrying out tests at ward level but there is also the ability to monitor biochemical changes in the patient and adjust drug treatment accordingly.

MAINTAINING THE COMFORT OF THE PATIENT

Nursing measures alone are not always sufficient to achieve maximum functioning of body systems and therefore comfort. Nevertheless, it is always better to try simple remedies in non-emergency situations before resorting to the use of medicines. Moreover, the start of a course of drug therapy does not indicate the discontinuation of these measures. In other words, medicines do not *replace* nursing care. Some examples may be cited:

- analgesics
  - maintaining good communication
  - giving the patient reassurance
  - careful positioning
  - promoting sleep
  - applying local heat or massage
- laxatives
  - increasing fluid intake
  - providing high-fibre foods
  - encouraging mobility
  - maximising the gastrocolic reflex
  - providing privacy for toilet purposes
- hypnotics
  - creating peace of mind
  - making a comfortable bed
  - ensuring a quiet, undisturbed environment
  - avoiding caffeine-containing drinks late at night.

In some patients unavoidable side-effects arise as the result of taking medicines, and precautions therefore have to be taken to minimise these side-effects. Certain groups of drugs are predictable in the nature of the effects they produce. For example:

• *Strong analgesics*. Drugs such as diamorphine make patients feel sick and this can be especially distressing postoperatively or, for example, following myocardial infarction when stress should be kept to a minimum. It is common practice for an anti-emetic to be prescribed for use at the same time.

• *Sedatives*. Patients may become disorientated as well as drowsy. It may be necessary to erect bed sides and advisable to position the patient's bed within view of the nursing staff, especially at night. Outpatients should be advised to avoid alcohol and not to drive or operate machinery.

• *Diuretics*. These are given early in the morning so that urinary frequency has worn off by the middle of the day, allowing freedom of activity for the remainder of the day. Incontinence of urine can be precipitated (as can falling) in an attempt to reach the toilet in time. In geriatric wards with large numbers of dependent patients, arrangements may be made to administer diuretics slightly later to fit in with the number of staff available to provide the necessary assistance with toileting. Where applicable, patients should be told what to expect, be shown some means of summoning assistance and should have their bed positioned close to the toilet or have a commode placed at the bedside.

• *Oral iron preparations*. These colour the stools black and the patient should be warned accordingly. This can be especially alarming to a patient who has a history of passing blood in the stools and mistakes the discoloration for a recurrence of bleeding.

Many patients, in spite of having serious conditions and receiving powerful medication, remain relatively well. Their appearance, however, may be deceptive and nurses must be forever vigilant in detecting the onset of an adverse reaction.

DISPOSAL OF TIME-EXPIRED AND UNWANTED MEDICINES

In general, doses of medicines removed from their original container for administration to a patient should not be returned to that container. An unopened ampoule may be returned to the box, but great care should be taken to ensure that the ampoule is replaced in the correct box.

The disposal of unwanted medicines must comply with the 'duty of care' legislation (see p. 19). The clinical pharmacist and community pharmacist will advise and help to ensure compliance with local policies. The disposal of cytotoxic drugs requires particular care (see p. 353) as does the disposal of Controlled Drugs (see p. 17). The contents of partially used ampoules should be flushed down a sink with running water.

DISPOSAL OF SHARPS

Accidental inoculation with infected blood as a result of needlestick injury presents a major risk to the healthcare worker (BMA 1990). Sharps injuries can give rise to the transmission of the human immunodeficiency virus (HIV), hepatitis B virus, hepatitis C, and other blood-borne diseases. Injuries which do not involve contaminated blood – for example, those which arise when drugs are being drawn up – carry with them fewer hazards but are nevertheless considered important because of the possible entry of infection through the punctured skin. Responsibility for safe practice rests with the employee through the Health and Safety at Work Act 1974 and the employer through the Control of Substances Hazardous to Health Regulations 1988.

One particularly important procedure in clinical practice is the disposal of needles. Re-sheathing of needles must not be attempted, and no attempt should be made to try to detach the needle from the syringe prior to disposal. The combined syringe and unsheathed needle should be carefully placed in a sharps bin immediately after use. It is the personal responsibility of the individual using the sharp to dispose of it safely. Sharps containers should be sealed when three-quarters full. There should be a sufficient number of them to allow this to happen. In any case, no attempt should be made to press down the contents of a sharps container to create room for more. Sharps containers should be carried by their handles and placed in a secure place prior to ultimate disposal by incineration or other high-temperature system. Although free sterile syringes and needles are available to people who abuse drugs, the risks of pilfering from sharps containers should not be overlooked. Access by patients (especially by children) to sharps containers must be prevented. Policies must be in place to deal with needlestick injuries if they occur. The prospect of the availability of retractable syringes is good news.

KEEPING RECORDS

A prescription sheet and recording sheet should be raised for all inpatients and, on discharge or transfer, filed with the patient's case records whether or not entries have been made. In hospital, all medicines must be entered on the patient's prescription sheet including any lay medicines the doctor has authorised the patient to continue to receive. On each occasion a medicine is administered, a record to this effect is made and signed or initialled as appropriate by those involved. When a medicine which is due is not given for whatever reason, or a medicine is given earlier than prescribed or only part of the dose is given the appropriate recording should be made.

EVALUATING AND REPORTING BACK

Maintaining effective drug therapy cannot be assured without some form of feedback by the nurse to the prescriber. A medicine may make the patient feel nauseated every time it is taken, or a patient may report gaining little benefit from it. On the positive side, it is equally important to note that a patient is, for example, sleeping better or breathing more easily as the result of medication. Observing and reporting *any* new clinical features following the start of a course of drug therapy are an essential part of the nurse's role. As the result of the evaluative process, the medicine may be discontinued, exchanged for another, continued as before, or continued with some alteration to the prescription.

REFERENCES

British Medical Association (BMA) 1990 A code of practice for the safe use and disposal of sharps. BMA, London, p 1

Control of Substances Hazardous to Health Regulations 1988 Statutory Instrument No. 1657. HMSO, London

Crooks J, Clark C E, Caie H B, Mawson W B 1965 Prescribing and administration of drugs in hospital. Lancet i:373

Department of Health (DoH) 1988 Guidelines for the safe and secure handling of medicines. DOH, London

Health and Safety at Work Act 1974 HMSO, London

Roper N, Logan W W, Tierney A J 1996 The elements of nursing: a model for nursing based on a model of living, 4th edn. Churchill Livingstone, Edinburgh, p 36

FURTHER READING

Shepherd M 2002 Medicines: 2 Administration of medicines. Nursing Times 98(16):45–48

Shepherd M 2002 Medicines: 3 Managing medicines. Nursing Times 98(17):43–46

CHAPTER CONTENTS

8

Calculations

INTRODUCTION

With the development of clinical pharmacy services and the introduction of patient-specific medicines, the overall need for nurses to undertake calculations in connection with the administration of medicines and other pharmaceutical products has declined. Situations, however, still arise where nurses need to perform basic calculations, and these they must be able to do accurately and with confidence. Apart from the need to calculate how to obtain a particular dose for an individual patient, a sound understanding of SI (Système International) units of mass (weight) and volume as well as percentages is essential if medicines are to be used safely and effectively. Whenever possible the need to perform calculations should be avoided by appropriate use of the pharmaceutical service, not because the nurse is lacking in the necessary skills, but so as to improve accuracy of dosage. In paediatric practice for example, it is much better to use a paediatric dosage specially dispensed for the purpose than to attempt to obtain the required dose from a product intended primarily for adult use, although, on occasions, there may be no practical alternative to this approach. It is against this background that the following paragraphs should be studied.

SI UNITS

The international system of units for mass and volume is as follows:

Mass	1 kilogram (kg)	= 1000 grams
	1 gram (g)	= 1000 milligrams
	1 milligram (mg)	= 1000 micrograms
	1 microgram (μg)*	= 1000 nanograms (ng)*
Volume	1 litre	= 1000 millilitres (mL)
	1 millilitre	= 1000 microlitres (μL)

* It should be noted that these abbreviations must not be used in prescription writing because of the possibility of confusion with other abbreviations.

The mole and the millimole (mmol)

The strength of a pharmaceutical preparation used in electrolyte replacement therapy is normally expressed in millimoles per tablet or millimoles per given volume of solution. In addition, the strength of a solution will be expressed as a percentage.

A millimole is one thousandth of a mole, which is the molecular weight of a substance expressed in grams. Nurses will not normally be expected to calculate millimoles from first principles but may have to calculate how much of a given solution to measure to obtain a particular dose.

PERCENTAGES

The strength of a pharmaceutical product may be expressed as a percentage, meaning parts per 100 parts. This is expressed in four ways:

- *Percentage weight in volume (% w/v).* The expression 5% w/v indicates that 5 g of active ingredient is present in 100 mL of product.
- *Percentage weight in weight (% w/w).* The expression 5% w/w indicates that 5 g of active ingredient is present in 100 g of product.
- *Percentage volume in volume (% v/v).* The expression 5% v/v indicates that 5 mL of active ingredient is present in 100 mL of product.
- *Percentage volume in weight (% v/w).* The expression 5% v/w indicates that 5 mL of active ingredient is contained in 100 g of product.

EXPRESSING THE STRENGTH OF ACTIVE INGREDIENT(S)

Solid dose forms

In most cases the strength of the active ingredient(s) present in each tablet or capsule will be expressed on the label of the product in grams, milligrams or micrograms, e.g. amoxicillin 250 mg. Quantities of less than 1 gram should always be expressed in milligrams; thus, the expression 500 mg is used and not 0.5 g. Similarly, quantities of less than 1 milligram should always be expressed in micrograms. This approach should always be followed when prescribing, recording the administration of, ordering or dispensing medicines. This reduces the need to use the decimal point, which, if incorrectly placed, can lead to massive errors in drug administration. The need for the decimal point to be used remains when doses such as 37.5 mg are required.

Strengths of active ingredients in some dosage forms are expressed in units of activity, e.g. heparin, interferon and some vitamins.

Products used for electrolyte replacement therapy, in addition to a strength of active ingredient being given in grams or milligrams, will also have the strength quoted in millimoles (mmol). A slow-release potassium chloride tablet, for example, contains 600 mg of potassium chloride or 8 mmol each of K^+ and Cl^-.

Liquid oral dosage forms

The amount of active ingredient per given volume is given for the strength of preparations such as antibiotic syrups. An ampicillin syrup will bear a label stating that the product contains 250 mg in 5 mL, or a paediatric digoxin elixir contains 50 micrograms in 1 mL. It is in connection with the administration of liquids (oral and parenteral) that calculations are often required.

Liquid parenteral dosage forms

Small-volume injections

Two main approaches will be encountered depending on the volume of the product:

- Small-volume injections will normally bear a label expressing the strength of the product in a manner similar to that used for oral liquids. For example, an injection will be shown to contain 25 mg per 1 mL but care should be taken to note the volume contained in each ampoule since, if the ampoule contains 2 mL, the amount of active ingredient in 2 mL is 50 mg.
- The strength of injections of local anaesthetics, such as, lidocaine (lignocaine) are commonly expressed as a percentage w/v.

On the label of parenteral products for electrolyte replacement therapy (large- or small-volume) the strength is frequently expressed as a percentage, mass per given volume, and mmol per given volume.

Examples

A strong sterile solution of potassium chloride contains potassium chloride 15% w/v or approximately 2 mmol each of K^+ and Cl^- per 1 mL.

The molecular weight of potassium chloride (KCl) is 74.55. 1 mole is therefore 74.55 grams. It follows from the definition that *1 millimole* is contained in:

$$\frac{74.55}{1000} \text{ g of KCl} = 0.07455\,\text{g} \text{ or } 74.55\,\text{mg}.$$

A 15% w/v solution contains 15 g per 100 mL
or 15 000 mg per 100 mL
or 150 mg per 1 mL

or $\frac{150}{74.55}$ millimoles per 1 mL

or 2.01 mmol *each* of K^+ and Cl^- per 1 mL.

For practical purposes, a figure of 2.0 mmol would be used.

Sodium chloride intravenous infusion contains sodium chloride 0.9% w/v or 0.15 mmol each of Na^+ and Cl^- per 1 mL.

The molecular weight of sodium chloride (NaCl) is 58.45. 1 mole is therefore 58.45 grams. It follows from the definition that *1 millimole* is contained in:

$$\frac{58.45}{1000} \text{ g of NaCl} = 0.05845 \text{ g} \quad \text{or} \quad 58.45 \text{ mg}.$$

A 0.9% w/v solution contains 0.9 g per 100 mL

or 900 mg per 100 mL

or 9 mg per 1 mL

or $\frac{9}{58.45} = 0.154$ millimoles per 1 mL

or 0.154 mmol *each* of Na^+ and Cl^- per 1 mL.

For practical purposes, a figure of 0.15 mmol would be used.

The strength of adrenaline (epinephrine) injections is still frequently expressed as 1 in 1000. This indicates that 1 gram of active ingredient is contained in 1000 mL of product. Of more value to the nurse is the fact that 1 mL of the injection contains 1 mg of adrenaline (epinephrine).

When a product is supplied in an ampoule or rubber-capped vial as a dry powder for reconstitution before use, the label will give the amount of dry powder contained in it. When reconstituting such products prior to injection the total volume produced by adding the diluent to the powder must be known if part of the total dose contained in the ampoule or vial is to be administered.

The strength of certain biological materials, such as insulin and heparin, is expressed in units of activity per given volume, e.g. 100 units per 1 mL (insulin) or 5000 units per 1 mL (heparin).

Large-volume parenteral products

Labels on containers of large-volume infusion solutions will generally give information on the strength of the product in percentage terms. For example, solutions of sodium chloride may contain 0.9% w/v, or a glucose infusion may contain 5% w/v. Solutions for electrolyte-replacement therapy will also contain information on the number of millimoles of given electrolytes per given volume.

Other pharmaceutical products

The strengths of products such as lotions, sterile topical solutions, ointments, antiseptic solutions, etc., will generally be expressed as a percentage, i.e. liquid preparations as a percentage w/v, solid or semi-solid preparations as a percentage w/w. When very dilute antiseptic solutions are in use, the strength may be expressed as the number of parts of active ingredient in a given volume of solution, e.g. 1 in 5000, 1 in 2000. In the first example, 1 gram of the active ingredient is contained in 5000 mL of product; in the second case 1 gram is contained in 2000 mL of product.

MAKING A CALCULATION

Two different approaches may be used: either a method based on first principles or a method involving the use of a simple formula. In practice, the nurse may feel more confident using one of these methods rather than the other. For the purposes of checking a more complex calculation it is worthwhile using both methods.

Example

A dose of 50 mg of a drug is required. The product available on the ward contains 200 mg in 5 mL.

Method 1 (first principles)
First, calculate the amount of drug in 1 mL of product, that is:

$$\frac{200}{5} = 40 \text{ mg}.$$

The product available therefore contains 40 mg in 1 mL. For a dose of 50 mg:

$$\frac{50}{40} \times 1 \text{ mL} = 1.25 \text{ mL}.$$

Answer: 1.25 mL must be measured.

Method 2 (formula)
This is based on simple proportion and uses the following formula:

$$\frac{\text{Dose required (mg)}}{\text{Strength available (mg)}} \times \begin{array}{l}\text{Dose volume (mL) of}\\ \text{available product}\end{array}$$
$$= \text{Volume (mL) containing the required dose.}$$

$$\frac{50}{200} \times 5 = \frac{50}{40}$$
$$= \frac{5}{4}$$
$$= 1.25 \text{ mL.}$$

Answer: 1.25 mL would be measured.

As a simple memory aid it may be helpful to think of the formula as 'want'/'got'. This of course is no substitute for a clear understanding of this method of calculating.

Solid dose forms

Calculations involving solid dose forms will generally cause few problems, but as with all calculations, the need for accuracy cannot be overstated. Sometimes there will be no alternative but to subdivide a tablet or to give a number of tablets to obtain the prescribed dose.

Example 1

The dose required is 50 micrograms, but the product available contains 100 micrograms.

It is obvious that the tablet must be divided to obtain the required dose since the product available is twice the strength of the dose required. A general formula can be used in situations of this kind.

It is essential that the strengths are expressed in the same units, in this case micrograms.

$$\frac{\text{Dose required}}{\text{Strength available}} \times 1 = \begin{array}{l}\text{Proportion of original dosage}\\ \text{form to give required dose}\end{array}$$

$$\frac{50}{100} \times 1 = \frac{1}{2} \text{ tablet required.}$$

Example 2

The dose required is 100 micrograms, but the product available contains 25 micrograms.

$$\frac{\text{Dose required}}{\text{Strength available}} \times 1 = \text{Number of tablets required}$$

$$\frac{100}{25} \times 1 = 4 \text{ tablets required.}$$

Example 3

A dose of 50 micrograms is required, and the tablets available are labelled 0.1 mg.

On some occasions it is necessary to convert fractions of a milligram into micrograms. This should rarely be required, since, for quantities less than 1 milligram, the doctor should use micrograms in writing the prescription and the label on the container should bear the strength of the product expressed in micrograms. Unfortunately, situations may arise where the dose is expressed in micrograms and the product available is labelled in milligrams, or vice versa.

The formula dose (required/strength available) × 1 can again be used, but the dose required and strength available must be expressed in the same terms, in this case micrograms:

1 milligram = 1000 micrograms

or

1.0 milligram = 1000.0 micrograms

(Decimal points would not normally be required here; they are introduced to aid explanation.)

Moving the decimal point one place to the left on each side of the equation, we get:

0.1 milligram = 100 micrograms

Using the formula:

$$\frac{\text{Dose required}}{\text{Strength available}} = \frac{50}{100} \times 1 = \frac{1}{2} \text{ tablet required.}$$

Example 4

A dose of 0.05 mg is prescribed, and the strength of the product is expressed as 100 micrograms.

Before proceeding it is necessary to convert 0.05 mg into micrograms:

1 milligram = 1000 micrograms
0.1 milligram = 100 micrograms
0.05 milligram = 50 micrograms (÷2)

The calculation is completed as before.

Oral liquids

Calculations involving liquid dosage forms are essentially similar to those for solid dosage forms, being based on either the first principles method or the formula.

Example 1

The dose required is 200 mg but the product available contains 250 mg in 5 mL.

From first principles:

If there are 250 mg in 5 mL, then 1 mL contains 50 mg. So, for a dose of 200 mg:

$$\frac{200}{50} \times 1\,\text{mL} = 4\,\text{mL required.}$$

Using the formula:

$$\frac{\text{Dose required (mg)}}{\text{Strength available (mg)}} \times \begin{matrix}\text{Dose volume (mL) of}\\ \text{available product}\end{matrix}$$

i.e.

$$\frac{200}{250} \times 5 = 4\,\text{mL required.}$$

The required dose is contained in 4 mL of the available product. It is important to note that the dose required and the strength available must be expressed in the same units, in this case milligrams.

Example 2

It is required to give a dose of 45 mg but the product available contains 30 mg in 5 mL.

From first principles:

If there are 30 mg in 5 mL, then 1 mL contains 6 mg.

For a dose of 45 mg:

$$\frac{45}{6} \times 1\,\text{ml} = 7.5\,\text{mL required.}$$

Using the formula:

$$\frac{\text{Dose required (mg)}}{\text{Strength available (mg)}} \times \text{Dose volume (mL)}$$

$$= \begin{matrix}\text{Volume (mL) to be measured to give}\\ \text{required dose}\end{matrix}$$

i.e.

$$\frac{45}{30} \times 5 = \begin{matrix}7.5\,\text{mL must be measured}\\ \text{to give the required dose.}\end{matrix}$$

Parenteral products

A similar approach to calculations is applicable here.

Example 1

The dose required is 50 micrograms but the strength available is 500 micrograms in 2 mL.

$$\frac{\text{Dose required } (\mu\text{g})}{\text{Strength available } (\mu\text{g})} \times \begin{matrix}\text{Dose volume (mL) of}\\ \text{available product}\end{matrix}$$

$$= \text{Volume (mL) containing the required dose}$$

i.e.

$$\frac{50}{500} \times 2 = \begin{matrix}0.2\,\text{mL of the available}\\ \text{product required.}\end{matrix}$$

The figures obtained by this means can (and should) always be checked by a second nurse, using first principles.

The strength available is:

500 micrograms in 2 mL,

or ÷2, i.e., 250 micrograms in 1 mL,

then ÷5, i.e. 50 micrograms in 0.2 mL.

It will be obvious that a sound knowledge of SI units and decimals is essential if these simple calculations are to be performed accurately. As with solid-dose forms, it may be that the dose required is contained in a multiple of the standard dosage form.

Example 2

The dose required is 7.5 mg but the strength available is 5 mg in 5 mL.

$$\frac{\text{Dose required (mg)}}{\text{Strength available (mg)}} \times \begin{matrix}\text{Dose volume (mL) of}\\ \text{available product}\end{matrix}$$

$$= \text{Volume (mL) containing the required dose}$$

i.e.

$$\frac{7.5}{5} \times 5 = 7.5\,\text{mL contain the required dose.}$$

Checking from first principles, product available contains:

5 mg in 5 mL

or ÷5, i.e. 1 mg in 1 mL.

So, for a dose of 7.5 mg, 7.5 mL of the available product is required.

Example 3

The dose required is 17.5 g but the strength available is 5% w/v, i.e. it contains 5 g in 100 mL.

To calculate how to obtain the 17.5 g dose required the general formula can again be used:

$$\frac{\text{Dose required}}{\text{Strength available}} \times \text{Dose volume (mL)}$$

$$= \text{Volume (mL) needed to obtain the required dose.}$$

In this situation the formula is expressed as follows:

$$\frac{\text{Amount of active ingredient required (dose) g}}{\text{Amount of active ingredient in grams per 100 mL of solution available}} \times 100\text{ mL}$$
$$= \text{Volume (mL) to give dose required}$$

i.e.

$$\frac{17.5}{5} \times 100 = 350\,\text{mL required.}$$

Again, the calculation can be checked from first principles:

A 5% w/v solution contains 5 g in 100 mL

or ×3, i.e. 15 g in 300 mL

or ÷2, i.e. 2.5 g in 50 mL.

So, 17.5 g is contained in 350 mL.

Example 4

A strong solution of potassium chloride contains 2 mmol each of K^+ and Cl^- in each mL. Calculate the volume required to obtain a dose of 10 mmol of K^+.

$$\frac{\text{Dose required}}{\text{Strength available}} \times \text{Dose volume (mL)}$$
$$= \text{Volume (mL) to give required dose}$$

i.e.

$$\frac{10}{2} \times 1 = 5\,\text{mL required to give a dose of 10 mmol } K^+.$$

Example 5

Heparin injection contains 5000 units per mL. Calculate the volume required to obtain a dose of 3000 units.

$$\frac{\text{Dose required}}{\text{Strength available}} \times \text{Dose volume} = \text{Volume (mL) to give required dose}$$

i.e.

$$\frac{3000}{5000} \times 1 = 0.6\,\text{mL required to give 3000 units.}$$

Topical antiseptics

Although antiseptic solutions are commonly produced in a ready-to-use form, calculations may still be required in connection with the dilution of antiseptics.

Example

Chlorhexidine is available as a 5% concentrate, and 1 litre of a 0.05% w/v solution is required for use as an irrigation.

Again, the general formula can be used, on this occasion using the percentages:

$$\frac{\%\text{ required}}{\%\text{ available}} \times \text{Volume required (mL)}$$
$$= \text{Volume of concentrate required to be diluted to 1 litre}$$

i.e.

$$\frac{0.05}{5} \times 1000 = 10\,\text{mL.}$$

So, 10 mL of a 5% w/v solution must be diluted to 1000 mL to give a 0.05% w/v solution.

Calculations involving reconstitution of injections

When an injection has to be reconstituted from a powder before use, it should be noted that the resulting volume is in excess of the volume of diluent added, owing to the displacement effect of the powder. This must be taken into account if a dose less than that contained in the vial is required.

Example

A vial contains 500 mg but the dose required is 200 mg.

The addition of 5 mL diluent yields a volume of 5.25 mL when drawn into the syringe. In this case it is useful to use the general formula:

$$\frac{\text{Dose required (mg)}}{\text{Strength available (mg)}} \times \text{Dose volume (mL)}$$
$$= \text{Volume (mL) to be measured}$$

i.e.

$$\frac{200}{500} \times 5.25 = \text{2.1 mL required to obtain a dose of 200 mg.}$$

Dosage calculations involving body surface area

In certain specialised forms of therapy (e.g. cytotoxic drug therapy) drug dosage is based on body surface area. The patient's body surface area is determined from a table (nomogram) using the patient's body weight and height. For example, if a patient's height is

190 cm and body weight is 90 kg, reference to the nomogram indicates that the patient's body surface area is 2.3 m^2. A typical dosage regimen for doxorubicin is 60 mg per square metre of body surface area given intravenously every 3 weeks. For a patient with a body surface area of 2.3 m^2, a dose of 60×2.3 mg (138 mg) would be given every 3 weeks.

FURTHER READING

Gatford J D, Anderson R E 1998 Nursing calculations, 5th edn. Churchill Livingstone, Edinburgh

Lapham R, Agar H 1995 Drug calculations for nurses: a step by step approach. Arnold, London

CHAPTER CONTENTS

9

Oral, parenteral and transdermal administration of medicines

ADMINISTRATION OF MEDICINES BY MOUTH

For the majority of patients, the most convenient and acceptable method of receiving medication is by mouth. Most medicines taken by mouth are intended to be swallowed, and are referred to as *oral medicines*. Others, known as *sublingual*, are specifically for dissolving under the tongue; some, known as *buccal*, are for holding against the mucous membranes of the cheek.

Oral administration

Tablets, capsules and liquid preparations are relatively easy to administer and are suitable delivery systems for drugs that are effective when given orally. If a tablet or capsule sticks in the oesophagus it can cause irritation to the point of ulceration of the mucosa, especially with drugs such as ferrous salts. Small tablets are generally easy to swallow. Larger uncoated tablets may present problems; torpedo-shaped coated tablets are more patient-friendly. To ensure complete transit from mouth to stomach, tablets and capsules should be swallowed with a large drink, ideally when standing. Where this is not possible, the patient should be in the sitting position (Channer 1985). Effervescent tablets are dissolved in water prior to administration.

Administering oral solids

Patients have their own preferences as to the order in which they will take their medicines. For example, they may wish to take unpleasant tasting ones first or those that for some reason cause them a problem. Patients who have difficulty swallowing tablets may be assisted in a number of ways:

- A drink beforehand moistens the mouth and gets the swallowing process started.

• Where the tablet is large and is scored, it may be split in two or even four. A specially designed tablet splitter may be helpful. Some tablets are not designed to be split, and attempts to do so could lead to an inaccurate dose being administered. If, for any reason, the tablet is unsuitable, the pharmacist should be asked to advise.

• In certain instances the tablet may be crushed using a mortar and pestle or specially designed tablet crusher. Enteric-coated or sustained-release formulations must not be split or crushed since this could destroy the properties of the tablet and cause gastric irritation or premature release of the drug into an incompatible pH.

• Some patients find it helpful to place the tablet at the back of the tongue, take a draught of water and tilt the head back before swallowing. This stimulates the back of the tongue and produces a swallowing reflex.

• For those who cannot swallow tablets or capsules, a liquid form of the medicine may be available.

• For dysphagic patients, consideration of the viscosity of an oral liquid medicine is important. Patients with swallowing difficulties may be able to swallow a more viscous preparation than a very mobile liquid.

Whenever possible, patients should put the tablet or capsule into the mouth themselves. By observing patients attempting to take a tablet and assessing their capabilities generally, the nurse can decide how best to present further medicines. The methods employed are:

- taking directly from a spoon, medicine measure or palm of the hand
- picking up using the thumb and forefinger.

However, some difficulties are encountered with each of these methods. For example:

- A spoon is not advisable for patients with any degree of tremor.
- Medicine measures are not designed with the size of an adult's nose in mind.
- Unless the medicine measure is completely dry, tablets can adhere to the measure and may be lost.
- Tablets or capsules may be dropped or may stick to the hand if moist.
- Intention tremor and stiff joints may make picking up difficult or impossible.

In general, patients who are elderly, frail, poorly sighted or confused, are helped if the tablets are placed in a row on the medicine tray accompanied by a glass of water or a suitable beverage. In this way they are more likely to see what they are to take – the colour of the tablets and the number. They can then safely pick each one up themselves and so retain some degree of independence. Hemiplegic patients find this a helpful method, especially when more than one tablet has to be taken. Using the unaffected hand, they require to break down the process. For example:

- Pick up glass, take drink, lay down glass.
- Pick up first tablet, place in mouth.
- Pick up glass, take drink, lay down glass.
- Pick up next tablet ... and so on.

White tablets may be overlooked when they are laid out on a white tray and so care must be taken to ensure that none has been missed. If the tray is used in this way, it must be washed before and after use.

Care must be taken, particularly where there is facial paralysis, to ensure that the tablets are swallowed and not retained in the side of the mouth. Patients who do not want to take their tablets are sometimes known to retain the tablet between the gum and the cheek until the staff are out of sight and then reject the tablet, often into the bed.

An adequate volume of fluid, for example at least 100 mL, ensures transport into the gastrointestinal tract. Apart from personal tastes and preferences, the choice and volume of liquid to be used will depend on a number of factors. Clearly, for patients on restricted fluids the volume may be critical. Milk may inhibit the absorption of some drugs, and acidic fruit cordials tend to cause capsules to swell – which may make swallowing more difficult. Improved formulations are a help in disguising the taste of many drugs but children of all ages may welcome the traditional 'spoonful of sugar'.

If a patient rejects part of a dose or vomits after swallowing a dose of medicine, the doctor should be informed of this along with the time lapse between drug administration and emesis or rejection. Vomitus should be retained for examination of drug content.

Administering oral liquids

• All liquid medicines should be thoroughly shaken before use and measured at eye level in a good light using a suitably designed measure, i.e. a measure with clear graduations that is convenient to pour into.

• When pouring a liquid medicine, the bottle is held with the label uppermost so that any drips will not deface the label.

• Viscous suspensions, syrups, etc., can be more completely administered if taken from a suitable graduated spoon rather than from a medicine measure. A standard 5 mL spoon should normally be used.

However, medicine spoons of different designs are available, the choice depending mainly on acceptability to the patient. Care should be taken not to overfill a medicine spoon when administering a viscous preparation.

- The formulation of liquid medicines presents many problems, not least of which is to achieve an acceptable taste. If particular problems are experienced, the clinical pharmacist should be consulted, as dilution or alternative formulation may be available.
- It is necessary to ensure that soluble (effervescent) tablets are completely dissolved prior to administration but an excessive volume should not be used since this could make the resulting solution less acceptable to the patient.
- Where the medicine is presented in powder form to be reconstituted (unstable antibiotics), the date of reconstitution or expiry should be marked on the bottle. The diluent and volume to be used will be specified on the label. If further dilution of the reconstituted medicine is required, this should be undertaken only in the pharmacy.
- Reconstituted medicines will normally require storage in a refrigerator, and it is very important to shake the bottle well prior to administration.
- When liquids are being instilled in the mouth from a dropper, a separate bottle and dropper are used for each patient.
- In some instances a specially designed oral syringe may be useful, for example in paediatrics or where specially potent oral liquid medicines are in use. Graduated droppers are supplied for use with high-dose oral morphine preparations.

The administration of oral medicines is summarised in Box 9.1

Box 9.1 Administration of oral medicines

Documentation
- Prescribing and recording sheet

The medicine
- Oral solids (tablet, capsule, lozenge, granules)
- Oral liquids (mixture, suspension, emulsion, linctus)

The nurse and the patient
- Identification of patient
- Explanation given to patient

Technique
- The nurse's hands should be socially clean
- Wherever possible, the patient should be in an upright position
- Whenever possible, patients should put the medicine into the mouth themselves
- The nurse should witness the medicine being taken
- If required, any fluid taken should be recorded on the patient's fluid balance chart
- Any medicines rejected should be retained

Problems
- Irritation of gastrointestinal tract
- Aspiration of the medicine
- Staining of teeth and lips

Sublingual administration

First-pass metabolism is avoided when drugs are given by the sublingual route (i.e. under the tongue) since the drug passes directly into the general blood circulation via the blood vessels on the under surface of the tongue. Sublingual tablets are uncoated ready for absorption. Once the tablet has been placed under the tongue, the patient should keep the mouth closed and refrain from swallowing saliva for as long as possible as this contains the drug which will be absorbed. As absorption through the oral mucosa is rapid; the effects of the drug become apparent within a minute or two.

Tablets to be given by this route must be prescribed as such. The method of administration is simple – requiring no liquid and demanding little effort from the patient. The cooperation of the patient is necessary, however, and a clear explanation of this method of administration should be given. Although no harm will ensue if the tablet is swallowed, the patient will benefit from the drug *only* if it is taken sublingually. The ease with which drugs can be given by this route can be used to advantage in postoperative patients and in those who are terminally ill, where swallowing of tablets can be a problem. The sublingual route is also useful when there is risk of symptoms arising unexpectedly and when a rapid effect is wanted, such as in angina pectoris. Patients who are prescribed glyceryl trinitrate tablets for prevention of anginal attacks should be advised to carry with them a small supply of the tablets at all times. The expiry date (8 weeks after *opening*) should be carefully noted on the label of the container. Once individual patients realise which activities tend to precipitate an attack, they should get into the habit of placing the tablet under the tongue just before embarking on any of these activities. When the tablet is used to alleviate an anginal attack, it should be taken immediately the pain is experienced and retained under the tongue until the pain is relieved, after which any of the tablet remaining is spat out. This may help to prevent headache caused by cerebral vasodilatation which often follows administration of this drug. Sublingual medication may also be administered in the form of an aerosol spray (see p. 190).

Buccal administration

When a tablet is to be held in the mouth against the mucous membranes, the term 'buccal' may be used. It refers to the area high up between the upper lip and the gum where the dosage form is left to dissolve. Tablets for buccal administration are uncoated to facilitate absorption. Glyceryl trinitrate is available as a buccal tablet (2 mg). The site chosen should be varied to reduce the risk of dental caries.

Medicine rounds

In spite of an increase in self-administration, the majority of medicines in hospital are still administered consecutively to groups of patients in the form of a medicine round (Box 9.2).

Box 9.2 Medicine round

Documentation
- Kardex system or individual prescribing and recording sheet at each patient's bedside or in document trolley

The medicine
- Mainly oral medicines (possibly medicines for inhalation also)
- Stored in alphabetical order according to approved name
- Individual locked medicine cabinet or trolley locked to wall when not in use
- Unlocked trolley never left unattended
- Sufficient spoons, medicine measures, oral syringes, etc., available

The environment
- So far as possible, uninterrupted

The nurse and the patient
- Each patient greeted and accurately identified

Technique
- Nurse works systematically according to local circumstances
- After use, non-disposable items washed, sticky bottles wiped and trolley/individual cabinet restocked as appropriate

Hazards
- Medicine(s) given to wrong patient
- Interruptions leading to error
- Medicines given too soon or much later than the time prescribed
- Misappropriation of medicines from unsupervised trolley/individual cabinet

ADMINISTRATION OF MEDICINES BY INJECTION

Medicines should only be administered by injection when no other route is suitable because of their hazardous nature. Where there is no alternative but to use this method, every precaution must be taken to minimise the risks involved (see Table 9.1). There are a number of reasons, however, why some medicines require to be administered by this method. For example:

- they may not be absorbed when given by mouth (gentamicin)
- they may be destroyed in the stomach (insulin)
- rapid first-pass metabolism may be extensive (lidocaine (lignocaine))
- a fast onset of action may be required in an emergency
- very precise control over dosage may be needed
- because the patient is unable, for whatever reason, to take the medicine by mouth
- to achieve high drug plasma levels.

Since the routes used for administering injections do not involve the gastrointestinal tract, drugs prepared for injection are often described as for *parenteral* use.

Presentation of medicines for parenteral use (small-volume injections)

The presentation of drugs for parenteral use requires the application of technological expertise. Wherever possible, injections should be available in a ready-to-use form (CRAG 2002). Where the injection is in a ready-to-use form (i.e. where no diluent or reconstitution is required) and there are no health and safety risks to the operator or the environment, it should be drawn up in the near-patient area. Such injections should be administered to the patient immediately. Sterility and stability of the drug must be ensured but, at the same time, the user of the product must be able readily to access the container to remove the contents for administration. Glass containers continue to be the first choice (since glass is a relatively inert product) especially for smaller-volume injections. Plastic materials are now the norm for packaging larger-volume infusions. Such containers are more user-friendly than heavy, breakable glass bottles. Table 9.2 summarises the characteristics of the containers in common use, and draws attention to particular aspects of their use. It is the duty of all health professionals to check each container for integrity and any special features before use.

The medicine for injection may on some occasions be presented in a rubber-capped multidose vial, especially

Table 9.1 Hazards associated with injections

Risk/cause	Possible outcome	Prevention
Contamination		
Dirty preparation area	Local sepsis	Keep preparation areas clear and clean
Unwashed hands	Septicaemia especially if patient is immunocompromised	Wash hands using chlorhexidine gluconate handwash before and after preparing injection
Unswabbed vial tops		Swab rubber-capped vials using alcohol swab and allow to dry
Aerosolisation		
Spraying the atmosphere with injection solution	Reduced sensitivity to the medication	Inject equivalent volume of air to volume of injection required Attach sheathed needle to syringe when expelling air from syringe
Needlestick injury		
Resheathing needles	Hepatitis B HIV	NEVER replace sheath on needle
Incorrect disposal of needle	Localised infection	Always use sharps receptacle for disposal of needles Do NOT overfill sharps receptacle
Nerve damage		
Improper siting of injection	Paralysis of a limb	Select appropriate site avoiding large nerve(s)

Table 9.2 Characteristics of containers for small-volume injectable products

Container/material/use	Description of container	Method of use/notes
Glass ampoule made of special quality glass that does not react with contents. Size range 0.25–50 mL. (Plastic ampoules are now used for certain products.) Normally contains solutions ready for use, but may contain a sterile powder for reconstitution	Body containing drug, narrow constriction leading to neck. The constriction is often marked with a white ring which indicates the place where the neck is to be snapped off to enable the contents to be accessed Some ampoules have colour-coded rings on the neck of the ampoule which are a help in avoiding mix-ups. These coloured rings must not be used to identify the product	After shaking down any solution that has entered the neck of the ampoule, the neck is wiped with an alcohol swab to remove any surface contamination and then snapped off using an ampoule sleeve to protect the fingers from glass spicules and/or any sharp edges Less commonly it may be necessary to make a scratch on the ampoule with a small file prior to following the procedure outlined above. Ampoule-opening devices of various designs are available Since glass ampoules cannot be resealed it follows that the containers are for single use only. Any unwanted contents must be discarded Plastic ampoules are accessed by twisting off a tab on the neck of the ampoule or by direct penetration with a needle at a site indicated on the ampoule
Glass rubber-capped vial (RCV). Used for solutions for injection and sterile powders for reconstitution	Squat glass container, closed with a rubber plug which is held in place by a metal ring. The exposed rubber surface is generally covered with a protective pull-off metal or plastic disc	The disc is removed, the exposed surface is swabbed with an alcohol swab, allowed to dry and the container accessed by penetration with a suitable needle. The required dose of drug is removed or the required volume of the appropriate reconstituted fluid is added prior to removal of the dose. (It is vitally important to follow the instructions regarding reconstitution and to ensure that the powder is dissolved before withdrawing the dose) RCVs are capable of being used as multidose containers since the rubber plug is self-sealing if correctly used. However, RCVs should be used as multidose containers only if the stability of the contents permits this and there is a suitable antimicrobial preservative present in the formulation. As with the use of ampoules and other containers, all sharps must be safely disposed of after use

where the dose is variable. The self-sealing rubber closure must be thoroughly cleaned with an alcohol swab and *allowed to dry* prior to puncturing it with a needle. Great care is essential in calculating what portion of the total volume is required. To facilitate withdrawal of fluid, the plunger of the syringe is first withdrawn and air injected, the volume of air being the same as the volume of fluid to be withdrawn. It is customary to change the needle after drawing up the injection and before injecting the patient in case particles of rubber are retained inside the needle. Another good reason is that when a needle is inserted through the rubber cap, it may become dulled or the needle coating that helps it glide through the skin may be removed (Beyea & Nicoll 1996). Besides, because of the high risk of needlestick injury when re-sheathing a needle, the practice of using a new needle for administering the injection to the patient is strongly advised.

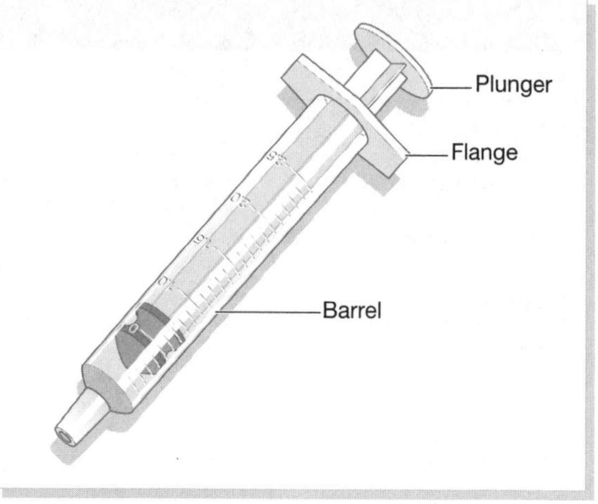

Figure 9.1 Syringe.

Reconstitution of medicines for injection

The medicine may be presented in powder form and require reconstitution. Most often this is done using Water for Injections but in certain instances special diluents may be required. It should be recognised that the addition of 1 mL of diluent to 250 mg of a drug will produce a volume in excess of 1 mL. Normally this is of little consequence but may be important if a fraction of the total content of the vial is to be administered. For emaciated patients the volume of reconstituting fluid should be the minimum compatible with the physical and other properties of the drug, e.g. solubility, and any possible local irritancy should be taken into account. Once the contents of a multidose vial have been reconstituted, the vial must be dated and stored in the refrigerator. On occasion it may be desirable to combine two drugs in the same injection. This may present problems, e.g. physical/chemical incompatibility in the syringe and in the management of any subsequent drug reaction. The prime considerations here should be the safety and comfort of the patient. Clearly, comfort for the patient should not be allowed to detract from safety in drug therapy. The advice of the prescriber and clinical pharmacist will often be helpful in resolving these difficult situations.

Syringes

A syringe consists of a barrel and a plunger (Fig. 9.1). The barrel is graduated. The plunger has a rubber stopper attached. Syringes are available in various sizes, e.g. 2 mL, 5 mL, 10 mL, 20 mL. The choice of syringe is made according to the volume of medication to be injected. It should be noted, however, that insulin must always be measured using an insulin syringe. The tip of a syringe can vary, with the *concentric* Luer tip being the one used for subcutaneous and intramuscular injections. It is also used for introducing medication via an already-sited intravenous cannula. For direct intravenous injections, the *eccentric* Luer tip is used to allow the needle to lie within the vein wall without puncturing the distal wall. The Luer tips of syringes interlock to an international standard with needle hubs. Disposable syringes are made of a plastic material which is compatible with most substances to be injected. There are one or two exceptions, however. Paraldehyde, for example, should be administered using a glass syringe since it dissolves plastic and rubber on prolonged contact. Syringes are individually sealed in a sterile pack. Before use, a check should be made that the seal has not been broken. Once a syringe has been removed from its pack, the utmost care is required to prevent contamination of the tip of the syringe.

Needles

A needle consists of a hub and a cannula (Fig. 9.2). The cannula is hollow and is made of strong flexible steel that has been siliconised to assist penetration. For the same reason, the tip of the cannula is bevelled. Different types of needle have a different bevel. A shorter bevel encourages minimal penetration, as is required in an intradermal injection. A longer bevel allows easier deep penetration, as needed for an intramuscular

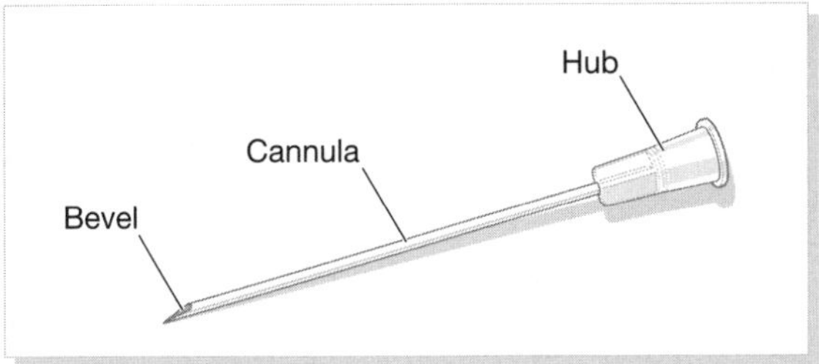

Figure 9.2 Needle.

injection. The gauge of the cannula is an indication of its diameter. The higher the gauge, the finer the bore. Higher gauges are used for 'watery' solutions and make for less painful injections. Low gauges are essential for injecting viscous (syrupy) solutions. Needle lengths also vary. Selection of length depends on the route of the injection as well as the patient's age and physical build. There is evidence to suggest that the use of a longer needle with a wider bore creates fewer local reactions in the vaccination of children (Diggle & Deeks 2000). Each needle is enclosed in a removable guard and individually sealed in a sterile pack. Before use, a check should be made to ensure that the pack has not been damaged. Once a guard is removed, the needle should be in one of two places only – in the ampoule or vial containing the medication, or in the patient.

For *drawing up any injection* from a glass ampoule, it is important to use a needle with a bore that is 21 gauge or smaller to filter out any shards of glass that may have entered the ampoule (Shaw & Lyall 1985).

For *administering subcutaneous injections*, a short fine-bore needle is used. For adults, this may be ⅝ inch (16 mm), 25 gauge; ½ inch (12 mm) 26 gauge; or ⅜ inch (10 mm) 27 gauge.

For *administering intramuscular injections*, the needle used has to be sufficiently long to reach deep into the muscle so as to increase the speed of effect and to reduce the likelihood of the drug seeping back along the needle track. For adults a 1½ inch (40 mm), 21 gauge (0.8 mm) needle is normally used. In severely emaciated adults and in small children a 1 inch (25 mm), 23 gauge (0.6 mm) needle may be used.

When drawing up and injecting drugs with a known potential to cause sensitivity reactions, disposable gloves should be worn to prevent possible contact with the skin and the development of a sensitivity reaction. The special precautions which require to be taken when handling cytotoxic drugs are given in Chapter 22.

Routes of administration

The routes most commonly used for administering injections are:

- subcutaneous (into the fatty layer beneath the skin)
- intramuscular (into skeletal muscle)
- intravenous (into a vein).

Intravenous medicines given by direct venepuncture are administered only by a doctor. A nurse who has undertaken specific training and is in possession of authorisation to do so may administer intravenous medication where venous access has already been established. In clinical practice there is widespread use of the intravenous route for the administration of drugs such as antibiotics and diuretics. However, some drugs still require to be given by either the subcutaneous or intramuscular route, and therefore nurses must maintain the skills involved.

The *subcutaneous* route is generally used for administering small doses of non-irritating, water-soluble substances. Drugs commonly given subcutaneously include:

- insulin
- heparin
- hyoscine
- vaccines.

The *intramuscular* route is used for administering irritating drugs, oily solutions and aqueous suspensions.

Drugs commonly given intramuscularly include:

- analgesics
- anti-emetics
- corticosteroids.

Rate of absorption

The rates at which drugs are absorbed and take effect after subcutaneous or intramuscular injection depend on two factors. These are the local blood circulation and the nature of the drug solution or suspension. Subcutaneous absorption occurs chiefly through the capillaries and is much faster compared with absorption following oral medication but usually slower than intramuscular absorption because of muscle tissue's excellent blood supply. Absorption following intramuscular injection may be speeded up by massaging the area of injection. However, insulin-dependent diabetics are discouraged from massaging the site vigorously, in an attempt to preserve the state of the capillaries. An inflamed or oedematous site should be avoided when administering subcutaneous or intramuscular injections so as to prevent a worsening of the inflammation/oedema and consequently a delay in absorption. In states of shock, blood flow to the skin and superficial muscle may be greatly reduced, thus reducing the absorption of drugs from these sites. In this case intravenous injection should be used.

Volume

When preparing an injection, the nurse should give consideration to the volume which may be effectively accommodated in one site. Apart from the route to be used, the patient's age and physical build are factors which will influence the decision. Normally the following would apply:

- For *subcutaneous injections* no more than 2 mL should be injected at one site.
- For *intramuscular injections* the volume injected at any one site should normally be no more than 3 mL. Where a volume in excess of 3 mL is to be given, two separate sites may have to be used. No more than 1 mL should be given into the deltoid muscle.

Site

The sites most commonly used for *subcutaneous* injections (Fig. 9.3) are as follows:

- middle outer aspect of the upper arm
- middle anterior aspect of the thigh
- anterior abdominal wall below the umbilicus.

The back and lower loin may also be used. The sites most commonly used for *intramuscular* injections are as follows:

- upper outer quadrant of the buttock (Fig. 9.4)
- anterolateral aspect of the mid-thigh.

(The deltoid muscle is used for hepatitis B and influenza vaccines.)

It is vital that the injection is confined to one of these areas to avoid damage to the sciatic nerve and to avoid penetrating a major blood vessel.

Rotation of the sites used for subcutaneous and intramuscular injections helps to reduce the likelihood of irritation and improves absorption. Rotation *within* the sites is also important. Patients who, for example, have to repeatedly self-administer subcutaneous injections may be taught to visualise a clock-face on the site and systematically work round it. Where nurses are repeatedly administering injections, the site used on each occasion may be plotted on a diagram held at the bedside. Before administering any type of injection, the skin should be inspected on each occasion. Lesions, such as birthmarks, moles or scars, and inflamed or oedematous sites should be avoided.

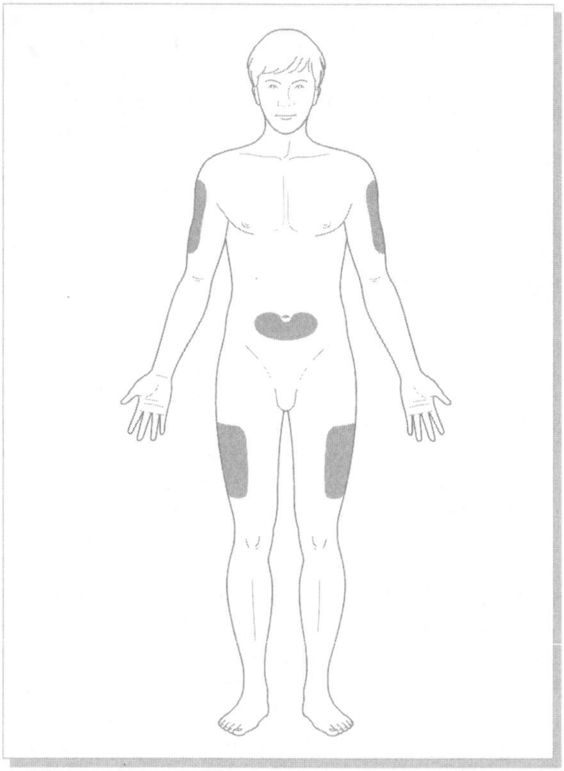

Figure 9.3 Sites for administering subcutaneous injections.

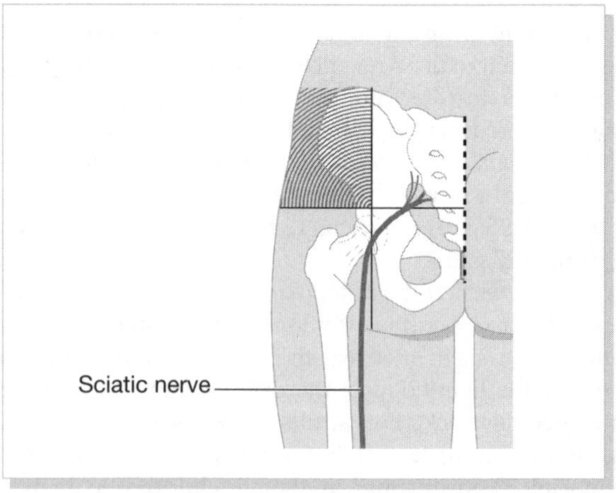

Figure 9.4 Upper outer quadrant of the buttock (shaded area).

Skin preparation

In spite of now quite old research findings, old habits die hard. It is not necessary to use an alcohol swab to clean the skin prior to the administration of injections (Dann 1969). Torrance (1989) cites two studies which prove this point. One describes a series of 1078 injections given by all routes without any skin preparation and which resulted in no case of systemic or local infection being recorded. The second was a study of 7000 insulin injections given to a group of diabetic patients without skin cleansing, with no infection noted. Lipids in the epidermis provide an antibacterial barrier, so that removal of the lipids may encourage bacterial colonisation (Torrance 1989). Clinical evidence suggests that no harm will be caused by pricking the skin *so long as it is socially clean*. Contaminated skin will need preparation to produce a low bacterial count. In this case the site should first be made socially clean followed by a 30-second rub using an 'alcohol swab' (alcohol swabs contain 70% alcohol and a disinfectant such as chlorhexidine). The skin should then be allowed to dry before proceeding so that the antiseptic does not cause irritation by being injected into the tissues. In immunosuppressed patients, the skin must be cleansed in this way, as this group of patients may become infected by inoculation of a relatively small number of pathogens.

Angle

The angles at which the needle is directed for subcutaneous and intramuscular injections are illustrated in Figure 9.5. It is common practice for subcutaneous injections of, for example, heparin or insulin, to be given into the abdomen at an angle of 90° using, for example, a 0.33 mm (gauge) × 13 mm (length) needle. An angle of between 45° and 90° may be used when a 0.5 mm × 16 mm needle is preferred.

Irritant or staining substances

The injection may be known to irritate the tissues and stain the skin if it is allowed to seep along the needle track to the epidermis (e.g. iron sorbitol injection). To prevent this, several precautions should be taken. After the syringe is filled, the needle is changed so that the substance is contained in the syringe only and is less likely to drip from the tip of the needle as it penetrates the skin. To reduce pain as well as the risk of staining, the injection is made deep into the muscle of the upper outer quadrant of the buttock. The arm and thigh do not allow for the depth required and so should not be used. A 21 gauge needle is suitable but it is important that it is long enough to reach the muscle. As a rule of thumb a 1½ inch (40 mm) needle will do for most normal-sized adults. Obese patients (e.g. >90 kg) will require a 2 inch needle. The so-called Z-track technique must be used. This technique involves displacement of the skin and subcutaneous tissue laterally prior to injection (Fig. 9.6). The injection is made slowly and steadily. Before withdrawing the needle, 10 seconds should be allowed to elapse so that the

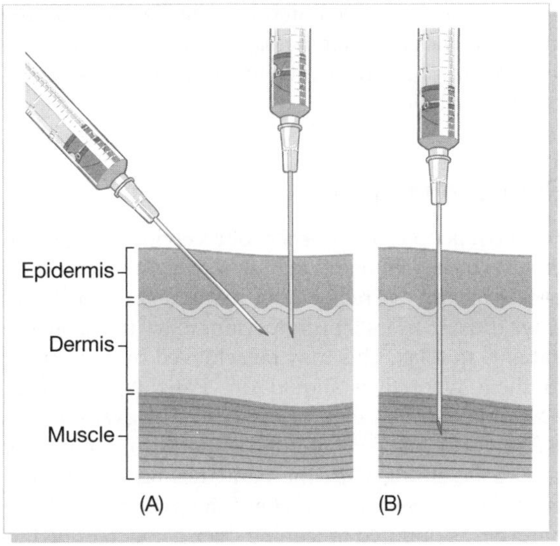

Figure 9.5 Angles for the administration of (A) subcutaneous and (B) intramuscular injections.

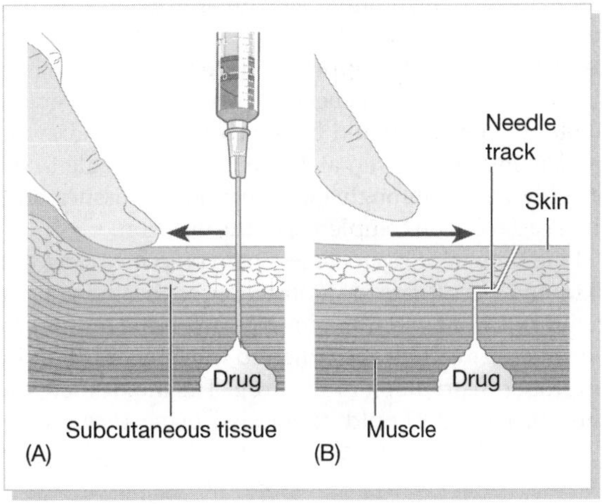

Figure 9.6 Z-track technique.

muscle mass can accommodate the volume of the injection. The site is not massaged, otherwise the medication may be forced into the subcutaneous tissue, causing irritation.

Reduction of pain

For most people, the prospect of receiving an injection of any kind is not one that they relish. Pain caused by injections can be reduced in a number of different ways (Box 9.3). First, it is important to try to encourage patients to relax. This may be achieved by explaining to them what they should do. Patients should be positioned so that they are at ease. For example, for *subcutaneous injections* into the upper arm, the patient should be sitting with the hand resting on the iliac crest; for *intramuscular injections* the patient should be lying *on*, as opposed to leaning over, a couch or bed.

When the buttock is the chosen site for intramuscular injection, administration may be made less painful by asking the patient to adopt the prone position and to point the feet inwards. Internal rotation of the femur helps to relax the gluteus maximus muscle. Alternatively, the patient may lie on one side with the lower leg extended and the upper leg flexed.

As a general rule, whenever an injection is to be given at 90°, the needle should be inserted (and withdrawn) *quickly*. Injections given at 45° require the needle to be steadily *pushed* through the skin into the tissues and then eased out on completion of the injection.

Fine-bore needles create less pain on puncturing the skin and necessitate slow injection of the fluid. Pain can result from injecting too large a volume of fluid at one site or injecting the drug too quickly, resulting in improper distribution of the drug. The medication, on the other hand, should be injected using *slow, steady pressure* at a rate of about 10 seconds per millilitre (Beyea & Nicoll 1996). The skin may be cooled using a volatile spray such as ethyl chloride. A further possibility is to use a local anaesthetic agent such as EMLA cream (see also p. 464).

Subcutaneous administration may be carried out by means of a high-pressure jet of liquid, using an injector which delivers an accurate dose without the aid of a needle. This technique may be useful in mass inoculation programmes. There is a reduction in pain to the patient and no risk of needlestick injury. The risk of transmitting blood-borne infections by this method should be carefully considered.

Use of the Z-track technique (see p. 75) may also reduce the discomfort associated with intramuscular injections since there is less likelihood of the medication leaking into the subcutaneous tissue by this method.

Box 9.3 Summary of methods for reducing pain associated with injections

- Use fine-bore needle where possible
- Do not exceed 3 mL of fluid at one site
- Rotate the sites
- Consider using skin coolant or local anaesthetic cream
- Consider using Z-track method for IM injections
- Be prepared to listen to view of experienced patient
- Explain benefits of the injection
- Encourage patient to relax
- If appropriate, ask patient to turn foot inwards
- Insert needle *quickly*
- Inject medication *slowly*
- Withdraw needle *quickly*

Administration

The process of checking a medicine for injection against the prescription is the same as for the administration of any medicine. Hands must be washed thoroughly using chlorhexidine gluconate solution at the start and finish of the procedure. Asepsis must be maintained throughout since puncturing the integument provides easy access for pathogenic microorganisms. Every effort must be made to encourage the patient to relax and to minimise pain as far as possible. Extra support will be required for patients suffering from needle phobia. Careful disposal of syringes and needles is of great importance.

The procedure for administering a *subcutaneous* injection is outlined in Box 9.4. Patients may be taught to self-administer medication by this route (see p. 73). The procedure for administering an *intramuscular* injection is outlined in Box 9.5.

Patients with haematological conditions such as leukaemia, in which the platelet count is likely to be low, must never be given intramuscular injections because of the high risk of bleeding into muscle tissue because of its rich blood supply.

Administration of subcutaneous insulin

The development of a very short (13 mm), fine-bore (0.33 mm) needle which comes already attached to an insulin syringe is more acceptable than equipment previously available for the self-administration of insulin. It is nevertheless as important as ever to reach the correct layer of tissue, namely, subcutaneous fat, on every occasion, and not to administer the insulin intramuscularly

Box 9.4 Administration of subcutaneous injection

Documentation
- As for intramuscular injection

The medicine
- As for intramuscular injection

The environment
- Patient seated or in bed
- Privacy, warmth, comfort

The nurse and the patient
- Patient identified
- Explanation given to patient
- Patient assisted into supine position if abdomen is the chosen site
- Patient's skin cleanliness assessed

Technique (drawing up the injection)
- As for intramuscular injection (see Box 9.5)

Technique (administering the injection)
- Nurse ensures hands thoroughly washed
- Chosen site for injection exposed
- Skin pinched up between thumb and forefinger
- *For 90° angle,* syringe held in 'pencil grip'; *for 45° angle,* syringe 'cradled' across all four fingers and steadied with thumb
- *For 90° angle,* needle *stabbed* through skin; *for 45° angle,* needle with bevel uppermost *pushed gently* through the skin
- Skin released
- Fluid injected *slowly* and *steadily*
- Needle *gently* withdrawn
- Site gently compressed for a few seconds until any oozing stops
- Patient made comfortable
- 'Sharps' carefully placed in disposal bin

Hazards
- Abscess formation

Box 9.5 Administration of intramuscular injection

Documentation
- Prescribing and recording sheets

The medicine
- Ampoule or vial containing prescribed drug
- Ampoule of Water for Injections (or other diluent) if necessary for reconstitution

The environment
- Patient in bed or on couch
- Privacy, warmth, comfort

The nurse and the patient
- Patient identified
- Nurse explains the procedure and indicates how the patient may assist
- Patient assisted into lateral or prone position
- Patient's skin cleanliness assessed

Technique (drawing up the injection)
- Nurse ensures hands are thoroughly washed
- Contents collected into body of ampoule by flicking ampoule with fingers
- Neck of ampoule wiped with alcohol swab
- Ampoule snapped at constriction using swab to protect fingers (or by using a plastic sleeve)
- Syringe assembled; 21G needle attached
- Care taken to prevent needle from touching anything unsterile
- Syringe filled
- New guarded needle attached
- Air bubbles expelled from syringe by:
  - holding it perpendicular at eye level in a good light
  - pulling plunger back slightly
  - tapping syringe with fingers to collect small bubbles into one
  - pushing plunger until liquid fills needle
- Final volume checked

Technique (administering the injection)
- Nurse ensures hands are washed just prior to administration if involved in positioning patient, and on completion of procedure
- Nurse ensures sufficiently large area of patient's buttock exposed to allow selection of exact site for injection while maintaining maximum privacy
- Fold of skin and tissue stretched taut or tissues pulled to one side (Z-track)
- Syringe held using 'pencil grip'
- Needle inserted *quickly*
- Plunger withdrawn slightly to verify that needle has not penetrated blood vessel (if blood appears, needle withdrawn and injection repeated at another site using fresh dose, syringe and needle)
- Fluid injected *slowly*
- Needle withdrawn *quickly*
- Site gently compressed for a few seconds until minor seepage stops
- Patient made comfortable
- 'Sharps' carefully placed in disposal bin

Hazards
- Abscess formation
- Nerve damage
- Injecting medication into large blood vessel

or by the intradermal route by mistake. Failure to reach the subcutaneous layer leads to altered rates of absorption and poor diabetic control. The recommended method is to pinch up the skin and, using a gentle stabbing technique, to inject at an angle of 90°. Such advice is thought to be important in thin diabetic patients, especially men, who it has been found may have less depth of subcutaneous fat than the length of the shorter needles in use, resulting in the administration of an intramuscular injection and not a subcutaneous one (Spraul et al 1988).

Patients receiving outpatient treatment for certain ongoing conditions are encouraged to self-administer subcutaneous medication where possible. Examples include the administration of insulin and interferon. Alternatively, a family member may be taught to do this. In either situation, the teaching skills of nurses will be called upon as will their role in providing encouragement.

Administration of subcutaneous heparin

In order to reduce the great risk of bruising leading to pain and unsightliness, a modified injection technique is recommended for the administration of subcutaneous heparin (Conaghan 1993). Efforts are directed at minimising the physical trauma which can be caused before, during and after the giving of an injection. Dann (1969) has shown that, in most patients, there is no need to clean the skin with an antiseptic. Besides, the use of an alcohol swab leads to vasodilatation and encourages bleeding. Vigorous rubbing or pinching of the skin may damage capillaries (Koivistov & Felig 1978). The preferred site is the abdomen because of the greater depth of subcutaneous fat, although abdominal surgery may limit the available area. Brenner et al (1981) claim that using an angle of 90° leads to fewer bruises. In addition, the amount of movement of the needle throughout the procedure should be kept to a minimum (McGowan & Wood 1989/90). It is recommended that a roll of tissue be *lifted* before inserting the needle. It is also generally thought that the plunger should *not* be withdrawn prior to injecting as this can lead to negative pressure and the formation of a haematoma. Once the needle has been removed, only light pressure over the injection site using cotton wool is necessary to stop any backflow of blood from the injection site.

Intravenous injection

Administering a drug directly into a vein avoids all complications of drug absorption and, as a result, an effective blood level of the drug can be achieved in a matter of seconds. The intravenous route is used:

- in emergency situations such as shock and status asthmaticus
- to administer general anaesthetic agents (e.g. propofol)
- for larger volumes (e.g. 5–20 mL)
- where the preparation has irritant properties (e.g. cytotoxic drugs)
- where subcutaneous or intramuscular injections would cause intolerable pain (e.g. aminophylline).

Intravenous injections may, however, be associated with a number of complications such as:

- a haematoma caused by puncturing through, instead of into, the vein
- necrosis caused by the drug escaping into the surrounding tissues when the needle slips out of the vein and is simply lying in the tissues
- phlebitis at the injection site resulting from a high concentration of an irritant agent, repeated injections or prolonged administration
- because of rapidity of action, intoxication or death if an error is made when calculating or measuring the dose.

As has been stated earlier, administration of medicines by direct venepuncture may be carried out only by a doctor, although nurses who have received special training and have been authorised to do so may administer intravenous drugs through an already sited cannula. A list of those drugs recommended for administration by medical staff only will be available within each trust. Irrespective of who administers it, the prescribing doctor is accountable for the effects of the medication.

It is important that all nurses understand how the procedure is carried out so that they can, if called upon, play a supporting role. The standard approach to prescribing, administering and recording medicines is followed. To reduce the risk of introducing microorganisms into the bloodstream, it is essential that the hands are washed, sterile equipment used and an aseptic technique practised. The patient should be given an explanation of what is to be done and should be in a comfortable position with the site to be used exposed. A vein in the elbow or the back of the hand is normally used. With the help of a tourniquet, the vein is distended to allow access. If indicated, the site of injection is swabbed with a suitable antiseptic and allowed to dry. A syringe with an eccentric nozzle and a 1 inch (25 mm) 20 gauge needle with an intravenous

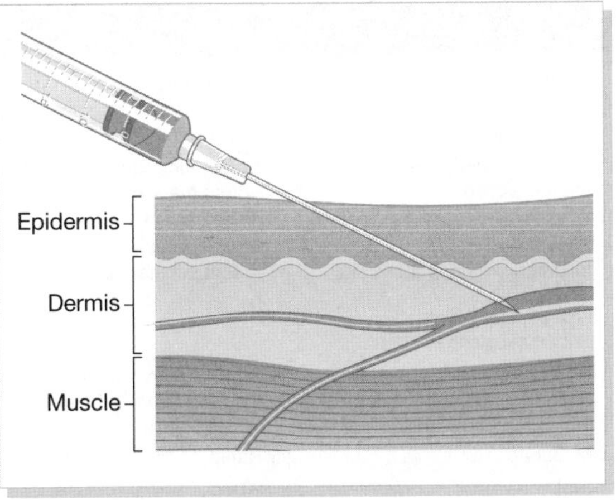

Figure 9.7 Intravenous injection.

bevel are used for giving an intravenous injection. All air bubbles are expelled from the syringe and the needle filled with drug. Holding the syringe in line with the vein, the needle with the bevel up is pushed through the skin into the vein in the direction of the heart (Fig. 9.7). Before injecting, the position of the needle must be verified by gently pulling the plunger. If no blood is aspirated, the needle must then be withdrawn and another attempt made. After releasing the tourniquet and making an initial injection of 0.1 mL, there should be a pause of at least 30 seconds to observe the response before the remainder is slowly injected (up to 10 minutes). It is dangerous to give a rapid intravenous injection as this exposes tissues and organs such as the heart and brain to high concentrations of a drug which has been poorly diluted with blood. A drug solution injected over 2 minutes will be 60 times more dilute than if injected over 2 seconds. After completing the injection, a sterile swab should be placed over the injection site, the needle slowly removed and gentle pressure maintained to avoid a haematoma.

Alternatively, intravenous drugs may be administered intermittently via the side inlet of an indwelling intravenous cannula or into the administration set of an intravenous infusion by means of a three-way stopcock or multiple-inlet device. If there is not a continuous fluid infusion to keep the cannula patent, a dilute heparin solution should be injected before and after the drug is administered to prevent blood from clotting in its lumen.

A summary of common routes for injection is given in Table 9.3.

Other routes of injection

Although parenteral administration is normally accomplished by subcutaneous, intramuscular or intravenous routes, occasionally other routes are used to deliver a drug to a particular tissue or organ.

Intra-arterial injection

This route is sometimes used to inject or infuse drugs into an artery supplying the affected organ if the drugs are rapidly metabolised or systemically toxic. Cytotoxic drugs for the treatment of local neoplasms or radio-opaque substances used in arteriography may be injected in this way.

Intra-articular injection

In inflammatory conditions of the joints, particularly rheumatoid arthritis, corticosteroids are given by intra-articular injection to relieve inflammation and increase joint mobility. Insoluble, long-acting compounds such as triamcinolone hexacetonide are used. Corticosteroids should not be injected into infected joints. Tissues or joints injected with corticosteroids have an increased susceptibility to infections. It is therefore essential to observe full aseptic precautions when making these injections.

Intradermal (intracutaneous) injection

Intradermal injections are small-volume injections of the order of 0.02–0.1 mL, given with a tuberculin syringe and a 16 mm, 26 gauge needle. The most common site used is the anterior aspect of the mid-forearm to allow for ease of inspection. The injection is given just under the skin, holding the syringe about parallel to the skin. The technique is most commonly used for the administration of certain diagnostic agents such as tuberculin PPD and skin testing solutions in the diagnosis of allergy. As the potential allergen is slowly injected a small weal forms. The needle is slowly withdrawn and the site is not massaged, in an effort to reduce interference with the formation of the weal.

In testing for allergy a distinct benefit in *not* cleansing the skin beforehand is that there is no risk of causing irritation which could interfere with the interpretation of the result. The local reaction is assessed 24–72 hours later by measuring its diameter.

Intrathecal injection

It is sometimes necessary to administer some drugs intrathecally if they have poor lipid solubility and as a result do not pass the blood-brain barrier (see p.119). In the treatment of meningitis, water-soluble antibiotics are administered by the intrathecal route to achieve adequate concentration in the cerebrospinal fluid (CSF). Drugs administered by this route include

Table 9.3 Summary of common routes for injections

	Subcutaneous	Intramuscular	Intravenous
Definition	Beneath the skin	Into muscle	Into a vein
Indications	Drug would be destroyed in stomach if taken orally Self-administration desirable	Oral medication cannot be tolerated/used	Emergency situations Irritant medication Anaesthetics
Contraindications	Shock Inflamed or oedematous site	Emaciation Inflamed or oedematous site Shock Low platelet count Irritant substance	Poor venous access Irritant substance
Who may administer	Registered nurse Student nurse under supervision of registered nurse	Registered nurse Student nurse under supervision of registered nurse	Registered nurse who has received specialist training
Relative rate of onset of action	Slow	Moderate	Rapid
Maximum volume at one site	2 mL	3 mL	20 mL
Sites (commonest)	Outer aspect of upper arm Anterior aspect of thigh Abdominal wall, i.e. below umbilicus	Upper outer quadrant of buttock Anterolateral aspect of mid-thigh	Forearm Back of hand Antecubital fossa at elbow
Needle: • length • gauge	 ⅝ inch (16 mm) 25G ½ inch (12 mm), 26G if abdomen used	 1½ inch (40 mm) 21G	 1 inch (25 mm) 20G
Angle	45–90° to the skin	90° to the skin	As near to parallel to the skin as possible
Hazards	Abscess formation	Nerve damage Abscess formation Injecting into large blood vessel	Cardiac embarrassment caused by very rapid administration Haematoma Extravasation Phlebitis/thrombophlebitis Air or particle embolism Localised infection Septicaemia

Box 9.6 Examples of drugs given intrathecally [Doses adjusted in accordance with patient's needs (under specialist supervision)]

Baclofen
Bupivacaine
Diamorphine
Gentamicin
Methotrexate

antimicrobial drugs, the choice of which will depend on the results of bacteriological examination of the CSF and toxicity. Doses have to be very carefully calculated and are much smaller than would be given by other routes since the volume of distribution is much reduced compared with systemic administration. Reduced doses are given to infants and children.

In addition to antimicrobial drugs, certain antimetabolites, diagnostic agents, skeletal muscle relaxants, opioids and anaesthetics may be administered intrathecally (see Box 9.6). A product specially prepared for intrathecal use should be used. In some instances, intrathecal therapy may be supplemented by a course of the drug given by intramuscular or intravenous injection.

Technique. Drugs for intrathecal injection are normally injected between lumbar vertebrae 3 and 4 into the subarachnoid space of the spinal cord as part of the procedure of lumbar puncture. The role of the nurse is directed towards careful positioning of the patient, assisting the doctor in maintaining an aseptic technique and providing the patient with support and encouragement throughout the procedure.

It is vitally important to maintain full asepsis in this procedure because of the risk of infection being introduced into the CNS. Great care has to be taken with all the procedures involved. In view of the potential hazards involved in the intrathecal injection of drugs, whenever possible, the drug should be supplied in a form that is ready to use without further manipulation.

In any event, the injection – as well as being sterile – must not contain particulate matter. A sterile, disposable bacterial filter (0.22 micrometre) must be used between the syringe and needle as a final safeguard for the patient.

Since drugs injected intrathecally come into immediate, direct contact with nervous tissue, the consequences of inadvertent injection of drugs intended for administration by other routes may be catastrophic for the patient (see also p. 344).

INTRAVENOUS INFUSION

When large volumes of fluid (50 mL upwards) require to be administered over a prolonged period, the most effective method is intravenous infusion. The indications for intravenous infusion are:

- when a patient cannot take oral medication
- when a rapid response is required
- to maintain or restore blood volume
- when a drug is inactivated in the gastrointestinal tract
- when there is a problem of absorption from the gut
- to supply electrolytes or nutrients
- when it is important to control plasma levels of a drug
- to administer irritant substances, for example, cytotoxic agents
- in life-threatening infections where it is vital to establish high concentrations of antibiotics in the tissues.

Intravenous infusions are normally packed in plastic containers and delivered to the patient via an intravenous administration set (Fig. 9.8) attached to an intravenous cannula (Fig. 9.9) which has been inserted into the patient's vein. Because of the considerable risk of introducing infection directly into the bloodstream, the infusion fluid, all parts of the administration equipment and any dressings used must be sterile.

Although introducing an intravenous cannula and establishing the free flow of the infusion are the doctor's responsibility, registered nurses (and midwives) who are appropriately trained may also carry out this procedure. The care of the patient before and after the procedure, and the satisfactory maintenance of the intravenous line, rests with the nurse.

Before assembling an intravenous line, it is important to read and carefully check the label of the infusion container against the fluid prescription. This should be carried out by a registered nurse or by a student nurse under the supervision of a registered nurse. Local

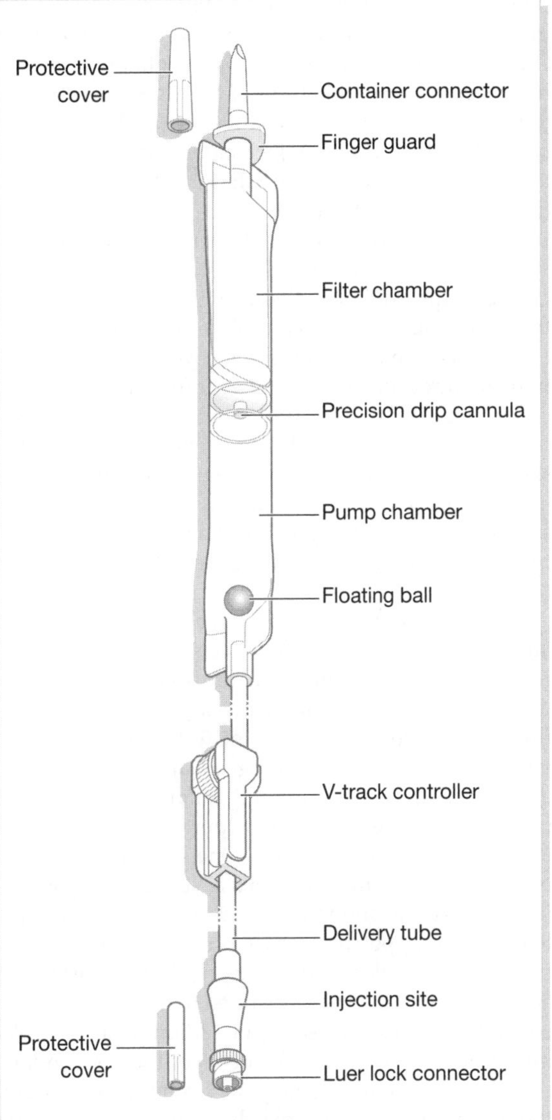

Figure 9.8 Intravenous administration set.

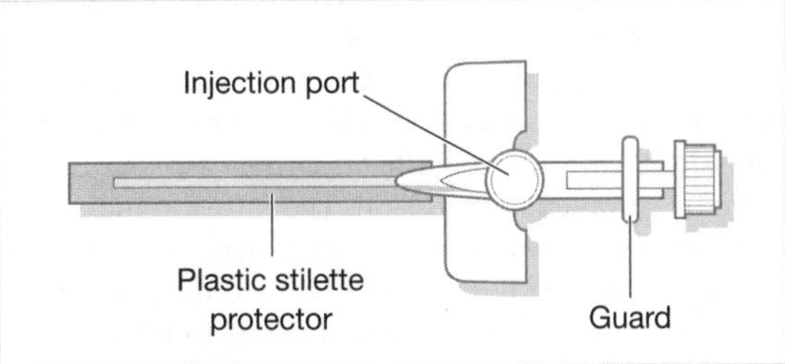

Figure 9.9 Intravenous cannula.

policy may dictate that two members of staff are to be involved at all times. The expiry date should be checked. The batch number of each container is always recorded so that in the event of an adverse reaction to the infusion the offending containers may be identified and withdrawn. The container should also be inspected to ensure it has no flaws and that the fluid is clear and free from particulate matter.

The entry port of the container is pierced by the spike of the appropriate administration set, the filter chamber squeezed to fill the set with fluid, air removed from the tubing and the control clamp closed. The free end of the administration set is covered by its sheath until required for use. Once an infusion container is connected to an administration set, the risk that exists of contamination through any of the points of entry should be recognised. The container is hung on an intravenous infusion stand which should be adjusted so that the container is just less than a metre above the cannula insertion site to achieve the optimum flow rate (Auty 1989).

The flow rate is adjusted by means of a roll clamp attached to the tubing. Where accurate control of flow rate is essential, an automatic infusion system may be used which pumps solutions at a preset rate. As the fluid runs through the administration set, the container empties and, in so doing, collapses.

Adjuncts are sometimes used with this system, e.g. a calibrated burette may be incorporated in the system into which the infusion drips. One or more drugs can be added to the burette and this is very useful, particularly in neonatal and intensive care units, for intermittent infusion of potent drugs in precise volumes. Drugs may be slowly injected through an additive port in the administration set or can be added to minibags usually containing either glucose 5% or sodium chloride 0.9% intravenous infusion. The contents of these secondary containers are infused using a Y administration set, three-way tap or non-return valve. This method may be used to give a higher intermittent blood level of a particular drug than would be achieved if the drug were added to the larger primary container, or to avoid an incompatibility with a drug which may already be present in the primary container.

Drugs commonly given by intravenous infusion include antibiotics, lidocaine (lignocaine), heparin and potassium chloride. Cytotoxic drugs are frequently given by intravenous infusion. The infusion maintains a steady blood level of the drug over a prolonged period of time and the patient is spared the pain of frequent injections. The addition of drugs to intravenous infusion fluids presents a number of hazards (e.g. resulting from interaction between the drug and the infusion fluid). Drugs should not be added to blood, plasma, lipid emulsions, saturated mannitol solutions, sodium bicarbonate solutions, amino acid solutions or dextran solutions because these infusion fluids are particularly likely to be degraded.

In addition to interactions, the fluid infused can be contaminated by microorganisms if admixtures are not carried out under strict aseptic conditions. Ideally, these additions should be made by pharmacy staff using laminar air flow cabinets in aseptic rooms and administered within 12–24 hours. Complications such as thrombophlebitis (a venous condition in which there is damage to the endothelium as the result of inflammation of the vein accompanied by formation of a blood clot) may arise at, and spread beyond, the site of cannula insertion. This results from physical or chemical irritation often related to the duration of the infusion or the type of fluid infused. Glucose is mildly acidic and, on autoclaving, a small quantity is broken down to hydroxymethylfurfural and these two factors appear to cause a higher incidence of thrombophlebitis when glucose infusions are given. Blood for transfusion should never be mixed with any drug or solution other than sodium chloride 0.9% because of the danger of interaction. If a unit of blood is preceded by a solution such as glucose, agglutination may result. To avoid this, the administration set should be flushed with sodium chloride 0.9% solution or changed.

The standard procedure for prescribing, checking and recording the administration of medicines similarly applies to intravenous infusions. It is important that an outline of the procedure is explained to patients in advance and that they are given the chance to have their toilet needs met. A change into a garment with wider sleeves may be required to ensure that the infusion flow is unobstructed. If possible, whichever arm/hand will make things easier for the patient should be used. The patient should be comfortable, with the site of introduction of the fluid exposed and well lit. Some pain is usually experienced with the insertion of a needle, and many patients appreciate having the support and encouragement of the nurse at this time.

The commonest sites of introduction are the forearm, the back of the hand and the antecubital fossa at the elbow. In an emergency, a vein in the foot or the external jugular vein may have to be used. A large straight vein, preferably at the junction of two veins and not running over a joint, is the one of choice.

The insertion of an intravenous cannula should be regarded as a minor surgical procedure. This, together with the fact that a cannula is to be lying in the vein for possibly several days, means that asepsis is an important objective. The prevention of microbial contamination begins with the appropriate handwashing technique. Careful preparation of the skin is important prior to insertion of the cannula. Although clipping extra-long hairs with scissors facilitates the subsequent removal of adhesive tape and is acceptable, shaving the skin is not recommended since it produces tiny abrasions which may become infected. Any visible dirt is washed from the area with soap and water.

Before completing the preparation of the skin, the venous outflow is blocked and the vein distended by applying pressure above the site. This may be achieved in one of three ways:

- the use of a tourniquet
- the use of a sphygmomanometer cuff inflated to 100 mm of mercury
- with the help of an assistant, making sure not to apply too great pressure as this may occlude the arterial supply.

The vein can also be made more prominent in different ways. For example:

- asking the patient to open and close the fist
- gently tapping the vein
- immersing the hand in hot water.

Increased venodilatation can also be achieved using glyceryl trinitrate applied in the form of a cream or transdermal patch (see p. 88) distal to the site of cannulation 20–30 minutes before venepuncture is performed.

Finally, the site is rubbed firmly for at least 30 seconds using a 70% alcohol swab and allowed to dry before puncturing the skin. Any further finger contact with the vein should be avoided.

Intravenous cannulae of different gauges are available. A small-gauge cannula (e.g. 19G) is sufficient for the delivery of most therapy and limits both the size of the wound and the incidence of intravascular complications. When viscous fluids are to be administered, a large-gauge cannula (e.g. 18G) is required. If a blood transfusion is likely to be required, the cannula introduced at the start of the infusion must be of large gauge (e.g. 16G).

The cannula is checked to ensure that it is patent and has no obvious defects. With the bevelled edge uppermost, the cannula is firmly entered under the skin a short distance away from the vein, always pointing the cannula proximally towards the heart. It is then gently pushed into the vein making sure to enter the plastic covering on the needle as well as the needle itself into the vein. Some types of cannula show a flash of blood at the hilt of the needle indicating that the needle, but not necessarily the plastic cannula, is in the vein. The tourniquet is then removed and simultaneously the needle withdrawn and the plastic cannula gently advanced into the vein. A well-sited cannula should introduce with little or no resistance. The tubing of the administration set is quickly attached. Gentle pressure on the vein proximal to the cannula tip prevents a leakage of blood through the cannula.

When a small vein is used, the tubing may be attached earlier so that the cannula advances, while at the same time infusing fluid through it, thus displacing the walls of the vein. The control clamp is released and the flow rate observed. Subcutaneous swelling around the cannula indicates that it is not in the vein and must be removed.

The cannula is secured using either a sterile gauze dressing or a semi-occlusive transparent dressing. The adjacent tubing is taped so as to prevent any pull on the cannula. A light conforming bandage promotes the patient's comfort. A splint may be applied and is essential if the cannula has been positioned over a joint.

On completion of the procedure the patient should be made comfortable with the arm supported on a pillow, if required. Personal requirements such as a drink, tissues, sickness basin, reading material, etc., should be placed within reach. The call bell should also be to hand and instruction in its use given.

A regimen of fluids to be infused is prescribed by the doctor. The rate of flow required (i.e. the number of drops per minute) can be calculated on the basis that for solutions using a standard administration set 1 mL equals 20 drops (15 drops per mL for blood or blood components using a blood administration set), that is:

$$\frac{\text{Volume of fluid (mL)} \times 20}{\text{Duration (min)}} \text{ drops/min.}$$

Thus, for 500 mL of fluid to be run through in 4 hours the number of drops per minute is:

$$\frac{500 \times 20}{240} = 41.66 \text{ rep.}$$

For working purposes, this figure may be regarded as 42.

Alternative methods of introducing an intravenous line are either by surgically cutting down on a vein and introducing the cannula under direct vision (e.g. when no veins are visible or patent) or by means of a central venous line (e.g. for prolonged feeding or for central venous pressure measurement). Both of these techniques are specialised procedures which are undertaken by experienced medical staff.

Throughout the ongoing administration of the infusion, the nurse's responsibilities are as follows.

Observing the patient

Each time the patient is attended by the nurse the patient's colour, respirations and general demeanour should be observed. An elevated temperature is noteworthy. Any apparent abnormality or change in the patient's condition should be reported to the nurse-in-charge or doctor.

Observing the infusion

A check is made that the infusion is running at the prescribed rate and that the container still has enough fluid in it. The nurse must anticipate the point when the container requires to be changed and estimate how much time will be required to get the next container checked and ready for use.

If the infusion is not running, a systematic list of checks should be made (Fig. 9.10).

When an infusion pump is in use, an alarm signals that the infusion is complete.

Observing the cannula site

The nurse must be alert to any:

- redness
- swelling
- leakage
- complaints from the patient of pain at or radiating from the cannula site.

Keeping accurate records

The following records must be maintained:

- fluid prescription sheet
- fluid balance sheet
- nursing care plan and progress notes.

Providing nursing care as required

Even the most able patient requires some assistance when one limb is not fully functional. Indeed, patients are to be discouraged from trying to be too independent as this can create movement of the cannula in the vein, especially one which crosses a joint, causing a mechanical phlebitis. Assistance with changing position, toileting, dressing, cutting up food, etc., will often be required.

Reporting abnormalities

Although the infusion is established by a doctor, the doctor depends on the nurse to notify him/her of any changes in the patient's condition, either of a localised or generalised nature, and any difficulties encountered with the infusion. To reduce the risk of infection it is normally recommended that administration sets be changed after 3 days (Band & Maki 1979, Josephson et al 1985, Maki & Ringer 1987). However, sets should be changed directly following blood transfusion and, in the case of parenteral nutrition, daily.

The hazards associated with intravenous infusion may be localised or systemic and are potentially very dangerous.

Local hazards are:

- thrombophlebitis
- infection
- extravasation.

Systemic hazards are:

- septicaemia
- cardiac embarrassment caused by too rapid rate
- allergic reaction to fluid or drug
- air or particle embolism.

Consequently, checking procedures, asepsis, careful observation and prompt reporting are vitally important.

The use of infusion systems

Infusion systems are used to deliver fluids (including emulsions), electrolytes and drugs in solution by the intravenous (and subcutaneous) route. They have become increasingly sophisticated and widely used over the past 20 years. This trend will continue in the years ahead. In common with other drug-delivery systems, infusion systems have all the key features outlined in Box 9.7.

The indications for the use of an infusion system include the need to maintain or restore blood volume, to deliver electrolytes and/or nutrients, and to administer drugs, especially those agents which are highly irritant and cannot be administered by other, more accessible routes. Infusion systems also provide the capability to control very accurately drug administration (e.g. cytotoxic therapy) over time, especially when a powered device is used.

Infusion systems relying on gravity

These infusion systems rely on gravity alone to provide the infusion pressure. It follows that the infusion

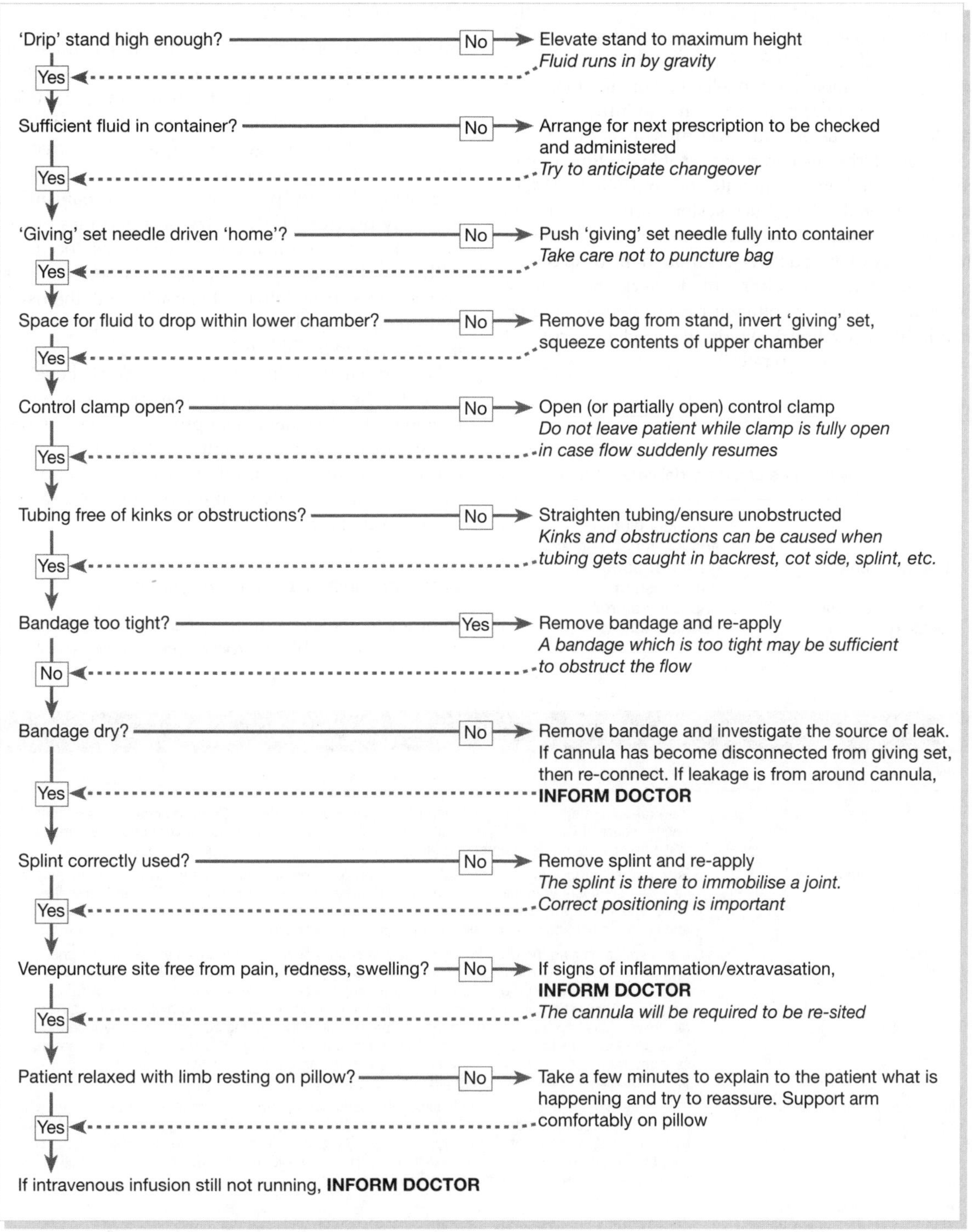

Figure 9.10 What to do when an intravenous infusion stops.

container must be placed at a suitable height above the infusion site. Drip-rate control is achieved by a simple mechanical clamp on the delivery tube. A drop sensor on the drip chamber monitors the rate of infusion. Such a device does not monitor resistance to infusion (leading to underinfusion) but overinfusion is effectively controlled. Drip-rate controllers enable the flow rate to be selected in drops per minute and controlled by identically powered valves. Such systems are acceptable in low-risk situations. A number of factors will influence the accuracy of drug delivery. Although the drop counting is accurate, the volume of delivery may not be (see p. 83). The use of volumetric controllers (calibrated in millilitres per hour) avoids the need to carry out calculations on the drip rate.

Box 9.7 Key features of a drug-delivery system

Structure	–	containers/tubing/administration set, etc.
Energy source	–	gravity or powered pump system
Control mechanism	–	drip-rate controller
Delivery port	–	needle/cannula

Powered infusion pumps

Infusion devices, such as infusion pumps and syringe drivers, are powered items of equipment which are capable of delivering fluids/drugs in a controlled manner in line with clinical requirements. Pumps have a number of advantages over gravity-powered systems. Notably, resistance to flow can be overcome by increasing delivery pressure. Safety mechanisms are normally provided if the entry port becomes blocked or displaced – normally referred to as 'occluded'. Although the use of powered pumps does enable safe and accurate drug delivery to be achieved, the risks of malfunction must be recognised. The range of devices is summarised in Table 9.4.

Unfortunately, although giving great benefit to patients, the use of infusion systems is not without problems. Poor management procedures, lack of training and inadequate documentation have in many cases contributed to significant patient morbidity and mortality. Table 9.5 gives an indication of the range of problems that can arise.

Safe management of infusion systems

In order to achieve safe use of infusion systems, it is necessary to establish procedures which ensure that

Table 9.4 Powered devices

Device	Notes
Drip-rate pumps	Flow rate set in *drops per minute*, peristaltic pump powers system. Such devices have few controls. The pressure of fluid in the line is not detected and occlusion detection is very poor. As a result, these pumps are not recommended for use at present
Volumetric pumps	Flow rate set in *millilitres per hour.* Various safety features are present, e.g. alarm to signal empty infusion container, air in line, occlusion, etc. These pumps are useful for medium and large flow rates, and for large-volume infusions. They can employ many different methods for accurate delivery, and nurses must know the details for the pumps they will use
Syringe pumps	A syringe containing the drug in solution is placed in a device which drives the plunger of the syringe at a predetermined rate. These devices are useful for low-volume/high-accuracy drug delivery. Syringes may be up to 60 mL. The volume is delivered in *mm/hour or mm/24 hours.* Heparin, cancer chemotherapy and analgesia are commonly administered by this method. As with all devices, it is important to set up the equipment correctly, e.g. the correct size of syringe must be used and located securely in order to ensure accurate delivery. Miniature syringe pumps accepting syringes from 2 to 10 mL which are battery operated can be used to achieve low rates of delivery, e.g. for insulin, and for ambulatory patients
Patient-controlled analgesia pumps (PCA)	These devices provide for patient initiation of doses of a pain-relieving drug. Controls are built in to prevent over-use by the patient. Pumps for ambulatory use are similar but lighter for ease of carrying by the patient. A variety of programming options are available; loading dose, continuous infusion with or without bolus can be achieved. It is important to avoid free-flow (siphonage) of solution, especially where patient supervision is minimal
Other devices, e.g.	
(a) pumps for the administration of anaesthetic agents (see Ch. 29)	These pumps are designed for the specific purpose of administering anaesthetic agents
(b) pumps using an elastomeric membrane	These disposable devices are 'powered' by an elastomeric membrane which contracts as a result of pressurisation caused by the filling process. They provide a simple method of administration especially suitable for home therapy

control is exercised at all stages from procurement of the equipment to use in patient care. A safe system will incorporate the following features:

- The structures and procedures established have the overall aim of reducing hazards to patients.
- Clear responsibilities for the choice of equipment and subsequent procurement are established, along with lines of accountability and responsibility. As few types of pump as possible should be used. They should be of the correct type and there should be adequate supplies of them. Extra sockets and cabling may have to be supplied. Operational manuals should always accompany items of equipment.
- A multidisciplinary committee is designated to oversee all aspects such as procurement, audit and monitoring, clinical/operational procedures and the effective communication of hazard warnings.
- Training needs are identified and met. Policy and procedure manuals should be readily available and kept up to date.
- Strong links are established with the local Drug and Therapeutics Committee and other medicine management arrangements within the health authority. Infusion devices are used within the community and so policies that recognise this dimension must also be established.

Technical support

Technical staff play a vital role in carrying out a regular maintenance programme on all infusion devices. 'Imported' pumps, for example any that have been donated, should be checked before use. The functioning of all equipment sent for repair should be checked before its return to the clinical area. Technical staff also play an important advisory role in the day-to-day use of such equipment.

Table 9.5 Examples of problems that can arise with infusion pumps

Type of error	Causes
Human error	Wrong rate/volume Failure to allow for priming volume Altered default settings Selection of inappropriate/wrong pump Incorrect loading (leading to occlusion or siphoning) Faulty pump in service Spillage of fluid (resulting in electric shock)
Equipment malfunction	Spontaneous failure Damage to equipment Flat battery Defect in set or bag Frequent alarms (staff start to ignore)
Other	Infiltration of tissues with fluid Patient or relative tampers with rate

Role of the nurse – infusion devices

All clinical staff involved in the management of patients with an infusion device have specific responsibilities but the responsibility for ongoing safety and comfort of the patient most definitely falls to the nurse. The potential for things to go wrong is very considerable and the nurse's responsibilities are numerous. Knowledge of the principles involved is vital and continuing evidence of clinical competence must be demonstrated. Attendance at in-service training sessions as well as personal updating are therefore imperative.

The responsibilities of the nurse looking after patients with infusion devices may be summarised as follows:

- being able to choose the most suitable pump by considering:
  - risk to the patient of:
    overinfusion
    underinfusion
    uneven flow
    high delivery pressure
    inadvertent bolus
    extravascular infusion
  - delivery parameters:
    infusion rate and volume required
    accuracy required (long and short term)
    alarms required
    ability to infuse into site chosen (venous, arterial, subcutaneous)
    suitability for infusing given drug (viscosity, half-life)
  - environmental features:
    ease of operation
    frequency of observation and adjustment
    type of patient (neonate, child, very sick)
    mobility of patient (battery operation needed?)
    (Medical Devices Agency 1995).
- using the administration set recommended by the pump manufacturer
- ensuring that all connections are tight but not overtight
- getting solutions, medications, rates and readings checked
- avoiding siphonage by positioning the device at the correct height
- keeping the alarm (where fitted) on and heeding it when it sounds

- ensuring that the medication is being administered
- checking the device every hour (in hospital) and on arrival at and departure from a home visit
- being observant at all times – of the patient, the infusion, the device and the documentation
- remembering there is a patient attached to the infusion who requires reassurance
- keeping lines free from obstruction and, where more than one are in use, taping the lines (at both the pump end and the cannula end)
- keeping all parts of the equipment clean (removing fluid from pump if spilled)
- handling equipment carefully so as to avoid damage
- reporting abnormalities/discrepancies in rate at once
- NEVER attempting to 'catch up' on the rate
- changing all components of the system every 24 hours
- recharging battery-operated devices by connecting to the mains supply
- labelling faulty equipment/reporting faults
- checking equipment on return from repair before next use
- instructing patients in the safe handling of portable equipment.

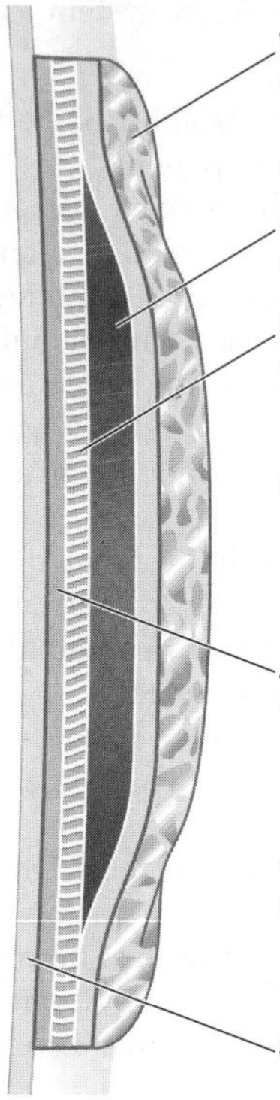

Waterproof backing foil
• enabling patients to shower, bathe or swim
• simple to apply
Drug reservoir
• containing glyceryl trinitrate
Rate limiting membrane
• consisting of a polymer film specifically permeable to glyceryl trinitrate
• prevents overdosage in patients with highly permeable skin and ensures that drug reservoir is not depleted in such patients
Adhesive layer
• comprising hypo-allergenic pressure-sensitive adhesive which ensures firm contact between the patch and the skin
• water resistant
• contains 8% of the drug to act as a priming dose thus ensuring rapid onset of action

Figure 9.11 Transdermal drug-delivery system (rate-controlling membrane type).

TRANSDERMAL ADMINISTRATION

Although most preparations are applied topically to give a local effect, the topical route can also be used to achieve a systemic effect. This is the transdermal route of administration. Drugs administered in this way avoid first-pass metabolism by the liver (see p. 118). The best known is glyceryl trinitrate used in the prophylaxis of angina. Where flexibility of dosage is required this may be achieved with the application of an ointment containing 2% glyceryl trinitrate. Magnitude and duration of effect are directly related to the amount of ointment applied. It is therefore possible by this method to titrate the dosage against the clinical presentation of the patient. To obtain the optimum dosage, 12 mm (0.5 inch) of ointment is applied on the first day, followed by 12 mm increments on each successive day until headache occurs; this length is then reduced by 12 mm. A graduated paper scale facilitates measurement of the dose. When applied to the skin the ointment is covered with a simple dressing. It is not rubbed in. This is a messy procedure and thus not commonly used.

A more sophisticated transdermal drug delivery system is the transdermal self-adhesive patch. Patches containing a reservoir of glyceryl trinitrate (see Fig. 9.11) are specially designed to achieve a prolonged and constant release of the drug. The main clinical indication for glyceryl trinitrate patches is in the prophylaxis of angina pectoris. The patches have also been used in the prophylactic treatment of phlebitis and extravasation, secondary to long-term venous cannulation.

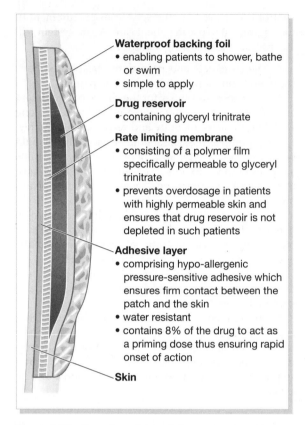

Patches are available from which the average amount absorbed in 24 hours is either 5 or 10 milligrams. One patch is applied every 24 hours to a hairless area to ensure that it sticks well. The anterior or lateral chest wall is recommended, although the upper arm or shoulder are other suitable sites. The site should have been washed and thoroughly dried, although not powdered, before applying the patch.

The sachet in which the patch is packaged should be torn rather than cut open otherwise the patch might be damaged. Without touching the sticky surface (which contains some medicament), the backing is removed and the patch applied – pressing firmly for about 5 seconds to ensure complete contact. The patch is then sealed to keep out air or water by running the finger round its edge. A different area should be used each day to avoid skin irritation. Patients who are to be self-administering a transdermal drug for the first time should be counselled in its use. Tolerance to glyceryl trinitrate can develop. There is evidence to suggest that this may be countered by intermittent therapy.

Several other drugs may be administered by this route. For example, a hyoscine patch to prevent motion sickness is placed behind the ear 5–6 hours before travelling and replaced after 72 hours, if necessary, by a patch behind the other ear; estradiol used in hormone replacement therapy is applied to unbroken areas below the waistline (not on or near the breasts or under waistband) and is replaced after 3–4 days. Nicotine transdermal patches are available for weaning addicted smokers off their nicotine dependence. Fentanyl patches are widely used in palliative care.

The transdermal route of administration offers many advantages to the patient and the nurse since it is non-invasive and convenient. However, the technology involved in developing and producing transdermal systems results in a relatively high-cost product. While the number of drugs that can be administered transdermally is gradually expanding there are many problems to be overcome before a clinically effective product can be introduced. Not least of these problems is the efficient barrier to systemic absorption provided by the skin itself.

REFERENCES

Auty B, 1989 Choice for instrumentation for controlled IV infusion. Intensive Therapy and Clinical Monitoring 10(4):117–122

Band J, Maki D 1979 Safety of changing intravenous delivery systems at longer than 24-hour intervals. Annals of Internal Medicine 90:173–178

Beyea S C, Nicoll L H 1996 Administering IM injections the right way. American Journal of Nursing 96(1):34–35

Brenner L R, Wood K M, George D 1981 Effects of alternative techniques of low-dose heparin administration on haematoma formation. Heart Lung 10(6):657–660

Channer K 1985 Stand up and take your medicine. Nursing Times 81(28):41–42

Clinical Resource and Audit Group (CRAG) 2002 Preparation of medicines for injection – good practice statements. Draft. CRAG, Edinburgh

Conaghan P 1993 Subcutaneous heparin injections – bruising. Surgical Nurse 6(2):25–27

Dann T C 1969 Routine skin preparation before injection: an unnecessary procedure. Lancet ii:96–97

Diggle L, Deeks J 2000 Effect of needle length on incidence of local reactions to routine immunisation in infants aged 4 months: randomised controlled trial. British Medical Journal 321(14 Oct):931–933

Josephson A, Gombert M E, Sierra M F et al 1985 The relationship between intravenous fluid contamination and the frequency of tubing replacement. Infection Control 6:367–370

Koivistov V A, Felig P 1978 Is skin preparation necessary before insulin injection? Lancet i:1072–1073

McGowan S, Wood A 1989/90 Administering heparin subcutaneously: an evaluation of techniques used and bruising at the injection site. Australian Journal of Advanced Nursing 72:30–39

Maki D G, Ringer M 1987 Evaluation of dressing regimens for prevention of infection with peripheral intravenous catheters. Journal of the American Medical Association 256(17):2396–2403

Medical Devices Agency 1995 Infusion systems. Device Bulletin MDA DB 9503. Department of Health, London

Shaw N J, Lyall E G H 1985 Hazards of glass ampoules. British Medical Journal 291:1390

Spraul M, Chateleau E, Kovmovlidov J et al 1988 Subcutaneous or nonsubcutaneous injection of insulin. Diabetes Care 11:733–736

Torrance C 1989 Intramuscular injection. Part 2. Surgical Nurse 2(6):24–27

FURTHER READING

Dougherty L 1992 Intravenous therapy. Surgical Nurse 5(2):10–13

Lawson T 2002 Guide to simple and safe local steroid injections. Prescriber 13:48–55

Mallett J, Dougherty L (eds) 2000 The Royal Marsden Hospital manual of clinical nursing procedures, 5th edn. Blackwell Science, Oxford

CHAPTER CONTENTS

10

Clinical governance and safety in the use of medicines

INTRODUCTION

Safety is a patient's right and the obligation of all health professionals (Barach & Moss 2001). Systems of healthcare provide a framework within which individual patient care is provided. The concept of clinical governance provides overall guidance to all healthcare staff on the need for high standards in all aspects of patient care. This should be seen as a background to this chapter.

CLINICAL GOVERNANCE/ QUALITY STRATEGY

Clinical governance is defined by Scally & Donaldson (1998) as 'a framework through which NHS organisations are accountable for continually improving the quality of their services and safeguarding high standards of care by creating an environment in which excellence in clinical care will flourish.' Health professionals have always worked within their own professional guidelines and relied on their employer to provide facilities, equipment and other resources to enable them to practise safely and effectively. No systematic methods of improving the quality of service were available until the concept of clinical audit was introduced to the NHS in the 1990s. Despite some success within the audit approach, it became clear that sustained progress in improving the quality of care could only be achieved by establishing a quality strategy and by a change in the culture of the NHS (see Box 10.1). Well-publicised failures in the NHS in the late 1990s have given added impetus to the need for change. Attitudes at all levels within the NHS have come under intense public scrutiny. Professional bodies and their members must now revalidate all aspects of the quality of care for which they are responsible. Effective leadership at all levels is essential so that the planning for quality services on the basis of the objective criteria can take place. Implicit in

Box 10.1 Quality strategy for NHS

Standards
- National Institute for Clinical Excellence (NICE) and Health Technology Board for Scotland (HTBS)
- National service frameworks

Local duty of quality
- Clinical governance
- Controls assurance

Assuring quality of individual practice
- NHS performance procedures
- Annual appraisal
- Revalidation

Scrutiny
- Commission for Health Improvement
- Education inspection visits

Learning mechanisms
- Adverse incident reporting
- Learning networks
- Continuing professional development

Patient empowerment
- Better information
- New patient advocacy service
- Rights of redress
- Patients' views sought
- Patients' involvement throughout NHS

Underpinning strategies
- Information and information technology
- Research and development
- Education and training

the need to improve the quality of patient care is the need to ensure that safe systems of work are in place throughout the particular organisation.

A report from the USA shows that 44 000–98 000 unnecessary deaths result each year from a range of preventable errors in hospitals in the USA (Weingart & Wilson 2000). A study from Australia produced even higher error rates. No comparable studies have been carried out in the UK, but it is reasonable to assume similar error rates. Unfavourable comparisons have been made between the safe systems used in the aviation industry and those used in the medical professions. Nolan (2000) places great emphasis on the need to design systems that can help prevent errors and to make them detectable. This aspect is further discussed on page 101.

Human error is often a contributory factor in drug errors, but inadequate systems of drug management may also be implicated. Reason (2000) outlines the distinguishing features of a 'high reliability' organisation. In such organisations, human error is expected and systems are put in place to enable the workforce to keep errors to a minimum, to recognise errors when they occur and to cope with the consequences of error. Built into this approach is the need to use each error as a learning experience and to change systems accordingly.

All the key elements are designed to interact with the overall aim of improving the quality of care within the NHS. Clinical governance at local level is supported by the national structures and mechanisms outlined in Box 10.1. Without the supporting framework at national level, clinical governance has only limited potential to improve the overall quality of patient care. Safe and effective systems of medicine management play a very significant role in patient care.

ERRORS IN THE MANAGEMENT OF MEDICINES

With the ever-increasing complexity of drug therapy and the need for many patients to receive multiple drug therapy, the potential for errors in the administration of medicines is great. Indeed, one of the highest risk areas of nursing practice is the administration of medicines (Scholz 1990). A busy, moderately sized hospital might need 5000–10 000 individual doses each day (Ferner 1995). A medical ward with 30 beds may have as many as 60 products in use at any one time and could keep in stock a range of 200 medicinal products, excluding lotions, sterile fluids, etc. Factors other than complexity of therapy also contribute to errors in the administration of medicines.

An error in the administration of medicines may be, at best, inconvenient for the patient or, at worst, catastrophic. In order to gain a balanced perspective it is necessary first to form a working definition of an error. This is best done by considering how, in practical terms, the overall objective of drug therapy (i.e. therapeutic benefit for the patient with minimal adverse effects) is most likely to be achieved. The assumption is made that the prescriber has taken all relevant factors into account before prescribing and that the choice of drug, dose, route, etc., is appropriate in every respect. To achieve therapeutic benefit for the patient it is obviously essential to ensure that *the right dose of the right drug is administered at the right time by the right route.* Adherence by all healthcare staff to recognised drug procedures is clearly a prerequisite at all times.

Adverse drug reactions and interactions (see Ch. 13) should be avoided if at all possible. However, if an adverse drug reaction is unavoidable, the effect on the patient should be minimised. It therefore follows that monitoring of the patient is essential. All adverse reactions to drugs should be reported to the prescriber.

A drug error can be defined as *any act of commission or omission that militates against the achievement of the*

Table 10.1 Issues linked with drug errors

Stage/source	Some issues
Manufacturer/distributor issues faulty product	Full and prompt recall of affected product Investigation/corrective measures Costs involved may be significant to supplier/NHS Loss of confidence by purchasers
Prescriber's error	May go undetected by pharmacy Error in administration may result Systems need to be reviewed Improved training for prescriber Professional relationships 'strained' Medical approach to drug errors may be less formal than in the other professions (unless serious consequences for the patient are involved) In errors resulting in a fatality, manslaughter charges may have to be faced
Pharmacist's error	Misinterpretation of prescriber's intentions Errors in compounding/dispensing Pharmacy system may need to be reviewed (including training issues) Professional disciplinary action may be taken against the pharmacist(s) involved
Nurse's error	Damage to professional relationships Loss of trust by patient/doctor The potential for damage to the nurse's confidence and professional future should not be underestimated. Every effort must be made to avoid loss of the nurse's self-esteem Clear distinction needs to be made between the failure of an individual or failure of the system
Patient's error	This aspect is discussed in detail in Chapter 11

therapeutic or diagnostic objectives, i.e. benefit for the patient. Such acts may relate to one or more of the practical aspects discussed above. It is obvious that it is not possible to comply to the letter with *all* aspects of medicine administration throughout *all* courses of drug therapy for *all* patients. Clearly, it is essential that, on every occasion, the correct dose of the correct drug is administered by the correct route. However, it must be recognised that it is often not possible to administer all medicines exactly at the time indicated on the prescription, owing to the time required to complete a medicine round. This is technically an error but will seldom be of clinical significance. There are occasions, however, when the timing of the administration of certain medicines is of vital importance to the patient such as, for example, with preoperative medication. Whatever the pressures, every effort must be made to eliminate errors by maintaining the highest possible standards of practice.

The definition given above is something of an oversimplification, since it does not reflect all the factors that may contribute to a drug error. Indeed, it is probably impossible to develop a definition which does include all the factors and issues that may contribute to or arise from a drug error. This is because drug administration is a multidisciplinary process that may well involve a chain of events (a 'cascade') from manufacturer, distributor, the prescriber, the pharmacist, hospital managers in all disciplines, the nurse and possibly the patient. Table 10.1 outlines some of the issues for health professionals (and others) who may become involved in a drug error or its consequences.

Sources of errors

A number of significant potential sources of drug errors are outlined in Table 10.2. It is hoped that by providing this overview, the complex and interactive nature of drug errors will be demonstrated. Seldom will a drug error arise because of the actions or inactions of one individual. A 'cascade effect' is often seen.

The prescriber

Full responsibility rests with the prescriber to state clearly and without ambiguity the medicines the patient is to be given. Well-designed prescribing documents undoubtedly contribute to more accurate drug therapy. However, adherence to the prescribing policy is essential if errors are to be avoided irrespective of the sophistication of the system used. Bad handwriting is probably the commonest potential source of error. Confusion between product names which look alike, especially when badly written, is a well-recognised source of error, e.g. co-codamol, co-codaprin, and other approved names with the co-prefix. Even when clearly written these words have a similar shape. Unofficial abbreviations for medicines are always open

Table 10.2 Potential sources of drug errors

Source of error	Prescriber	Pharmacist	Nurse	Patient/carer
Non-adherence to set procedures	✓	✓	✓	
Communications failures	✓	✓	✓	✓
Failure to comply with drug administration procedures	✓		✓	✓
Failure to review/cancel prescriptions	✓	✓	✓	
Transcription of information	✓	✓	✓	
Pressure on staff time, interruptions	✓	✓	✓	
Inadequate training on drug administration procedures	✓		✓	✓
Use of unofficial abbreviations, non-standard terminology	✓	✓	✓	
Inadequate policies and procedures. Poorly designed documents	✓	✓	✓	
Misinterpretation/lack of information on purposes of therapy	✓	✓	✓	✓
Calculation of doses	✓	✓	✓	
Failure to identify product correctly, mis-reading labels	✓	✓	✓	✓
Confusion with drug names; generic and proprietary products	✓	✓	✓	✓
Poor labelling/packaging		✓		
Lack of pharmaceutical services; failure to act on pharmaceutical information/advice	✓		✓	✓
Drug interactions	✓	✓	✓	
Known drug allergy	✓	✓	✓	
Chemical incompatibility – drug additives to parenteral fluids	✓	✓	✓	
Complex drug regimens – variable doses, non-standard intervals	✓	✓	✓	✓
Improper use of equipment, including infusion pumps	✓	✓	✓	✓
Lack of availability of drugs – borrowing	✓		✓	✓
Failure to identify patient correctly	✓	✓	✓	
Patient non-compliance				✓
Rejection of treatment				✓
Use of medicines brought into hospital by patient	✓	✓	✓	✓
Special dosage regimens at extremes of age	✓	✓	✓	✓
Clinical trials – inadequate information	✓		✓	
Involvement of a 'third party' – possible confusion of roles	✓	✓	✓	✓
Disincentives to report errors, leading to continued weakness in systems	✓	✓	✓	
Unauthorised manipulation of dosage form, e.g. crushing slow-release tablet	✓	✓	✓	✓

to misinterpretation and should not be used. Those who prescribe, dispense and administer medicines should never accept badly written instructions.

The omission of essential information (e.g. the strength of the drug) may result in assumptions being made about what is required. Where cancellation of a prescription lacks precision, the medicine may continue to be given to the possible detriment of the patient.

Electronic prescribing and dispensing systems have the potential to improve the overall quality of prescribing. Such systems are no substitute for effective training and teaching of all staff involved in the use of medicines.

Maxwell & Walley (2002) contrast the training programme available to nurse prescribers (see p. 46) with the minimal time currently available for teaching medical students the skills needed to use medicines safely. It is hoped that the General Medicine Council will provide clear directions to the UK medical schools about the need for the learning and assessment of the skills needed to use medicines safely, effectively and cost-effectively (Maxwell & Walley 2002). Although the optimum use of medicines can only be achieved by effective team working, the prescribing process is clearly fundamental. If this process is flawed, the patient is highly unlikely to gain benefit from the therapy.

The pharmacist

Errors in the administration of medicines may be due directly or indirectly to failures in the pharmaceutical service. As with clinical departments and wards, standards and procedures in pharmaceutical departments are designed to ensure that, as far as possible, errors are eliminated. Nevertheless, errors can and do occur which may be due to failures to meet standards and, on some occasions, to lack of effective communication with the prescriber or nurse in charge of a ward or department.

Errors or omissions in the labelling of medicines may cause difficulty, which may lead to an incorrect dose or even a wrong drug being administered. There has been much debate about colour coding of labels and containers, but there can be no substitute for *reading* the label at all times. Coloured rings on ampoule necks may help to identify a 'rogue' ampoule in a box or on a tray.

On occasion, medicines may be required when a full pharmaceutical service is not available. This could result in delay in administering a medicine, which may have serious consequences for the patient.

Regrettably, medicines may be supplied to wards with minimal background information as to the actions, uses or dosage of the product. Ward staff may then have to rely on their own limited information sources, especially if a comprehensive drug information service is not available. On fairly rare occasions a product or particular batch of a product may have to be withdrawn from use because of a fault or suspected fault. In such circumstances pharmaceutical staff must ensure the rapid communication of accurate information to wards and departments concerned.

When products are issued to wards for use in connection with a clinical trial it is very important that sufficient information be made available (without breaking any code) to the medical and nursing staff to enable the product to be used safely. The interest and cooperation of nurses are gained when the background to, and reasons for, a clinical trial are explained. It is also helpful if the results of the work are discussed with those participating.

The role of the pharmacist in drug therapy may be described as that of 'safety net and overseer'. Any failure to discharge this role has serious implications for the safety and well-being of the patient. The community pharmacist has legal liabilities for personal injury caused by medicinal products (Ferguson 1997).

The nurse

Nurses are responsible for the safe and accurate administration of medicines to most inpatients and to their patients in the community. In order to discharge this responsibility the nurse must interpret the prescription, select the correct medicine and make a record of the administration.

The administration of medicines is the culmination of research, development, manufacture, prescribing and dispensing. Although the skills and resources that have gone into producing a medicine are of great benefit to patients, the patient is now dependent on the nurse's skills. The responsibility to ensure safe and accurate administration of a medicine to a patient irrespective of the patient's circumstances should never be underestimated.

Identification of the patient

In a study of 79 drug errors, 12.7% were due to the medicine being given to the wrong patient (Gladstone 1995). The bracelet is, as yet, the best method developed for identifying patients. However, it is only as safe as those who apply it and refer to it. While every precaution may be taken to include accurately the information on the bracelet, and to attach the bracelet carefully to the right patient, problems can still arise. Sometimes a bracelet has to be removed – for example, when an intravenous infusion is being set up – and it may not be replaced. The patient, unwittingly, may remove the bracelet, or may do so while on weekend leave. The writing on the bracelet may become indistinct with the passage of time. Even when the bracelet remains satisfactorily in position, reference must be made to it. Of course, it was never intended that the bracelet should take the place of effective communication between nurse and patient, or that it would obviate the need for regular updating of staff on the patients under their care.

There can be no doubt about the need for identification bracelets to be used in paediatric units, intensive care units, theatres and in all acute areas where patients are unable to identify themselves. Areas that may pose particular difficulty are care of the elderly units and psychiatric wards. Patients in these wards may understandably have feelings of resentment at being 'labelled'. In addition, staff may feel that this procedure militates against their efforts to reduce any feelings patients may have of being institutionalised and that they know their patients anyway.

Regularly updated passport-size photographs (attached to the prescription sheet) are often used as a more sympathetic aid to patient identification. In any event, health authorities must devise workable policies which are in patients' best interests.

Errors in calculations

There is now increasing recognition of the major difficulties young people in the UK from differing backgrounds are having with simple arithmetic (Reid 1996,

Clare 1997). With less emphasis placed on the subject in schools and the widespread use of calculators, this is a real cause for concern in nursing. Particular problems relate to the use of quantities less than one milligram. Efforts to convert 0.125 mg into micrograms have resulted in gross overdosage of digoxin in paediatric practice. It has been suggested that there might be a place for calculators in assisting those who have such difficulty. If the individual's lack of numeracy is so severe as to call for this level of assistance, there must be grave doubts as to whether a calculator could be used safely. Indeed, the improper use of such equipment may be another source of error. Calculators have a place but should probably be used only to make a final check.

Use of inadequate equipment/unorthodox use of medicines

Measures for liquid medicines with indistinct markings cannot safely be used. This is especially important in paediatric practice where potent liquid medicines are often used. Oral syringes must be used.

Using medicines in an unorthodox way may also lead to errors. Some tablets are designed to be broken if a fractional dose is required. Other tablets are not so designed; an attempt to break or divide such a product will almost certainly result in the administration of an incorrect dose. Similarly, the crushing of a modified-release tablet will destroy the essential properties of the formulation, any benefit to the patient being lost. Errors may arise because of the attempted use of an unsuitable presentation such as a very large capsule or tablet which a patient may be unable to swallow.

Error reduction/avoidance

Given that drug errors often arise as a result of a series of failures by the health professionals involved, it follows that programmes designed to improve matters must have the active support of prescriber, pharmacist, nurse and hospital managers. The assumption should not be made that actions by members of one profession acting alone will be all that is required to eliminate or reduce errors. Recognition of the need to improve the safety of healthcare is now apparent at the highest levels of government, both in the UK and USA. The National Patient Safety Agency has been set up in the UK and the Agency for Health Care Research and Quality in the USA has received additional funding to promote research on the safety of patients (Barach & Moss 2001). Healthcare leaders have embraced patient safety but it is only within the teams delivering patient care that real advances in patient safety can be made.

The nurse manager

The nurse who is in overall charge (nurse manager/ward sister/charge nurse) is accountable for the maintenance of standards of medicine administration in the ward.

Insisting on accurate prescribing practice is one of the most demanding aspects of the role. It will be to the benefit of both the nurse manager and the patients to make it known that failure to meet the standard is unacceptable.

It is important to ensure that up-to-date relevant information on drugs is readily available at ward level. All wards and departments should have an up-to-date copy of the British National Formulary and local formularies. Clear lines of communication must be established with clinical pharmacists and medicine information services.

Whenever possible, the nurse-in-charge should avoid delegating the administration of medicines to nurses who are unfamiliar with the identity of patients in the ward. Examples include nurses who have recently been appointed to the ward, have just returned from a period of absence or have been sent to assist on a temporary basis from an agency or from another ward. It is important also to assign appropriate members of staff to the administration of medicines. It is irresponsible to ask nurses to participate in the administration of medicines unless they have been taught the theoretical aspects of it. Although in other aspects of care the role of nursing auxiliaries/assistants has developed in recent years, their involvement in relation to the administration of medicines remains as before, i.e. to see that the patient has a drink with which to take the drug, to help the patient into a suitably comfortable position to take the drug and to report to the person conducting the drug round if for any reason the patient fails to take the drug.

Although care assistants in residential homes may be involved in issuing medicines from previously prepared medicine distribution systems, the responsibility for interpreting the prescription and dispensing the medicines totally rests with the community pharmacist.

In some nursing homes, in the absence of a second registered nurse, it may be necessary for a care assistant to check Controlled Drug stock, but a care assistant is not permitted to participate in the administration of the drug.

Efforts should be made to discourage discussion with patients' visitors or visiting members of staff during procedures involving the administration of medicines. It may be useful to display a notice on the medicine trolley – 'DO NOT DISTURB' – with the intention of minimising interruptions during administration of medicines.

In the event of duplications in patients' names in a ward, staff and the patients concerned must be alerted. The nurse in charge must also ensure that identification bracelets/photographs are renewed and replaced as necessary.

Great emphasis is rightly placed on the need for the accurate administration of medicines, but it is also essential to ensure that medicines are discontinued when a course of treatment is complete. Where an instruction to discontinue therapy has been given, and where it is clear that the medicine does not constitute replacement or other long-term therapy, the continuing need for the medicine should be questioned. Prime responsibility for discontinuation of treatment must rest with the prescriber.

All staff are required to keep accurate and legible records (NMC 2002), which includes those used in drug administration. Prescribers should be asked to re-write prescription sheets when they become untidy or when the use of two prescription sheets concurrently could be obviated. 'Kardex' or similar holders for prescribing and recording documents should be kept in good repair and the order of sheets should be re-arranged to correspond with the movement of patients within the ward. Nursing staff must adopt a safe and efficient system of storing all medicines and withdraw medicines which are no longer required. Advice from pharmacy staff on appropriate levels of ordering, expiry dates, etc., and on any other aspects of stock management is readily available. In situations where drug regimens remain unchanged for long periods of time every effort must be made to prevent complacency.

Teaching the administration of medicines should relate to the procedure only and not to the pharmacological aspects. It is safer when administering medicines to concentrate fully on the procedure and to leave the discussion of uses, actions, side-effects, etc., for a more appropriate time. Since teaching and learning are demanding of time and effort and not without risk for both the clinical supervisor and the person being supervised, it is advisable to limit the experience to a few patients, preferably ones with whose care the learner is already involved.

The administration of medicines should be kept high on the list of priorities in a ward. The nursing staff's awareness of medicines in use in their ward may be increased by referring to patients' prescription sheets in conjunction with the giving of a verbal report on the patients, for example, at the changeover of staff. If time permits, a separate reporting session specifically about the medicines in use and any related difficulties that the patient or nurse may be having with them can be valuable to the nurse-in-charge as well as to more junior nursing staff.

Consideration should also be given to the timing and number of medicine rounds required. Standardised systems of prescribing and administration should allow room for flexibility to meet the needs of individual patients. For example, special account may need to be taken of the timing of administration to patients suffering neurological conditions such as Parkinson's disease. Such flexibility, of course, must reflect the need for effective drug therapy.

Clinical pharmacy services (see p. 23) should be fully utilised. Any special needs of the ward will become apparent to the clinical pharmacist but there is no substitute for active cooperation with the pharmacist. A climate of passive acceptance of any service is not conducive to achieving the highest standard of care for patients.

The senior nurse manager

The continuing need to promote safe practice and in so doing reduce drug errors is the responsibility of those involved in policy making, management and education as well as those in clinical practice.

Nurse managers spend time allocating staff to meet service commitments. Along with the many other demands which they try to meet, greater consideration should be given to staff levels needed at the main medicine round times or when pre- and postoperative medications are to be given.

The extent to which two nurses should be involved in the administration of medicines continues to exercise the minds of nurse managers and nurses in clinical practice.

Practitioners whose names are on the Nursing and Midwifery Council register (including midwives) are considered competent to administer medicines on their own, and are responsible for their actions in so doing. The involvement of a second person in the administration of medicines with a registered practitioner needs to occur where that practitioner is instructing a student nurse. The patient's condition or other circumstances as locally determined may also make it necessary to involve a second person. Where two persons are involved, responsibility still attaches to the senior person.

Community nurses have, of course, always administered medicines single-handed. Currently, however, it is common for hospital policies to require that two nurses be involved in the administration of medicines, one of whom is a registered nurse. The possible advantages

Box 10.2 The advantages and disadvantages of involving two nurses in the administration of medicines in hospital

Advantages
- Presence of second nurse provides an additional check which should improve patient safety by reducing drug errors.
- Presence of second nurse helpful if calculations of drug dosage are required.
- Patient feels reassured that a second person is involved in checking the medicine.
- Provides important learning situation for procedures of medicine administration.
- Impact of interruptions can be minimised since the medicine round can probably be continued by one nurse.
- Some patients understandably wish to ask questions about their medicines during rounds. This may be difficult for one nurse to cope with, although even if two nurses are present some complex questions may have to be noted for answering later.
- Improved security of medicines during medicine rounds.
- Any emergency arising during the medicine round can be dealt with more promptly.

Disadvantages
- Blurring of responsibility leading to confusion and perhaps error.
- Student nurse may be reluctant to 'challenge' a trained nurse, assuming that the trained nurse is always right.
- May provide false sense of safety in medicine administration.
- Medicine round may take longer because of double checking.
- Dilution of professional responsibility.
- In some situations, e.g. night duty, staffing levels make it impracticable for two nurses to be routinely involved in medicine administration, leading to delay.

and disadvantages of this approach are summarised in Box 10.2. It should be noted that there is little evidence in the literature to confirm or otherwise the views expressed – which is not surprising since a valid comparative study would be very difficult to undertake with so many variables to influence the outcome.

Clearly, the advantages and disadvantages outlined in Box 10.2 do not carry equal weight, but will serve as a frame of reference when local policies are being formulated. As with other aspects of nursing care, the procedure to be adopted will always be chosen with the best interests of the patient in mind.

The need for two nurses to be involved in the administration of medicines to children is a generally agreed principle.

Equipment and siting of fixtures used in the management of medicines, such as drug trolleys, medicine cupboards and refrigerators, should be chosen with care so that the particular needs of the ward are satisfied. Nurse managers should always be prepared to take time to consult with practising clinical colleagues as to their requirements. Guidance from the pharmacist should also be sought. Policy makers must ensure that the systems of medicine management, including prescribing and recording documents, reach the required standard, are of suitable design and are relevant to the drug therapy used in all wards. With increased opportunities for healthcare professionals to design and produce documents within their own clinical area, the required standard may not always be reached. Mechanisms are needed to ensure that there is an effective means of updating the design of or introducing new prescription sheets and associated documents in such a way that the needs of all practitioners are fully met.

Continuing education on the subject is essential for all trained nursing staff along with updating of nurses returning to work after some years' absence. Attendance at regular in-service lectures and seminars on medicine administration should be given a very high priority.

There is also considerable scope for operational research into many aspects of medicine management. Nurse managers have a duty to encourage their staff in this direction.

Nurse managers must ensure that procedures applicable in the event of errors in medicine administration are not seen as threatening by nurses or a deterrent to the reporting of errors.

Apart from actions taken by individuals or within a particular profession, it is essential to ensure that an active multidisciplinary Drug and Therapeutics Committee keeps under review all aspects of medicine management and issues guidance when necessary. The establishment of a post of medication safety officer should be considered.

The patient

Whenever possible, the active cooperation of the patient is essential in order to achieve the therapeutic benefit of a course of drug treatment. Nurses and their medical colleagues should never take the patient's cooperation for granted or expect this to be given automatically. The patient's right to question or even reject treatment must be respected. However, nurses must play their part in ensuring that, if a patient does decide to reject a particular treatment, this decision is reached on the basis of a full understanding of the implications for the patient's health and well-being. It would obviously be unfair to attribute the patient's action or lack of action as a source of drug errors, but in some situations the patient will bear some responsibility if the treatment fails. The not uncommon occurrence of finding tablets in the patient's bed or under the cushions of a chair may or may not indicate failure on the part of the patient. This may be the first indication the nurse has that all is not well. Needless to say, great tact and perception may be needed to establish the true cause of this rejection. The role of the patient in the management of medicines is further discussed in Chapter 11.

Care must be taken when using medicines brought into hospital by patients on admission. Such medicines dispensed for individual patients may have been inappropriately stored in the patient's home. Labels may have been altered or removed, causing difficulty in identifying the contents of a container. It may be appropriate to use patients' own medicines when they are in hospital (see Ch. 3), but the responsibility for doing so should not be undertaken lightly. All available means, including clinical pharmacy services, must be used to validate the patient's own medicines before using them in hospital. This may involve seeking information from patients and/or their carers. As patient packs are now the norm, the use of patients' own medicines during hospitalisation is often a worthwhile option.

Aspects of the role of the patient in safe and effective use of medicines is discussed further in Chapter 11.

Error reduction/avoidance checklist

Patient (see also Ch. 11)

- Pay particular attention to identification of the patient.
- Take extra care at extremes of age. With individual exceptions, the risks to infants and the very old are greater – partly because of the effects of the drugs but also because these patients may be unable to speak for themselves.
- Be especially careful when patients are mobile and where large groups of patients are sitting about at random, e.g. in day rooms.
- Whenever possible, increase involvement of patients in their own drug therapy.

Prescription

- Consider benefits of electronic prescribing systems.
- Use correct documentation and report any inadequacies in the documentation design/layout.
- Develop/update documentation in line with changes in practice.
- Follow the policy and do not accept inadequate, unclear instructions.
- Avoid prospective prescribing whenever possible. If this is necessary, ensure directions are clear.
- Avoid use of unofficial abbreviations and chemical symbols/nomenclature.
- Take particular care with similar-looking drug names.
- Complex calculations should be checked by a second person.
- Be alert to sudden changes in dosage.
- If it appears that a dose has to be made up of several tablets/ampoules, check carefully that all is in order.
- Pay particular attention to doses expressed in micrograms or units.
- Pay particular attention to doses of drugs that alter key physiological parameters, e.g. insulin injections.
- When two nurses are involved in the administration of medicines, read out the details of the prescription and the label so that each is aware of the other's interpretation of them. Also, when administering a medicine for which a calculation has to be made, make the calculations independently before making comparison.
- Ask/check/ask again if not satisfied. While wishing to trust colleagues, do not passively take the word of a senior member of staff as necessarily correct.
- Report at once any suspicions you may have that all is not in order regarding the prescription.

Medicine

- Ensure correct storage of medicines, e.g. do not mix different ampoules in the same container.
- Do not alter any labels on containers of medicines and other pharmaceutical products.
- Do not remove drugs from containers unless for administration to the patient.
- Any medicine removed from its container and not used should be disposed of safely.
- Report any apparent abnormalities to the supplier or senior colleague, e.g. changes in size, shape, colour of a product.
- Use the correct dosage form, e.g. request a supply of 5 mg tablets rather than try to divide a 20 mg tablet.
- Where there is no intravenous reconstitution service available and this task has to be undertaken by nursing staff, ensure correct volume of correct diluent is used. (This applies equally to the reconstitution of liquid oral dosage forms.) If in

any doubt, always ask advice from the pharmacy department.
- Drugs intended for intrathecal use must be supplied in a presentation that ensures correct administration.
- Use the correct equipment, e.g. measures, syringes.
- Ensure that mechanical equipment is maintained/serviced on a programmed basis.
- Be aware of drug interactions, e.g. drug–drug; drug–food.
- Be aware of any drug that could interfere with laboratory tests.
- Avoid drug incompatibility, e.g. when adding drugs to intravenous fluids. Use pharmacy-based services whenever possible.

All staff

- Be observant. Here is the distinction between seeing and observing. The ability to take in an overview of a chart or the contents of the medicine trolley/cupboard as well as the details of one prescription or one product has to be developed.
- When a telephoned order for medicines is unavoidable write the message down and repeat it to the caller.
- Ensure adequate flow of information to other clinical departments. Diagnostic tests may be influenced by patients' current or previous drug therapy.
- Report/discuss/seek views of colleagues, especially if the safety of the patient is involved, e.g. unexplained side-effects of a drug.
- When two nurses are involved in administering medicines, the more experienced nurse should check the decisions, calculations and actions of the less experienced nurse.
- Whenever possible, reduce the ward medicine inventory by encouraging the adoption of a ward formulary or prescribing policy.
- Read the literature and keep up to date; ask for more information if it is not provided.
- Make full use of pharmacy services, especially ward/clinical pharmacy service and drug information services.
- Encourage the development of a questioning, enquiring attitude at all levels.

Ward managers

- Encourage by all practical means adherence to drug policy.
- Integrate verbal report on current ward drug therapy with nursing report.
- Provide suitable drug information source at ward level, e.g. BNF, Data Sheet Compendium.
- Eliminate borrowing of medicines between wards and departments.
- Reduce interruptions during the administration of medicines.
- Ensure equipment available for medicine administration is suitable in all respects.
- Improve procedures for checking medicines prior to administration.

Senior managers

- Encourage the development of ward prescribing policies, reduction of ward medicine inventory.
- Make careful choice of new equipment. Establish regular in-service education for nurses on all aspects of drug therapy.
- Develop clinical pharmacy services.
- Improve nurse staffing levels.
- Ensure nurses have the necessary skills and knowledge relating to the use of medicines.
- Establish educational programmes for junior hospital doctors on procedural aspects of ward medicine management including prescribing.
- Promote research/clinical audit into all aspects of medicine use.
- Examine and, if necessary, improve procedures for dealing with errors in the administration of medicines.

However accurate and detailed the prescribing, however efficient the pharmaceutical service, however effective the nursing management, there can be no substitute for the greatest care and attention to detail when a medicine is being administered. Understandably, the nurse who undertakes the final act feels in a very vulnerable position. This is because the administration of a medicine is so 'visible' and so final. The medicine has actually been taken by the patient or injected into the patient's tissues. At this stage any second thoughts are not capable of being translated into action (other than reporting the error or suspected error). Unlike written prescriptions, doses actually given cannot be changed. This situation should be recognised by all those who prescribe and dispense medicines and by those who draw up policy and procedure documents.

In designing safe systems for the management of drugs it is important to assess the levels of risk involved. It is quite unacceptable to accept different standards but it must be recognised that the risks involved in administering complex parenteral chemotherapy are greater than the oral administration of a simple analgesic.

Table 10.3 Risk management (IV administration of chemotherapy as an example)

Phase	Questions	Answers
1. Identification of risk	What could go wrong? How could it happen? What would be the effect?	Incorrect dose/route/complex regimes Inadequate information/documentation Failure of treatment, adverse drug reaction
2. Analysis of risk	How often is it likely to happen? Cost if it does happen? How severe if it does happen?	Confining use of chemotherapy to specialist unit helps in this matter Potentially very high Outcome potentially catastrophic for patient
3. Control of risk	How can risks be eliminated? How can risks be avoided?	Reduce complexity. Provide drugs in patient-specific presentations. Improve staff training
	How can they be made less likely? How can they be made less costly?	Use of protocols. Use best available technology. Use automated processes. Manage change effectively

Managing risk has three main components: the identification of risk; the analysis of the risks involved; and most importantly the control of risk. Table 10.3 outlines how these principles could be applied to medicine administration. By applying risk management techniques it is possible to analyse drug errors in a systematic way. Following such an approach provides the basis for the establishment of safe systems of working.

Prevention of errors

Unfortunately, errors in the administration of medicines can never be completely eliminated (Ferner 1995). In recognition of the risks involved in the administration of medicines, a preventive approach has been used in an effort to help nurses avoid making errors (Downie et al 1997). The use of up-to-date documents outlining the requirements and responsibilities at national, health authority and trust levels is essential. Access to written texts, which include the safe and effective use of medicines as well as their pharmacological properties, should be created. The use of an open learning programme on calculating medicine dosages has allowed students to learn in private and at their own pace (Mackenzie, unpublished work, 1996). Links between healthcare professionals and between service and education personnel help to ensure that records used in relation to the management of medicines and the content of policies and procedures are constantly reviewed.

Dealing with medication errors/incidents

In the past, drug errors were universally viewed in the same way by senior nursing staff and disciplinary action was often taken against offenders for their mistakes. The belief was that this was necessary to protect the patient. Such action is thought to do the exact opposite (Goodall 1993). Indeed, the fear of being disciplined may actually do the patient harm if the nurse is too frightened to ask for help (Arndt 1994). Punitive measures may also lead to under-reporting of drug errors (Cooper 1995). Over the years, there has been a gradual move towards a more positive approach. It is now considered important to make the distinction between human error caused by, for example, pressure of work and negligence or reckless practice (NMC 2002). Every effort must be made to develop an open culture where errors and near misses can be openly discussed and lessons learned. If considered appropriate, an anonymous reporting system may be established, but a system that guarantees confidentiality may be preferred. There is also the view that training should be provided for those involved in an error and support given to restore self-confidence (Williams 1996). One approach being used with student nurses who have been involved in a medication error/incident is based on the application of clinical risk management. The steps of risk management include identification, analysis and control of the risks involved (DoH 1993) (Table 10.3). Consideration of any financial implications (and this may be taken to include social costs) is also included. The teaching of subjects such as the management of medicines is, in effect, directed at managing the risks attached to the procedures involved. In the event of an error taking place, the steps of risk management are revisited but this time in relation to the specific incident. Risk management is thus used in a cyclical way to help identify knowledge deficits or misunderstandings on the part of the student as well as those areas which would benefit from greater emphasis or clarification in future teaching. Both student and teacher thus stand to benefit. Whichever way drug errors are investigated, it is vitally important to have a structured approach to the investigation process. An excellent approach has been described which should ensure that lessons from an incident can be learned, especially about the organisational factors involved (Vincent et al 2000).

Facing up to drug errors, or any other errors in delivering healthcare, is not easy for either health professionals involved in direct patient care or for those in managerial roles. It is encouraging to see the development of a much more frank and open approach to medical errors as a whole. In the USA a report from the Institute of Medicine (1999) has received widespread attention from the media and even at presidential level. Comprehensive action is being taken in the USA which must surely act as a model for healthcare leaders in the UK. There are encouraging signs that the problem of drug errors in particular is being addressed in the UK. Leape & Berwick (2000) provide us with encouragement in this challenging area of professional activity. 'When given the opportunity to help, when the barriers of shame and punishment are removed, doctors, nurses, pharmacists and others eagerly work to improve safety, implementing best practices or developing new ones.'

Patient safety must be approached by all the professions involved on a joint basis. Lessons can be learned from other industries (Helmreich 2000), but above all, we must learn from our patients and avoid the long-established 'the doctor/nurse/pharmacist knows best' cliché.

REFERENCES

Arndt M 1994 Nurses' medication errors. Journal of Advanced Nursing 19:519–526

Barach P, Moss F 2001 Delivering safe healthcare. British Medical Journal 323:585–586

Clare J 1997 Survey shows Britons simply can't add up. The Daily Telegraph, January 17

Cooper M C 1995 Can a zero defects philosophy be applied to drug errors? Journal of Advanced Nursing 21:487–491

Department of Health (DoH) 1993 Risk management in the NHS. DoH, London

Downie G, Mackenzie J, Williams A 1997 Help nurses avoid drug errors. Pharmacy in Practice (November): 539–543

Ferguson P R 1997 The legal liability of the community pharmacy for personal injury caused by medicinal products: liability for negligence. Pharmaceutical Journal 258:133–135

Ferner R E 1995 Is there a cure for drug errors? Editorial. British Medical Journal 311:463–464

Gladstone J 1995 Drug administration errors: a study into the factors underlying the occurrence and reporting of drug errors in a district general hospital. Journal of Advanced Nursing 22:628–637

Goodall C 1993 Crimes (and misdemeanours). Nursing Standard 7(20):46–47

Helmreich R L 2000 On error management: lessons from aviation. British Medical Journal 320:781–784

Institute of Medicine 1999 To err is human: building a safety health system. National Academy Press, Washington DC

Leape L L, Berwick D M 2000 Safe healthcare: are we up to it? British Medical Journal 320:725–726

Maxwell S, Walley T 2002 Using drugs safely. British Medical Journal 324:930–931

Nolan T W 2000 System changes to improve patient safety. British Medical Journal 320:771–773

Nursing and Midwifery Council (NMC) 2002 Guidelines for records and record keeping. NMC, London

Reason J 2000 Human error: models and management. British Medical Journal 320:768–770

Reid T 1996 Official: young British workers cannot count. The Sunday Telegraph, September 29

Scally G, Donaldson L J (1998) Clinical governance and the drive for quality improvement in the new NHS in England. British Medical Journal 317:61–65

Scholz D A 1990 Establishing and monitoring an endemic medication error rate. Journal of Nursing Quality Assurance 4(2):71–85

Vincent C, Taylor-Adams S et al 2000 How to investigate and analyse clinical incidents. Clinical Risk Unit and Association of Litigation and Risk Management protocol. British Medical Journal 320:777–781

Weingart S N, Wilson R M 2000 Epidemiology of medical error. British Medical Journal 320:774–777

Williams A 1996 How to avoid mistakes in medicine administration. Nursing Times 92(13):40–41

FURTHER READING

Adcock H 2001 Learning from medication errors. Pharmaceutical Journal 267:287–289

Audit Commission 2001 A spoonful of sugar. Medicines management in NHS hospitals. Audit Commission, London

Buisson J 2001 Number plates for medicines – a new way of reducing medication errors. Pharmaceutical Journal 267:286

Editorial 2001 Compulsory guidelines aim to stop intrathecal chemotherapy disasters. Pharmaceutical Journal 267:707

Fradgley S, Pryce A 2002 An investigation into the clinical risks in the use of patients' own drugs on surgical wards. Pharmaceutical Journal 268:63–67

Halligan A, Donaldson L 2001 Implementing clinical governance: turning vision into reality. British Medical Journal 322:1413–1416

Hughes C M 2000 Drug formularies: a basic bibliography. Prescriber 11:16–117
Kendall M J 2002 Therapeutics needs to be better taught. British Medical Journal 324:792
Kravitz R L, Melnikow J 2001 Engaging patients in medical decision making. British Medical Journal 323:584–585
Moscrop A 2001 Expert patients will help to manage chronic disease. British Medical Journal 323:653
NHS Executive 1999 Controls assurances standards for medicines management. DoH, London
Nursing and Midwifery Council (NMC) 2002 Guidelines for the administration of medicines. NMC, London
Runciman B, Merry A 2001 Improving patients' safety by gathering information. British Medical Journal 323:298
Scott H 2002 Increasing numbers of patients are being given wrong drugs. Editorial. British Journal of Nursing 11(1):4
Various authors 2001 Medical errors. British Medical Journal 322:1421–1425
Various authors 2000 Theme editions. British Medical Journal 320(7237)

USEFUL WEB SITE

Drug errors: www.medicine-errors.org.uk

CHAPTER CONTENTS

11

The role of patients and carers in medicines management

INTRODUCTION

The Bristol inquiry which examined many failures on the part of cardiac surgeons and others, made numerous recommendations regarding the importance of health professionals treating all patients as partners by regarding them as 'equals with different expertise' (Coulter 2002). Key recommendations in the report of the inquiry are given in Box 11.1.

Although these recommendations were made following major failures in the provision of paediatric cardiac surgery services, the principles involved can be used to encourage greater responsiveness to the needs of patients by all those involved in the provision of drug therapy. Healthcare professionals carry out many functions that help to ensure a good outcome of a patient's drug therapy. However, without the active participation of the patient (and parents or carers) optimal results of the treatment may not be achieved. The recommendations in Box 11.1 provide the necessary broad guidance for health professionals which, if followed, will help to ensure the achievement of an effective partnership with patients' concordance. Involving patients more in decision-making has many benefits, not least in

Box 11.1 Bristol inquiry report recommendations (Bristol Royal Infirmary Inquiry 2001)

- Involve patients (or their parents) in decisions
- Keep patients (or their parents) informed
- Improve communications with patients (or their parents)
- Provide patients (or their parents) with counselling and support
- Gain informed consent for all procedures and processes
- Elicit feedback from patients (or their parents) and listen to their views
- Be open and candid when adverse events occur

improving patient safety. Prescribing errors could be reduced by actively involving patients in their own care (Coulter 2002). It is recognised that to achieve this, resource implications will have to be met and cultural and technical barriers overcome (Coulter 2002). Electronic access by patients to a range of relevant information may be the way forward (Coulter 2002). Patients may also become involved in the training of those involved in the provision of healthcare. The concept of the 'expert patient' is being developed. Selected patients suffering from a chronic disease are given short training programmes in anatomy, physiology and the disease process. Drawing on this training and, above all their own experiences, patients are then able to provide inputs on a range of matters into the training of medical students, doctors and other healthcare professionals.

The key recommendations of the Bristol inquiry and the implications of these should be kept in mind when reading this chapter.

COMPLIANCE OF THE PATIENT

An essential component for the successful outcome of any treatment plan, drug or otherwise, is the patient's compliance with the prescriber's advice and directions. The compliance of a patient can be defined as the 'extent to which the patient's behaviour coincides with medical or health advice' (Sackett 1976). The term 'patient compliance' is often considered to be unsatisfactory, since it has overtones of coercion or compulsion and does not include any reference to treatment outcome. Alternative, less-threatening terms that have been proposed include 'therapeutic alliance' and 'treatment adherence' (Blackwell 1976). More recently the term 'concordance' has been introduced but this has not yet come into wide use (Royal Pharmaceutical Society of Great Britain 1997). For the purposes of this discussion the term 'patient compliance' will be used because it is capable of definition and it can be measured. At no time will the term be used here with any implications of coercion of the patient.

Nurses in both community and hospital practice are well placed to help patients comply with the medical advice and instructions they are given regarding drug treatment. Often, the nurse is the only health professional who has continuing contact with the patient over long periods. As a result, the nurse is able to gain an understanding of the patient's difficulties, offer advice and monitor compliance.

NON-COMPLIANCE OF THE PATIENT

Some indication of the extent of non-compliance can be obtained when surveys are undertaken on the vast quantities of drugs returned to pharmacies by patients and unwanted prescribed medicines collected during 'medicine amnesty' campaigns. (This may also be a sign of poor management of repeat prescriptions.)

Many studies have been published which demonstrate in detail the extent of non-compliance with directions regarding drug treatment. In long-term therapy, compliance is often inadequate. Patients taking antiepileptics achieved a 76% compliance level which fell to 39% when the dosage schedule was changed from 8-hourly to 6-hourly (Cramer 1989). With short-term therapy the position may generally be better. Studies by Donabedian & Rosenfeld (1984) and Mushlin (1972) showed that up to 75% of patients complied with their directions. Few studies relate the extent of non-compliance to the failure to achieve the desired therapeutic outcome. Nevertheless, non-compliance should always be considered as a possible reason for the failure of treatment.

Measurement of non-compliance

Many difficulties are presented when measuring or assessing patient compliance. The methods available vary from the basic tablet count to the use of electronic monitoring devices (Punchak et al 1992), and the measurement of the drug (or metabolite) in body fluids. The methods available are listed under two headings: first, methods that are normally available to the nurse, and second, those methods which require considerable technical back-up and are applicable only in structured investigations into patient compliance.

Methods of compliance assessment available to the nurse

- General impressions of the patient's understanding of the drug regimen.
- Tablet counts at suitable intervals.
- Physiological markers, e.g. pulse rate in digoxin therapy.
- Visible presence of drug or metabolites in urine or faeces, e.g. rifampicin produces a reddish discoloration of the urine.

Methods of compliance determination

- Chemical methods of determination of metabolites in body fluids.
- Measurement in body fluids of pharmacologically inert chemical markers added to the medicine.
- Medication monitors that record the withdrawal and time of withdrawal of a dose from the container.

- The presence of some drugs detected by chemical analysis of the patient's hair.
- Electronic devices incorporated into containers which record the date and times the containers were opened or used (eye drop bottles).

Significance of non-compliance

Does it matter that some patients fail to take their medicines as prescribed? There can be no simple answer to this question. Failure to comply may delay a patient's restoration to full health (failure to complete a course of antibiotic therapy), or may be life-threatening (inappropriate use of a corticosteroid by an asthmatic patient). Failure to take anti-rejection therapy following renal transplantation can be catastrophic, both for the patient and the service. Failure to take HIV therapy can mean the difference between life and death. Non-compliance with therapy for diabetes could have very serious consequences for the patient. The extent of non-compliance must also be taken into account since it may well be that for a particular regimen an 80% compliance level by the patient may be adequate to achieve the desired therapeutic outcome. No general rules can be established. The whole situation must be assessed, since, in many cases, the patient's condition will vary – and thus the patient's need for medication will also change. Intelligent non-compliance has been described by Weintraub (1976) as occurring when patients either reduce the dose or stop taking a medicine altogether. The reasons for this behaviour may, when examined, be quite rational, such as the adjustment of a drug dose in response to the occurrence of side-effects.

Factors in non-compliance

Many factors have been identified as contributing to patient non-compliance. Haynes (1979) cites more than 200 factors, ranging from doctor–patient relationships to the colour and taste of the prescribed medicine. The factors involved can be classified into three main groups:

- personal factors
- social factors
- factors directly related to the medicines.

Rarely, if ever, will non-compliance be due to a single factor. Often it will be attributable to a number of interacting factors. Table 11.1 lists the factors which contribute to non-compliance.

Occupational therapists have an important role to play in advising on the use of the various aids available. While the provision of an aid to compliance will help many patients, equally, the mere provision of an aid without more supportive action is unlikely to achieve anything.

The practical problems discussed above, although often contributing to non-compliance according to the strict definitions given, may also jeopardise the safe management of medicines by the patient, e.g. child-resistant closures, once removed, may be left off, with consequent loss of security. Many patients find more unfamiliar presentations, such as suppositories and pressurised aerosols, difficult to use properly.

The patient's response

Many highly motivated patients, their carers, health personnel and social workers develop their own DIY compliance aids. A number of approaches have been reported (Williams 1979). The most common is probably the setting out of individual doses, in advance, in household containers such as egg cups, ice trays, egg boxes and the like. Sellotape has been used to stick tablets and capsules to suitable fixtures in the kitchen or living room to act as a reminder that the dose is due. To help the patient select the right medicine, labels on containers are often supplemented by lay terms such as 'water tablets', 'sleeping tablets', 'heart tablets', etc. Instructions on labels may also be modified, additional labels being added often using large print or symbols to reinforce the dosage instructions. The timing of a television programme may be used by some patients as a signal that a dose is due. A variety of charts, calendars, etc., have also been used to assist the memory.

It would appear that many of these ingenious aids are of assistance to some patients and such self-help should not normally be discouraged. Equally, however, there can be no doubt that in some situations the 'home-made' devices will be a further source of problems which may not always be recognised by the patient. By transferring tablets from the original well-closed container, product security and stability will often be lost. For example, if glyceryl trinitrate tablets are not stored in a well-sealed glass container the volatile active ingredient will be lost. Some products (e.g. omeprazole capsules) absorb moisture from the atmosphere and should always be stored in the original packaging.

Nurses, pharmacists and doctors can learn from patients' coping strategies since these may highlight inadequacies in the service provided. Expert patients in particular (see p. 109) can provide health professionals with valuable insights on many aspects of drug therapy.

Table 11.1 Factors contributing to non-compliance

Factor	Comment
Personal factors	
Patient's belief as to value of therapy	
Ethnic aspects	May conflict with mainstream western medicine
Relationship with health personnel involved	Patient's faith in prescriber, especially, often influences outcome
Ageing process	Loss of recent memory, physical disability, etc. may contribute to non-compliance
Some psychiatric illnesses	Schizophrenia, for example, may bring particular problems
Pressures of a busy life	Especially hard to comply when several daily dosage intervals are involved
Poor understanding of regimen	
Limited knowledge of condition	
Social factors	
Isolation	May arise from a breakdown in the family structure
Deprivation	Some patients have to contend with a difficult journey to the surgery or pharmacy. Older people often have to contend with multiple deprivation, and are more vulnerable when things do go wrong with their medicine-taking
Poverty	Patients who cannot afford prescription charges will probably need help and guidance not only with use of medicines but with the Social Security system also
Factors directly related to medicines	
Tablets	Large tablets may be difficult to swallow; very small tablets may be difficult for a patient with stiff fingers to pick up
Liquid medicines	Liquid medicines may have an unpleasant taste, colour or 'feel' in the mouth. Many liquid medicines that are used by older patients are formulated for children. Highly coloured, sweet, sickly flavours are generally not very acceptable to older patients, even if children find them acceptable, which often they do not. Measuring liquid medicines will be difficult for many patients, as will shaking a 500-mL glass bottle of liquid medicine which may weigh almost 1 kg
Topical preparations	Stiff ointments may be difficult to use or there may be difficulty squeezing creams or ointments out of a tube. Products that stain the patient's linen, shower or bath may prove unacceptable
Packaging	Child-resistant closures are difficult for many people, although the use of these has reduced accidental poisoning of children significantly
Labelling	Labelling systems have been improved with the introduction of machine-printed labels for all dispensed medicines, but the small print on some labels may be impossible for some patients to read
Prophylactic medicines	Medicines prescribed for prophylaxis may not always be taken as prescribed because the patient does not feel the benefit directly
Unpleasant side-effects	Unpleasant side-effects, such as headache, nausea, etc., may, undoubtedly, be a cause of non-compliance

METHODS FOR IMPROVING PATIENT COMPLIANCE

Before embarking on a course of action designed to improve patient compliance, two main questions must be borne in mind. First, does the patient really need drug therapy or is some other form of therapy more appropriate? Second, will improved compliance assist in the achievement of the therapeutic objective(s)? For instance, it may well be that improved compliance will result in an unacceptable level of side-effects. It is also vital to determine the real causes of non-compliance and to ensure that any strategies decided upon are within the patient's capabilities, otherwise further problems will be created for the patient.

The available methods can be considered as follows:

- involving the patient in decision-making and if possible, the prescribing process (see p. 6)
- improving presentation (labelling and packaging) of dispensed medicines (see Table 11.2)
- providing aids to compliance (see Table 11.2)
- providing patient education and counselling (including the provision of patient information leaflets, in the form of package inserts and/or other suitable specially designed material)
- encouraging pre-discharge self-administration of medicines
- using financial incentives.

Table 11.2 Methods for improving patient compliance

Presentation of dispensed medicines	
Appropriate containers and closures	Plastic, lightweight bottles with a cleft for ease of handling by an arthritic patient may be useful. Containers used for tablets should generally be at least the 32 mL size for ease of handling. Plastic containers are generally preferred by patients
	Screw caps that can be easily removed have obvious advantages (Le Gallez et al 1984) for some patients, although there is great need to ensure that containers fitted with such closures are stored out of the reach of children
Improved labelling	A wide variety of labelling systems are available, each of which is designed to provide the information required for the patient in a clear unambiguous way
	Ideally the label of a dispensed medicine should bear the following information:
	Full instructions about the drug and its required frequency Approved name of product and strength Name and address of dispensing pharmacist Date of dispensing Quantity dispensed Expiry date of product Lay term (e.g. water tablets) Warning – keep out of reach of children Any special storage instructions Any special precautions in use For external use only and/or other appropriate warnings
	Illustrations Large print Braille
	The needs of patients whose command of English is minimal will require attention. Labels written in their mother tongue will be required. The needs of the illiterate must be recognised and dealt with in a sympathetic way. Pictorial labels have been developed and these may prove useful in some situations
Aids to compliance	
Aids in the management of solid dosage forms	The 'Dosett' tray has certain special features, notably the Braille markings and a detailed labelling facility on the reverse. Other compartmentalised trays of the 'Wiegand' type are useful since each compartment can be labelled with the contents and any special instructions. The 'Pill Minder' has some degree of 'child resistance' unlike the other trays described above. Other products available include the 'Medidos' system which has the advantage of being highly portable since each daily tray can be carried separately
	Combination products (e.g. diuretic with potassium) may prove useful, since the number of tablets to be taken daily is reduced. Compliance packs (calendar packs) are also made available for some products (e.g. oral contraceptives)
Aids in the management of liquid dosage forms	Measuring liquid medicines with the standard medicine spoon may prove difficult for many patients. Several alternative measuring devices are available
	Blind patients may find a special measuring device helpful
Other aids in the management of medicines	A long-handled ointment applicator has been developed for patients with physical disabilities
	A device (Opticare) to aid the instillation of eye drops is available which helps the patient to aim the drop and squeeze the eye drop bottle (Fig. 26.4, p. 421)
	Other devices for eye drop instillation include Easidrop for aiming and Autodrop for aiming and squeezing

In some situations a combination of strategies may be required, the patient being given a suitable aid and counselled as to the importance of therapy. While there is no sure way to identify the potential defaulter, it is essential to make every effort to identify the high-risk patient.

Education and counselling

Patient groups are becoming increasingly active on a range of issues relating to drug therapy. Availability of treatments and the need for more information about prescribed medicines are key issues. Along with their professional colleagues, nurses can play a key role in ensuring that patients have sufficient knowledge to enable them to manage their prescribed medicines safely and effectively and thus achieve therapeutic benefit. Herxheimer (1976) has outlined the knowledge needed by patients, or by those responsible for their day-to-day care, in terms of questions to the prescriber – see Box 11.2.

In certain situations, such as when providing palliative care, it may not be appropriate to give the patient

Box 11.2 Herxheimer's questions to the prescriber

What for and how?
- What kind of tablets are they and in what way do you expect them to help?
- How should I take them? How many and how often?
- Will I be able to tell whether they are working?
- How do I keep them?

How important?
- How important is it for me to take these tablets?
- What is likely to happen if I do not take them?

Any side-effects?
- Do the tablets have any other effects that I should look out for?
- Do they ever cause any trouble?
- Is it alright to drive when I am taking them?
- Are they alright with other medicines I may need?
- Will alcohol interfere with them?
- What should be done if someone takes too many?

How long for?
- How long will I need to continue with these tablets?
- What should be done with any left over?
- When will I need to see you again?
- What will you want to know at the time?

all the information listed in Box 11.2, but the list of questions does give much useful guidance to nurses, pharmacists and prescribers.

Patient information leaflets

Patient information leaflets are available which are used to supplement and reinforce the counselling of patients (see Box 11.3). These range from general information on a particular condition and associated drug therapy to information packages designed to meet the needs of an individual patient. A study by George et al (1983) found that patients who received a leaflet were more likely to be completely satisfied with the treatment and with the information they had been given. It is vitally important that the information given to patients by different health workers is complementary and does not give rise to confusion.

Education packages

Nurses working in the community can play a wider educational role by presenting talks to organised groups in the community on aspects of the safe use of medicines. The topics covered by the talks would naturally be selected in line with the interests and needs of the group. In some situations, however, a structured presentation in the form of a tape–slide or video package may be appropriate. As an example of this approach,

Box 11.3 Examples of areas explained in a patient information leaflet

- Name of medicine
- What is in your medicine
- What your medicine is for
- What to consider before taking your medicine (e.g. other conditions you may suffer from, allergy)
- How to take your medicine
- What to do if you take too many tablets
- What to do if you miss a tablet
- Undesirable effects you may experience
- How to look after your medicine (including storage)

audio-visual packages have been developed for groups interested in the care of older people (Graves Organisation 1984, 1989). An outline of the content is as follows:

- demographic aspects
- extent of use of medicines by older people
- physiology of the ageing process
- factors that cause older people to have difficulty managing their medicines
- practical help in medicine management available to older people.

SELF-ADMINISTRATION OF MEDICINES

A valuable opportunity to improve patient compliance may be presented during a period of inpatient care by instituting a programme of self-administration of medicines. Such methods of medicine administration have been used over the years with particular emphasis on the needs of patients in wards providing rehabilitation, care for older people and care for patients with a mental illness. It is recognised that self-administration systems can be used to advantage in acute wards (Bird 1988). The advantages claimed for systems of self-administration include improved patient compliance on discharge from hospital arising from better understanding of the medication(s) and more appropriate timing of medicine administration than can be achieved by the traditional 'medicine round'. Nurses and other professional colleagues may be anxious about the risks that self-administration of medicines may cause, particularly as regards the safety and security of medicines in the ward environment. However, the adoption of a well-structured system will eliminate risk to a very large extent. Well managed self-administration systems are essential to ensure both patient safety and the achievement of the desired therapeutic outcome. Self-administration systems may be useful when patients use their own

Box 11.4 Essential components of a system for the self-administration of medicines

- A system which has been fully documented and agreed by all responsible authorities.
- Full patient information made available and the patient's consent obtained.
- A detailed protocol which includes:
  - assessment of the patient
  - stages of the process once it has been confirmed that the patient is suitable for self-medication and wishes to undertake this detailed documentation including the prescription sheet, a record of self-administration, a record of checks made on the patient's compliance, and any other records of action taken to assist the patient
  - clear guidelines on the role of the healthcare professionals involved, especially nurses and clinical pharmacists.

prescribed medicines during their hospital stay (see p. 24). The essential components of a system for self-administration of medicines are outlined in Box 11.4.

A number of methods of medicine management have been used to facilitate self-administration of medicines. In limited circumstances, patients can be given a small supply of certain medicines to keep in their bedside cabinet, or patients can be encouraged to ask for their medicines from the medicine trolley or treatment room cupboard. A system that gives the patient full involvement and control is based on using a small lockable medicine cabinet attached to the bedside locker. Access to the medicines is given according to the patient's abilities and needs. Patients who have been shown to be capable of managing their medicines well and whose needs are quite specific may be given the key to the medicine cabinet for the period of their inpatient treatment. In other situations, the key may only be made available to the patient at specific times/intervals.

Opportunities to assess and improve patient compliance are presented at all stages of the self-administration process. The stages are summarised in Box 11.5 together with a brief discussion of patient compliance issues.

If at any stage difficulties are identified it may be necessary to review the arrangements, which could include discontinuation of the plan or reverting to an earlier stage of the process. This should seldom prove to be necessary if the assessment and checks are made with due care and sensitivity. Patient self-administration of medicines is playing an increasing role in helping patients to achieve good compliance and resulting benefits from their medication.

Box 11.5 Stages in self-administration of medicines

Stage 1: Patient assessed
Patient's knowledge of the medication can be assessed and a general idea of degree of compliance can be established. At this stage any special needs patient may have can be identified, e.g. need for compliance aid.

Stage 2: Patient given access to bedside medicine cabinet under nurse's supervision
Process of assessment can be continued, frequency and nature of any checks on patient's compliance can be determined on a multidisciplinary basis. Value of any aid to compliance can be evaluated.

Stage 3: Patient given key to medicine cabinet and allowed to self-administer with only limited supervision/checks
Further information/education on patient's medicines can be given at this stage as patient's confidence develops.

Stage 4: Patient allowed to self-administer with reduced level of checks (say, weekly) on compliance
During this stage patient can be prepared for discharge and any remaining problems resolved.

CLINICAL EFFECTIVENESS, CLINICAL AUDIT AND CLINICAL GOVERNANCE

(see Ch. 10)

Apart from the need to ensure safe drug therapy it is essential to achieve the best possible outcome for the patient. While there can be no substitute for expert professional judgement and relevant experience, guidance to clinicians is increasingly being made available in the form of clinical guidelines. Clinical guidelines must include standards and outcomes. The Scottish Royal Colleges and other agencies in the UK, working with specialist groups and clinicians with special interests using clinical audit techniques, have developed agreed guidelines which providers of healthcare are encouraged to use. Guidance from NICE and the HTBS is increasingly relevant. In many instances it may be necessary to change the way in which services are provided as a result of considering available evidence and information. Changes made to services must be monitored and assessed to show that the changes introduced have resulted in improvements to patient care. The techniques of clinical audit are used as a means of reviewing clinical practices. Clinical audit is defined as 'a clinically-led initiative which seeks to improve the quality and outcome of patient care through structured peer review whereby clinicians examine their practices and results against agreed explicit standards and modify their practice where indicated' (NHS Executive, 1996 as cited by National Centre for Clinical Audit 1997). The National Centre for Clinical Audit (NCCA) has been established to promote all aspects of clinical audit. In particular, the NCCA seeks to facilitate best practice in healthcare by promoting multidisciplinary clinical audit. Treatment with drugs is capable of structured examination by clinical audit techniques. Examples where clinical audit has been used to evaluate drug therapy include information for elderly patients being discharged on warfarin therapy (Kane et al 1995) and influencing temazepam capsule and buprenorphine prescribing in general practice (Long et al 1995). The achievement of safe and effective drug treatment will continue to challenge health professionals in the years ahead. It seems certain that clinical audit will be a key tool capable of application in many different situations and often with minimal resources, other than the commitment of those involved.

Financial incentives

In a review of the literature, Giuffrida & Torgerson (1997) found that, in 10 out of 11 studies reviewed, patient compliance was improved with the use of financial incentives. The incentives included cash, vouchers, lottery tickets or gifts. The studies examined were carried out in the USA, and it is not clear whether similar beneficial results could be achieved in other countries. Since patient non-compliance generates additional costs, it may be that provision of financial incentives would be cost-effective in certain situations. Further research is required in different environments, but it would be essential to ensure that any aspect chosen for study was capable of effective monitoring of patient compliance. In the present climate within healthcare in the UK it does not seem likely that a financial approach to improving patient compliance will be followed.

THE ROLE OF SOCIAL WORK HOME CARERS IN THE ADMINISTRATION OF MEDICINES

The emphasis on care in the community has resulted in home carers becoming involved in aspects of the administration of medicines on behalf of their clients. The level to which the home carer becomes involved will be a matter for local social services departments to determine. In any event, most home carers will from time to time be required to provide their clients with assistance with their medicines. This assistance could range from helping with the taking of medicines to the disposal of unwanted medicines.

Box 11.6 Contents of training programme for home carers

- Introduction
- Learning objectives
- Roles and responsibilities
- Taking the medicine – what happens next?
- Risk factors associated with medicines
- Types of medication (formulations)
- Ordering, collection, storage and disposal of medicines
- Dispensing labels – how to take the medicine
- Additional administration instructions – what do they mean?
- Ambiguous labels – or none at all
- Adverse effects of medication
- OTC medicines – what can be bought in a shop?
- Documentation:
  - medicines chart
  - recording sheet
  - medicines disposal form
- Medicine administration practice
- Professional help and advice
- Case scenarios
- Good practice points

In order that the role can be discharged safely and effectively, locally recognised training programmes will be beneficial. An outline of what might be included in such a training programme is indicated in Box 11.6.

The training programme defines levels of responsibility in accordance with the needs of clients. Some clients will take full responsibility for their prescribed (and other) medicines. Other clients may need minimal assistance, e.g. ordering, collection and disposal of medicines. In some situations, more assistance will be required, for example the carer may administer an oral dose or may assist in the use of topical preparations. In all situations, the level of input by the home carer will be clearly defined by supervisors and other social work or health professionals (e.g. community nurse). The home carer may need to be aware of any medicines the client may purchase.

Home carers can play a vital role in helping to ensure that their clients gain the full benefit of their medication and can also alert colleagues to any developing problem.

MEDICINES IN SCHOOLS

A significant number of children attending mainstream schools need to take medication during the school day. It is vitally important to ensure that the necessary medication is made available in such a way that the pupil's education is not disrupted. Cooperation between parents/guardians and school authorities is required to ensure this. Cooperation between NHS and education authorities is also essential to ensure systems are put in place to facilitate the safe management of medicines in schools. The overall aim of any system must be to ensure that pupils with medical needs are able to benefit fully from their education. Key elements of a safe system of medicine management for mainstream schools are outlined below. (In special schools it will be necessary to make arrangements that reflect the particular needs of the pupils. However, the following key elements will also apply.)

1. Set up an individual care plan or incorporate this in a pupil's other written plan, e.g. personal learning plan.
2. Ensure cooperation of staff and meet any training needs. (Legal position of staff and school may need clarification.)
3. Involve parents/guardians in the provision of information on the pupil's medical condition and supply of the necessary medicines.
4. Involve NHS and school health service in such matters as local protocols/procedures and the training needs of staff involved in medicine administration.
5. Establish good working relationships with local general practitioners, nurses, pharmacists and other healthcare professionals.
6. Work within guidance of the local education authority.
7. Set up and document care policy/procedures. Such procedures should be applied flexibly, with sensitivity and must preserve confidentiality.
8. Put in place procedures for dealing with mild and severe allergic reactions, and other special situations, e.g. asthma. Ensure arrangements for calling emergency services are well known to all staff.
9. Establish procedures for the administration of medicines including the recording of the administration of all medicines. (Consent of the pupil or parent/guardian must be secured.) The principles of medicine administration are those that apply to the administration of a medicine by a health professional (see Ch. 7). However, the information available within the school may not be as comprehensive as the information available to a health professional.
10. Ensure arrangements for medicines management are in place for out-of-school activities.
11. Ensure safe storage of all medicines at all times. Stocks held should be limited to essential needs only. Disposal of unwanted medicines must be in accordance with local guidance. Inhalers must be readily available on the basis of need.
12. Observe basic hygiene procedures, e.g. in the use of topical preparations and inhalers.
13. Strike the right balance between making medicines available to pupils who need them and the safety of all pupils.
14. Prescribed medicines help many people to live a normal life. The whole aim of medicine management procedures in schools must be to ensure that pupils derive benefit from their medicines, which in turn will enable them to benefit fully from all their educational opportunities.

REFERENCES

Bird C A 1988 Taking their own medicine. Nursing Times 84(45):28–32

Blackwell B 1976 Treatment adherence. British Journal of Psychiatry 129:513–531

Bristol Royal Infirmary Inquiry 2001 Learning from Bristol: the report of the public inquiry into children's heart surgery at the Bristol Royal Infirmary 1984–1995. The Stationery Office, London

Coulter A 2002 After Bristol: putting patients at the centre. British Medical Journal 324:648–651

Cramer J A 1989 How often is medication taken as prescribed? A novel assessment technique. Journal of the American Medical Association 261:3273–3277

Donabedian A, Rosenfeld L S 1984 Follow-up study of chronically ill patients discharged from hospital. Journal of Chronic Disorders 14:847–862

George C F, Nicholas J A, Waters W E 1983 Prescription information leaflets: a pilot study in general practices. British Medical Journal 287:1193–1196

Giuffrida A, Torgerson D J 1997 Should we pay the patient?: review of financial incentives to enhance patient compliance. British Medical Journal 315:703–707

Graves Organisation 1984 Older people and their medicines. Tape–slide presentation

Graves Organisation 1989 Medicines and older people. Videotape presentation

Haynes R B 1979 Factors contributing to patient non-compliance. In: Haynes R B, Taylor D W, Sackett D L (eds) Compliance in health care. Johns Hopkins University Press, Baltimore, pp 1–7

Herxheimer A 1976 Sharing the responsibility for treatment. Lancet ii:1294

Kane J, Hamilton S J C, McDonald J 1995 An audit of information provision regarding patients discharged on warfarin therapy from a hospital geriatric department. Clinical Resource and Audit Group. The Scottish Office, Edinburgh

Le Gallez P, Bird H A, Wright V et al 1984 Comparison of 12 different containers for dispensing anti-inflammatory drugs. British Medical Journal 288:699–701

Long K, Thorburn A W, Kidd K 1995 Influencing temazepam capsule and buprenorphine prescribing in general practice. Clinical Resource and Audit Group. The Scottish Office, Edinburgh

Mushlin A I 1972 A study of physicians' ability to predict patient compliance. Master's thesis. Johns Hopkins University, Baltimore

National Centre for Clinical Audit (NCCA) 1997 Information for better healthcare. NCCA Publications, London

Punchak S S, Goodyer L I, Miskelly F G 1992 Recent developments in electronic monitoring aids in assessing compliance with medication. Hospital Pharmacy Practice 2(3):167–169

Royal Pharmaceutical Society of Great Britain 1997 From compliance to concordance. Royal Pharmaceutical Society, London

Sackett D L 1976 Introduction. In: Sackett D L, Haynes R B (eds) Compliance with therapeutic regimens. Johns Hopkins University Press, Baltimore, p 1

Weintraub M 1976 Intelligent and capricious non-compliance. In: Lasagna A (ed) Compliance. Futura, Mt Kisco, New York, p 39

Williams A 1979 The role of the pharmacist in improving compliance in the elderly patient. Proceedings of the Guild of Hospital Pharmacists 6:1–22

FURTHER READING

Aronson J K, Hardman M 1992 Patient compliance. British Medical Journal 305:1009–1011

Bird C A 1990 Patient self-medication. Surgical Nurse 3(1):22–26

Bloom B S 2001 Daily regimen and compliance with treatment. British Medical Journal 323:647

Cameron C 1996 Patient compliance: recognition of factors involved and suggestions for promoting compliance with therapeutic regimens. Journal of Advanced Nursing 24:244–250

Chief Administrative Pharmaceutical Officers' Group (Scotland) 1992 Medicine self-administration guidelines.

Davis S 1991 Self-administration of medicines. Nursing Standard 5(15/16):29–31

Ferguson T 2002 From patients to end users: quality of online patient networks needs more attention than quality of online health information. British Medical Journal 324:555–556

Grills A 1997 An assessment of the pharmaceutical needs of the blind and partially sighted in Dumfries and Galloway. Pharmaceutical Journal 259:381–384

Holloway A 1996 Patient knowledge and information concerning medication on discharge from hospital. Journal of Advanced Nursing 24:1169–1174

Ley P 1981 Professional non-compliance: a neglected problem. British Journal of Clinical Psychology 20:151–154

Ley P 1988 Communicating with patients. Improving communication, satisfaction and compliance. Psychology and medicine series. Croom Helm, London

Nyatanga B 1997 Psychological theories of patient non-compliance. Professional Nurse 12:331–334

Pharmacy Community Care Liaison Group 1997 Medicines in schools. Implementing good practice in mainstream schools – a guide for pharmacists. Pharmaceutical Journal 258:69–71

Presentation to Parliament by the Secretaries of State for Health, Social Security, Wales and Scotland by Command of Her Majesty 1989 Caring for people: community care in the next decade and beyond. Cmnd 849. HMSO, London

Raynor D K T, Britten N 2001 Medicine information leaflets fail concordance test. British Medical Journal 322:1541

Runciman B, Merry A 2001 Improving patients' safety by gathering information. British Medical Journal 323:298

Scottish Executive 2001 The administration of medicines in schools. Scottish Executive, Edinburgh

Skene L, Smallwood R 2002 Informed consent: lessons from Australia. British Medical Journal 324:39–41

Stockwell Morris L, Schulz R M 1992 Patient compliance – an overview. Journal of Clinical Pharmacology and Therapeutics 17:283–295

USEFUL WEB SITE

The expert patient – a new approach to chronic disease management for the 21st century: www.doh.gov.uk/whatsnew

SECTION 2

General principles of pharmacology

SECTION CONTENTS

CHAPTER CONTENTS

12

Pharmacokinetics and pharmacodynamics

PHARMACOKINETICS

Patients rely on nursing staff and pharmacists to ensure that medicines are administered appropriately. It is essential that nurses have a sound understanding of what happens to a drug following administration. Pharmacokinetics is the term used to describe how the body handles a drug over a period of time, including how the body absorbs, distributes, metabolises and excretes the drug (Fig. 12.1). These processes influence the effectiveness of the drug because, in order for a drug to be effective, it must be available at the site of action in the correct concentration. In the simplest terms pharmacokinetics can be described as what the body does to the drug, as opposed to pharmacodynamics which is what drugs do to the body.

ABSORPTION

Except for the intravenous route, a drug must be absorbed across cell membranes before it enters the systemic circulation. The oral route is the one most commonly used for drug administration. Most drugs are absorbed by diffusion through the wall of the intestine into the bloodstream which is aided by the very large surface of the gut wall (see Fig. 15.1). The rate of absorption also depends on the lipid-solubility of the drug. Drugs are normally formulated to make them as lipid-soluble as possible to enable them to cross the cell membranes of the intestinal wall. However, sometimes a drug's low lipid-solubility is used to good effect since it reaches the colon largely unabsorbed, e.g. aminosalicylates for use in ulcerative colitis and the antibiotics vancomycin and neomycin. In these examples, the aim is to get the drug into the lumen of the colon for therapeutic purposes while avoiding systemic absorption. A few drugs are absorbed by active transport processes. Iron, levodopa and fluorouracil are examples of drugs actively transported across the intestinal mucosa.

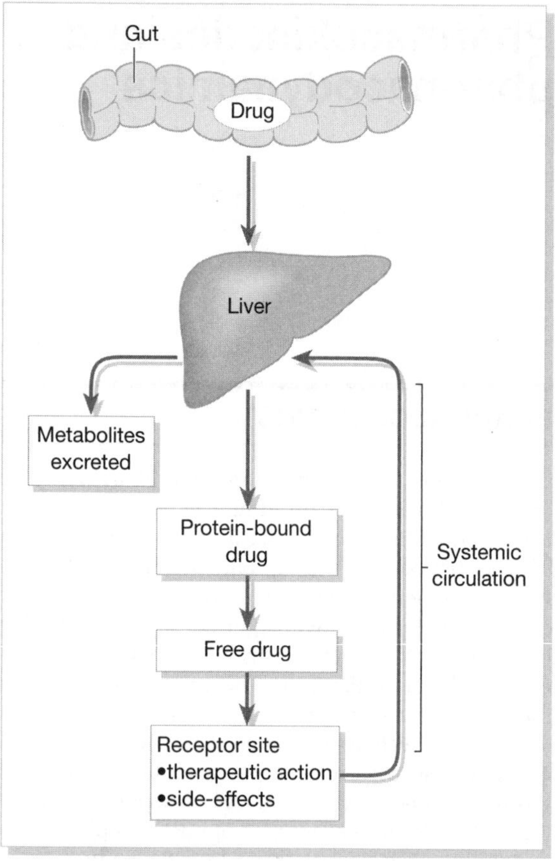

Figure 12.1 Absorption, distribution, metabolism and excretion of an oral drug.

The presence or absence of food in the stomach can affect the rate and amount of drug absorbed. Penicillins, erythromycin and rifampicin are examples of drugs which are better absorbed on an empty stomach and should be given half an hour before meals. Absorption of drugs from the gastrointestinal tract may be complete or incomplete. This can be influenced by the lipid-solubility of the drug and as a result the rate it crosses cell membranes, the rate at which the stomach empties and the presence or absence of food in the stomach.

Following absorption from the gastrointestinal tract, drugs are transported via the portal vein to the liver before reaching the general circulation. Many drugs are broken down (metabolised) as they pass through the liver so that only a proportion of the amount absorbed reaches the general circulation to be carried to the site of action. This is called the first-pass effect. Some drugs show a very significant first-pass effect. Examples include glyceryl trinitrate, which is often given sublingually resulting in absorption through the mucosa, and lidocaine (lignocaine), which is given by injection, in both instances bypassing the portal circulation. The manufacturers will, of course, be aware of the first-pass effect and, where drugs are affected by this, they will have tailored the dose accordingly in order to ensure a therapeutic effect.

DISTRIBUTION

When a drug enters the bloodstream it is rapidly diluted and transported throughout the body. Movement from the blood to tissues is influenced by a number of factors which can greatly affect the resultant drug action. Plasma proteins, particularly albumin, can bind many drugs. Only the *unbound* fraction of the drug is free to move from the bloodstream into tissues to exert a pharmacological effect. The bound drug is pharmacologically inactive because the drug–protein complex is unable to cross cell membranes. It provides a reserve of drug since the complex can dissociate and quickly replenish the unbound drug as it is removed from the plasma. The degree of protein binding will thus affect the intensity and duration of a drug's action.

In addition, if a patient suffers from a disease in which plasma proteins are deficient (e.g. liver disease, malnutrition), more of the drug is free to enter the tissues. A normal dose of a drug could then be dangerous because so little is bound by available protein, thus increasing the availability of unbound drug.

In practice, changes in the protein-bound drug, resulting in increased levels of unbound drug, are important only for highly-bound drugs with a narrow therapeutic index, such as warfarin or phenytoin. The term narrow therapeutic index is used to describe drugs where the toxic level is only slightly above the therapeutic range and a slight increase in unbound drug may therefore result in toxic symptoms. It is important therefore that the nurse has an awareness of these drugs and knowledge of the symptoms which the patient may show should toxic levels be reached.

Drugs diffuse out of the plasma into tissue spaces and some enter cells and spread through the total water of the body. The total body water represents about 0.55 litres/kilogram. Thus the more widely a drug diffuses, the lower will be the concentration produced by a given dose. Factors which affect the rate and extent of distribution are cardiac output and regional blood flow. If the patient is nursed in a warm environment this will help to maintain a better blood circulation and improve drug distribution, an important factor in patients receiving antibiotics. Similarly, inflamed tissues have increased vascularity

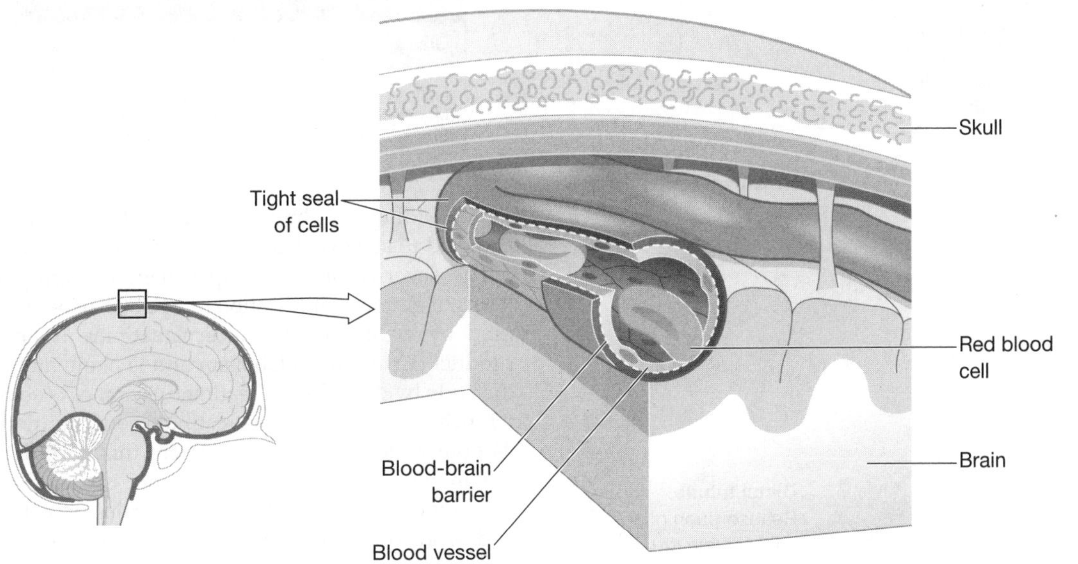

Figure 12.2 Blood–brain barrier.

and permeability which lead to an increased rate of passage of drugs, especially antibiotics.

TRANSFER BARRIERS

The CNS is surrounded by a specialised membrane consisting of the blood–brain and blood–cerebrospinal fluid barriers (Fig. 12.2). This membrane is highly selective for lipid-soluble drugs, e.g. the penicillins diffuse well into body tissues and fluids but penetration into the cerebrospinal fluid is poor, except when the meninges are inflamed. Chloramphenicol, because of its lipid-solubility, is one of the few antibiotics which reaches the cerebrospinal fluid in appreciable concentrations. Dopamine in the treatment of Parkinson's disease cannot be given in this form since it does not cross the blood–brain barrier. It is administered orally as the precursor, levodopa, which is absorbed, crosses the blood–brain barrier, and is broken down to dopamine by the enzyme dopa decarboxylase.

During pregnancy the placenta provides a barrier between mother and fetus. Some drugs (e.g. chlorpromazine and morphine) cross it relatively easily, while others (e.g. suxamethonium chloride) are not transferred. Since fetal liver and kidney are unable to metabolise or excrete drugs, and the fetus is likely to be more sensitive to them, drugs must be used with caution in pregnancy and, in general, few are used.

METABOLISM AND EXCRETION

Some drugs such as atenolol, digoxin and captopril are water-soluble and are readily eliminated by the kidney without prior metabolism. However, many drugs require to be changed into a form that can be readily eliminated by the body and this process is called metabolism.

Most drugs are very lipid-soluble and this enables them to cross cell membranes or the blood–brain barrier in order to reach their site of action. If a lipid-soluble drug is filtered by the kidney it is largely reabsorbed from the distal tubule (Fig. 12.3) and retained in the body. Metabolism increases the water-solubility of the molecule and aids its elimination. Most metabolism takes place in the liver but it can also be carried out in other organs including the gut wall, lungs, kidney and in the plasma.

In the process of metabolism, drugs may be broken down or combined with a chemical. This is brought about by substances called enzymes. The nurse should be aware that the rate at which this occurs in the liver can vary. If the liver cells are damaged or the circulation to the liver is reduced as in cardiac failure, the

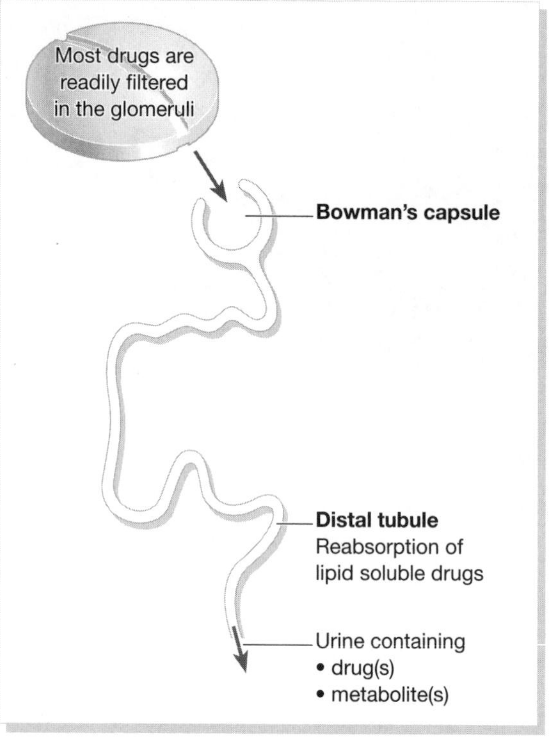

Figure 12.3 Filtration of drugs through the kidney.

inactivation process may be slowed and a lower dose of drug would be indicated.

Pharmacogenetics

Pharmacogenetics is the study of the influence of heredity on the pharmacokinetics of drugs and the pharmacodynamic responses to them. The rate of metabolism for the same drug may vary between individuals because of genetic or racial factors. Hydralazine and isoniazid are inactivated by acetylation, a process involving enzyme action. Acetylation proceeds at different rates in different individuals, over half the population being slow acetylators and the remainder fast acetylators. The fast acetylators will require a higher dose than the slow acetylators in order to receive an equivalent therapeutic effect.

Renal disease

When drugs or their breakdown products are excreted through the kidneys, excretion will be delayed if the kidneys are damaged by disease, and accumulation can occur. Kidney function is also reduced in old age. Since renal impairment results in a decreased capacity of the kidney to eliminate drugs, dosages must be adjusted to achieve drug therapeutic plasma levels.

Table 12.1 The three grades of renal impairment

Grade	Glomerular filtration rate
Mild	20–50 mL/min
Moderate	10–20 mL/min
Severe	< 10 mL/min

The severity of renal impairment is expressed in terms of glomerular filtration rate (GFR), usually measured by creatinine clearance. Creatinine is an end-product of muscle metabolism and is eliminated from the body by the kidney. Creatinine clearance is obtained by measuring the plasma creatinine concentration in a 24-hour collection of urine. Where this is difficult to obtain, the serum creatinine clearance is used. Normal creatinine clearance is 100–120 mL/min for both men and women. Renal impairment is divided into three grades, as shown in Table 12.1. Renal function declines with age, and many elderly patients have a glomerular filtration rate of less than 50 mL/min.

If the glomerular filtration rate is only 50% of normal, the time for a drug to be eliminated in an unchanged form by the kidney, will be doubled. The dose can be adjusted either by being halved or by giving the normal dose at double the time intervals.

The BNF provides guidance on the use of an extensive list of drugs where there is mild, moderate or severe renal impairment.

DOSE–EFFECT RELATIONSHIP

Safe and effective therapy can be achieved only with doses which produce optimal concentrations of a drug in the plasma and target tissues. Smaller doses will be ineffective, while larger doses will not increase the benefits and may have toxic effects. Between the minimal dose which gives the required therapeutic response and the dose at which toxic symptoms appear is a dose range called the therapeutic dose range. Some drugs have a narrow range, whereas others have a wide therapeutic range.

After administration of a drug, its plasma level rises; the more rapidly the drug is absorbed, the faster its plasma level rises (Fig. 12.4).

As drug absorption decreases, and distribution, metabolism and excretion rates increase, the curve reaches its peak. It then descends, as elimination occurs more rapidly than absorption. As previously noted, the route of administration influences the time taken for the drug to reach maximal concentration. This is

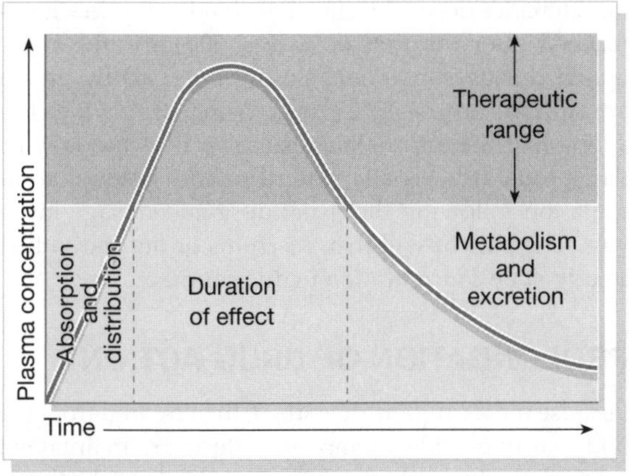

Figure 12.4 Effects of absorption, distribution, metabolism and excretion on the plasma concentration of an administered drug.

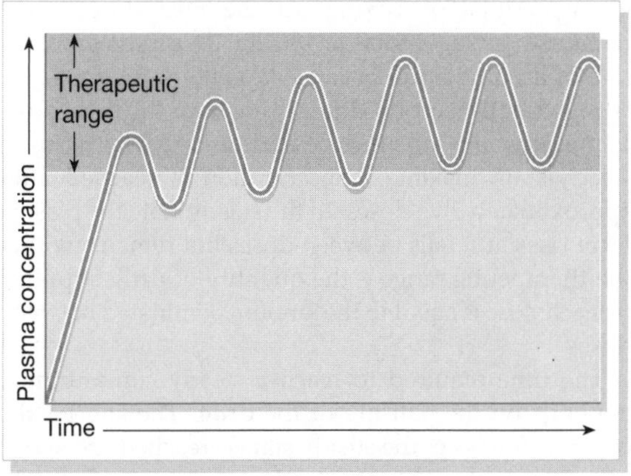

Figure 12.5 Concentration of drug after repeated dosage.

fastest with an intravenous injection, and slower with intramuscular and subcutaneous injections, and oral doses.

As the dose of a drug is increased, its therapeutic effect increases as more receptors are occupied. Eventually the dose is reached that produces a maximal effect when all the receptors of the target organs are occupied by drug molecules. Increasing the dose further will therefore not increase the therapeutic effect.

HALF-LIFE OF DRUGS

The rate at which drugs are eliminated from plasma is commonly expressed in terms of the drug's half-life (t½). This is the time required for the concentration of the drug in the plasma to decrease to one-half of its initial value.

The plasma concentration of a drug at one half-life is 50% of its initial value, at two half-lives 25%, at three half-lives 12.5%, at four half-lives 6.25% and at five half-lives just over 3%. Thus, most of a drug (almost 97%) is eliminated in five half-lives, regardless of the dose or route of administration. This rule of thumb can be applied in calculating the time required to elapse when discontinuing one drug and starting another which may interact if given in conjunction with the first. It is also useful in estimating how long it will take a toxic plasma concentration (after overdosing) to clear the body.

Half-lives of different drugs vary widely, e.g. the t½ of theophylline is 3 hours, the t½ of aspirin is 6 hours, of metronidazole 9 hours, of digoxin about 36 hours, and that of phenobarbital is about 5 days. A short half-life may result from extensive tissue uptake, rapid metabolism or rapid excretion, and a long half-life may be the consequence of extensive plasma protein-binding, slow metabolism, or poor excretion. The knowledge of half-lives of drugs is essential in determining the intervals between drug doses.

Certain conditions can be treated with a single dose of medication (e.g. analgesics for a headache). Many conditions, however, require continuous drug action (e.g. diabetes mellitus, infections, arthritis). This can be achieved through the administration of repeated doses at regular intervals. In such therapy the second, third and subsequent doses will add to whatever remains of the previous dose, causing gradual accumulation until stable concentrations are maintained (Fig. 12.5).

The level of drug in the plasma rises after absorption, reaches its peak, then falls to minimal effective concentration. Administration of the next dose raises the drug concentration to a peak. The concentration falls as the drug is metabolised and excreted, then rises again after the next dose. If the interval between doses is too long, or the dose too small, the plasma concentration will have fallen below the therapeutic range before the next dose is given. As a result, the drug concentration is within the therapeutic range only for short intervals.

If a drug is administered too frequently or in too high a dose, the plasma concentration will rise above the therapeutic range and may give rise to toxic effects. In theory, the optimal dosage interval between drug administrations is equal to the half-life of the drug. Initially, the drug accumulates in the body. If 100 mg of drug is given with a half-life of 6 hours, when the second dose of 100 mg is given 6 hours later, 50 mg of the original dose will still be present in the body – giving a total of 150 mg. After a further 6 hours, 75 mg will remain when the third dose of 100 mg is administered, giving a total of 175 mg. At the next dose, 88 mg remains – giving a total of 188 mg. As can be seen, the rate of accumulation becomes less between doses, i.e. 50 mg after the second dose, 25 mg after the third dose, 13 mg after the fourth dose and, in practical terms, a steady-state maximal concentration is reached after approximately five doses. In the steady state the plasma level rises and falls between doses but remains within the therapeutic range – the quantity of drug supplied by each dose is equal to the amount eliminated between doses.

The time required to reach a steady concentration depends on the half-life of the drug. The shorter the half-life, the faster the steady state is reached, irrespective of the route of administration. Aspirin, with a half-life of 6 hours, will reach equilibrium in five half-lives, i.e. 30 hours.

A dosing interval equal to the half-life of a drug may be impractical for drugs with very short half-lives. Penicillin would have to be given every 30 minutes. This would be inconvenient (if not impossible) for the patient and would lead to poor compliance. Penicillin, however, has a wide therapeutic range, and high doses are relatively non-toxic, so that much higher doses can be given every 6–8 hours compared with the dose that would be given every 30 minutes. This ensures that the therapeutic level in the blood is maintained until the next dose. Short half-life drugs, such as lidocaine (lignocaine), which have a narrow therapeutic range, must be given by intravenous infusion since larger doses given infrequently would cause toxic effects.

Most drugs obey a simple relationship between steady-state concentration and dose. Usually the dose and steady-state concentration are directly proportional: if the dose is doubled, the steady-state concentration doubles. For some drugs (e.g. phenytoin, aspirin), however, the rate of clearance decreases with increasing serum concentrations. When dosages of these drugs are increased, steady-state concentrations increase more than expected. There are also drugs (e.g. disopyramide, sodium valproate), with the opposite effect, i.e. clearance increases with increasing concentration. In these cases, increased dosages will produce a smaller than expected increase in steady-state concentration.

LOADING DOSE

In certain conditions it is desirable to reach an effective level of drug in the blood without waiting for accumulation to take place (e.g. if a patient has an infection and requires antibiotic treatment). This can be achieved by giving the patient an initial dose which is twice the maintenance dose. The effective blood concentration is reached after the first dose (e.g. 500 mg) and maintained during subsequent dosing intervals by giving appropriate doses (e.g. 250 mg). With a drug which has a long half-life this regimen is impractical and may be dangerous. It is usually better to allow gradual accumulation following the usual dose and dosage intervals. The patient will then reach his or her individual steady-state concentration in due course.

PROLONGATION OF DRUG ACTION

Because most drugs are absorbed, then cleared from the body fairly quickly, therapeutic effects are maintained for a relatively short time. In order to prolong the therapeutic effect, the drug must be administered either frequently or by constant infusion. It may be desirable to reduce the frequency of dosage, for example, where compliance is poor, or to simplify regimens, where a number of drugs are being administered. Either or both may be achieved by regulating the release of the active drug from the dosage form in order to maintain therapeutic plasma concentrations (Fig. 12.6).

Absorption can be delayed and the drug's action correspondingly prolonged in a number of different ways. In local anaesthesia with lidocaine (lignocaine), the addition of adrenaline (epinephrine) causes constriction of local blood vessels, thus delaying absorption of the anaesthetic and prolonging its local effect. Delay can also be achieved by giving the drug as a suspension (e.g. insulin zinc suspension) which is absorbed slowly (depot therapy).

In certain instances, extremely slow absorption may be desirable. In psychiatric practice, long-acting preparations can be used to avoid frequent drug

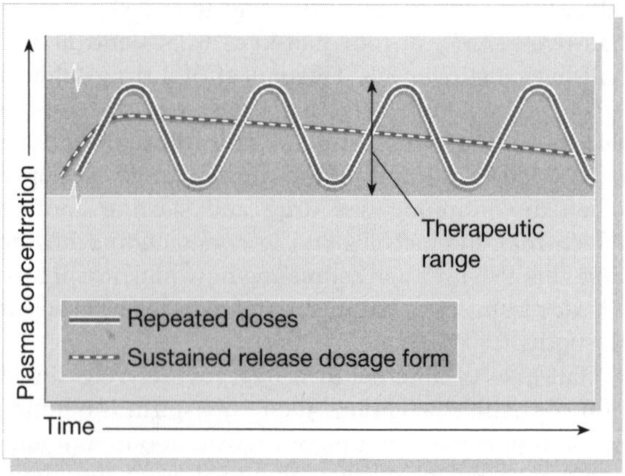

Figure 12.6 Prolongation of drug action.

administration to patients who find it difficult to remember, or who refuse to take their medications by the oral route. The introduction of oily injections of fluphenazine ensures that non-compliant chronic schizophrenic patients can be treated satisfactorily by single intramuscular injections at 2- to 5-weekly intervals. Similarly, long-lasting contraception can be achieved with depot injections of progestogen.

Some longer-acting oral preparations

The sustained release of a drug can be achieved in a number of ways, as discussed below.

Coated granules

The active drug is contained in small granules packed in a gelatin capsule. Some granules have no coating and dissolve immediately. Other granules have coatings of varying thickness of materials such as waxes. The granules with thin coatings will dissolve and release the drug faster than those with thicker coatings. It is possible therefore for the active drug to be released over a longer period of time and a steady plasma level to be maintained by one dose instead of three or four individual doses of the conventional preparation.

Multilayer tablets

Sustained action can be achieved by manufacturing tablets which consist of a number of layers or several coats. The drug is dissolved immediately from one layer or the outer coat and more slowly from succeeding layers or coats.

Matrix preparations

The active ingredient is distributed throughout an inert wax or plastic matrix. The drug is slowly leached out of this network and its action may be sustained for up to 24 hours. A variation of this involves the active substance being embedded in a tablet surrounded by a porous coating. The pores are filled with water-soluble crystals which dissolve on contact with aqueous liquids allowing the active ingredient to be released in a controlled manner by diffusion through the pores.

Miniature osmotic pump

A novel method of achieving oral controlled release of a drug is the miniature osmotic pump. The traditional tablet structure is replaced by a tablet-sized structure made up of a semipermeable membrane which encloses the active drug and the osmotic driving agent. This system is used to provide a controlled release of salbutamol in the treatment of asthma and related conditions. As with other controlled-release products it is important to explain to patients that the tablet must be taken whole with a glass of water and not chewed or crushed.

Controlled-release oral dosage forms may be more convenient than conventional preparations because they require less frequent administration thus improving the patient's compliance. In addition, the gastric mucosa is exposed to a lower concentration of drug than would have been the case with immediate-release products. This may be important when the drug causes irritation or bleeding of the gastrointestinal tract. However, in practice, the results obtained from controlled-release dosage forms may be far from ideal and may vary between patients. The contents of sustained-release preparations may not be released completely and may tail off, giving therapeutic concentrations initially, but only subtherapeutic concentrations prior to the next dose.

PHARMACODYNAMICS

Pharmacodynamics is the process by which specific drug dosages produce biochemical or physiological changes in the body. In the simplest terms pharmacodynamics can be described as what drugs do to the body, as opposed to pharmacokinetics which is what the body does to drugs.

MECHANISMS OF DRUG ACTION

In certain cases the medicine will bring about a normal physiological response where it is a replacement for a deficiency, for example:

- levothyroxine is taken orally in hypothyroidism
- insulin is injected subcutaneously in diabetes mellitus
- hydroxocobalamin is injected intramuscularly in the treatment of pernicious anaemia
- ferrous salts are taken orally to treat anaemia due to iron deficiency
- electrolytes in aqueous solution may be administered orally in cases of severe diarrhoea.

More frequently, however, drugs act by affecting either biochemical or physiological processes in the body or by controlling changes in these processes brought about by disease. One way this is achieved is by affecting receptors.

Receptor agonists and antagonists

The term 'receptor' can be used to mean any clearly defined target molecule with which a drug molecule has to combine in order to produce a specific effect. Receptors will interact only with those drugs that are exactly compatible structurally (Fig. 12.7). When the drug binds to the receptor a complex is formed which may produce two results. First, activation of the receptor may occur, producing a specific result (receptor agonist). The second type of effect is where a drug binds with a receptor preventing a naturally-occurring substance within the body combining with the receptor. In this way the normal response is blocked (receptor antagonist).

Receptor agonists can be used to alleviate a variety of conditions, examples of which are detailed below.

1. Beta$_2$-adrenoceptor agonists. The main effect is a bronchodilator action directly on the β_2-adrenoceptors of smooth muscle, providing relief in asthma sufferers. Examples include terbutaline, salbutamol and rimiterol.
2. Sumatriptan is a 5-HT$_1$ (hydroxytryptamine) agonist which is used in the treatment of migraine. Headaches that are a prominent feature of migraine are believed to result from excessive dilatation of extracerebral cranial arteries, arteriovenous shunts, or both. Sumatriptan is a novel selective agonist which blocks these mechanisms.
3. In Parkinson's disease, dopamine production in the brain is greatly reduced. Bromocriptine can be administered to alleviate this condition since it acts as a direct agonist, stimulating dopamine receptors. It has another action since it mimics the action of dopamine on the pituitary, which inhibits prolactin release and, as a result, lactation is suppressed.

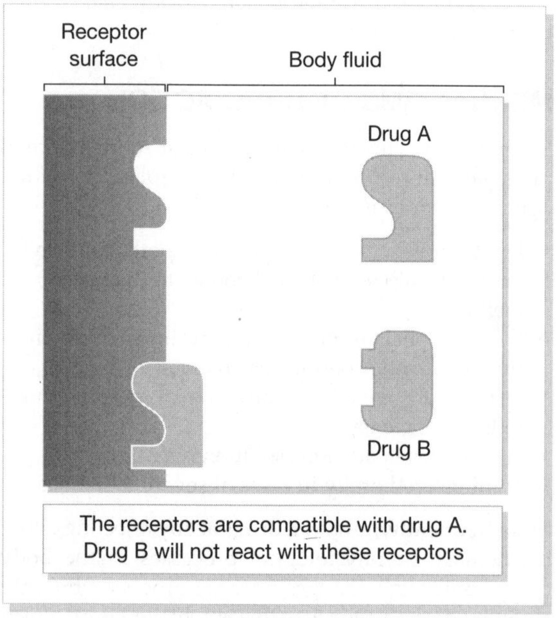
Receptor surface
Body fluid
Drug A
Drug B
The receptors are compatible with drug A. Drug B will not react with these receptors

Fig. 12.7 Drug–receptor interaction.

Receptor antagonists, by preventing a naturally occurring substance combining with the receptor, produce therapeutic outcomes as illustrated by the following examples.

1. 5-HT$_3$ receptor antagonists. The major sites responsive to emetic stimuli are in the gut and in the brain, areas which are rich in 5-HT$_3$ receptors. Ondansetron is a potent 5-HT$_3$ receptor antagonist and, as such, blocks the emetic reflex responses.
2. Beta$_1$-adrenoceptor antagonists. Atenolol blocks the β_1 actions of noradrenaline (norepinephrine) released from cardiac sympathetic stimulation and of circulating adrenaline (epinephrine). It is used to treat angina pectoris and hypertension. In angina pectoris, β-receptor antagonists reduce the force and contraction of the ventricle, resulting in a reduction in cardiac oxygen consumption, relieving anginal pain.
3. H_1 histamine receptor antagonists. There are two classes of histamine antagonists: H_1 receptor antagonists and H_2 receptor antagonists. The term 'antihistamine' conventionally refers to the H_1 receptor antagonists such as promethazine and terfenadine. They are used mainly to block the actions of histamine released during hypersensitivity reactions.
4. H_2 histamine receptor antagonists. Histamine has numerous actions, including a powerful stimulant effect on gastric secretion. Selective antagonists have been developed which have proved potent in blocking the stimulant action of histamine on the acid-secreting parietal cells of the stomach. H_2 receptor antagonists such as cimetidine and ranitidine are capable of reducing gastric acid secretion by 70% or more.

Enzyme inhibitors

An enzyme is a protein which can promote or accelerate a biochemical reaction with a substrate. When the enzyme mistakenly identifies the drug as being the substrate, a drug–enzyme interaction occurs. This interaction could increase or decrease the rate of a biochemical reaction.

1. Carbidopa/benserazide. In Parkinson's disease, levodopa is given as the precursor to dopamine since it crosses the blood–brain barrier, which dopamine is

unable to do. It is then broken down to dopamine by dopa decarboxylase. However, dopa decarboxylase is present in the gut and liver – resulting in the breakdown of a proportion of the levodopa before it enters the brain. By combining the levodopa with either carbidopa or benserazide, which inhibit the action of dopa decarboxylase, the breakdown of levodopa is reduced and a lower dose can be given.

2. Vigabatrin. Gamma-aminobutyric acid (GABA) inhibits the spread of seizure activity by blocking synaptic transmission. GABA is metabolised by the enzyme GABA transaminase (GABA-T). The action of vigabatrin in the treatment of epilepsy is to inhibit GABA-T irreversibly, thus preventing the breakdown of GABA. The action persists until new enzyme is synthesised.

3. Neostigmine. Neostigmine is used in the treatment of myasthenia gravis. Acetylcholine is broken down by the enzyme cholinesterase. Neostigmine inhibits the action of cholinesterase, allowing an accumulation of acetylcholine at the muscle motor end-plate, thereby alleviating the block in neuromuscular transmission which occurs in this condition.

4. Omeprazole. Omeprazole reduces secretion of gastric acid by inhibiting an enzyme called H^+K^+-adenosine triphosphatase (the so-called gastric proton pump). This enzyme is responsible for the final stage in the production of acid in the parietal cells of the gastric mucosa. It pumps protons out from the cell into the gastric lumen in exchange for potassium ions. Once in the lumen the protons (hydrogen ions) meet up with chloride ions to form hydrochloric acid.

Drugs affecting transport processes

This mechanism of action can apply both to drugs introduced to the body and substances synthesised by the body.

1. Thiazide diuretics. The thiazide diuretics decrease the reabsorption of sodium in the renal distal tubule. This results in an increased excretion of sodium and water.

2. Probenecid. In gout there is an increase in the amount of uric acid in the body. Probenecid inhibits the transport of organic acids across epithelial membranes. The reabsorption of uric acid from the renal tubule is blocked by probenecid, resulting in an increased secretion and relief from the symptoms of gout.

3. Insulin. Insulin has a number of actions, one of which is to promote the transport of glucose into cells. This action results in a rapid fall in glucose levels in the blood in relieving hyperglycaemic diabetic coma.

Chemotherapeutic agents

In cancer chemotherapy, cytotoxic drugs act by interfering with cell growth and division. Ideally, a drug is required to have a selective action on all abnormal, rapidly dividing cells found in cancerous conditions, with no toxic effect in normal cells. Such a drug is not yet available since currently used drugs attack normal growing cells as well as malignant cells. All cells which are synthesising deoxyribonucleic acid (DNA) go through a cycle which has several different phases. Different cytotoxic drugs act at different phases of the cell cycle:

- methotrexate inhibits the formation of folic acid, which is important in the synthesis of DNA
- bleomycin damages DNA.

In infective disease an increasing number of drugs affect bacteria and other microorganisms:

- penicillins and cephalosporins inhibit synthesis of bacterial cell walls
- nystatin and amphotericin act by increasing the permeability of cell membranes of invading organisms
- chloramphenicol and erythromycin inhibit bacterial protein synthesis.

Miscellaneous

There are a significant number of drug actions which can be classed under this heading:

1. Antacids such as aluminium hydroxide and magnesium hydroxide have a direct neutralising effect on acid and reduce gastric acidity.

2. Ion-exchange resins such as calcium polystyrene sulphonate are used to remove excess potassium in mild hyperkalaemia. The sodium in the ion-exchange resin exchanges for potassium, which is removed from the body as the resin passes through and is excreted.

3. Desferrioxamine chelates ferrous iron in the treatment of iron poisoning.

4. Potassium citrate makes the urine alkaline and relieves the discomfort of cystitis in lower urinary tract infections.

DRUGS AT THE EXTREMES OF AGE

Drugs in pregnancy

During the first 2 weeks of human gestation the fertilised ovum is already sensitive to drugs and, after this, drugs may produce congenital malformations in the first trimester in the fetus. The time of greatest risk is between the 3rd and 11th weeks of pregnancy when differentiation of organs occurs. The development of the embryo is very rapid, with continuous changes resulting from cell division, cell migration and cell differentiation. Each organ and each system undergoes a critical stage of differentiation at a precise period of prenatal development, e.g. the heart from day 20 to day 40, and limbs from day 24 to day 46. It is during this time that specific gross malformations can be produced by particular drugs.

Complete closure of the palate occurs in the fetus at 8 weeks, differentiation of the external genitalia between the 4th and 5th month, and further differentiation of the nervous system from the 4th month until after birth. Drugs administered around these times may interfere with the normal development of the genitalia and nervous system.

As a general principle, drugs should not be administered to a woman during pregnancy unless the potential benefit to the mother outweighs the risk to the fetus. However, serious illness can occur during pregnancy, and complications of pregnancy often need to be treated with drugs so that administration cannot always be avoided. The mother may suffer from a chronic condition which requires continuous medication. For example, patients with hypothyroidism require regular doses of levothyroxine. Although the placenta is relatively impermeable to levothyroxine, adequate replacement in hypothyroid patients is extremely important as it has been shown that children of women who had inadequate replacement therapy scored lower in tests of mental and fine motor development when compared to the offspring of women with adequate replacement therapy.

The transfer of drugs across the placenta is accomplished in a similar manner to the distribution of drugs in body organs and tissues. Most drugs cross the placenta by simple diffusion from an area of high concentration to an area of low concentration. Biochemical and physiological changes occur in women during pregnancy and, therefore, drug distribution, metabolism and excretion may be altered. Metabolism of drugs in the maternal liver is reduced during pregnancy and an increase in plasma volume in conjunction with a reduction in albumin content may increase the amount of free drug in the plasma. Since the fetus is in equilibrium with the maternal circulation, drugs and metabolites which readily cross the placenta and enter the fetal circulation will also be in equilibrium and will then pass back into the mother's circulation when cleared by the fetus.

Care must be taken when drugs are administered shortly before term or during labour since these may not have been cleared from the fetus before birth. A drug can no longer pass from the fetal to the maternal circulation after the umbilical cord has been clamped, and this may cause adverse effects on the neonate after delivery owing to problems of metabolism and excretion. If treatment is required, drugs preferred are those which have been used extensively. New or untried drugs should be avoided when an alternative with a known 'safe' history is available.

Antibacterial drugs may be used in pregnancy for the treatment of maternal infection. The penicillins are probably the safest antibiotics for use in pregnancy. Tetracyclines are irreversibly incorporated into fetal teeth resulting in discoloration and a tendency to develop dental caries. Although the benefits of antiepileptics to the mother may outweigh the risk to the fetus, there is an increased incidence of congenital malformation in infants born to mothers receiving antiepileptic drugs. There is no evidence that general anaesthetics are harmful to the fetus provided that maternal hypotension and respiratory depression are avoided.

Although a great deal of work is now being done on the adverse effects of drugs administered during pregnancy, the effects of many drugs on the fetus have yet to be determined. Much of the work has been done on laboratory animals, which may react differently to humans. In addition, studies conducted in humans are usually retrospective and it is difficult to attribute adverse effects on the fetus to a particular drug.

Drug treatment should be avoided whenever possible during pregnancy, especially during the first trimester and prior to delivery. Care should also be taken in administering drugs to women of childbearing age as major harmful effects of drugs on the fetus will be produced very early in pregnancy, possibly before the woman realises she is pregnant.

Drug therapy in the young

All children, and particularly neonates, differ from adults in their response to drugs. The immaturity of organs involved in drug metabolism and excretion may alter not only the pharmacokinetics but also the toxicity of many drugs. Great variability exists in absorption, protein-binding, distribution, metabolism and excretion according to age and weight, and important differences have been observed in premature neonates, full-term babies and older children. These differences become more complex where congenital anomalies or disease states exist.

Absorption of drugs

Gastrointestinal tract. The absorption of drugs from the gastrointestinal tract is influenced by the pH of the stomach contents and also by gastric emptying time. The pH of the stomach at birth is 6–8 but falls to 1–3 in the first 24 hours. (In premature neonates this fall does not occur because the acid-secreting mechanism has not fully developed.) The pH then returns to between 6 and 8 for 10–15 days, since no more acid is secreted during this period. This relatively neutral pH of the stomach contents may result in higher blood levels of drugs such as penicillin because of reduced chemical decomposition resulting in increased availability for absorption. The adult value of gastric pH (approximately 3) is gradually reached between 2 and 3 years of age.

The gastric emptying time may be as long as 6–8 hours in neonates, reaching adult values at 6–8 months. This prolonged emptying time may have an important influence on the absorption rate of orally administered drugs.

Intramuscular injection. The absorption rate of drugs following intramuscular injection is influenced by the changes in muscle blood flow which occur in the first days of life and by vasoconstriction resulting from temperature change or circulatory insufficiency.

Skin. Percutaneous absorption is greatly increased in neonates and young infants who have thin, well-hydrated skin. This increased permeability has led to toxic effects associated with the use of hexachlorophene soaps and powders, and preparations containing salicylic acid. The dangers of absorption of corticosteroids from topical preparations are also widely recognised (see p. 447).

The binding of drugs by proteins

Neonates have reduced plasma protein binding of various drugs. This is because of a reduced plasma protein concentration and because neonatal albumin has a lower binding capacity for drugs than that of adults. These factors may vary in their effects and may lead to drug toxicity. On the other hand, the dose of digoxin required in infants is high compared to that for adults. An average daily maintenance dose for adults is 3–5 micrograms/kg body weight, whereas in infants it is 10–25 micrograms/kg. This higher dose is required because the digoxin has a lower binding affinity for digoxin receptors in the myocardium of neonates. In addition to reduced plasma protein binding, another factor affecting drug distribution is the total body water in neonates – which is 70%, compared to the adult value of 55%.

Hepatic metabolism of drugs

Drug metabolism by the liver can occur in a number of ways, for example by acetylation or by conjugation. In the newborn the necessary enzyme systems are developed to varying extents. Conjugation involving glucuronidation is deficient in some newborn infants. A number of drugs, including chloramphenicol, are metabolised in this way. Grey syndrome (abdominal distension, pallid cyanosis, circulatory collapse) may follow excessive doses of chloramphenicol in neonates with immature hepatic metabolism. This deficiency in metabolism disappears in the first or second week of life.

Excretion of drugs

At birth, all aspects of renal function are diminished but become comparable to that in adults between 6 months and a year. Full-term babies have a reduced glomerular filtration rate compared to adults. Compounds which are not extensively metabolised and depend on renal function for excretion are eliminated more slowly in neonates. The maintenance dose must be adjusted depending on the child's kidney function, increasing as the kidney function develops. On the other hand, drugs such as diuretics which depend on the glomerular filtration to produce a therapeutic effect will require a higher dose at birth when the creatinine clearance is approximately 20 mL/min, but at age 1 month, when the clearance rate is 60 mL/min, the dose would be reduced accordingly.

Drugs in breast milk

Breast milk is the only food the infant needs for the first 4–6 months of life. There are many benefits to be gained from breast-feeding. The composition of human milk is tailored to organ development and growth, and some protection against infection is obtained; compared with cow's milk, there is less likelihood of food allergy and it is more digestible. The advantages for the nursing mother, in addition to maternal bonding, are a lower cost compared with substitute products and convenience.

The contact of the baby's sucking serves to keep prolactin levels high and may delay subsequent pregnancy. Prolactin secretion can be altered by drugs. It is decreased by levodopa and bromocriptine and increased by phenothiazines, methyldopa and theophylline. The production of milk can be affected by diuretics. Bendroflumethiazide (bendrofluazide) has been shown to stop lactation. Spironolactone, however, can be used safely.

Although most drugs are excreted to some extent in breast milk, the significance of their effects depends on the amount excreted in the milk. The newborn metabolise and excrete drugs very inefficiently. Preterm infants are at greater risk than others but the risk decreases as renal and hepatic functions mature. Since infants have poorly developed renal and hepatic functions, they may be particularly sensitive to the accumulation of drugs. Where possible, drugs should be avoided during breast-feeding and mothers should be warned of the possible dangers of self-medication.

Because of their potential toxicity, a number of drugs are absolutely contraindicated while the mother is breast-feeding. These include antithyroid drugs, radioactive isotopes, lithium, chloramphenicol, ergot alkaloids and most anticancer drugs. If some form of drug treatment is essential, then alternatives to these must be used or breast-feeding must be stopped. A number of other drugs are to be avoided or used with caution. For example, atropine may cause intoxication in sensitive infants and calciferol, in high doses, may cause hypercalcaemia in the infant.

If drugs (e.g. penicillins) are secreted in milk in relatively low concentrations, the advantages of breast-feeding probably outweigh the marginal risks involved. Many drugs (e.g. cephalosporins) known to be excreted in breast milk do not appear to produce adverse effects in the infant.

Generally, the mother should breast-feed prior to taking medication. When a nursing mother takes a drug which is potentially hazardous to the infant, breast-feeding may be temporarily discontinued where a single dose or short course is involved. Attention should be paid to the half-life of the drug. In this situation breast milk should be expressed regularly to maintain lactation, and then discarded.

When drugs are prescribed for a nursing mother, a number of principles are adhered to by the doctor, and the nurse should be aware of these principles:

- never prescribe a drug unless it is essential
- use the safest drug where alternatives are available
- use the lowest effective dose for the shortest possible time.

If there is no alternative to drug therapy and the principles above are adhered to, adverse effects on the baby should not occur. The mother may need reassurance and general guidance so that she is alert for any recognisable effects on the baby.

Appendix 4 of the BNF gives specific guidance on drugs to be avoided, or to be used with caution in pregnancy. As with all prescribing, risk/benefit issues must be taken into account. For example, the benefits of treatment of severe asthma with corticosteroids outweigh the risk. Risks of teratogenicity must always be considered, as must the possibility of drug interactions.

As more medicines become deregulated (see p. 27), care must be taken to ensure that a pregnant woman receives good advice on the use of medicines that can be purchased without prescription (over-the-counter medicines – OTC). Community pharmacists are well placed to advise women; indeed, there is a professional responsibility to ensure, as far as is practicable, that sales of medicines are made within agreed protocols which are designed to protect the purchaser.

Drugs in older people

It is wrong to view older people as a homogeneous group, all of whom are suffering from several coexisting disease processes. However, there is no doubt that, as the ageing process continues, there is an increasing likelihood that drug treatment will be required. The physiological changes that occur with ageing have an impact on the distribution and metabolism of drugs.

Distribution of drugs in the body

In most older people, total body mass, lean body mass and total body water decrease; total body fat increases. These changes in body composition can affect a drug's concentration in the body. A water-soluble drug is distributed primarily in the aqueous parts of the body and lean body tissue. Because an older person has relatively less water and lean tissue, more of the water-soluble drug stays in the blood which leads to increased blood concentration levels. As a result, dosage reduction may be required.

The older patient has a higher proportion of body fat, and more of a fat-soluble drug is distributed to the fatty tissue. This produces misleadingly low blood levels and may cause dosage to be incorrectly increased. The fatty tissue slowly releases stored drug into the bloodstream and this explains why a fat-soluble sedative may produce a hangover effect.

A decrease in albumin results in a reduction in the plasma protein binding of some drugs (e.g. phenytoin, warfarin). More non-bound drug is available to act at receptor sites and may result in toxicity. In these cases a dose reduction should be considered.

Metabolism of drugs in older people

Hepatic metabolism of some drugs would appear to be altered as a consequence of the ageing process which results in a reduction of liver blood flow and a reduction in liver mass. General rules cannot be formulated, but for some drugs it appears that decreased hepatic metabolism does result in longer half-life of the drug.

Renal excretion of drugs in older people

Whereas the effect on drug action of reduced hepatic metabolism is difficult to predict, the effect of reduced renal excretion is more readily determined. Glomerular filtration rate by the age of 80 may have fallen to less than 50 mL/min. Drugs or active metabolites of those which are excreted mainly in the urine will require to be administered in lower dose, particularly those with a narrow therapeutic index, e.g. warfarin, digoxin, lithium, phenytoin and carbamazepine. Tetracyclines are best avoided in older people because, in the presence of poor renal function, they accumulate, causing nausea and vomiting, resulting in dehydration and further deterioration in renal function.

FURTHER READING

Bradley J R 1997 Renal disorders. Hospital Pharmacist 4(6):137–139
Cadman B 1996 Drug induced liver disease. Hospital Pharmacist 3(2):31–35
Kelly J 1995 Pharmacodynamics and drug therapy. Professional Nurse 10(12):792–796
McGavock H 2001 Getting a drug to its site of action: distribution. Prescriber 12(19):29–32
McGavock H 2001 Getting a drug into the body: absorption. Prescriber 12(18):39–47
Walker D 1999 How relevant is drug metabolism to prescribing. Prescriber 10(19):139–142

CHAPTER CONTENTS

13

Adverse drug reactions and drug interactions

INTRODUCTION

An adverse drug reaction (ADR) has been defined by the World Health Organization as 'any response to a drug which is noxious, unintended and occurs at doses used for prophylaxis, diagnosis and therapy.' All pharmaceutical preparations are potentially harmful and this is a key reason why many medicines are strictly controlled and only available on prescription. The safe use of medicines is an important issue for nurses, pharmacists, doctors, regulatory authorities, the pharmaceutical industry and the public. Health professionals have a responsibility to their patients who themselves are increasingly aware of problems associated with drug therapy. It is essential that the practising nurse has a knowledge of the adverse effects of drugs and how to recognise and prevent them. The special roles performed by nurses give them a unique opportunity to help reduce the incidence of ADR and to minimise their impact on patients.

A tragic event occurred in the early 1960s which involved a hypnotic called thalidomide. This drug proved to be teratogenic, and many babies with congenital limb defects were born to mothers who had taken this preparation in early pregnancy. This major disaster led to the establishment of regulatory agencies which enforce rigorous testing and evaluation of drugs prior to the granting of a product licence and subsequent marketing. In addition to these processes, detection and recording of adverse drug reactions that occur when the drug is in use are of vital importance. A well-established reporting system enables ADRs to be reported to the Committee on the Safety of Medicines (CSM). Both prescribed and non-prescribed medicines are included in this system. Yellow reporting forms for ADRs are included in the BNF.

Classification

The simplest classification of adverse drug reactions is into types A and B.

Type A reactions

Type A reactions to drugs include augmented responses which are undesirable. Examples include hypoglycaemia with a sulphonylurea and postural hypotension with an antihypertensive drug. Many type A reactions arise from secondary pharmacological effects of a drug, such as anticholinergic effects with antihistamines and tricyclic antidepressants. Type A reactions are usually dose-dependent and predictable and are often recognised before a drug is marketed.

Type B reactions

Type B reactions are unrelated to the drug's pharmacology and are generally unrelated to dosage. Although comparatively rare they often cause serious illness and may result in death. These reactions are often caused by pharmacogenetic and immunological mechanisms. Genetic differences in the population can result in altered drug metabolism, e.g. fast and slow acetylators (see p. 120).

Allergic reactions are immunologically mediated effects. They vary from rash and angio-oedema to life-threatening bronchospasm and hypotension associated with anaphylaxis. Features of these reactions are that there is often a delay between the first exposure to the drug and the occurrence of the subsequent adverse reaction, very small doses of the drug may trigger the reaction once allergy is established and the reaction disappears on withdrawal. Documenting of allergic reactions for individual patients is important in order to avoid future exposures to the allergen.

Other predisposing factors

Age may be a factor and the very old and the very young are more susceptible to adverse drug reactions. In older people the incidence of multiple and chronic diseases is increased, resulting in increased reliance on medication. This results in a higher incidence of adverse drug reactions because of increased drug exposure and also age-related pharmacokinetic changes. Drugs which commonly cause problems in older people include hypnotics, diuretics, non-steroidal anti-inflammatory drugs, antihypertensives, psychotropics and digoxin. All children and particularly neonates differ from adults in the way they handle and respond to drugs. Hazardous drugs in neonates include chloramphenicol and morphine. A specific example of concern in children is Reye's syndrome with aspirin. Children under 16 years of age should not take aspirin.

Pharmacovigilance

As part of the stringent conditions for granting a product licence to a newly developed drug, clinical trials with patients must be carried out to assess the efficacy and adverse effects of the product. On average around 1500 people will have taken the product and only the common adverse effects will have been experienced. Type B reactions which occur to a lesser extent may not be identified. Exclusion criteria for those taking part in the trial may mean patients with multiple disease states, children, older people and pregnant women are excluded or are not well studied. In addition the effect of long-term use will be unknown. Post-marketing surveillance or pharmacovigilance is therefore essential in detecting uncommon reactions.

DRUG-INDUCED GASTROINTESTINAL DISORDERS

Adverse drug reactions frequently affect the gastrointestinal tract. This is understandable when one considers that this is the most common route for medication and, in addition, the vast range of medicines now available which are taken orally. Nausea and vomiting is one of the commonest adverse effects experienced by patients. However, in many cases symptoms soon resolve with continued use. Where this is not the case, a lower dose or an alternative preparation may need to be considered, otherwise a concurrent anti-emetic may be required. If nausea and vomiting are severe, treatment may have to be stopped.

Non-steroidal anti-inflammatory drugs (NSAIDs) including aspirin are very widely used but have a potential to damage the gastrointestinal tract. NSAIDs are administered to reduce pain and inflammation, particularly in arthritis. This is achieved by inhibition of synthesis of certain prostaglandins. However, it appears that they also inhibit prostaglandins which are protective to tissues, resulting in irritant effects on the gastric epithelium.

Adverse drug reactions including abdominal pain, nausea, diarrhoea and dyspepsia are experienced. NSAID-induced erosions can result in bleeding and perforation of the stomach and duodenum. The following guidance can help minimise the risk from NSAIDs.

- Where an NSAID is indicated, one with a lower incidence of side-effects should be the first choice, e.g. ibuprofen.
- The lowest effective dose should be used. The maximum recommended dose should not be exceeded.
- No more than one NSAID should be used at any one time.

Table 13.1 Examples of drugs causing adverse drug reactions

Adverse drug reaction	Examples of drugs
Dry mouth	Anticholinergics, antihistamines, CNS stimulants, ribavirin, tricyclic antidepressants, phenothiazines
Metallic taste	Metformin, metronidazole, zopiclone
Taste disturbance	ACE inhibitors, penicillamine, terbinafine
Oesophageal reflux	Anticholinergics, calcium-channel blockers, opioids
Nausea and vomiting	Cytotoxics, levodopa, opioids, quinolones, ribavirin
Diarrhoea	Antibiotics, colchicine, gold compounds, misoprostol, proton pump inhibitors
Constipation	Anticholinergics, antihistamines, diuretics, iron preparations, opioid analgesics, tricyclic antidepressants, verapamil

- The patient's medication should be regularly reviewed and NSAIDs stopped or changed to a safer product where possible.
- Patients should be counselled on how the drug works, the dose to be taken and side-effects to expect. They should be advised to consult their doctor without delay where signs of internal bleeding occur, e.g. blood-stained vomit or black tarry stools.

Table 13.1 provides details of several of the more commonly experienced gastrointestinal adverse effects (dry mouth, taste disturbance, oesophageal reflux, nausea and vomiting, diarrhoea and constipation) and examples of drugs causing these.

DRUG-INDUCED MENTAL HEALTH DISORDERS

Drug-induced mental health disorders are relatively common. Most adverse psychiatric effects of drugs are classified as type A reactions as they are dose related or predictable, although a few are idiosyncratic type B reactions. Psychiatric symptoms are also a common feature of withdrawal reactions which can occur after certain drug therapy is stopped, particularly when it is stopped abruptly. For example, rapid withdrawal of benzodiazepines may cause rebound insomnia and anxiety.

The risk of an individual experiencing a psychiatric reaction to a drug is greater if mental illness is present or has been experienced in the past. Other associated factors include alcohol or drug abuse. Drugs implicated in psychiatric reactions can cause more than one effect. For example, phenytoin can cause delirium, hallucinations and psychosis.

Table 13.2 Drugs associated with drug-induced mental disorders

Condition	Examples of drugs associated with the condition
Depression	Ciprofloxacin, beta-blockers, calcium-channel blockers, benzodiazepines, levodopa, carbamazepine, phenothiazines, rivastigmine, corticosteroids, disulfiram, levetiracetam, isotretinoin, mefloquine
Psychosis	Quinolones, anticholinergics, antiepileptics, disulfiram, ganciclovir, levodopa, mefloquine, zolpidem
Mania	Baclofen, bromocriptine, corticosteroids, levodopa
Delirium	Anticholinergics, antiepileptics, antipsychotics, corticosteroids, disulfiram, lithium, opioids
Confusion	Diazepam, carbamazepine, mexiletine, omeprazole, spironolactone

Psychiatric conditions

Psychiatric conditions arising as a result of adverse drug reactions include depression, psychosis, mania, confusion and delirium. Depressive reactions to drugs may vary from mild mood changes to more severe adverse effects such as sleep disturbances, loss of appetite and suicidal ideation. Where a drug is suspected of causing depression, resolution of symptoms on withdrawal will confirm diagnosis. Psychosis is characterised by delusions, hallucinations and distorted personality. As adverse effects of drugs, these are more common in older people. The effects are usually dose related and resolve on discontinuation.

Mania is characterised by an elevated mood and also rapid speech, overactivity, insomnia and disinhibition. Drug-induced mania is uncommon and affected patients usually have a history of mood disorder. Drugs linked to this include levodopa and corticosteroids. The suspected drugs should be discontinued and manic symptoms treated with an antipsychotic.

Patients suffering from acute confusional state have a short attention span, appear bewildered and have difficulty following commands. Delirium is characterised by disorientation and reduced attention and the patient may be frightened, restless and hostile. Most drug-induced confusional states resolve on withdrawal of the drug. Anticholinergics are recognised as causing delirium, disorientation, confusion and visual hallucinations. Table 13.2 lists drugs associated with drug-induced mental disorders.

DRUG-INDUCED SKIN DISORDERS

Drug-induced skin eruptions are likely to be the most frequent adverse reaction seen by a nurse since approximately 30% of reported drug reactions involve the skin.

Erythematous eruption

This is a skin rash characterised by erythema (abnormal flushing of the skin) and is the most common type of drug-induced skin reaction. Erythematous rashes may be morbilliform (resembling measles) or maculopapular, i.e. consisting of macules (distinct flat areas, mostly discoloured) and papules (raised lesions). Early reactions start within 2 or 3 days of the administration of the drug and occur in previously sensitised patients, i.e. patients who have built up antibodies after receiving the drug on a previous occasion. In the late-type reaction the hypersensitivity develops during administration. The peak incidence is around the 9th day but rashes can occur as late as 3 weeks after starting treatment. A high incidence of erythematous rashes can be expected during or following treatment with penicillins, gold salts and non-steroidal anti-inflammatory drugs.

Pruritus

Pruritus may be the first sign of drug hypersensitivity and should act as an early warning for more severe skin reactions, such as those seen with gold therapy. Anal pruritus can be produced as a contact allergy following the local administration of ointments and suppositories.

Urticaria

Urticaria is referred to as 'hives' or 'nettle rash' and is an acute or chronic allergic reaction in which red weals develop. The weals itch intensely and may last for hours or days. Sometimes urticaria affects areas other than the skin, causing swelling of the tongue, lips and eyelids. This serious variety is called angio-oedema and requires urgent medical attention. Only acute urticaria is likely to be drug-induced, occurring straight away or shortly after the administration of a drug to a sensitised patient, and can be regarded as the cutaneous manifestation of anaphylaxis. Urticaria may arise following treatment with, for example, penicillins, vaccines, indometacin, imipramine, aspirin, dextrans and X-ray contrast media.

Erythema multiforme

The lesions are erythematous maculopapules affecting the hands and feet more than the trunk. They appear over a few days and fade within 1 or 2 weeks. Lesions, which may be 1–2 cm after 48 hours, can reach a size of up to 10 cm with the centre becoming cyanotic – a characteristic 'iris' or target-shaped lesion. Involvement of the mucosa is common. The drugs most likely to cause erythema multiforme are penicillins, phenytoin, carbamazepine, NSAIDs and gold salts.

Toxic epidermal necrolysis

This condition usually starts a few weeks after the start of treatment with the drug concerned. It is characterised by a redness of the whole skin with widespread exfoliation. Causes include captopril, carbamazepine, gold salts and thiazide diuretics.

Lichenoid eruptions

In lichenoid drug eruptions the characteristic wide, flat, mauve pimples of lichen planus skin disease are present but can be associated with papular, scaling and eczematous lesions. The lesions are found mainly on the forearms, neck and between the thighs. Drugs which can cause this condition include phenothiazines, carbamazepine, gold salts, NSAIDs, penicillamine and thiazide diuretics.

Erythema nodosum

The lesions are painful subcutaneous nodules usually limited to extremities and may be preceded by transient erythema. Although not commonly drug induced, erythema nodosum has been observed in women taking oral contraceptives. Other suspect drugs are drugs with a sulphonamide component, salicylates, penicillins and gold salts.

Photosensitivity

Increased sensitivity to light may be produced by thiazide diuretics, tetracyclines, chlorpromazine, promazine, carbamazepine, naproxen and amiodarone. Patients should be warned to avoid exposure to strong sunlight.

DRUG-INDUCED BLOOD DISORDERS

Like other adverse drug reactions, those affecting the blood can be divided into type A and type B reactions. Type A reactions can be predicted from the therapeutic action of the drug. Bone marrow suppression by cytotoxic drugs is a common type A effect.

The nurse has a role in advising patients prescribed high-risk drugs to seek urgent medical attention should they develop signs or symptoms suggestive of haematological adverse drug reactions. Patients will often present with a sore throat, mouth ulcers, rash, malaise, fever, bruising or bleeding. For some high-risk drugs, the risk is such that regular monitoring of the blood count is advised. These include amphoteracin, clozapine, gold therapy, penicillamine, phenytoin, sulfasalazine and zidovudine.

Drugs can cause blood dyscrasias by acting at different stages of haemopoiesis from the stem cell through to the mature cells – red cells, white cells and platelets. Aplastic anaemia, agranulocytosis and thrombocytopenia are blood dyscrasias which can occur.

Aplastic anaemia

In aplastic anaemia there is suppression of red cells (anaemia), white cells (leucopenia) and platelets (thrombocytopenia) resulting from suppression of bone marrow function (hypoplasia). This condition may persist despite drug withdrawal. The presenting features are anaemia, infection and bleeding giving rise to the main symptoms of weakness, fatigue and pallor.

Agranulocytosis

Leucopenia is the term used to describe a reduction in total white cell count but agranulocytosis is more common. This is a selective reduction in granulocytes which include neutrophils, eosinophils and basophils. In agranulocytosis the absence of neutrophils in the blood results in the patient being very susceptible to serious infection. Common symptoms of acute neutropenia include fever, sore throat and painful mucosal ulcers. Any drug that might be implicated should be stopped immediately. In most cases there is spontaneous recovery within 2 weeks of drug withdrawal.

Drugs strongly associated with agranulocytosis are listed in Table 13.3.

Table 13.3 Examples of drugs associated with aplastic anaemia, agranulocytosis and thrombocytopenia

Drug group	Drugs
Antipsychotics	Chlorpromazine, clozapine
Antiepileptics	Carbamazepine
Antibacterials	Chloramphenicol, co-trimoxazole, sulphonamides, cephalosporins, penicillins
Antithyroid drugs	Carbimazole, propylthiouracil
Anti-inflammatory drugs	Indometacin, phenylbutazone
Rheumatic disease suppressants	Gold, penicillamine, sulfasalazine

Thrombocytopenia

Thrombocytopenia is defined as a reduction in platelet count to less than 150×10^9/L. The main presenting feature is haemorrhage which is most commonly seen in the skin, resulting in purpura and petechiae; also nosebleeds (epistaxis) and bleeding from the gums. The mechanism of drug-induced thrombocytopenia is either as a result of reduction in platelet production due to suppression of the bone marrow or an immune reaction. This results in the production of antibodies which reduce the lifespan of platelets in the circulation from 7–10 days to several hours. Table 13.3 lists the drugs most commonly associated with thrombocytopenia.

Cessation of the drug responsible is often sufficient to restore the platelet count within several days. Platelet transfusions may be required if the count is very low. Future exposure to the likely causative drug should be avoided.

DRUG-INDUCED NEUROLOGICAL DISORDERS

Many drugs have the potential to cause adverse effects on the central nervous system (CNS). Headache is a common symptom. Vasodilators such as nitrates, calcium-channel blockers and hydralazine may precipitate a vascular headache but tolerance to this effect usually occurs and the nurse should encourage patients to continue with therapy. Table 13.4 lists drugs commonly associated with headache, particularly on initial therapy.

Table 13.4 Drugs which may cause headache

Drug group	Examples
Antidepressants	Lofepramine, trazodone, venlafaxine
Antipsychotics	Clozapine, risperidone
Anticonvulsants	Gabapentin, lamotrigine, phenytoin, vigabatrin
NSAIDs	Indometacin, naproxen, piroxicam
Nitrates	Glyceryl trinitrate, isosorbide mononitrate
Anti-arrhythmics	Amiodarone, digoxin, metoprolol, verapamil
Ulcer-healing drugs	Proton pump inhibitors, ranitidine
Antidiabetic drugs	Glipizide
Diuretics	Bumetanide, furosemide (frusemide), spironolactone
ACE inhibitors	Enalapril, lisinopril
Calcium-channel blockers	Amlodipine, nimodipine

ADVERSE REACTIONS – CENTRAL NERVOUS SYSTEM

Nausea and vomiting

Chemotherapeutic agents may cause the release of 5-HT (see p. 246) in the small intestine, initiating a vomiting reflex by activating 5-HT receptors. In addition, 5-HT may be released in the brain – which promotes emesis centrally. The emetogenic effect of cancer chemotherapy varies according to the dose and combination of drugs used. High-dose cisplatin therapy is highly emetogenic. Carboplatin is also emetogenic but less so than cisplatin. Other drugs cause gastrointestinal side-effects by a more direct irritant effect on the gut.

Dizziness

Dizziness is a symptom which can arise from most centrally acting drugs, especially on initiation and at higher doses. The nurse's awareness of drugs which cause dizziness (see Table 13.5) will help to prevent falls.

Tinnitus

This refers to any noise, such as ringing, in the ears. The reaction is dose related and the dose must be reduced or the drug stopped. Tinnitus caused by salicylates is an indication of a toxic reaction.

Drowsiness

Some medicines have special labelling requirements because they cause drowsiness, for example: 'This drug may cause drowsiness. If affected, do not drive or operate machinery. Avoid alcoholic drink'. Drowsiness is a common effect of many drugs that act on the central nervous system.

Table 13.5 Examples of drugs associated with dizziness

Class of drug	Examples
Antidepressants	Amitriptyline, clomipramine, sertraline, venlafaxime
Antipsychotics	Haloperidol, trifluoperazine
Drugs in Parkinson's disease and parkinsonism	Orphenadrine, trihexyphenidyl
Anticonvulsants	Gabapentin, lamotrigine, phenytoin, vigabatrin
Opioids	Buprenorphine, diamorphine
NSAIDs	Indometacin, piroxicam
Anti-arrhythmics	Metoprolol, mexiletine, verapamil
Ulcer-healing drugs	Proton pump inhibitors, ranitidine
Diuretics	Bumetanide
ACE inhibitors	Enalapril, lisinopril
Calcium-channel blockers	Amlodipine, nifedipine

Parkinsonism

Parkinson's disease, due to a decrease in dopamine production, is characterised by tremor, rigidity and a poverty of spontaneous movements. Drug-induced parkinsonism resembles Parkinson's disease and occurs to varying degrees in patients treated with antipsychotic drugs. The phenothiazines (e.g. trifluoperazine, fluphenazine), the butyrophenones (e.g. haloperidol) and the diphenylbutyl piperidines (e.g. pimozide, fluspirilene) are associated with a higher incidence of extrapyramidal effects. Drug-induced parkinsonism is reversible on dose reduction or drug withdrawal. Other drugs which have been implicated in parkinsonism include prochlorperazine, metoclopramide and tricyclic antidepressants.

ALLERGIC EMERGENCY (ANAPHYLACTIC SHOCK)

This is a life-threatening reaction with abrupt onset caused by exposure of sensitised individuals to specific allergens. The mechanism in susceptible individuals involves the production of IgE antibody directed against the antigens. IgE binds to the surface of the mast cells and basophils. Subsequent exposure to antigen triggers the release of various substances, predominant among which is histamine. This causes:

- vasodilatation
- increased capillary permeability
- tissue oedema.

These changes give rise to:

- hypotension
- urticaria
- erythema of face and neck.

The reaction develops rapidly, reaching a maximum within 5–30 minutes. Individuals who experience an anaphylactic reaction may have a personal or family history of allergy.

In a severe reaction the signs and symptoms are:

- pallor or cyanosis with weakening pulse
- skin cold and clammy to touch
- swelling of the glottis
- bronchoconstriction
- feeling of faintness
- loss of consciousness.

Other less serious features include:

- nasal congestion
- rhinorrhoea
- hoarseness.

Death from anaphylactic shock is due mostly to respiratory tract obstruction resulting from laryngeal oedema and bronchoconstriction. The incidence of these serious reactions is low, but in their rarity lies danger.

Common causes include:

- drugs, particularly if given by injection
- blood products
- insect stings
- desensitising agents
- certain foods (nuts, fish, shellfish).

The following groups of drugs are most commonly implicated:

- vaccines
- antibiotics, particularly penicillins
- desensitising solutions
- heparin
- anti-inflammatory analgesics
- neuromuscular blocking drugs
- hydroxocobalamin (rarely)
- cytotoxic drugs.

Anaphylaxis is more likely to occur as the result of an injection than from taking an oral preparation.

Prevention

The following actions may help to prevent an anaphylactic reaction:

- Ask the patient if he/she has suffered any previous reaction to drugs.
- Ask the patient if he/she is taking drugs currently, including both prescribed and non-prescribed drugs.
- Ask the patient if he/she has suffered from previous allergies such as asthma, hay fever, eczema.
- If in doubt, discuss with the doctor or other colleague before giving the drug.
- Consider giving a small, test dose and carefully observe the patient before giving the full dose.

Treatment

This takes the form of drug therapy and is directed towards antagonising the effects of chemical mediators, and preventing the further release of mediator substances.

First-line treatment includes laying the patient flat then restoring the blood pressure by administering 0.5–1 mL of adrenaline (epinephrine) 1 in 1000 (0.5–1 mg) by the intramuscular route as quickly as possible. This is repeated every 10–15 minutes until improvement in the blood pressure occurs.

Adrenaline (epinephrine) inhibits the release of mediator chemicals from mast cells, limiting the severity of anaphylaxis. It also stimulates the β_2 receptors in bronchial smooth muscle, causing bronchodilatation. Where there is a severe reaction, the adrenaline (epinephrine) injection is followed by chlorphenamine (chlorpheniramine) given by slow intravenous injection and continued for 24–48 hours to prevent a relapse. This is an antihistamine or H_1-receptor blocking drug. The effect of this is to block the H_1-receptor-mediated actions of histamine, reducing vascular permeability and bronchospasm.

Corticosteroids such as hydrocortisone or prednisolone are of no value in the immediate treatment of anaphylaxis as onset of their therapeutic effect takes several hours. They are, however, very useful in preventing further deterioration in severely affected patients by inhibiting the release of inflammatory mediators and suppressing inflammatory reactions. Some patients with severe allergy to insect stings may be advised to carry an adrenaline (epinephrine) inhaler or syringes pre-filled with adrenaline solution.

Peanut allergy

Peanut allergy is probably the most common cause of food anaphylaxis. Peanuts are widely used as both ingredients in processed foods and readily identified peanut products such as peanut butter and roasted peanuts. Peanut oil has wide application as an industrial lubricant and as an ingredient in healthcare products e.g. Naseptin cream, arachis oil enema and cosmetics. Nurses need to be aware and check the patient is not a known allergy sufferer.

The allergen is contained in the protein but has been identified in cooking oils. Avoidance of exposure to the allergen is very difficult but people with a known allergy must take every precaution to avoid exposure by checking carefully the foodstuffs they consume and not experimenting with unknown foods. This is vitally important since the allergen is very potent and mere traces can cause severe problems. The anaphylaxis caused by peanuts (and other nuts) is characterised by circulatory collapse and hypotension. Loss of consciousness, shock and cardiac disturbances may occur. As with other allergies, oedema of the larynx, epiglottis and pharynx may cause suffocation leading to death.

Treatment of peanut anaphylaxis follows accepted practice for the treatment of other allergies. Milder reactions are treated with antihistamines, and adrenaline (epinephrine) is used for severe reactions. Prefilled adrenaline syringes should be carried by those with a history of severe reactions.

ROLE OF THE NURSE IN ADVERSE DRUG REACTIONS

The nurse in liaison with the doctor and pharmacist can play an important role in identifying adverse drug reactions or situations where these may occur and as a result may be able to reduce the incidence or severity of these occurrences. Factors involved in this include:

- recognising where a patient has had a previous allergic reaction and ensuring that there is not an exposure to the allergen which caused the reaction
- identifying drugs which are known to produce predictable dose-related adverse effects and avoiding their use where an equally effective and safer alternative is available
- checking that patients are not unnecessarily exposed to risk through use of unrequired drugs, disregard for warnings, special precautions or contraindications
- ensuring that patients receive patient information leaflets and counselling on the correct use of their medicines.

The role of the nurse in relation to adverse drug reactions may be summed up as anticipating and avoiding reactions and recognising and responding to any that arise. A sound knowledge of the principles of pharmacology and ready access to current data on medicines are essential if the nurse is to play a full part in anticipating those situations where an adverse reaction to a drug is likely. A thorough initial history of medicine taking and any previous experience of side-effects should be taken. Nurses are trained to be active listeners. Adverse drug reactions may be avoided or at least minimised by following the manufacturer's or pharmacist's instructions. For example, gastrointestinal effects may be avoided by the simple action of taking the medicine with food. Midwives can advise women at what stage in their pregnancy medicines, if they must have them, may be safely taken. Warning patients and/or relatives of possible adverse effects should be done in such a way, however, that they receive sufficient information without at the same time being put into a state of alarm.

To fulfil their role in this field, nurses must not only be observant but must also be able to make connections between their observations and the treatment being given. In any unexplained illness, they should always consider the possibility of an adverse reaction to the medicines the patient is receiving. Particular care should be taken in this regard in relation to older people since the incidence of adverse drug reactions tends to increase with age as a result of metabolic and excretory processes becoming impaired. Having noted signs which they suspect may be linked with the medicines being taken, nurses must know how to respond appropriately. At one extreme, they may simply require to advise the patient to 'wait and watch'; at the other, immediate action may be called for, including the instigation of appropriate resuscitative measures. Finally, nurses must be able to report and record accurately their observations, any significant symptoms described by the patient and any decisions made or advice given.

TREATMENT OF POISONING

At the extreme end of the adverse drug reaction spectrum is poisoning. The treatment of acute poisoning, either intentional or accidental, presents a major challenge to clinical staff. Careless storage of medicines and household products is a common cause of accidental poisoning in children. Natural products, leaves, berries, etc. may also be implicated. Intentional poisoning is a complex subject. Self-poisoning may be undertaken by people determined to end their life. However, in some cases the ingestion of a poisonous substance, often a medicinal product, may be a 'cry for help' or form part of a manipulative personal situation. Many social factors contribute to the tragic situations that can arise, e.g. poverty, alcoholism, drug abuse and social deprivation.

The management of a patient who has been poisoned, whatever the cause or circumstances, must be directed towards the maintenance of respiration and circulation. Seldom are the symptoms of poisoning highly specific, but many clues are available to the observant doctor or nurse. Tablets may be found in the victim's possessions or at the scene of the tragedy. Family members and/or friends may be able to give useful information. The first priority of treatment is to maintain the patient's vital functions. If necessary, laboratory tests to determine the exact nature of the poison are undertaken at an appropriate time. National Poisons Centres provide back-up, advice and guidance on clinical management in special situations. Key aspects in the treatment of poisoning are as follows:

- maintenance of respiration – physical methods
- maintenance of circulation – physical methods and drug treatment

- maintenance of body temperature – physical methods
- maintenance of fluid and electrolyte levels in accordance with biochemical tests
- removal of the poisons (gastric lavage/emesis/active elimination)
- inactivation of the poisons – use of activated charcoal to adsorb the poison
- correction of metabolic complications, e.g. metabolic acidosis.

Once the acute situation has been dealt with and the patient assessed it may be necessary to call in specialised psychiatric help.

Some poisons have specific antidotes, but there can be no substitute for general supportive measures outlined above. An outline of the agents available for the treatment of poisoning is given in Table 13.6. These agents will be used together with general supportive measures.

In considering the treatment of acute poisoning, it is important to recognise the place of prevention, especially in children. Some useful guidelines for parents are given in Box 13.1.

DRUG INTERACTIONS

The term interaction can be applied to the effects that drugs, food and other substances can have on the action

Box 13.1 Guidelines on the prevention of child poisoning for parents or guardians

- Keep medicines locked away
- If your medicine is stored in a fridge, fit a safety lock to the door
- Teach children not to play with medicines
- Never share medicines
- Warn children not to swallow anything unfamiliar
- Never pretend that medicines are sweets
- Dispose of medicines at the pharmacy

If you think your child has swallowed a medicine or poison:

- Get the child to the nearest accident and emergency department as soon as possible
- Take the drug container with you so that the doctor knows what has been taken
- Do not try to make the child sick
- If the child is unconscious, lay on one side to ease breathing and stop choking

Table 13.6 Treatment of poisoning

Agent/method	Uses/indications
Acetylcysteine	This drug is given by IV infusion in the treatment of paracetamol poisoning. The dose is determined by reference to plasma paracetamol levels. Treatment with acetylcysteine is designed to reduce the often fatal liver damage caused by paracetamol ingestion in high doses. Treatment must be commenced as soon as possible after ingestion. If a period of more than 24 hours has passed after ingestion the liver damage will be irreversible
Charcoal (activated)	Used to bind poisons, thus reducing absorption. A single dose of up to 50 g reduces absorption, and repeated doses of activated charcoal enhance the elimination of certain drugs after absorption
Desferrioxamine	This is a specific antidote for iron poisoning. The drug acts by chelating the iron. Administration is by mouth, IM injection, or IV infusion, depending on the patient's condition
Dicobalt edetate	This is a specific antidote used in the treatment of cyanide poisoning
Dimercaprol	In poisoning by metals such as gold and mercury. Also in poisoning by arsenic and antimony
Haemoperfusion and haemodialysis	These techniques may be used in severely poisoned patients particularly in the treatment of salicylate and barbiturate poisoning
Ipecacuanha	Used to induce emesis. Available as a specially made up elixir for oral administration. Must be used with care, but is preferred to other emetics such as common salt (sodium chloride)
Methionine	Given orally in paracetamol poisoning. This may be a useful approach where hospital treatment is not readily available
Naloxone	Naloxone is a specific antidote for opioid overdosage. The IM, IV or SC routes can be used, the dosage being determined in accordance with the patient's needs, e.g. 2 mg in 500 mL as an IV infusion, the rate of infusion depending on the patient's condition
Penicillamine	Copper and lead poisoning by oral administration
Pralidoxime	With atropine in the treatment of organophosphorus poisoning by IM or slow IV injection
Sodium calcium edetate	The treatment of lead poisoning by IV infusion
Sodium nitrate and sodium thiosulphate	Used in combination in the treatment of cyanide poisoning

of a drug. When two or more drugs are administered at the same time they may exert their effect independently or they may interact. This may result in the action of one drug being more potent or being reduced because of an effect by the other drug. Many drug interactions are harmless, and a particular drug combination may cause harm to only a small proportion of individuals who receive it. The drugs most often involved in serious interactions are those with a narrow therapeutic range (e.g. aminoglycosides, phenytoin) and those where the dose must be closely monitored according to the response (e.g. anticoagulants, antidiabetic drugs). Patients at increased risk from drug interactions include those with impaired renal and liver function, and the elderly because of changes in physiology due to ageing and also because older people are prescribed proportionately more drugs than younger people.

Drug interactions can be considered under three main headings:

- chemical interactions
- pharmacokinetic interactions
- pharmacodynamic interactions.

Chemical interactions

These may occur in a number of situations, especially where drugs are reconstituted prior to administration either in large or small volumes. The use of a Central Intravenous Additive Service (CIVAS) will help to minimise problems but if reconstitution has to be carried out at ward level, the manufacturer's instructions must always be followed and the correct diluent used. For example, amphotericin must be diluted in glucose 5% injection with a pH greater than 4.2. Care must be taken when calcium salts and phosphate are added to an intravenous infusion since above certain concentrations a precipitate is formed. Appendix 6 of the BNF gives a list of suitable infusion vehicles to be used in specific circumstances.

Mixing of drugs in a syringe prior to administration can cause a chemical interaction. Such admixtures may facilitate ease of administration, e.g. in a syringe driver, but pharmaceutical advice should always be taken to help to avoid harmful clinical interactions, particularly if the contents of the syringe become cloudy or opaque.

Pharmacokinetic interactions

These occur when one drug alters the absorption, distribution, protein binding, metabolism or excretion of another, thus increasing or reducing the amount of drug available to produce its pharmacological effects.

Absorption

Antacids and binding agents such as colestyramine may impair absorption of a drug from the gastrointestinal tract by binding the drug, e.g. iron, tetracycline. Other drugs such as metoclopramide may influence the gut transit time and hence the absorption of other drugs. In many cases this influences the rate of absorption rather than the amount absorbed (extent). Most of these interactions have a low level of clinical significance and can be managed by separating the administration of each drug.

Protein binding

Many drugs bind to plasma protein, particularly albumin. At any one time there is an equilibrium between bound drug (attached to protein) and free drug. In general, the bound fraction is unavailable for activity, and the effect of the drug is exerted by the free fraction.

Protein displacement interactions occur where two drugs compete for the same binding site and one or both is displaced. This increases the concentration of free drug, but this is usually compensated for by increased excretion. The effect is usually transient and of minor importance. There may be exceptions, for example if the excretory mechanisms are unable to cope with the increased load (e.g. in renal or hepatic impairment) or if the therapeutic margin of the drug is so narrow that even transient increases can be damaging.

Phenylbutazone alters metabolism as well as protein binding of warfarin, potentially resulting in prolonged disturbances of anticoagulant control.

Lithium levels which are within the therapeutic range in a patient stabilised on lithium and a diuretic may be upset during illness which alters fluid and electrolyte balance.

Metabolism

Many drugs are metabolised in the body, principally in the liver. The result of metabolism may be inactive metabolites which are excreted (usually in bile or urine), or active metabolites which contribute to the effects of the drug. Some drugs (pro-drugs) are inactive until metabolised to their active form.

There are a number of enzyme systems which metabolise drugs and the most important is called the cytochrome P450 system. Interactions involving enzyme systems fall into two main categories.

Enzyme induction. Certain drugs may cause enzyme induction, increasing the level of a particular enzyme. Drugs which are metabolised by this enzyme will therefore be broken down more quickly. Griseofulvin potentiates the enzymes which break down warfarin, and rifampicin potentiates those which break down oestrogens and progestogens. The latter interaction is important where the patient is taking oral contraceptives since these will be broken down more quickly resulting in an increased risk of pregnancy occurring.

Enzyme inhibition. Enzyme inhibition results in a lower level of enzymes resulting in an accumulation of the drug which is metabolised by these particular enzymes. Examples of enzyme inhibitors are allopurinol, erythromycin, clarithromycin, fluconazole and ketoconazole.

Renal excretion

Drugs are eliminated through the kidney by both glomerular filtration and active tubular excretion. Competition can occur when drugs share the active transport mechanisms in the proximal tubule. Probenecid delays the excretion of all penicillins and some cephalosporins, which leads to their increased plasma levels. A combination of aspirin and methotrexate leads to a risk of toxicity from increased levels of methotrexate because of competition for tubular secretion. NSAIDs can reduce glomerular filtration rate especially during stress and can reduce elimination of renally excreted drugs. Figure 13.1 summarises pharmacokinetic influence in drug interactions.

Pharmacodynamic interactions

These are interactions between drugs which have similar or antagonistic pharmacological effects or side-effects. They may be due to competition at receptor sites, or occur between drugs acting on the same physiological system. They are usually predictable from a knowledge of the pharmacology of the interacting drugs; in general, those demonstrated with one drug are likely to occur with related drugs. They occur to a greater or lesser extent in most patients who receive the interacting drugs.

These interactions occur between drugs which have similar or antagonistic pharmacological effects or side-effects.

Interactions at receptor sites

These interactions occur when two drugs act on the same site either antagonistically or synergistically.

Antagonism. An example of this, which is therapeutically beneficial, is the reversal of the effects of opiates by naloxone.

Synergism. Aminoglycosides enhance the effect of non-polarising muscle-relaxant drugs such as atracurium.

Sedation with anxiolytics and hypnotics is enhanced by many other drugs with sedative properties, including some antihistamines, antidepressants and antipsychotics. Few of these interactions are hazardous and some may be beneficial in patients for whom a sedative effect is appropriate.

Interactions between drugs affecting the same system

Acetazolamide, carbenoxolone, corticosteroids and corticotropin interact with thiazide diuretics, furosemide (frusemide) and bumetanide, causing increased urinary potassium loss resulting in hypokalaemia. Antihypertensive drugs are potentiated by hypnotics, tranquillisers and levodopa which produce hypotension as a side-effect.

Interactions due to altered physiology

These interactions can occur in a number of ways, e.g. carbenoxolone and corticosteroids antagonise the effect of antihypertensive drugs because of fluid retention.

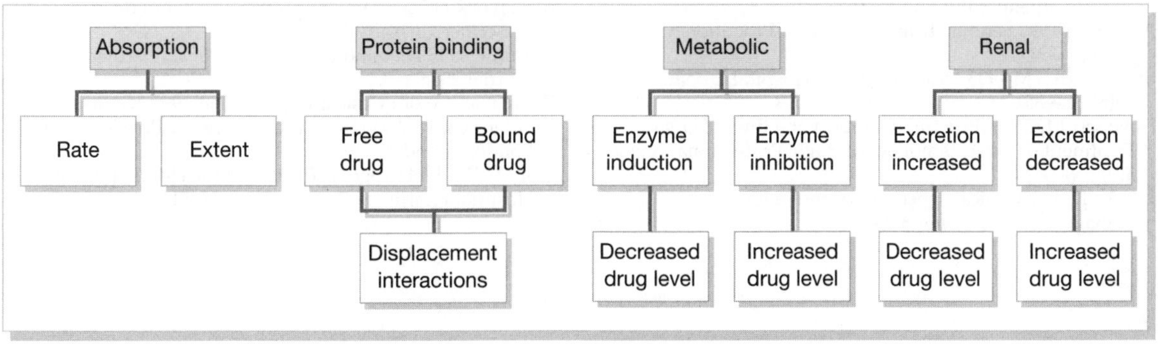

Figure 13.1 Pharmacokinetic interactions.

Potassium-losing diuretics may give rise to digoxin toxicity because of increased potassium loss.

Drug interactions with alcohol

Alcohol can interact with many drugs. It has a depressant effect on the nervous system and when administered concurrently with CNS depressants the effect is additive. Alcohol increases the risk of death from an overdose of these drugs. The vasodilator effect of alcohol increases the postural hypotension of antihypertensive drugs. It can cause postural hypotension with peripheral vasodilators (e.g. pentoxifylline (oxpentifylline)) and anti-anginal drugs (e.g. nitrates, verapamil). This interaction can also occur with metronidazole and procarbazine. Some alcoholic drinks contain tyramine. If this is taken along with monoamine oxidase inhibitors such as phenelzine or tranylcypromine there is a risk of a hypertensive crisis. People who abuse drugs may be especially at risk from 'cocktails' of drugs with alcohol.

Minimising drug interactions

Avoid combinations of drugs where possible

If the potential hazards of adding an interacting drug to existing therapy outweigh any benefit, then the patient may have to be denied the new therapy.

However, in most cases, an alternative can be found which does not interact in the same manner. If there is no alternative to the 'new' drug, then perhaps the existing therapy can be changed.

The choice of an alternative may depend on whether or not an interaction is a 'class' effect which is likely to apply to any drug with a similar mode of action and/or chemical structure. For example, cimetidine is known to inhibit the metabolism of carbamazepine, phenytoin and valproate and in this case ranitidine may be considered as an alternative.

Adjust the dose

If the net effect of an interaction is to increase or reduce the effect of one or more drugs, then modification of the dose of one or both may compensate for this. If a patient on lithium therapy is commenced on an NSAID, the excretion of lithium is reduced, resulting in higher plasma levels. A reduction in dose will compensate for this. Dose modification may be necessary on discontinuation of a drug as well as at introduction.

Dose adjustment can also involve a change to the timing of doses so that plasma concentrations of one drug are relatively low when the second is given. This may or may not be effective depending, for example, on the half-life of each drug.

Monitor the patient

Whatever course of action is taken in the face of a potential interaction, it may be prudent to monitor the patient more closely for a realistic period after change of therapy.

FURTHER READING

[Anonymous] 1996 Drugs and alcohol: harmful cocktails? Drug and Therapeutics Bulletin 34:36–38
[Anonymous] 1997 Drug-induced agranulocytosis. Drug and Therapeutics Bulletin 35(7):49–52
Aronson J 1993 Serious drug interactions. Practitioner 237:789–791
Breathnach S M 1993 Drug eruptions. Hospital Update 19(6):344–351
Davenport D 1993 Structured support at a time of crisis. Treatment of paracetamol overdosage. Professional Nurse 8(9):558–562
Davies R 1997 Clinical aspects of peanut allergy and management. Prescriber 8:23–28
Dawson M, Hodgson S L, Judd A 1997 Poisoning – common exposures and problems. Pharmaceutical Journal 4:111–115
McGavock H 2002 How to predict and avoid drug reactions. Prescriber 13(10):107–111
Mason P 1995 Diet and drug interactions. Pharmaceutical Journal 255:94–97
Royal College of Physicians of London 1997 Medication for older people, 2nd edn. Royal College of Physicians of London, London
Tully H P 1993 Iatrogenic disease in the elderly patient. Hospital Pharmacy Practice 3(3):138–144

CHAPTER CONTENTS

14

Autonomic nervous system

INTRODUCTION

The autonomic or involuntary nervous system conveys all outputs from the central nervous system to the rest of the body, except for skeletal muscle. It controls the activities of the gastrointestinal tract, the respiratory system, the urogenital system, the heart and vascular system, the eyes and various secretory glands. The autonomic nervous system consists of two divisions, and most organs are supplied by nerves from both of these divisions. They are called the sympathetic and the parasympathetic systems. Each organ controlled by the autonomic nervous system can be stimulated or inhibited according to physiological needs, and the functions of the sympathetic and parasympathetic nervous systems can be regarded as having basically opposite effects which counterbalance each other in order to maintain the body systems functioning smoothly.

ANATOMY

The sympathetic nervous system consists of a series of short nerve fibres (preganglionic fibres) from the thoracic and lumbar parts of the spinal cord passing to one of a chain of ganglia on either side of the vertebral column (Fig. 14.1). Here they form a synapse or junction, and other longer nerve fibres (postganglionic fibres) pass out to the smooth muscle of the visceral organs.

The preganglionic parasympathetic nerve fibres originate in the midbrain, medulla and sacral parts of the spinal cord. They synapse in ganglia situated either in or close to the innervated organ. Consequently, the postganglionic parasympathetic nerve fibre is much shorter than the postganglionic sympathetic fibre (Fig. 14.1).

Transmitters

When an impulse passes from the central nervous system along a preganglionic fibre and reaches a ganglion,

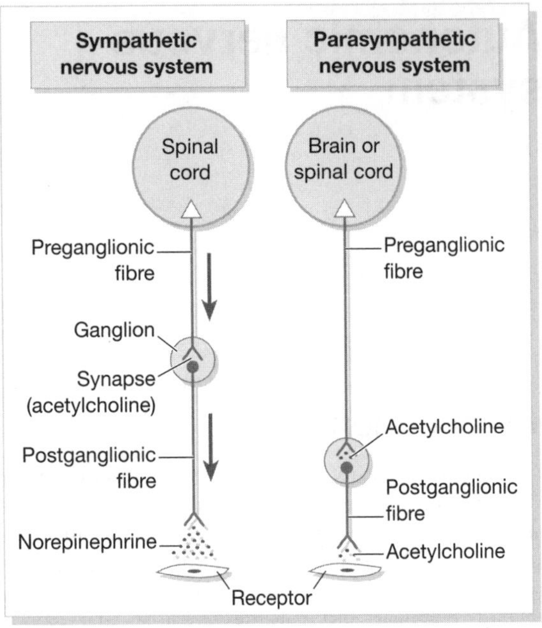

Figure 14.1 Neurotransmitter systems.

a messenger substance, acetylcholine, is liberated in order to carry the impulse across the ganglion to the postganglionic fibre. As soon as the impulse has passed, the released acetylcholine is immediately broken down by an enzyme, cholinesterase. The impulse continues along the postganglionic fibre and, in the case of parasympathetic nerves, acetylcholine is released when the impulse reaches the point where the nerve joins the organ concerned. The acetylcholine acts on a receptor to produce the necessary response. The response is limited in duration and intensity by the rapid destruction of the acetylcholine, as occurred in the ganglion.

A similar process takes place in the sympathetic nervous system up to the junction of the nerve and tissue but, instead of acetylcholine being released, the neurotransmitter is noradrenaline (norepinephrine) (Fig. 14.1). In addition, this is accompanied by a release of noradrenaline (norepinephrine) and adrenaline (epinephrine) from the medulla of the adrenal gland. These substances enter the systemic circulation and produce widespread effects since they can act on a number of receptors, i.e. α, β_1 and β_2. The noradrenaline (norepinephrine) may be broken down by monoamine oxidase or may be taken back up into the nerve ending by a reuptake mechanism. If this did not happen there would be continual stimulation of the receptors. This process is known as chemical transmission of nerve impulses. It is important to have an understanding of the processes involved because many drugs act by interfering with these processes.

Table 14.1 Commonly used terms

	Sympathetic nervous system	Parasympathetic nervous system
Agonists	Sympathomimetics	Parasympathomimetics
Antagonists	Sympatholytics	Parasympatholytics

Receptors

Receptors are generally termed according to the transmitter which activates the receptor, i.e. cholinergic receptors are activated by acetylcholine and noradrenergic receptors by noradrenaline (norepinephrine). A drug which acts on a receptor in a way similar to that of the transmitter is called an agonist; a drug which prevents the action of the transmitter at the receptor is an antagonist.

Some commonly used terms are given in Table 14.1.

Cholinergic agents are drugs that promote the function of the neurotransmitter acetylcholine. The cholinergics are also called parasympathomimetics because they produce effects that imitate parasympathetic nerve stimulation. Drugs which antagonise the effect of postganglionic parasympathetic nerve stimulation are called parasympatholytics.

Similarly, noradrenaline (norepinephrine) and drugs which mimic the effect of postganglionic sympathetic nerve stimulation are called sympathomimetics, and those which antagonise this effect are called sympatholytics.

SYMPATHETIC AND PARASYMPATHETIC NERVE STIMULATION

The activation of these two parts of the autonomic nervous system is of profound physiological importance. Often both systems act on the same organ (at different times) but produce opposite effects. In a healthy person the two parts of the system are in dynamic equilibrium in response to physiological needs. In order to understand how drugs affect the functioning of the autonomic nervous system it is necessary to know which organs respond to stimulation and which receptors are involved (Table 14.2).

EFFECT OF DRUGS ON THE AUTONOMIC NERVOUS SYSTEM

Drugs are administered in order to modify the activity of the autonomic nervous system. These drugs can act in a number of ways; they can:

- mimic the effect of sympathetic or parasympathetic stimulation

Table 14.2 Actions resulting from sympathetic and parasympathetic nerve stimulation

Organ	Sympathetic response	Sympathetic receptor type	Parasympathetic response
Heart	Rate and force of contraction increased	β_1	Rate and force of contraction decreased
Blood vessels			
skin	Vasoconstriction	α	Dilatation
skeletal muscle	Vasoconstriction	α	Dilatation
	Vasodilatation	β_2	
Lungs (bronchial muscles)	Relaxation	β_2	Contraction
Intestine			
motility and tone	Decreased	α and β_2	Increased
sphincters	Contraction	α	Relaxation
glands	No effect		Secretion
Urinary system			
bladder	Relaxed	β_2	Contracted
sphincter	Contracted	α	Relaxed
Eye			
pupil (radial muscle)	Dilatation	α	Constriction
ciliary muscle	Relaxation	β	Contraction
Salivary glands	Sparse, thick secretion	α	Profuse, watery secretion
Skin			
sweat glands	Secretion	α	No effect
Male sex glands	Ejaculation	α	Erection

- interfere with the enzymatic destruction of transmitters and thus potentiate the natural response
- block the receptor to the transmitter and reduce or negate the effect of the neurotransmitter (noradrenaline (norepinephrine) or acetylcholine).

Adrenaline (epinephrine) acts at a number of receptor sites and, following injection, various actions quickly become apparent:

- an increase in force and rate of the heart (β_1)
- an increase in systolic blood pressure due to increased output of blood by the heart (β_1)
- bronchodilatation (β_2).

Because adrenaline (epinephrine) is non-specific, its use is now restricted mainly to the treatment of anaphylaxis by intramuscular injection.

More selective drugs are now used in the treatment of various conditions, in order to reduce side-effects. Examples of the types of drug affecting the autonomic nervous system are listed in Tables 14.3–14.5. Many of the side-effects of these drugs are due to their ability to alter the equilibrium of the autonomic nervous system.

Table 14.3 Sympathomimetics

Drug	Receptor stimulated	Effect
Methoxamine	α	Causes vasoconstriction of peripheral blood vessels and is used to control blood pressure in anaesthesia
Dobutamine	β_1	Increases force of contraction of the heart in cardiac failure
Salbutamol Terbutaline	β_2	Bronchodilatation in asthmatics

Antimuscarinic/anticholinergic actions

The actions of a substance called muscarine were found to be similar to those of choline, a substance present in the body. However, the acetyl ester of choline, acetylcholine, also had muscarinic-like actions which were much more potent than choline. Responses to acetylcholine mimicked the effects of parasympathetic nerve stimulation. These actions of acetylcholine became known as muscarinic or parasympathomimetic actions.

There are many drugs that block the muscarinic actions of acetylcholine and other parasympathomimetic drugs. Most of the therapeutically useful drugs in this class block muscarinic receptors by competitive antagonism. They also block most of the responses evoked by stimulation of parasympathetic nerves.

Drugs that block muscarinic receptors are sometimes called anticholinergic drugs, although this is rather too

Table 14.4 Adrenergic blocking drugs

Drug	Receptor blocked	Effect	Side-effects
Terazosin	α	Causes vasodilatation – used in hypertension	Peripheral oedema
Sotalol	β_1 and β_2	Slows the heart and reduces cardiac output; used in hypertension and angina	Bradycardia, bronchospasm (acts on β_2 receptors in lungs)
Metoprolol Atenolol	Mainly β_1	As for sotalol	More selective – less likelihood of bronchospasm

Table 14.5 Drugs affecting the autonomic nervous system

Drug	Action	Side-effects
*Parasympathomimetics – these mimic the effect of parasympathetic stimulation**		
Pilocarpine	Contracts ciliary muscle, improving drainage and relieving pressure in the eye in glaucoma	Constriction of pupil, blurring of vision
Anticholinesterase drugs – these drugs block the enzyme responsible for the breakdown of acetylcholine, i.e. cholinesterase		
Neostigmine	Used to treat muscle weakness in myasthenia gravis	Salivation, sweating, gastric secretion, motility, diarrhoea
Rivastigmine	Maintains higher levels of acetylcholine which can relieve the symptoms of Alzheimer's disease in certain patients	Sweating, GI disturbances
Parasympatholytics (anticholinergics) – these drugs block the receptor and have an effect opposite to that of parasympathomimetics		
Hyoscine hydrobromide	Antispasmodic; used to dry excessive bronchial and salivary secretions	Hallucinations, ataxia; avoid in glaucoma
Ipratropium	Relieves bronchoconstriction	Dry mouth; avoid high doses in glaucoma

*Parasympathomimetics are contraindicated in hyperthyroidism (cause glands to secrete), peptic ulcer, bronchial asthma, bradycardia, hypotension and parkinsonism.

broad a term since it must logically include drugs that block responses to cholinergic nerves other than post-ganglionic parasympathetic nerves; furthermore, it wrongly implies an effect on acetylcholine production. Drugs of this type are related to the prototype drug, atropine, and may be called atropine-like drugs.

SECTION 3

Clinical pharmacology

SECTION CONTENTS

CHAPTER CONTENTS

15

Drug treatment of gastrointestinal disorders

DRUG TREATMENT OF DISORDERS OF THE GASTROINTESTINAL TRACT

Anatomy and physiology

The gastrointestinal tract (GIT) consists of a long, tubular structure extending from the mouth to the anus via the oesophagus, stomach and intestines. Its purpose is to digest, absorb and eliminate substances following the ingestion of food. The process of digestion is assisted by four accessory organs, namely, the salivary glands, liver, gall bladder and the pancreas.

Digestion

Food is digested both mechanically and chemically. Mechanical digestion results from voluntary and involuntary muscle action, i.e. nervous control; chemical digestion is produced by the action of enzymes and hormones. The digestive processes taking place in each section of the GIT are summarised in Table 15.1.

Absorption

The absorption of some nutrients begins in the stomach, and some absorption takes place in the large intestine. By far the most absorption, however, occurs in the small intestine (see Fig. 15.1). Table 15.2 summarises some aspects of the absorption of nutrient materials and drugs from the GIT.

Elimination

Undigested and unabsorbed foodstuffs, along with the bile pigments and bilirubin, are eliminated as waste from the body via the large intestine in the form of faeces. Defecation is the term used to describe the expulsion of faeces from the rectum and anal canal. Prior to the act of defecation, several physiological processes take place; these are shown in Box 15.1.

Table 15.1 Stages of digestion

Organ	Mechanical	Chemical
Mouth	Food taken in is masticated (chewed) by the teeth. The muscular action of the tongue and the presence of saliva convert the food into a moist bolus ready for swallowing	Saliva is produced by the salivary glands under the control of the autonomic nervous system. It consists of water and the enzyme salivary amylase. Salivary amylase converts cooked starches into maltose
Oesophagus	Bolus is propelled forward first by voluntary muscle action and then under autonomic nerve control	No chemical action initiated in the oesophagus
Stomach	The muscular layers produce a churning action and assist peristalsis. The semi-solid mixture produced is known as chyme	Stimulated by the hormone gastrin, gastric juice is produced by the gastric mucosa. It is composed of: • water, which liquefies food • hydrochloric acid, which acidifies food, kills microorganisms and converts the enzyme pepsinogen secreted by the parietal cells into pepsin, an essential factor in the digestion of protein • intrinsic factor, necessary for absorption of vitamin B_{12} • mucus, which, as a lubricant, protects the stomach wall from the harmful effects of hydrochloric acid and protein-digesting pepsin
Small intestine	Onward movement of contents by peristalsis and segmental movement	The hormones secretin and cholecystokinin-pancreozymin (CCK-PZ) stimulate the secretion of pancreatic juice which consists of: • water • mineral salts • enzymes: pancreatic amylase, which converts starches not affected by salivary amylase to sugars; lipase, which converts fats to fatty acids and glycerol; trypsinogen and chymotrypsinogen, which convert polypeptides into amino acids Stimulated by CCK-PZ, bile, secreted by the liver but stored in the gall bladder, passes into the duodenum after a meal has been taken. Bile consists of: • water • mineral salts • mucus • bile salts • bile pigment Bile is essential for the emulsification of fats and the absorption of vitamin K, and it colours and deodorises the faeces Intestinal juice is secreted by glands in the small intestine and consists of: • water • mucus • the enzyme enterokinase
Large intestine	Intermittent waves of peristalsis known as mass movement, often precipitated by the gastrocolic reflex following the entry of food into the stomach	No secretion of enzymes – the last phase of digestion depends on the presence of bacteria in the colon. Bacteria: • ferment foodstuffs in faecal matter, producing gases which form flatus • break down other nutrients and give faeces their distinctive odour • decompose bilirubin, giving faeces their characteristic colour • synthesise vitamins

The act of defecation is voluntarily assisted by contraction of the diaphragm and the muscles of the abdominal wall. Relaxation of the external anal sphincter finally allows the faeces to be expelled.

Disorders and their treatment

Dyspepsia

Duodenal and gastric ulcer disease are significant causes of morbidity and mortality in spite of the great advances made in both their diagnosis and treatment. Well-managed treatment will bring about control of these conditions. Maintenance therapy following healing of an ulcer is frequently required. The key diagnostic features of ulcer disease are localised epigastric pain and nocturnal pain. The pain is often relieved by food and antacids. In some patients the pain may be relieved by vomiting. Endoscopy is used to confirm the diagnosis. There are significant differences between gastric and duodenal ulcers; these are summarised in Table 15.3.

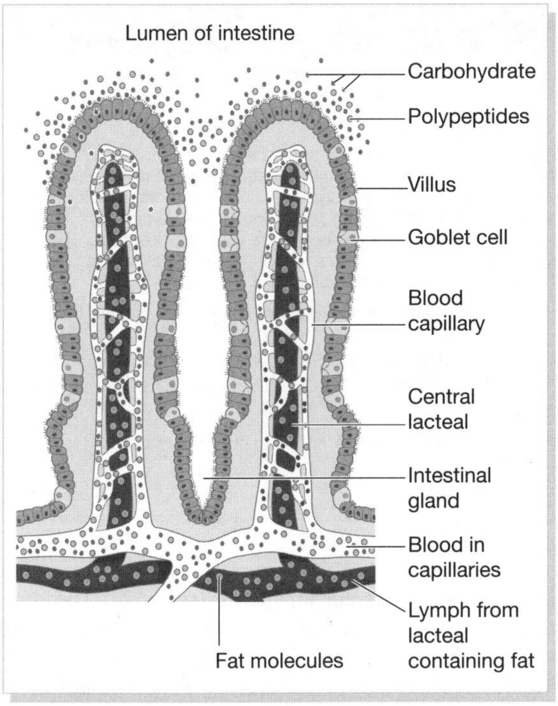

Figure 15.1 Absorption in the small intestine. (From Waugh A, Grant A 2001 Ross and Wilson Anatomy and physiology in health and illness, 9th edn. Churchill Livingstone, Edinburgh.)

Table 15.2 Absorption in the gastrointestinal tract*

Organ	Site of absorption	Substances absorbed
Stomach	Walls of the stomach. Systemic absorption influenced by acid environment and gastric emptying time	Water Alcohol Weak acids, e.g. aspirin, lipid-soluble non-ionised drugs
Small intestine	The villi and microvilli into the capillaries and lacteals. Largest gastrointestinal surface area for absorption. Alkaline environment may influence absorption of some substances	Carbohydrates as monosaccharides Proteins as amino acids Fats as fatty acids and glycerol Vitamins Mineral salts Some water (one-tenth only)
Large intestine	Predominantly the caecum and ascending colon	Water (remaining nine-tenths) Mineral salts, especially sodium Drugs not absorbed in small intestine may be absorbed to some extent

* Absorption of drugs from the GIT is very complex and may be affected by a range of factors, including dosage form, pH, gut motility, presence/absence of food and pathology.

Box 15.1 Physiological processes prior to defecation

Mass movement in pelvic colon
↓
Faecal matter enters rectum
↓
Rectal wall distended
↓
Pressure receptors in wall stimulated
↓
Nerve impulses transmitted to sacral cord
↓
Motor impulses transmitted back from cord via parasympathetic nerves
↓
Rectal muscles contract
↓
Pressure in rectum increases
↓
Reflex relaxation of internal anal sphincter
↓
Desire to defecate

Table 15.3 Peptic ulceration – a comparison

Gastric ulcers	Duodenal ulcers
Rare in patients under 40	Prevalence highest in patients over 60 but occur in all age groups
Pain relief following food intake short-lived	Pain relieved by food intake Pain generally worse before meals
Anorexia and nausea more prominent than in duodenal ulcers	
Gastric acid secretion may be normal or even below normal	Gastric acid is a major factor
Anti-secretory therapy produces healing but more slowly than with duodenal ulcers	Anti-secretory therapy often produces healing in 4 weeks Lesions smaller than in gastric ulcers
Healing can occur without active treatment	
Recurrence rate lower than with duodenal ulcers	Ulcers recur when therapy stopped
Helicobacter pylori infection present in 85% of cases	*Helicobacter pylori* infection present in 100% of cases
Very important to exclude gastric cancer in patients who present with symptoms of gastric ulcer	

The importance of accurate diagnosis cannot be overemphasised. Patients with alarm symptoms such as gastrointestinal bleeding, anaemia, jaundice, vomiting, severe pain and the presence of an epigastric mass need referral to a consultant gastroenterologist.

Table 15.4 Risk factors in dyspepsia

Acid	This is especially important in duodenal ulcer patients who often have twice as many parietal cells as normal subjects
Mucus	Reduced mucus production may be involved since the protective effect of mucus may be lost
Helicobacter pylori (*H. pylori*)	*H. pylori* has the ability to colonise human gastric mucosa, especially the distal antral region of the stomach. The bacteria are found on the mucosal surface and do not penetrate the underlying tissues. The organism stimulates an inflammatory response, and produces ammonia (an alkali) which protects the organism from gastric acid. The organism is widely distributed in the population and has a major role in dyspepsia. The mechanisms involved in acquiring *H. pylori* infection are not well understood. The presence of this organism can be confirmed by a breath test. Breath samples are taken before and after ingestion of an oral solution of ^{13}C urea. Laboratory analysis of the samples is required
Cigarette smoking	The smoking of cigarettes is a major risk factor; peptic ulcers in smokers heal more slowly and are more likely to recur than those in non-smokers
Drugs	Many NSAIDs (see p. 399) can cause serious gastric damage; the extent to which duodenal ulceration is caused by NSAIDs is still the subject of much debate and research
Stress	Stress has long been associated with dyspepsia
Foods	Some foods have been associated with dyspepsia – there is considerable variation between patients; avoidance of foods that cause problems is advocated
Hereditary factors	There is a proven hereditary component in duodenal ulcers

Risk factors in dyspepsia

The risk factors are summarised in Table 15.4.

In healthy people there is a balance between damaging forces (e.g. acid, smoking, drugs, stress) and protective and repair mechanisms. When these forces become out of balance, ulcers and erosions can occur.

Treatment of dyspepsia

Various aspects of treatment are as follows:

General measures. Control of smoking and drinking, and attention to diet (avoiding certain foods that the patient finds exacerbate symptoms).

Simple antacids. Examples include:

- aluminium hydroxide mixture
- magnesium-containing compounds
- combined antacid preparations
- magnesium trisilicate mixture or powder.

Antacids can interact with other drugs (see p. 132) and may cause the coating of enteric-coated tablets to break down in the stomach. Antacids do often provide rapid relief of dyspeptic symptoms but have no ulcer-healing properties.

Combination antacid products. Antacids may be combined with anti-foaming agents (dimeticone) which are claimed to be of value in flatulence. Alginates (derived from certain seaweeds) form a gel-like 'raft' which, when combined with sodium bicarbonate, is effective in reflux oesophagitis.

Atropine-like antisecretory agents. Antimuscarinic agents have little antisecretory effect in doses that are practicable due to atropine-like side-effects. The more specific antisecretory drugs, the H_2-receptor antagonists, are the basis of the treatment of peptic ulceration.

Histamine H_2-receptor antagonists (see p. 124). The introduction of cimetidine and ranitidine (and similar drugs such as famotidine) has played a major part in improving the treatment of peptic ulcer disease. Cimetidine is given orally in a dose of 400 mg twice daily or as a single dose of 800 mg at night. A 4-week course of treatment is given in duodenal ulceration, and a 6-week course in the treatment of gastric ulceration. Once healing has been achieved, a maintenance dose must be given over a long period. Ranitidine is also given orally, 150 mg twice daily or 300 mg at night. The side-effect profile of ranitidine is lower than that of cimetidine. The use of both these drugs has greatly reduced the need for surgical treatment of peptic ulcers. Parenteral forms of the drug are available for use in conditions where the oral route is inappropriate, for example when there is severe bleeding, for the prevention of stress ulceration in seriously ill patients and prophylactically in patients thought to be at risk from acid aspiration syndrome. Although these two drugs have similar properties there are significant differences (Table 15.5). Ranitidine has been combined with a bismuth compound to form a compound ranitidine bismuth citrate. This drug is used together with antibacterial agents in eradication therapy and to treat duodenal ulceration associated with *Helicobacter pylori*. A dose of 400 mg twice daily for 8 weeks is used to treat benign gastric ulceration. *Helicobacter pylori* eradication therapy (see p. 154) has replaced low-dose maintenance therapy with H_2-receptor antagonists. It should be noted that a number of H_2 antagonists are available without prescription from pharmacies. The indications for which these products may be sold are defined in the product licence.

Table 15.5 Similarities of, and differences between, cimetidine and ranitidine

	Cimetidine	Ranitidine
Mode of action	Selective histamine-H_2-receptor antagonist	As cimetidine
Indications	Peptic ulcer disease; Zollinger–Ellison syndrome	As cimetidine
Oral dose	400 mg twice daily	150 mg twice daily
Maintenance dose	400 mg at night	150 mg at night
Availability	Tablets, syrup; parenteral	As cimetidine – also granules
Contraindications and warnings	Dose reduced in patients with impaired renal function	As cimetidine
	Prolongs elimination of drugs metabolised by oxidation in the liver	Some changes (transient) have been reported in liver function
	May mask symptoms of gastric carcinoma	As cimetidine
	Some drug interactions, especially with oral anticoagulants and phenytoin (dosage reduction of these drugs may be needed)	Few drug interactions have been reported
	Rare reports of bradycardia and AV block	As cimetidine
	H_2-receptor antagonism may potentiate falls in blood cell counts caused by other factors, e.g. disease or other drug treatment	Leucopenia and thrombocytopenia have been rarely reported
	Gynaecomastia has been reported but is reversible on stopping treatment	Few reports with ranitidine

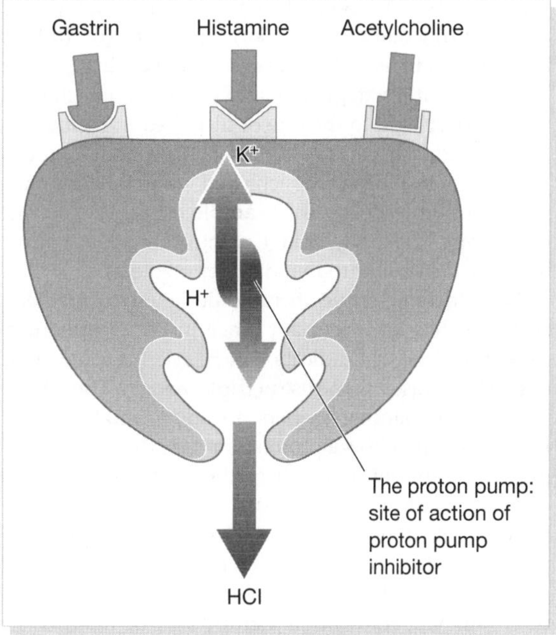

Figure 15.2 Parietal cell: proton pump.

Chelates and complexes. Tripotassium dicitratobismuthate is thought to act by an antibacterial action on *H. pylori*. Other actions attributed to this compound include the stimulation of the secretion of prostaglandin (a mucosal protective) and/or the stimulation of bicarbonate secretion. The usual dose is 2 × 120 mg tablets twice daily. Sucralfate (complex of aluminium hydroxide and sulphated sucrose) has only minimal antacid properties but is an effective treatment for both gastric and duodenal ulcer. The mode of action may be to protect mucosa from acid and pepsin attack. Side-effects include constipation, diarrhoea, dry mouth, aches and pains, and skin rashes.

Prostaglandin analogues (see also p. 402). Misoprostol is a synthetic compound similar to prostaglandin E_1. It acts by inhibiting acid secretion and it promotes the healing of both gastric and duodenal ulcer. It may be given to treat gastric ulceration caused by non-steroidal anti-inflammatory drugs (NSAIDs). Combination products (NSAID and misoprostol) are claimed to be safer than NSAIDs alone for 'at risk' patients, for example, older people.

Carbenoxolone. This drug improves the resistance of gastric mucosa to attack from acid. A combination of carbenoxolone, antacids and alginate is used for the treatment of oesophageal ulceration and inflammation. Carbenoxolone has significant side-effects, such as sodium and water retention, and hypokalaemia. It should be avoided in patients with cardiac problems.

Proton pump inhibitors. Esomeprazole, omeprazole, lansoprazole, pantoprazole and rabeprazole are effective drugs used in the treatment of both gastric and duodenal ulcer. These drugs are the treatment of choice in stricturing and erosive oesophagitis. Patients very much welcome rapid relief from the distressing symptoms of this condition.

The mode of action is based on the property of blocking the hydrogen–potassium adenosine triphosphate enzyme system (see Fig. 15.2) in the parietal cell. This is also a very effective treatment for Zollinger–Ellison syndrome (see below) and reflux oesophagitis. An oral dose of 20 mg daily for 4 weeks is often effective but can be increased in refractory cases to 40 mg daily. It should be noted that the degree of acid suppression achieved is directly related to the rate of ulcer healing. Omeprazole 20 mg daily can produce healing within 4 weeks. This rate of healing can be achieved with H_2 antagonists given in higher doses, for example, ranitidine 300 mg twice daily. The dosage range of the other proton pump inhibitors is similar to that of omeprazole.

Triple therapy. Triple therapy, designed to eradicate *H. pylori*, has an important place in the treatment of dyspeptic disease. Eradication of *H. pylori* is achieved in over 90% of cases by the use of triple therapy. The following regimens, amongst others, are advocated (see BNF). Each regimen utilises a proton pump inhibitor (acid suppressant) plus antibiotics. Treatment must be given for 4 days. Eradication therapy should not be given to patients with non-ulcer dyspepsia or oesophagitis. Chest pain caused by *H. pylori* infection may be difficult to distinguish from cardiac pain. If cardiac problems can be eliminated, eradication therapy may be helpful:

Omeprazole 20 mg twice daily (or lansoprazole 30 mg twice daily)
Clarithromycin 500 mg twice daily
Amoxicillin 1 g twice daily.

Or if allergic to penicillin:

Lansoprazole 30 mg twice daily
Metronidazole 400 mg twice daily
Clarithromycin 500 mg twice daily.

A 2-week dual therapy regimen using a proton pump inhibitor and a single antibacterial agent is inferior to triple therapy and should not be used. Factors such as acceptance by the patient, bacterial resistance, antibiotic allergy, local policies and cost are taken into account. Successful eradication therapy leads to long-term remission but reinfection can occur with *H. pylori*.

If the patient's symptoms persist, this may or may not indicate 'success' of the eradication therapy. If a breath test, carried out 4 weeks after the completion of a course of eradication therapy, indicates the continuing presence of infection, a second but different course of eradication therapy should be given. It is important to check patient compliance before commencing a second course of therapy.

Complications of duodenal and gastric ulceration

Bleeding is a serious complication of ulceration. If uncontrolled, ulceration develops and a blood vessel at the base of the ulcer is penetrated, resulting in serious blood loss. Up to 20% of patients may suffer a bleeding episode and may experience haematemesis and/or melaena. The loss of blood may cause cardiovascular shock which must be treated urgently. Blood transfusion and resuscitative measures will be needed together with the combined skills of both gastroenterologist and surgeon.

Role of the nurse in the care of the dyspeptic patient

In view of the nature of the condition it is essential to ensure that patients comply with treatment regimens, especially in eradication therapy. Compliance by the patient can be improved by explaining to the patient the nature of the condition and the need to take the medication regularly over a period of time. The tendency of some patients to discontinue therapy once the symptoms ease must be recognised and appropriate action taken, otherwise a serious relapse may occur. Some drugs (the bismuth compounds) may darken the tongue and blacken the faeces and it is important to warn patients accordingly. Other drugs used in the treatment of peptic ulcer disease have side-effects but these drugs are generally well tolerated. Dizziness, somnolence and fatigue have been reported with H_2-receptor antagonists.

Many patients who present with peptic ulcer disease are elderly and may have coexisting diseases such as diabetes or cardiovascular problems. Nurses, as well as providing care, can encourage patients to adopt a more healthy lifestyle such as improved dietary habits (avoid highly spiced foods, fatty foods and heavy meals in the evening), cessation of smoking and avoidance of stress. Weight reduction is also important. Excessive alcohol intake is very harmful. Patients with peptic ulcer disease may adjust doses of H_2 antagonists to control their symptoms. Some degree of freedom to adjust dosage (but not in eradication therapy) may be an acceptable part of the patient's care. However, primary carers should be alert for any tendencies the patient may have to increase the dose prior to a planned episode of over-indulgence. Patients receiving eradication therapy must avoid alcohol because of severe interactions.

The availability of H_2 antagonists and a wide variety of antacids over the counter may lead to difficulties if patients receiving prescribed medicines purchase additional medicines. Community nurses will need to be alert to any inappropriate or over-use of non-prescription medicines, especially anti-inflammatory pain-relieving medicines (see p. 35).

Zollinger–Ellison syndrome

This condition is characterised by severe and often intractable ulceration caused by very high levels of acid secretion. The high levels of acid result from the continuous stimulation of the parietal cells by the hormone gastrin. Abnormal amounts of gastrin are produced by a gastrinoma (tumour) often situated in the pancreas. In two-thirds of cases the tumour is malignant.

Treatment of Zollinger–Ellison syndrome
Treatment is with a proton pump inhibitor such as omeprazole. Doses are higher than those used in the treatment of gastric or duodenal ulcer.

- *Drug treatment.* Omeprazole 60 mg once daily initially, increasing up to 120 mg daily in 2 divided doses.
- *Surgical treatment.* Surgery and/or cytotoxic therapy may be valuable if the growth of secondaries is not advanced.

Gastro-oesophageal reflux disease (GORD) (heartburn)

Patients presenting with GORD complain of a 'burning sensation' which is often accompanied by severe pains in the chest which may be difficult to distinguish from cardiac pain. Many patients admitted to hospital for suspected myocardial infarction are found to be suffering from GORD. In other patients the diagnosis creates no difficulty, especially where symptoms occur after a meal. Peptic ulcer disease may coexist with GORD (as may cardiac disease) and it is also important to eliminate gastric neoplasm as a factor. Full diagnostic measures are used to establish the true nature of the patient's condition. Barium meal, endoscopic examination and oesophageal pH monitoring are cornerstones of differential diagnosis together with a full history of the patient.

Treatment of GORD
The patient's dietary habits must be attended to. Weight loss, smoking cessation and reduction in alcohol intake are also vitally important. The head of the patient's bed should be raised by 20 cm.

Since the pain of GORD is caused by refluxing of gastric contents onto very sensitive oesophageal mucosa, it follows that antacids are the first-line agents. Combinations of antacids with alginates are very useful. If reflux does occur, the stomach contents have been 'neutralised' to some extent and therefore are less likely to cause irritation. If simple antacid therapy does not provide relief, omeprazole, or an alternative proton pump inhibitor, should be considered. Proton pump inhibitors are more effective than H_2 antagonists and are the treatment of choice.

Metoclopramide may be useful since this drug improves gastric emptying times, stimulates small intestinal transit and increases the strength of the oesophageal sphincter contraction. Cisapride increases lower oesophageal sphincter pressure and improves oesophageal motor activity. The product licence for cisapride has been suspended because of rare but severe cardiovascular side-effects. Domperidone has actions similar to metoclopramide. If medical treatment fails (this is rare), consideration has to be given to surgical intervention.

Diarrhoea

The term diarrhoea is used to describe an increase in frequency, fluidity and/or volume of stools. It is a leading cause of death in underdeveloped countries. Chronic diarrhoea may occur in conditions such as malabsorption and malnutrition.

In the acute form of diarrhoea, dehydration can quickly develop – especially in infants and older people. Prevention and treatment of dehydration is vital. Fluid and electrolyte replacement takes priority in acute cases admitted to hospital. Abdominal cramp may be relieved by the use of an antispasmodic such as dicycloverine (dicyclomine), alverine and peppermint oil.

Simple gastroenteritis will usually resolve without the need for antibiotic treatment. Where there is systemic infection, systemic antibiotic treatment will be needed.

In acute diarrhoea, anti-motility drugs such as loperamide, codeine phosphate and co-phenotrope may offer some relief, along with fluid and electrolyte replacement, in adults. The management of chronic diarrhoea which occurs with specific disorders of the bowel appears in the relevant parts of this chapter.

Inflammatory bowel disease (IBD)

The most common presenting symptom of IBD is chronic diarrhoea. However, it is important to recognise that diarrhoea may be due to one of a number of causes. Infection often presents as a sudden episode of diarrhoea but more sinister causes of diarrhoea are IBD or neoplastic disease. Differential diagnosis is vitally important so as to ensure that the treatment instigated does not mask the underlying condition. The two main conditions are Crohn's disease (CD) and ulcerative colitis (UC). These conditions have similar features and yet are distinctly separate diseases (Table 15.6). Both diseases are relatively common; within a general practice of 2000 patients, about four will have some form of IBD.

Diagnosis of Crohn's disease and ulcerative colitis
Differential diagnosis relies on clinical examination (including endoscopy) supported by histological examination. Differentiation can be very difficult as both conditions can be mimicked by enteric infections and pseudomembranous colitis.

Table 15.6 A comparison of the main features of Crohn's disease and ulcerative colitis

Crohn's disease (also known as ulcerative enteritis)	Ulcerative colitis
Can affect any part of the GI tract from mouth to anus	Primarily involves large intestine
Most common sites are terminal ileum and ascending colon	
Rectum affected in approximately 50% of patients	Most patients have rectal involvement
Inflammatory process involves all layers of bowel	Inflammatory process mainly confined to mucosa
Presence of multiple granulomas	Multiple granulomas not seen
Clinical symptoms: bloody diarrhoea; anorexia; pain; fever; weight loss due to malabsorption	Clinical symptoms: similar to Crohn's disease but bloody diarrhoea very common; abdominal pain and fever more prominent; signs of malabsorption not seen
Strictures are common	Strictures very rare
Neoplastic changes may be seen in cases of extensive disease	

Drug treatment

Although the causes of IBD are not yet known, knowledge of the factors involved is increasing. Various theories have been put forward. The fact that corticosteroids and immunosuppressants are beneficial in the treatment of IBD lends support to the theory that these diseases are due to an immunological disorder. An infection and/or sensitising agents may be the 'trigger' for the immunological changes that occur in IBD. The pathogenesis of these conditions may be multifactorial with infection, genetic influences, diet and environmental agents combining in ways which are not fully understood. Prostaglandins (see p. 402) have been shown in animal studies to act with other agents such as histamine to alter lymphocyte function and increase vascular permeability. The treatments available do ameliorate the symptoms of IBD, which can be very distressing and debilitating. Table 15.7 gives an outline of the main drugs used in the treatment of UC and CD. In addition to drug treatment, attention must be given to diet, although direct links between diet and IBD are not clear. Foods that have a high residue content are best avoided.

Systemic manifestations of IBD are often seen. Joint disease (arthritis), skin problems (erythema nodosum), aphthous ulcers, eye disease (iritis), gallstones (patients with Crohn's disease of the ileum) and inflammation of the veins of the legs occur in UC.

Treatment given to control the GIT symptoms will help to resolve the systemic manifestations but specific local treatment may be required, for example for inflammatory eye conditions. Regular follow-up and review of medication are essential.

Irritable bowel syndrome (IBS)

Although not all sufferers present for investigation, as many as 20% of adults in the western world, mostly young and female, suffer from the functional disorder of the digestive system known as irritable bowel syndrome. The condition is characterised by abdominal pain (relieved by defecation), abdominal distension, loose frequent stools after the onset of pain, rectal mucus and a feeling of incomplete evacuation. The major presenting features are diarrhoea and constipation. As well as physical signs and symptoms, many IBS sufferers have high stress levels.

Before establishing that the patient does in fact have IBS, it is essential that more serious conditions of the bowel are excluded by studying the history and carrying out haematological investigations as well as sigmoidoscopy. These would include inflammatory bowel disease, infection, malabsorption and carcinoma of the colon.

The contribution that drugs can make to the treatment of IBS is limited. Treatment is directed at whatever is the predominant symptom. Considerable relief can be achieved from bulk laxatives (see Table 15.8) and antispasmodics, many of which can be bought over the counter. Antispasmodics fall into two main categories – antimuscarinics such as atropine, dicycloverine (dicyclomine), hyoscine and propantheline, and smooth muscle relaxants such as alverine, mebeverine and peppermint oil. Antimuscarinics in high doses may cause dry mouth, blurred vision, constipation and urinary retention. In certain individuals, there may be a place for anxiolytics and antidepressants.

Attention to diet is important. Regular meals with a rich fibre content are advocated. Exercise is to be encouraged. Some patients may benefit from alternative therapies such as homeopathy and psychotherapy. There is an extremely important placebo effect in IBS.

Constipation

Normal bowel habit is influenced by upbringing and culture. As a result, constipation is often interpreted in different ways. It arises from decreased colonic activity. Bowel contents pass slowly through the colon, becoming dehydrated and hard with loss of faecal volume. Decreased colonic activity can arise in old age and with immobility, and is often associated with a low dietary fibre intake and dehydration.

Table 15.7 Treatment of IBD

Drug	Dose/formulation	Notes
ANTIDIARRHOEAL AGENTS		
Codeine phosphate Loperamide	15–30 mg three or four times daily; 4 mg initially, then 2 mg after each loose stool with a maximum of 16 mg daily for 5 days	Reduce GI motility; antidiarrhoeal agents should not be used in patients with acute ulcerative colitis
Colestyramine	See page 199	Used for the treatment of diarrhoea in some patients with ileal Crohn's disease
CORTICOSTEROIDS		
Prednisolone	Variable dose depending on the condition; 10 mg three or four times daily is a typical dose given for 2–3 weeks. Above this level, side-effects may be troublesome	Small-bowel diarrhoea reduced by oral corticosteroids. Beneficial action thought to be due to anti-inflammatory and immunosuppressive action.Corticosteroids are especially useful in the acute phase of IBD
Budesonide	Available as 3 mg capsules in two formulations for the treatment of mild/moderate CD affecting the ileum or ascending colon. Two capsule formulations are available; both are controlled-release formulations. Budenofalk is a pH-sensitive formulation which has different release characteristics compared with Entocort CR. Comparative clinical trials are needed to determine the relative advantages of the formulations. In each case, the daily dose is 9 mg for up to 8 weeks. Dosage during the last 2 weeks of treatment should be reduced. The Entocort CR formulation is given as a once-daily dose. A budesonide enema is available (2 mg/100 mL). One enema at bedtime is given for 4 weeks	This corticosteroid has fewer adverse effects than prednisolone since it has less systemic bioavailability. Its activity is mainly topical since it has a high affinity for corticosteroid receptors. In clinical trials, budesonide achieved similar rates of remission to oral prednisolone but with a lower incidence of adverse effects
ANTIMICROBIAL AGENTS		
Metronidazole Tetracycline	Doses given in relation to body weight and carefully monitored by blood level determinations	Bacterial overgrowth in small bowel due to active Crohn's disease may cause diarrhoea which is amenable to treatment with antimicrobial agents in normal doses
Ciclosporin		Potent immunosuppressive drug (see p. 374). Place in treatment of refractory Crohn's disease remains to be further investigated
IMMUNOSUPPRESSIVE THERAPY		
Azathioprine	3 mg/kg body weight per day reducing to smaller maintenance dose according to response	Not first-line therapy but reserved for patients who are intolerant of or who do not respond to corticosteroids. Used to reduce corticosteroid dosage levels in patients with ulcerative colitis. Has been reported to induce remission in patients with Crohn's disease. Adverse effects limit its use (see p. 374)
Infliximab	For severe active Crohn's disease 5 mg per kg by IV infusion over 2 h, repeated at 2 and 6 weeks after the first infusion. Specialist supervision is essential	This drug is a monoclonal antibody active against tumour necrosing factor. Very careful monitoring is essential for signs of acute reactions. This treatment is reserved for patients with a disease state that is not treatable by conventional therapy (aminosalicylates and corticosteroids). The treatment is safe to use in combination with standard drugs
SALICYLATES		
Sulfasalazine	1–2 g four times daily in acute attack. Maintenance dose of 500 mg four times daily. Corticosteroids may be needed in the acute phase	Used for the treatment of active Crohn's disease and is the first-line agent of choice for maintenance therapy in ulcerative colitis. Combination of a salicylate and a sulphonamide. Salicylate part of compound has desired therapeutic effect; sulphonamide part associated with side-effects. An enteric-coated tablet may be useful for patients who are intolerant of the uncoated tablet. Topical sulfasalazine also available in the form of suppositories or retention enema. Drug colours the urine yellow and patients should be warned about this

(*continued*)

Table 15.7 *(continued)*

Drug	Dose/formulation	Notes
Mesalazine (5-aminosalicylic acid)	For acute ulcerative colitis 800 mg (two tablets) three times daily with corticosteroid therapy where necessary. Maintenance dose should be lowest that will maintain remission. 400 mg three times daily up to 800 mg three times daily may be required. A foam enema containing 1 g per metered dose is used for acute attacks affecting the rectosigmoid region; 2 g daily is administered for 4–6 weeks	Sulfasalazine is metabolised to sulfapyridine and 5-aminosalicylic acid, and it is thought that the sulfapyridine component is the major cause of side-effects. Mesalazine is the active component of sulfasalazine. Presented for use as a tablet coated with special resin designed to release active ingredient in the terminal ileum and colon. Suppositories of 250 mg and 500 mg also available for use in patients with distal disease. The drug should not be given to patients with renal impairment; large doses have been shown to cause renal damage in experimental animals. Should not be given to patients with salicylate intolerance. Anti-inflammatory effect not achieved if intestinal transit time rapid owing to diarrhoea
Balsalazide sodium	2.25 g three times daily for up to 12 weeks. 1.5 g daily for maintenance	This is a pro-drug of 5-aminosalicylic acid (5-ASA) It is designed to avoid the side-effects associated with the sulfapyridine portion of mesalazine. Side-effects due to the 5-ASA are not eliminated
Olsalazine	For acute mild ulcerative colitis 1 g daily in divided doses up to maximum of 3 g daily over 1 week. 250 mg twice daily will often maintain patient in remission	Compound which is combination of two molecules of 5-aminosalicylic acid (5-ASA). Specifically designed to reach the colon where the compound breaks down to release 5-ASA. Almost no systemic absorption of 5-ASA; therefore available to act topically on colonic mucosa. Side-effects reported similar to other salicylates; GI problems such as watery diarrhoea may occur
ELECTROLYTES AND FLUID	In accordance with the needs of the patient	The need for the correction of electrolyte imbalance arises from the profuse diarrhoea
IV NUTRITION	In accordance with the nutritional status of the patient	Impaired ability to absorb nutrients must be recognised and treated in both the short and long term

In considering the causes of constipation, a detailed drug history (including the use of OTC medicines) should be taken. Drugs with antimuscarinic activity (see p. 145) are especially liable to cause constipation. Constipation is often present in patients suffering from depression and confusional states. Certain metabolic disorders, such as hypercalcaemia and myxoedema, may also cause constipation. Constipation may occur when the call to stool is neglected. This has the effect of decreasing the sensitivity of rectal sensors. If the patient is too ill to respond to the call to stool or for some other reason is unable to respond, such as pressure of duties, the stimulus is gradually lost and the rectum becomes overloaded with faecal material.

All patients complaining of constipation should be carefully investigated so as to eliminate a more serious condition. Pain (arising from a malignant condition) on bowel evacuation may result in constipation. Whenever possible, constipation should be treated by attention to diet and exercise, and the encouragement of a healthy lifestyle. For example, the simple step of adding bran or other dietary products to food may be all that is required.

If drug treatment is required a wide range of products is available (Table 15.8). Laxatives may be classified into four main groups:

- Bulk-forming laxatives act by drawing water into the colon and thus help to expand and soften the faeces. The increased bulk stimulates receptors in the colonic mucosa which promote peristalsis. It is vital that there is a concurrent increase in fluid intake so as to avoid intestinal obstruction. These laxatives generally take a few days to work. Only where it is not possible to increase fibre in the diet should they be used.
- Stimulant laxatives increase intestinal motility by nerve stimulation. There is a risk of causing abdominal cramp, and long-term use may lead to colonic atony and hypokalaemia.
- Faecal softeners lubricate and soften the faeces thus easing their passage.
- Osmotic laxatives act by retaining fluid in the lumen of the gut by osmosis leading to a softening of the stools and stimulation of intestinal contractions.

Despite the 'homely' image of laxatives, it must not be forgotten that these are drugs with potentially serious

Table 15.8 Main laxative drugs

Drug	Dose	Notes
BULK-FORMING AGENTS		
Ispaghula husk	3.5 g twice daily with water	Important to ensure patient has good fluid intake to avoid intestinal obstruction. For ease of use can be made into a jelly
Methylcellulose	Available as 500 mg tablet. 3–6 tablets daily with 300 mL of water	Good fluid intake essential. Bulk-forming agents should be carefully swallowed with water and should not be taken immediately before going to bed
		An increase in dietary fibre is preferable to the use of bulking agents but this may not be possible when dietary intake is compromised (e.g. in older patients)
STIMULANTS		
Bisacodyl	5–10 mg orally at night. Also available as suppository	Like other stimulant laxatives, can cause local irritation and griping pain
Dantron	Available as co-danthramer (i.e. dantron 25 mg with poloxamer 200 mg in 5 mL). Normal dose 5–10 mL	Because of possible carcinogenic effects, reserved for use in older patients. Especially valuable where essential that bowel movements are not accompanied by straining. Also widely used in patients receiving opioids in palliative care
Docusate sodium	Orally up to 500 mg daily in divided doses	
Glycerol (glycerin)	Given in suppository form	Mild irritant
Senna	2–4 tablets, each containing 7.5 mg sennosides at night	Also used prior to radiological examination, endoscopy and surgery
Sodium picosulfate	Available as elixir containing 5 mg/5 mL. Dose: 5–15 mL at night	Indications similar to those of senna
FAECAL SOFTENERS		
Arachis oil	130 mL given as retention enema	Warmed before use. Used to soften impacted faeces. As with all enemas, should be used with caution in patients with intestinal obstruction and a history of peanut allergy
ISO-OSMOTIC LAXATIVES		
Macrogol solutions (polyethylene glycol)	Low doses of macrogol solutions help to increase bowel frequency and improve defecation. Stools are also softened	Contraindicated in a number of conditions, e.g. IBD
OSMOTIC LAXATIVES		
Lactulose (a disaccharide)	Available as an elixir containing 3.35 g in 5 mL. Initial dose 15 mL twice daily reducing when patient's condition warrants	Lactulose passes through the small intestine unchanged. It is broken down in the colon by bacteria to substances (acetic and lactic acids) which exert their osmotic effect in the gut lumen. May cause cramps and flatulence
Magnesium sulphate	5–10 g in water	Produces rapid bowel clearance (2–4 hours). Other magnesium salts also used, e.g. magnesium citrate and magnesium hydroxide
Phosphates	Sodium acid phosphate 12.8 g and sodium phosphate 10.24 g in the form of an enema (128 mL)	Contraindicated in patients with ulcerative or inflammatory bowel conditions. Local irritation may occur, and sodium absorption can cause problems in patients who have a low sodium requirement
Sodium citrate	Given in form of a microenema together with a surfactant	Small volume (5 mL) of these enemas makes for ease of use
LUBRICANTS		
Liquid paraffin		The long-term use of this may interfere with the absorption of fat-soluble vitamins (A, D and K). Lipid-aspiration pneumonia has been reported (inhalation of liquid paraffin following vomiting). Leakage of oil from the anus often occurs. There is some evidence that the long-term use of liquid paraffin may cause cancer of the large bowel. Liquid paraffin is no longer prescribed

adverse effects. Overuse of laxatives can cause hypokalaemia and an atonic non-functioning colon. Inappropriate use of laxatives in situations where the diagnosis of the cause of the constipation is inadequate can be very dangerous. Patient group directions may permit the prescription of laxatives by nurses. Nurses have an important role to play in advising patients about their use of laxatives. Laxatives should be used only where other measures have failed. These would include attention to the amount of dietary fibre (whole-wheat cereals, wholemeal bread and whole fruit), fluid intake and exercise. Attention to details such as the provision of warmth and privacy when attending to toileting needs and exploiting the gastrocolic reflex after breakfast can greatly assist the constipated patient. Where laxatives are indicated, patients should be encouraged to continue with these simple measures and to take only the recommended dose. There are, of course, very important indications for the use of laxatives on a routine basis especially in patients receiving opiates for palliative care.

Bowel-cleansing solutions

Prior to colonic surgery, radiological examination and colonoscopy, it is essential to ensure that the bowel is free of solid faecal matter. A range of preparations is available. Most are based on inorganic salts, such as phosphates, magnesium compounds and a combination of electrolytes. Patient counselling on the need for compliance with the regime and reconstitution of the powder is vitally important in achieving a good clearing of the bowel (see specialist literature for dosage details). There are a number of contraindications to the use of these products, in particular, known gastrointestinal disease (e.g. ulceration, obstruction and gastric retention). Congestive cardiac failure is also a contraindication to the use of these agents.

Haemorrhoids and other perianal conditions

Painful, itching and bleeding conditions of the perianal region are common. Usually the lesions are benign and may often be amenable to treatment by topical application of soothing, emollient, anti-inflammatory and anaesthetic agents, alone or in combination. The most common perianal condition is haemorrhoids. The condition may present in a variety of ways ranging from superficial bleeding to permanently prolapsed haemorrhoids. The causes of haemorrhoids are not fully understood but the condition is associated with congestion of the superior haemorrhoidal venous plexus. Surgical treatment or local injection with a sclerosing agent (oily phenol injection) may be required. Considerable relief can be obtained by the use of rectal ointments designed to relieve itching and pain. Application of the ointment is aided by using a rectal nozzle. In some cases a suppository with active ingredients similar to those of the ointments may be used. Some active ingredients of rectal ointments are listed in Table 15.9. Unprolapsed haemorrhoids may be treated by local injection of a sclerosant, usually phenol in an oily base.

Malignant disease (see Ch. 22)

DRUG TREATMENT OF HEPATIC DISORDERS

Anatomy and physiology

The liver can be considered as the 'chemical factory' of the body. It is the largest organ in the body, weighing up to 2.3 kg (range 1–2.3 kg). The liver has four lobes and occupies the greater part of the right hypochondriac region (see Fig. 15.3). The most obvious lobes are the right and left lobes. Closely associated with the liver are the organs of the gastrointestinal tract, large blood vessels and the gall bladder (see Fig. 15.4). At the microscopic level hepatocytes make up the lobules, which are just visible to the naked eye.

The liver carries out a great range of chemical functions which are essential to health. These functions are summarised in Table 15.10.

Liver diseases disrupt the functions of the liver, which may have profound consequences for the patient.

Hepatic disease

The main diseases of the liver are potentially life-threatening but unfortunately some are not very amenable to drug treatment. Drug treatment in combination with general supportive measures, and alteration to diet, can help to ameliorate symptoms.

Table 15.9 Active ingredients of rectal ointments and suppositories (often used in combination)

Ingredient	Normal strength in ointment	Action/notes
Allantoin	0.5%	Healing agent
Betamethasone*	0.05%	Anti-inflammatory
Bismuth compounds	Various	Mild astringent
Cinchocaine	0.5%	Local anaesthetic
Hydrocortisone*	0.5%	Anti-inflammatory
Lidocaine (lignocaine)	0.5%	Local anaesthetic; as with other anaesthetics, may be absorbed to produce toxic effects
Phenylephrine	0.1%	Vasoconstrictor
Prednisolone hexanoate*	0.19%	Anti-inflammatory
Zinc oxide	Range 10–18%	Mild astringent

* All corticosteroid topical preparations should be used for limited periods to avoid absorption and possible side-effects (see p. 447). A typical formulation for a rectal ointment is: betamethasone 0.05%, lidocaine (lignocaine) 2.5% and phenylephrine 0.1%; the base is usually of soft paraffin, which has a lubricant effect.

Hepatitis

Hepatitis may be caused by one of a number of viruses or by a toxic chemical, very often a drug. In both virus- and drug-induced hepatitis there is extensive cell damage throughout the liver, although there may be

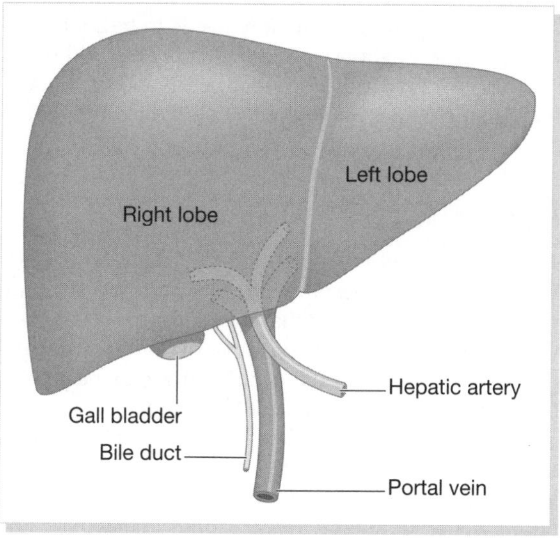

Figure 15.3 The liver.

Table 15.10 Functions of the liver

Main function	Outline of functions
Amino acid metabolism	Breakdown of certain amino acids to form urea; formation of uric acid from nucleoprotein
Bile production	Bile salts, pigments and cholesterol produced in liver cells
Carbohydrate metabolism	Glucose is converted to glycogen (after a meal), and glycogen is broken down to glucose to meet energy requirements (see also Ch. 20)
Detoxification processes	Drugs and other noxious substances (e.g. toxins produced by microorganisms); also metabolises ethyl alcohol taken in alcoholic drinks (see p. 163)
Fat metabolism	Fat is converted into a form which can be used by the body as an energy source
Heat production	Since a great number of chemical processes are carried out in the liver, heat is produced, which is the main source of body heat
Inactivation	A wide range of hormones are inactivated, e.g. insulin, thyroid hormones, sex hormones and aldosterone
Storage functions	Vitamins, both fat- and water-soluble, iron and copper; glucose in the form of glycogen
Synthesis	Vitamin A, non-essential amino acids and blood-clotting factors

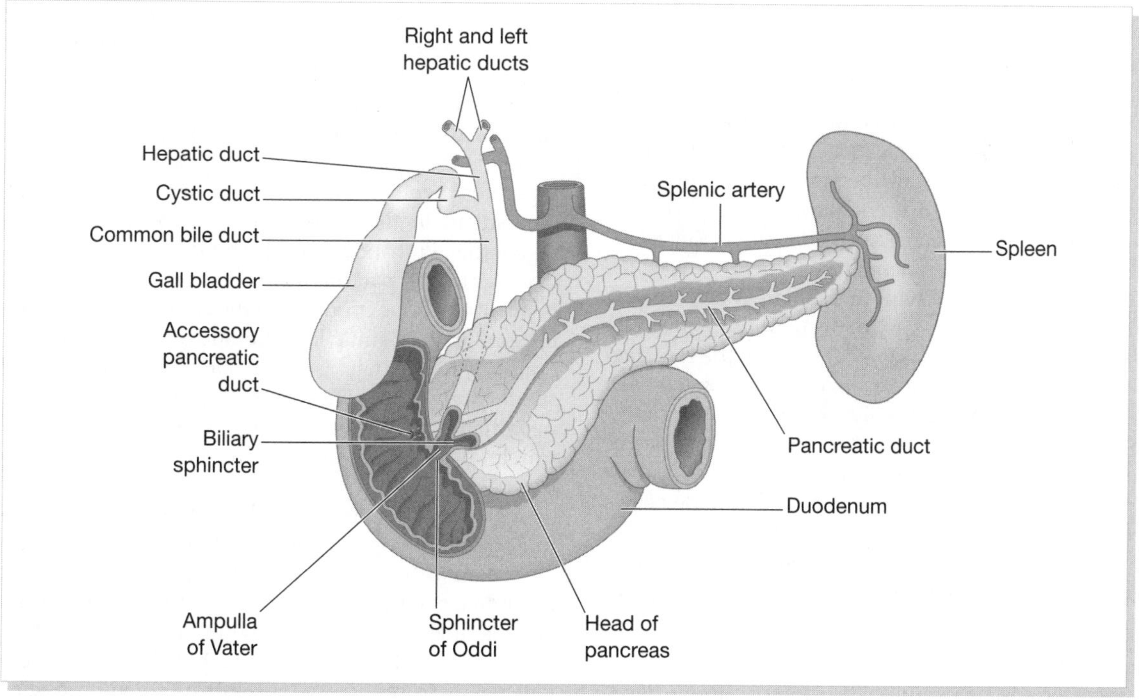

Figure 15.4 Associated organs.

variation in the extent of the damage in different lobes of the liver.

Hepatitis due to the A virus is associated with anorexia, nausea, malaise, fever and joint pain. The liver is tender and jaundice occurs as the fever abates. The virus is spread by the faecal–oral route, and contaminated food or drink may be involved. The course of the A infection generally lasts 3–6 weeks. A vaccine is available (see p. 365).

Hepatitis due to the B virus is a much more serious condition. The virus is spread by blood, secretions and sexual intercourse. In view of the seriousness of hepatitis B, special attention must be given to protecting people at particular risk. Health and other vulnerable workers should be protected by vaccination, and great care must be taken with all procedures involved in taking blood and other invasive techniques. Safe disposal of contaminated equipment is essential.

In both forms of infection the symptoms are similar although much more severe in the B form of the disease. Symptoms include chills, headache, general malaise, gastrointestinal disturbances and anorexia. Abdominal pain and dark urine will be followed by jaundice. Liver enlargement occurs and the liver is often tender.

Hepatitis C may be acquired via infected blood, plasma derivatives, unsafe sex and injecting drug abuse. It has an insidious onset with vague abdominal discomfort, anorexia, nausea and vomiting, and eventually jaundice.

Treatment of acute hepatitis

Care must be taken to determine the cause of the condition. It is particularly important to exclude drugs as a cause. If a drug is implicated (see p. 132) the treatment should be stopped and further exposure to the drug avoided. Exposure to toxic chemicals in the workplace must also be considered as a possible cause. Key elements of the treatment of hepatitis are dietary measures and bed rest. It is important to maintain a high-calorie diet although patients' gastrointestinal problems may restrict the range of foods they are able to tolerate. Bed rest is very important so as to avoid exhaustion to which the patient may be especially prone. Fluid and electrolyte therapy should be given in the acute phase of the condition. Corticosteroids may be of value for their appetite-stimulating properties although the side-effects of corticosteroids are so hazardous that their use should be minimised. All drugs with a potential to cause liver damage must be avoided, as must alcohol, a well-recognised liver toxin.

Treatment of chronic hepatitis

Corticosteroids are useful in the form of chronic hepatitis that is not due to viral infection.

Hepatitis B and hepatitis C viruses are major causes of chronic hepatitis. Interferon alfa is of limited use in the treatment of chronic hepatitis B and is contraindicated in decompensated liver disease. Lamivudine may be used as an alternative.

The antiviral agent ribavirin in combination with interferon alfa-2b may be of value in the treatment of chronic hepatitis C. Therapy needs to be continued for 6 months. Peginterferon alfa-2b may be used when ribavirin for any reason cannot be given but therapy with a single agent is less effective than combination therapy.

Hepatic failure

This is a very serious condition for which no specific treatment is available. Since the liver performs so many vital functions it follows that liver failure has very serious consequences. The usual cause of fulminant hepatic failure is an acute viral infection but it may be caused by drugs, pregnancy or Wilson's disease.

The symptoms of hepatic failure include cerebral disturbance. Encephalopathy arises from the accumulation of toxic substances in the blood which arise because the damaged liver cannot metabolise the range of chemical substances a healthy liver can cope with. A wide range of neurological symptoms are seen including restlessness, behavioural abnormalities, mania, drowsiness and coma. Jaundice develops and physical signs are abnormal. Mortality is age-related. Profound biochemical disturbances such as electrolyte disturbance, alkalosis and coagulation disorders are common during the course of the illness.

Treatment plans include general supportive measures together with measures designed to sustain the patient in the hope that the hepatic tissue will regenerate. Nutritional needs should be met with glucose orally or parenterally. Bacteria which produce toxic nitrogenous products in the colon should be suppressed with a suitable antibiotic such as neomycin orally. Neomycin is a non-absorbable antibiotic but small amounts may be absorbed over time to produce potentially dangerous side-effects. Infection and electrolyte disturbances must be treated and, if renal failure occurs, haemodialysis and other measures may be required. The physical and biochemical parameters must be monitored and corrective measures taken. Disorders of blood coagulation may lead to bleeding from the gastrointestinal tract. Ranitidine by intravenous injection may be required to control this. Lactulose (orally) is used to acidify the colonic contents so as to reduce the level of nitrogen-producing bacteria.

Cirrhosis of the liver

Cirrhosis is caused by alcohol abuse, chronic hepatitis or biliary cirrhosis. Alcohol has a direct toxic effect on the liver. A daily substantial intake over a number of years will result in cirrhosis. Women are at greater risk than men from a prolonged and regular intake of alcohol. Other causes of cirrhosis include certain metabolic disorders, viral infections and drugs. Obstruction in the biliary network may also cause cirrhosis. Cirrhosis of the liver has a number of clinical features. The presentation of the condition varies but often includes portal hypertension, blood disorders, ascites, circulatory changes and jaundice. Treatment of hepatic cirrhosis is based on attempting to halt the progression of the condition since there is no treatment that can reverse it.

Substance abuse (alcohol and/or drugs) must be dealt with by complete abstinence. A high-calorie diet is advisable together with bed rest. Fluid and sodium intake must be restricted. Diuretics should be used with care in conjunction with monitoring of electrolytes and blood urea.

A common complication of hepatic cirrhosis is bleeding from oesophageal varices. These are caused by portal hypertension. Various techniques are used to deal with this condition. Pressure can be applied to the varices by special tubes with inflatable 'cuffs', or surgical treatment can be used. Any treatment designed to arrest bleeding by constriction of the splanchnic arterioles may be useful. Vasopressin is given by intravenous infusion in a dose of 20 units over a period of 15 minutes.

Blood transfusions may be required to correct losses from recurrent bleeds. The possibility of injecting the varices with a sclerosing agent may be worth considering.

Since the liver plays an important part in the metabolism of drugs, it follows that drug choice/dosage for patients with liver disease must be given special consideration.

The treatment of malignant disease of the liver is discussed on page 342.

DRUG TREATMENT OF BILIARY TRACT DISORDERS

Anatomy and physiology

The gall bladder is attached to the posterior surface of the liver. Its function is to concentrate and store bile. Bile is secreted by the liver from where it passes into the gall bladder via the hepatic duct and cystic duct. The bile from the liver already contains bile salts, bile pigment and cholesterol. In the gall bladder, mucus and water are added. When fatty foods enter the duodenum, the hormone cholecystokinin is released which in turn causes the gall bladder to contract expelling its contents into the bile duct and thence to the duodenum.

Disorders and their treatment

The reasons for the formation of gallstones are not fully understood. They are made up of cholesterol although some gallstones contain a high proportion of calcium in the form of salts of bilirubin. Gallstones are frequently asymptomatic but can cause a variety of symptoms, including biliary colic or cholecystitis relieved by strong analgesia and treatment with antibiotics.

Treatment is by surgical removal often by laparoscopic cholecystectomy or, in the case of small stones, by the oral administration of ursodeoxycholic acid. This drug has no effect on large radio-opaque stones. Ultrasound is used as a non-invasive method of breaking up gallstones.

DRUG TREATMENT OF PANCREATIC DISORDERS

Anatomy and physiology

The pancreas is located in the abdomen with its head in the curve of the duodenum. It is both an exocrine and an endocrine gland. Its exocrine function is to produce pancreatic juice which enters the duodenum. Pancreatic juice contains enzymes involved in the digestion of carbohydrate, protein and fat. The pancreas also contains specialised cells known as the islets of Langerhans, which secrete insulin and glucagon (see p. 310).

Disorders and their treatment

The main conditions affecting the pancreas are pancreatitis (often caused by either gallstones or alcohol abuse), pancreatic tumours and failure of the organ to produce pancreatic (exocrine) secretions.

Pancreatitis may be acute or chronic. A necrotic process is established which often leads to infection and organ dysfunction. A severe attack requires urgent hospitalisation, and even patients with mild pancreatitis require supportive therapy in hospital. In the mild condition, intravenous fluids (crystalloids) are required and suitable analgesics will be needed. Antibiotic therapy may be required for coexisting infections. In severe cases, specialist care in a high dependency unit is required. Hypovolaemic shock must be dealt with by suitable (often large) volumes of crystalloids and colloids. Prophylactic antibiotics in high doses (cefuroxime and imipenem) may be worthwhile, since these penetrate pancreatic tissue. No specific drug treatment is available and prognosis is poor in patients who exhibit signs of both necrosis and infection. Surgical intervention to remove necrotic tissue will be required. Gallstones are dealt with by laparoscopic cholecystectomy. Chronic pancreatitis is treated using suitable analgesics and the control of metabolic complications (diabetes and fat malabsorption). Alcohol intake must be eliminated completely in all cases of pancreatitis.

Pancreatic enzyme deficiency states (exocrine secretions)

Where pancreatic enzyme secretions are absent or reduced, pancreatin is given by mouth. The deficiency state may be caused by cystic fibrosis, chronic pancreatitis or as a result of certain surgical procedures. Pancreatin (of porcine origin) is inactivated by gastric acid and heat. Drugs which reduce acid secretion (cimetidine or ranitidine) are given 1 hour before food, and heat should be minimised if pancreatin is to be added to food. Dosage of pancreatin is adjusted to meet the individual patient's needs. Stool consistency and frequency give a good indication of the need to adjust dosage levels. Preparations of pancreatin include granules and capsules containing protease, lipase and amylase. A range of strengths is available. A Committee on the Safety of Medicines (CSM) warning regarding the high-strength pancreatin preparations is in force, because of the possibility of the development of bowel strictures.

Pancreatic tumours

Pancreatic tumours range from benign to highly malignant. Most tumours develop in the head of the pancreas. Back pain, pruritus due to biliary obstruction, and appetite disturbances are presenting symptoms. Prognosis is poor. Surgery may be beneficial where the tumour is suitable for resection. Radiotherapy and chemotherapy are seldom helpful. The search continues for an effective treatment.

ADMINISTRATION OF RECTAL MEDICINES (Box 15.2)

Drugs can be administered via the rectum:

- in solid form, as a suppository which melts at body temperature
- as a solution, suspension or foam in the form of an enema.

Box 15.2 Administration of medications by the rectal route

Documentation
- Prescribing and recording sheet

The medicine
- Suppository or enema as prescribed

The environment
- Patient in bed
- Privacy, warmth, comfort
- Incontinence pad(s) to protect clothes and bedding
- Call bell to hand
- Commode positioned at bedside if appropriate

The nurse and the patient
- Patient identified
- Explanation given of what is involved and consent obtained
  Patient instructed to breathe through the mouth to relax the anal sphincter
- Patient assisted into left lateral position with head on one or two pillows, buttocks in line with edge of bed and knees drawn up towards chin

Technique
- Nurse ensures hands are socially clean before and after procedure
- Disposable gloves are worn for insertion of suppositories
- *Suppositories:*
  - suppository lubricated using, for example, 'KY Jelly' or tip melted in hot water as directed on packet
  - anus carefully located avoiding external haemorrhoids if present
  - suppository slowly and gently inserted – tapered end first when used to evacuate rectum; blunt end first when suppository to be retained
  - finger withdrawn smoothly
- *Enemas*
  - enema warmed then nozzle lubricated after air expelled
  - anus carefully located avoiding external haemorrhoids if present
  - enema nozzle inserted for 4–6 cm and then pack slowly rolled up to introduce contents
  - nozzle withdrawn gently
- Anal region wiped and patient left comfortable
- For evacuant medications, patients encouraged to postpone first urges to defecate and to make medication work; for retention medication, elevating foot of bed may help patient to retain medication

Hazards
- Local irritation
- Trauma

The rectal route may be utilised for local or systemic action when:

- drugs cannot be swallowed (e.g. because of vomiting, coma, stricture)

- drugs cause severe irritation of the upper gastrointestinal tract (e.g. indometacin)
- a prolonged action is desired (e.g. oxycodone)
- the drug must be delivered close to the site of the lesion(s) (e.g. corticosteroid).

The absorptive surface area of the rectum is small, although the blood supply is extremely efficient and therefore absorption can be rapid. However, the presence of faeces may slow absorption, and irritation may cause early evacuation. Laxatives are administered in order to evacuate the rectum and are retained there for approximately 20 minutes. All other drugs given rectally are for retention and are normally administered on retiring to bed so that they may be retained overnight. Before administering rectal medicines, the nurse should ensure the patient has no history of allergy. Arachis oil enemas are contraindicated in patients with nut allergy.

Given the option, perhaps more patients on long-term drug therapy would choose this route of administration. Where this is the chosen method, patients should be encouraged to insert suppositories themselves (e.g. paracetamol, diclofenac) and may be taught self-administration of a small disposable enema containing a soluble form of prednisolone in the treatment of colitis.

STOMA MANAGEMENT

Modern methods of stapling anastomoses in the rectum have resulted in fewer people requiring the formation of a stoma. Nevertheless nurses will encounter patients who have had a stoma operation performed recently as well as those they meet for other reasons who happen to have a stoma. Stoma care involves the active participation of a number of healthcarers, with the nurse taking a central part. The overall aim is to rehabilitate patients so that they may care for themselves within the framework of a near-normal way of life. However, there will be situations where self-care alone is inadequate, not because of any failing on the part of the patient, but because the patient's needs make it so. Many patients manage very well from day to day provided they have continual general support and access to specialist help and advice when they require it. Ostomists are individuals who happen to eliminate in a different way. Each, naturally, will have particular problems and individual methods of overcoming them.

Types of stoma

A stoma is usually created when it has been necessary to form a surgical diversion of faeces or urinary flow. There are three main types:

- An operation which necessitates removal of the rectum and sigmoid colon results in the formation of a *colostomy*. At this point in the intestinal tract, the faeces are generally well formed and evacuation is fairly predictable.
- When the large intestine has been entirely removed, or diverted, the stoma is made at the lower end of the small intestine and is known as an *ileostomy*. With this type of stoma, waste is looser because more of the intestine has been removed, or diverted, resulting in loss of reabsorptive capacity.
- In the treatment of certain bladder disorders, the ureters may be transplanted into a short segment taken from the ileum to form an *ileal conduit* or they may have been brought to the skin surface in the formation of a *urostomy*. Waste in these cases is urine.

In all forms of stoma, since no voluntary muscles are involved, the excretory flow cannot be controlled at will. Management therefore is directed towards modifying waste where this is possible and applying some form of device for its collection.

Diet

For those who have a colostomy or ileostomy, correct diet comes before anything else. The aim is to produce faeces which are as well-formed as possible without causing constipation. Sensible eating can help to achieve this aim and can minimise other problems for the ostomist (e.g. odour, flatus and excoriation of the skin). Dietetic advice is always available and aims to help the person find a diet which is as near normal as can possibly be managed. At first, a certain amount of experimentation may be required with food combination. In time, the person usually finds that most foodstuffs can be taken in moderation with a few exceptions. Wind-producing foods are soon identified. Highly spiced foods and onions are to be avoided as they can produce loose and odorous faeces, and much flatus. Pulse foods and Brussels sprouts can cause flatus and noise although not so much odour. The timing of liquid in relation to food is important. It is safer not to drink immediately before, during or until about half an hour after a meal, so as to avoid loosening the faeces. Fizzy drinks are to be avoided, and advice on which alcoholic drinks may be safely taken should be sought.

Odour

Odour is caused by either faeces or flatus, and therefore good dietary management helps to keep it to a minimum. Very careful hygiene is essential of course, although deodorants also may be used. Deodorant drops or powders are available for placing in the stoma appliance, although care should be taken not to allow liquid deodorants to touch the stoma or surrounding skin, otherwise they may cause severe irritation. Some ostomy bags have a small vent at the top for inserting deodorant liquid or have a charcoal filter incorporated. A deodorising spray may be used at the time of emptying the appliance and a deodorising air device may be placed as appropriate.

Appliances

All ostomists are entitled to free prescriptions for all their stoma needs and these may be obtained through a local pharmacy or a dispensing appliance contractor. Many of the items are listed in the Drug Tariff. It is advisable to liaise with the community pharmacist to ensure the availability of the correct product(s). No single appliance is suitable for all those who have a stoma, and this is reflected in the wide range of products currently available. The aim is to find a device which not only serves the purpose of satisfactorily collecting the waste but is discreet, rustle-free and acceptable. A detailed description of all the different appliances is beyond the scope of this book but there are several aspects which should be understood when considering appliances generally. Stoma bags may or may not be disposable and/or drainable. They are available either as one- or two-piece systems. One-piece appliances consist of a disposable collection bag complete with its own adhesive seal. Two-piece appliances comprise an adhesive flange to which a separate disposable collection bag may be fitted. The flange may be left attached for 3–4 days, while the bag is replaced as often as necessary.

The type and site of the stoma, manual dexterity and skin sensitising, all influence the choice of appliance. Many modern appliances involve the use of skin protectives such as hydrocolloid wafers which, because of their malleability, impermeability and skin-protection properties, provide a good skin seal. Microporous adhesives may also be used and are mostly well tolerated. A belt may be attached to some appliances for added support. Filler pastes are useful for filling dips and creases peristomally, thus making the surface level prior to putting on an appliance. These pastes must not be used on sensitive skin as they are spirit-based.

Many permutations of apparatus have been produced, and ostomists themselves make adaptations to suit their own needs.

The question of disposal of appliances and their contents is an important one for all concerned. Many patients dispose of the contents of the bag down the lavatory, and as it is flushed they 'sluice' the bag. The empty bag is then wrapped in newspaper and sealed with tape to make a small package. If this is disposed of among ordinary domestic waste in the usual way there will be no problem.

Skin protection

In the same way as a person who is paraplegic lives with the threat of pressure sores, the ostomist must constantly take care to prevent irritation and breakdown of the skin which surrounds the stoma. A routine of changing the appliance right to the skin will be followed by each individual. Care must be taken to remove plasters without tearing the skin. The area around the stoma is washed using cotton wool, for example, and warm, soapy water, taking care to remove all traces of faeces, mucus, and skin applications. It is important to rinse off all soap to reduce irritation and to pat the skin dry. Any traces of adhesive should be removed using an adhesive solvent. Additional applications of barrier cream and skin gel may be used for protection of the skin. Creams should be applied sparingly to a radius of about 10 cm from the stoma but not on the stoma itself.

Skin breakdown

In the event of the skin becoming red and weepy, adhesives may have to be temporarily replaced with some form of dressing. This may be left in position for several days with the appliance being placed on top of the dressing. Efforts should then be made to identify the cause of the excoriation. It may be that the motions are too loose, calling for a change in diet or a bulking agent. Changing the bag more promptly helps to reduce faecal contact with exposed skin. The size of the aperture may be too big, causing a similar problem, and may have to be reduced. Ideally there should only be about 0.5 cm of a gap between the stoma and the appliance. Antiseptic solutions tend to be painful when applied to sore skin, causing further irritation, and are best avoided in preference to soap and water, thorough rinsing with cool water, and careful drying.

Medicines and ostomists

Certain precautions have to be taken by doctors prescribing medicines for patients with an ileostomy or colostomy. Nurses should also be aware of these and other problems relating to medicines that may arise for the ostomist.

Patients with a colostomy

Constipation may be a problem for many colostomy patients and should always be borne in mind in their management. For the treatment of constipation, colostomy patients should increase their fluid intake or make some dietary adjustments in preference to taking medication. If this approach does not help then bulk-forming laxatives such as ispaghula husk or methylcellulose may be used. These act by increasing faecal mass, which stimulates peristalsis and effects expulsion of faeces provided sufficient fluid intake is maintained. These medicines are supplied in tablet and granule form. Tablets may be broken up and should be chewed with a little water half an hour before a meal. Liquids are then withheld until about half an hour after the meal. Because these preparations have a hygroscopic action, the timing of fluid is important, otherwise the medication absorbs fluid recently taken instead of the fluid content of the faeces. The granular form of agents such as methylcellulose is found by patients to be less manageable since there is a tendency for the granules to swell in the mouth and thus be difficult to swallow. Ispaghula husk is available in granule form in different flavours and when added to water makes an acceptable drink. Lactulose, which is an osmotic laxative, is another useful preparation in this situation as is the stimulant laxative senna.

Antacids. Those containing aluminium salts may cause the colostomy patient to become constipated.

Antidepressants. The anticholinergic effects of some antidepressants can lead to a number of troublesome side-effects, including constipation.

Opioid analgesics. Analgesics such as dihydrocodeine are especially constipating. Other opioid analgesics such as codeine and morphine may also be troublesome.

Patients with an ileostomy

Diarrhoea with subsequent loss of water and potassium is a very real threat to the ileostomist at any time, and may be exacerbated by taking medicines.

Digoxin. The improvement in renal perfusion which results from digoxin therapy may cause additional potassium depletion. Potassium supplements (preferably in liquid form) may be needed when digoxin therapy is indicated.

Diuretics. These should be avoided whenever possible owing to the risk of dehydration and potassium loss. If diuretic therapy is essential a potassium-sparing diuretic should be used.

Antacids. Magnesium-containing antacids tend to be laxative.

Iron preparations. The intramuscular route should be used instead of by mouth if it is vital that iron is given. Modified-release preparations should not be given.

Laxatives, enemas and bowel washouts. Any form of laxative or washout is contraindicated because of the severe risk of dehydration rapidly occurring.

Tablets. Those with slow-release properties are unsuitable. Such preparations are designed to release the drug from the tablet during its passage through the digestive tract over a period of 3–6 hours. In ileostomy patients this period is shortened, with the result that drug release may be incomplete, leading to underdosage. For this reason, if potassium replacement therapy is required, a liquid form is used to ensure full absorption of potassium.

Patients with ileostomy or colostomy

For any patient with an ileostomy or colostomy, oral antibiotics, oral iron preparations, and antacids containing magnesium salts should be avoided whenever possible because of the likelihood of diarrhoea. If necessary, concurrent intestinal sedatives such as codeine phosphate, loperamide or co-phenotrope may be given. Salt may have to be replaced in the form of oral rehydration salts, a glucose and electrolyte powder which requires to be reconstituted.

Conclusion

There can be no doubt that the formation of a stoma brings change to the individual's way of life. The prospect of such an operation for individuals and their families is a daunting one. With the practical and psychological support of a team of staff through the perioperative, rehabilitative and independent phases of stoma management, individuals have a very real chance of being able to pursue a career, raise a family, and resume many previously enjoyed activities. The role of the nurse is to help them to regain confidence in their ability to cope in order to lead a full life.

TREATMENT OF CHILDREN WITH GASTROINTESTINAL DISEASE

Many of the drugs discussed in this chapter are not licensed for the treatment of infants and children. Specialist advice is required in many instances especially as regards dosage, method of administration and duration of treatment.

FURTHER READING

Beckingham I J, Bornman P C 2001 ABC of diseases of liver, pancreas and biliary system: acute pancreatitis. British Medical Journal 322:595–598

Bennett J 2001 Oesophagus: atypical chest pain and motility disorders. British Medical Journal 323:791–794

Bornman P C, Beckingham I J 2001 ABC of diseases of liver, pancreas and biliary system: pancreatic tumours. British Medical Journal 322:721–723

Caestecker J D 2001 Oesophagus: heartburn. British Medical Journal 323:736–739

Calam J, Baron J H 2001 Pathophysiology of duodenal and gastric ulcer and gastric cancer. British Medical Journal 323:980–982

Fuchs G J 2001 A better oral rehydration solution? British Medical Journal 323:59–60

Gow P J, Mutimer D 2001 Treatment of chronic hepatitis. British Medical Journal 323:1164–1167

Harris A, Misiewicz J J 2001 Management of *Helicobacter pylori* infection. British Medical Journal 323:1047–1050

Harris H E, Ramsay M E 2002 Clinical course of hepatitis C virus during the first decade of infection: cohort study. British Medical Journal 324:450–453

Johnson C D 2001 ABC of the upper gastrointestinal tract: upper abdominal pain: gall bladder. British Medical Journal 323:1170–1173

Mayberry J 2001 Explaining inflammatory bowel disease to patients. Prescriber 12:30–38

Meenan J 2000 IBD: a guide to successful drug management. Prescriber 11:93–104

Spiller R C 2001 ABC of the upper gastrointestinal tract: anorexia, nausea, vomiting and pain. British Medical Journal 323:1354–1357

CHAPTER CONTENTS

16

Drug treatment of cardiovascular disorders

ANATOMY AND PHYSIOLOGY

The heart

The heart lies between the lungs, behind the lower sternum, in front of the oesophagus and above the diaphragm, on which it rests. It is roughly conical in shape with a base and an apex. It consists of four chambers: the right and left atria above, and the right and left ventricles below. The atria and ventricles are separated by, on the right side, the tricuspid valve and, on the left side, the mitral valve. The walls of the heart have three layers – outermost, a fibrous envelope called the pericardium, in the middle, a thick muscle known as the myocardium, and the innermost layer, a smooth lining called the endocardium (Fig. 16.1).

Venous blood returns from various parts of the body to the heart. It enters the right atrium via the superior and inferior venae cavae and passes through the tricuspid valve to the right ventricle. The right ventricle pumps the blood to the lungs, via the pulmonary artery. In the lungs the blood is oxygenated and carbon dioxide is removed. The blood then returns via the four pulmonary veins into the left atrium from where it passes through the mitral valve into the left ventricle. The left ventricle pumps the oxygenated blood through the aortic valve into the aorta and out into the body.

The heart derives its own blood supply from the two main coronary arteries which originate from the aorta just above the aortic valve.

The activity of the heart is rhythmical, consisting of contraction ('systole') and relaxation ('diastole'). The impulse to contract is generated by a microscopic area of specialised cardiac muscle – known as the sinoatrial (SA) node – situated at the junction of the superior vena cava and the right atrium. The wave of excitation spreads throughout the muscle layer of both atria causing them to contract, forcing blood into the ventricles. The impulse is picked up by another small mass of

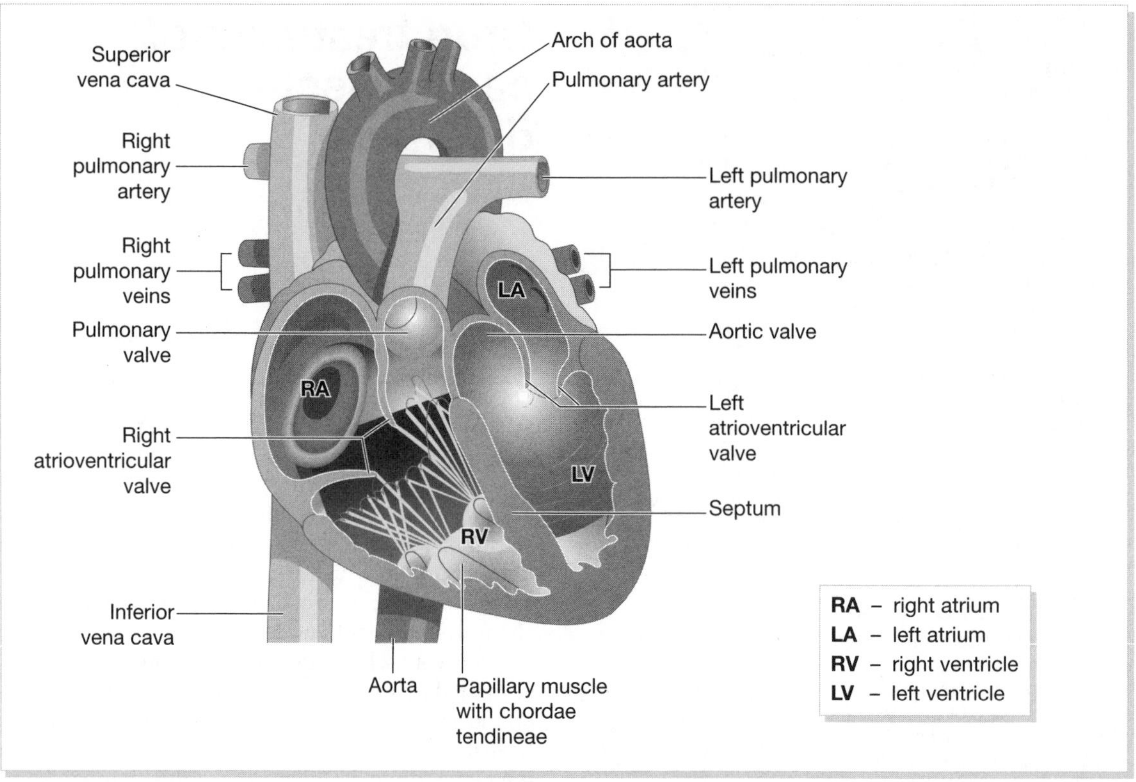

Figure 16.1 The heart. (From Waugh A, Grant A 2001 Ross and Wilson Anatomy and physiology in health and illness, 9th edn. Churchill Livingstone, Edinburgh.)

specialised cardiac muscle called the atrioventricular (AV) node situated in the septal walls of the right atrium. It is relayed by the fibres of Purkinje down the bundle of His and along the right and left branches, causing the ventricles to contract and drive blood into the pulmonary artery and the aorta. The heart then relaxes, refills with venous blood, and awaits the next stimulus for contraction. Although the heart initiates its own impulse to contract, the fine adjustments to its activity required to meet the body's constantly changing needs derive from the autonomic nervous system. Sympathetic nerves increase the heart rate and parasympathetic nerves slow the heart rate.

The SA node is normally the pacemaker for the heart because of its rapid firing rate of 60–100 electrical discharges per minute. Although the specialised cells at the AV node and at the bundle of His are also capable of spontaneously producing an electrical discharge and taking over control of the rhythm, they are normally required to do so only if the SA node fails or becomes unduly slow. The cells of the AV node emit discharges at 50 per minute and those of the ventricles at 40 or fewer per minute.

Every time the heart beats, approximately 70 mL of blood is pumped out of each ventricle. The heart rate is normally around 70 beats per minute. These two figures multiplied together are termed the cardiac output.

The blood vessels

The blood is transported round the body via the blood vessels which comprise arteries and arterioles, veins and venules, and capillaries. As a rule, arteries convey oxygenated blood and veins convey deoxygenated blood which has a high percentage of carbon dioxide. Arteries convey blood away from the heart; veins transport blood back to the heart. Capillaries are tiny blood vessels in the periphery of the arteriovenous system. It is through the capillary walls that oxygen and nutrients pass to the tissues and cells and waste products return from the cells into the circulation.

Like the heart, the walls of the blood vessels consist of three layers – the fibrous outer *tunica adventitia*, the middle muscular layer, the *tunica media*, and the smooth lining, the *tunica intima*. The outer coat of an artery allows it to stand open, whereas a vein collapses when it is cut. The proportion of muscle tissue depends on the size of the vessel, with much more in arteries than in veins. Some veins have valves which allow the blood to flow back to the heart but prevent flow in the opposite direction. The walls of the capillaries are only one cell thick; this readily facilitates gaseous and nutrient exchange.

POSITIVE INOTROPIC DRUGS

Cardiac glycosides

These drugs are used almost exclusively in two conditions:

- cardiac failure (see p. 201)
- cardiac arrhythmias (see p. 175).

Digoxin

In chronic congestive cardiac failure, digoxin is given to increase the force of myocardial contraction, hence increasing cardiac output for any given filling pressure. Digoxin is used in atrial flutter and fibrillation because it reduces conduction through the AV node and the bundle of His, allowing fewer of the excitatory transmissions from the atria to pass and hence slowing ventricular rate and restoring rhythm.

Mode of action. The actions of digoxin are complex and revolve around its ability to inhibit sodium transport out of cells through inhibition of the enzyme Na^+, K^+-ATPase, which allows increased intracellular myocardial calcium concentrations. This, in turn, improves contractility.

Pharmacokinetics. Digoxin may be given orally as either tablets or as a liquid preparation. It may also be given intravenously but this is relatively rare. Intravenous digoxin should always be given very slowly to minimise the risks of exposing the myocardium to localised high concentrations which may induce arrhythmias. It may be simpler to add the digoxin to an intravenous infusion of sodium chloride 0.9% and administer this by intravenous infusion pump over 1 hour. Since digoxin is 80% renally eliminated, the dose must be adjusted according to renal function in order to minimise the risks of toxicity. In the elderly, the renal clearance is lower than that in young healthy adults, so that a lower maintenance dose is required. The elimination half-life of digoxin in a patient with normal renal function is 36 hours – which means that up to 7 days may be required after any dosage alteration to ensure that a steady state has been reached.

Dose. Where patients have mild failure, a loading dose is not required and a satisfactory plasma concentration can be achieved over a period of about a week using a dose of 125–250 micrograms orally twice a day, which may then be reduced having special regard to renal function. Because of its long half-life, maintenance doses need be given only once daily. The maintenance dose in atrial fibrillation can usually be governed by ventricular response – which should not normally be allowed to fall below 60 beats per minute. If rapid digitalisation is required (i.e. very severe atrial fibrillation with very fast ventricular rate and danger or presence of other arrhythmias) digoxin may be given intravenously in a digitalising dose of 1–1.5 mg, preferably as an infusion over 2 or more hours (too rapid a rate is associated with nausea and risk of arrhythmias). Digoxin plasma concentrations are commonly measured and provide an indicator of toxicity and patient compliance. They relate only partially to the therapeutic effect because so many other factors can contribute to myocardial excitability, e.g. electrolyte concentrations, catecholamines and hypoxia, but generally:

1–2 micrograms/litre – therapeutic
$>$2 micrograms/litre – possibly toxic.

Complications of digoxin therapy. Digoxin treatment is particularly hazardous because the toxicity of digoxin is difficult to recognise and it has the potential to cause fatal arrhythmias. The drug's toxicity is more pronounced in the presence of metabolic and electrolyte disturbances (especially hypokalaemia, but also hypomagnesaemia, hypercalcaemia, alkalosis, hypothyroidism and hypoxia). The patient's renal function should be taken into account when deciding the digoxin dose in order to minimise the risk of toxicity. Excessive digoxin dose should be considered in any patient who is unwell or who has suddenly deteriorated. Important signs of toxicity are abdominal pain, nausea/anorexia, tiredness/weakness, diarrhoea, confusion and any change in vision, mobility or mood. Toxicity can often be managed by discontinuing therapy and correcting hypokalaemia if appropriate. Serious occurrences require urgent specialist management. Digibind, digoxin-specific antibody fragments in injectable form, is available for reversal of life-threatening over-dosage.

Interactions. Hypokalaemia predisposes to toxicity, so that diuretics used with digoxin should be either potassium-sparing or given with potassium supplements. Drugs such as amiodarone, verapamil or nifedipine may cause an increase in plasma digoxin concentrations and increase the risk of toxicity.

DIURETICS

Physiology of the kidney

Each kidney is made up of approximately one million nephrons, each nephron comprising a glomerulus and a proximal and distal tubule which are connected by the loop of Henle. The glomerulus consists of a group of capillaries and as the blood passes through these it is filtered. A large amount of water and dissolved salts is filtered from the blood and passes on to the tubules. In the tubules a selective reabsorption takes place. Glucose is normally completely reabsorbed. Water and electrolytes, including sodium, potassium, chloride and bicarbonate are selectively reabsorbed and pass back into the circulation. Urea, excess water, salts and other unwanted substances are excreted as urine. The exact amount of each substance excreted in the urine is controlled in order to maintain the composition of the body fluids at normal levels. The urine is further concentrated and, depending on the electrolyte balance, more sodium is absorbed in exchange for potassium. In the distal tubule, antidiuretic hormone (vasopressin) excreted by the posterior pituitary gland is an important controlling factor. Increased ingestion of water results in an increased urine flow. When water is absorbed from the GI tract, it causes the plasma to become more dilute and this, in turn, decreases the release of antidiuretic hormone (ADH) by the posterior lobe of the pituitary gland. Less ADH reaches the kidney and this causes the tubules to reabsorb less water so that more is excreted as urine.

Disease states resulting in oedema

In health the kidney maintains the composition of the blood within narrow limits. Disease can upset this delicate balance. Where the blood supply to the glomerulus is reduced because of impaired blood circulation, filtration slows. However, tubular reabsorption continues at the normal rate and excess water and salts accumulate in the body tissues, resulting in oedema. This can arise in cardiac failure. Oedema can also arise in renal disease (nephrotic syndrome) and cirrhosis of the liver.

Diuretics are used in the treatment of these conditions and also in the treatment of hypertension. They cause a net loss of sodium and water from the body by decreasing the reabsorption of sodium and chloride. Since a large proportion of the salt and water which passes into the tubule is reabsorbed, a small decrease in reabsorption can result in a marked increase in excretion.

Types of diuretic

There are a number of different diuretics which produce the same end result but through a different mode of action (Fig. 16.2). The following diuretics are considered:

- thiazide and related diuretics
- loop diuretics
- potassium-sparing diuretics.

Thiazide and related diuretics

Mode of action. Thiazide diuretics act by inhibiting the reabsorption of sodium and chloride in the distal tubule of the nephron, resulting in increased sodium, chloride and water secretion. There is also an increased secretion of potassium. The mode of action in relieving hypertension is unclear.

Pharmacokinetics. These diuretics are well absorbed orally and are excreted unchanged by the kidney. Compared with loop diuretics (see later) the potency is lower with a slow onset and longer duration of action. Since the duration of action is about 12 hours, a thiazide diuretic should be given in the morning.

Indications. Thiazide diuretics are used to treat hypertension and oedema resulting from cardiac failure, liver disease and nephrotic syndrome (see Table 16.1). In the management of hypertension a low dose of a thiazide, e.g. bendroflumethiazide (bendrofluazide) 2.5 mg daily, produces a near-maximal blood pressure-reducing effect with very little biochemical disturbance. Higher doses may cause more marked changes in plasma potassium, uric acid, glucose and lipids with no advantage in blood pressure control and should not be used. Optimal doses for the control of heart failure may be larger, and long-term effects are of less importance. Metolazone is particularly effective when combined with a loop diuretic. Profound diuresis may occur and therefore the patient should be monitored carefully.

Adverse effects. The most important adverse effects are hypokalaemia, hyponatraemia and dehydration. Hypomagnesaemia may also occur. Impotence is reversible on withdrawal of treatment. Competition with uric acid for secretion into the proximal tubule may cause hyperuricaemia and this may result in gout. Impaired glucose tolerance can occur. Hypotension, headache and dizziness may be experienced.

Hypokalaemia is a common side-effect of thiazide diuretics, particularly at higher doses. Combination products are available containing diuretic plus potassium, but the quantity of potassium is insufficient to correct hypokalaemia. Where potassium supplements are necessary these should be given routinely in tablet or liquid form. Alternatively, the addition of a potassium-sparing diuretic can alleviate the need for supplementation.

Interactions. Lithium excretion is reduced by thiazide diuretics. Dosages should be halved initially and

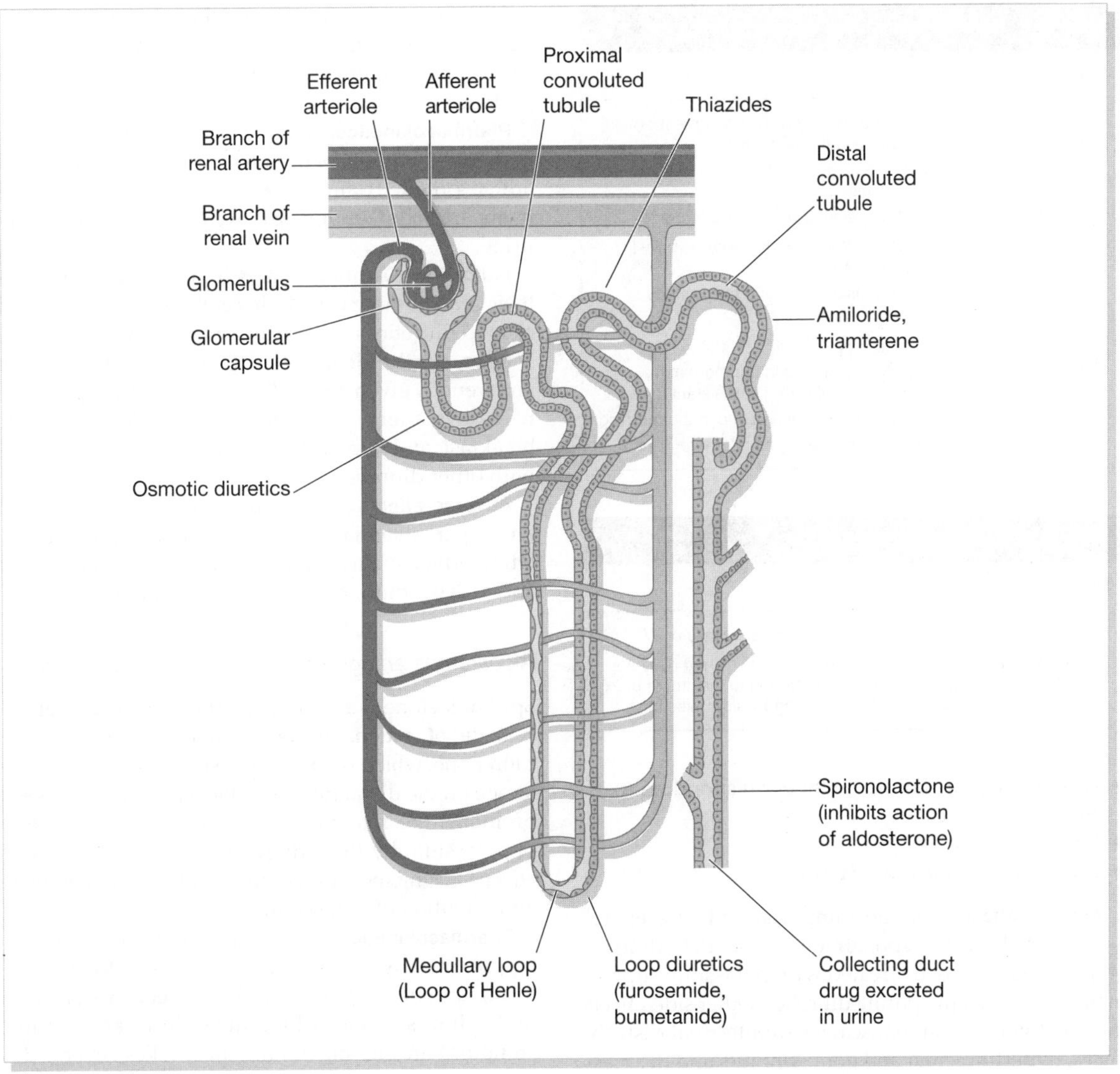

Figure 16.2 Sites of action of diuretics.

adjusted with careful monitoring of plasma concentration. Hypokalaemia potentiates the effects of digoxin and toxicity may result.

Loop diuretics

Mode of action. This group of diuretics gets its name because sodium and chloride reabsorption in the ascending limb of the loop of Henle is inhibited. In addition, potassium secretion in the distal tubule is increased (greater with furosemide (frusemide) than with bumetanide).

Pharmacokinetics. Bumetanide is almost completely absorbed after oral administration, while furosemide (frusemide) is 60–70% absorbed. Bumetanide is partially metabolised in the liver, and about 80% of a dose is excreted in the urine – 50% as unchanged drug. Furosemide (frusemide) is excreted primarily unchanged in the urine. Onset of action occurs in 30 minutes after an oral dose and within a few minutes of intravenous administration. The duration of action lasts between 3 and 6 hours after an oral dose.

Indications. The loop diuretics (see Table 16.2) are the most potent diuretics available. They are used in:

- pulmonary oedema (may arise due to left ventricular failure)

Table 16.1 Some commonly used thiazide diuretics

Drug	Dose
Bendroflumethiazide (bendrofluazide)	Oedema: initially 5–10 mg in the morning, daily or on alternate days Maintenance: 2.5–10 mg one to three times weekly Hypertension: 2.5 mg in the morning
Cyclopenthiazide	Oedema: 250–500 micrograms daily in the morning Hypertension: 250–500 micrograms in the morning
Indapamide	2.5 mg daily in the morning
Metolazone	Oedema: 5–10 mg in the morning to a maximum of 80 mg in resistant cases Hypertension: initially 5 mg in the morning Maintenance: 5 mg on alternate days

Table 16.2 Examples of loop diuretics

Drug	Dose
Bumetanide	1–5 mg once daily orally or IV
Furosemide (frusemide)	Oral: oedema, 20–80 mg daily Oliguria: 250 mg to maximum of 2 g IV: 20–50 mg by slow injection

- congestive heart failure no longer responding to thiazide diuretics
- hepatic disease
- acute and chronic renal failure.

Adverse effects. The most important adverse effects are hypokalaemia, hyponatraemia and dehydration. Hypokalaemia may be treated with potassium supplements or potassium-sparing diuretics. Other side-effects include hypotension, nausea, gastrointestinal disturbances, hyperuricaemia and gout. Tinnitus and deafness may occur with large parenteral doses and rapid administration, particularly with furosemide (frusemide).

Interactions. Hypokalaemia potentiates the effects of cardiac glycosides. Lithium excretion is diminished by furosemide (frusemide) and the dose should be halved. Furosemide (frusemide) also potentiates the nephrotoxic and ototoxic effect of the aminoglycosides.

Potassium-sparing diuretics

Mode of action. Amiloride and triamterene cause increased sodium and chloride excretion in the distal tubule resulting in an increase in water excretion. The secretion of potassium in the distal tubule is inhibited (unlike thiazide and loop diuretics). The potassium-sparing diuretics have weaker diuretic and antihypertensive effects than other diuretics, but they have the advantage of conserving potassium. For this reason they are often prescribed with thiazide or loop diuretics.

Pharmacokinetics. Following oral administration, approximately 50% of triamterene and 20% of amiloride are absorbed. Triamterene is extensively metabolised by the liver, but amiloride is excreted unchanged in the urine.

Indications. Amiloride and triamterene are used on their own or, more usually, in combination with thiazide or loop diuretics in the treatment of oedema.

Dose. Amiloride is given 10–20 mg orally, daily; triamterene is given 150–250 mg daily, reducing to alternate days after 1 week; taken in divided doses after breakfast and lunch; lower initial dose when given with other diuretics.

Adverse effects. The more common adverse effects are hyperkalaemia, dehydration and hyponatraemia. Other adverse effects include gastrointestinal disturbances, dry mouth, rashes, confusion and hypotension.

Aldosterone antagonist – potassium-sparing diuretic

Spironolactone is also a potassium-sparing diuretic.

Mode of action. Spironolactone is metabolised to canrenone, which is an antagonist of the action of aldosterone on the distal tubule of the nephron. Aldosterone promotes the retention of sodium and the excretion of potassium by the kidneys. Canrenone reverses this effect, causing increased excretion of sodium and water, and retention of potassium.

Pharmacokinetics. Spironolactone is well absorbed (approximately 70%). It is metabolised to its active form, canrenone, in the liver. The onset of action occurs in 2–4 hours. It has a long duration of action (up to 96 hours) and its maximum effect takes several days to occur.

Indications. This diuretic is used to treat fluid retention due to cardiac failure, the nephrotic syndrome and hepatic disease. In the first two conditions it is usually used in combination with a thiazide or loop diuretic. In oedema caused by excessive aldosterone activity, e.g. cirrhosis of the liver, primary aldosteronism, it counteracts these effects by competing with aldosterone for receptor sites.

Dose. Oral, 100–200 mg daily, increasing to 400 mg where required.

Adverse effects. Hyperkalaemia is the major risk, and potassium supplements must not be given with spironolactone as the body potassium could rise to a dangerous level. Gastrointestinal disturbances and gynaecomastia may occur.

General precautions to be observed in the use of diuretics

Caution must be exercised when administering diuretics to patients with impaired liver or kidney function and also in patients suffering from diabetes. The patient should always be observed for signs of fluid and electrolyte imbalance.

Diuretics can cause acute toxic reactions in patients to whom digitalis glycosides or non-depolarising muscle relaxants have already been administered, by depleting serum potassium. They also enhance the effects of antihypertensive drugs, e.g. methyldopa, hydralazine, and this enables the dose of these drugs to be reduced when treating hypertension.

The thiazides and loop diuretics can lead to potassium depletion. In these cases, potassium supplements may have to be given.

Potassium supplements

The potassium loss produced by certain diuretics may lead to a severe degree of hypokalaemia with its associated muscle weakness, mental disturbances, cardiac effects and increased risks of digitalis toxicity. Potassium supplements may have to be given with the thiazide and loop diuretics.

Potassium chloride in solution is poorly tolerated because of its nauseous effects and it is not often used. Slow-release preparations, e.g. Slow K, are well tolerated and are widely used. Apart from the use of diuretics, deficiency of potassium may occur for various reasons, for example ulcerative colitis, diarrhoea, vomiting, but the most common cause is diuretic therapy.

ANTI-ARRHYTHMIC DRUGS

Disorders of conduction

Under certain circumstances the cycle of contraction and relaxation of the heart may be disturbed. These disturbances are known as cardiac arrhythmias. There are several types of arrhythmia for which anti-arrhythmic drugs are used. An anti-arrhythmic drug is a drug which is used to control or correct abnormal rhythms of cardiac action. These drugs may be used for several different types of cardiac arrhythmia and it is essential that the specific type of arrhythmia is diagnosed by ECG prior to commencement of treatment.

Supraventricular arrhythmias

These are:

- atrial flutter
- atrial fibrillation
- ectopic beats
- supraventricular tachycardias.

As their name implies, these involve arrhythmias arising from above the ventricles and are normally tachyarrhythmias (i.e. faster than normal). The most common of these are atrial flutter and atrial fibrillation, which are often a result of ischaemic heart disease.

Atrial flutter. This is very rapid, but regular, contractions of the atria of the heart which the ventricles may follow accurately, producing a very fast, regular pulse.

Atrial fibrillation. This type of arrhythmia, which may develop following atrial flutter, involves very rapid (400–600 per minute) disordered contractions of the atria. This results in irregular stimulation of the AV node and, coupled again with AV block, a fast irregular pulse. Either of these conditions may lead (sometimes rapidly) to exhaustion of the myocardium, other arrhythmias and cardiac failure.

In both atrial flutter and atrial fibrillation, AV block develops because of, and its degree is determined by, the refractoriness of the bundle of His and the AV node. After each stimulation there is a period during which the fibres cannot be re-stimulated, and this is known as the 'refractory period'.

In atrial fibrillation and flutter, messages from the atria will reach the AV node during this refractory period and hence be missed. The length of the refractory period will determine how many atrial beats are blocked for each that is passed and hence the ventricles may contract only for every second, third, fourth or more atrial beats.

Ectopic beats. Ectopic beats, also called premature beats or extrasystoles, arise from a focus other than the pacemaker. They rarely require drug treatment but it should be remembered that they may precipitate other types of arrhythmia. In certain cases they do become troublesome and may be treated with β-adrenoceptor blocking drugs.

Supraventricular tachycardias. These tachycardias may arise for a number of reasons, e.g. following myocardial infarction, in patients with thyrotoxicosis or in patients suffering from Wolff–Parkinson–White syndrome. (This is a condition whereby impulses are conducted not only through the AV node but also through an anomalous pathway connecting the atria to the ventricles.) Paroxysmal supraventricular tachycardia (coming on in sudden bursts) does not usually require drug treatment and normal rhythm can often be achieved by, for example, respiratory manoeuvres, prompt squatting or pressure over one carotid sinus.

Ventricular arrhythmias

Ventricular tachycardia is potentially more dangerous than supraventricular tachycardias. These arrhythmias are common following acute myocardial infarction or can be precipitated by supraventricular tachycardias. A ventricular ectopic beat may initiate ventricular tachycardia followed by ventricular fibrillation with loss of cardiac output and death.

Bradycardia

Bradycardia is a slowing of the heart, is supraventricular in origin, and may occur, for example, following myocardial infarction or can be a side-effect of beta-adrenoceptor blocking drugs.

Anti-arrhythmic drugs are used to treat abnormal electrical activity of the heart (see Tables 16.3–16.6). These drugs limit cardiac electrical activity to normal conduction pathways and decrease abnormally fast heart rates. They may be classified in a number of ways:

- those that act on supraventricular arrhythmias (e.g. verapamil)
- those that act on both supraventricular arrhythmias and ventricular arrhythmias (e.g. disopyramide)
- those that act on ventricular arrhythmias (e.g. lidocaine (lignocaine))

Table 16.3 Treatment of supraventricular arrhythmias

Drug/drug group	Treatment
Adenosine	This drug causes rapid reversion of sinus rhythm of paroxysmal supraventricular tachycardias. It is given by rapid IV injection into a large peripheral vein. Dose: 3 mg over 2 seconds with cardiac monitoring. If required, this is followed by 6 mg after 1–2 minutes, then by 12 mg after a further 1–2 minutes. Adverse effects include transient facial flush, dyspnoea, light-headedness, choking sensation and nausea
Cardiac glycosides	Treatment of choice in slowing ventricular response in atrial flutter or atrial fibrillation (see p. 175)
Verapamil	Is usually effective for supraventricular tachycardias. An initial IV dose may be followed by oral treatment. It should not be injected into patients recently treated with beta-blockers because of the risk of hypotension and asystole

Table 16.4 Treatment of supraventricular and ventricular arrhythmias

Drug	Indications
Amiodarone	Used to treat tachycardia associated with the Wolff–Parkinson–White syndrome as it has an inhibiting effect on both the anomalous and normal conduction pathways. It should be initiated only under hospital or specialist supervision when used for treatment of other arrhythmias where previous treatments have failed, e.g. paroxysmal supraventricular, nodal and ventricular tachycardias, atrial fibrillation and flutter, and ventricular fibrillation
Beta-blockers	Act as anti-arrhythmic drugs for the control of inappropriate sinus tachycardia or supraventricular arrhythmias provoked by conditions of high catecholamine excretion, e.g. emotion, exercise or anaesthesia. They are also used to control tachycardias following myocardial infarction. They may be used in conjunction with digoxin to control the ventricular response in atrial fibrillation, especially in patients with thyrotoxicosis. Esmolol is a relatively cardioselective beta-blocker with a very short duration of action, used IV for the short-term treatment of supraventricular arrhythmias. Sotalol, a non-cardioselective beta-blocker with additional class III anti-arrhythmic activity, is used for prophylaxis in paroxysmal supraventricular arrhythmias. It also suppresses ventricular ectopic beats and non-sustained ventricular tachycardia
Disopyramide	Is very effective against ventricular extrasystoles and is also used for ventricular arrhythmias, especially where myocardial infarction is suspected or has been proven. It suppresses the frequency of ectopic ventricular beats as well as the frequency and duration of self-limiting bursts of ventricular tachycardia
Flecainide	It is of value for serious symptomatic ventricular arrhythmias and paroxysmal atrial fibrillation. It delays intracardiac conduction (should be initiated in hospital). Like quinidine, it may precipitate serious arrhythmias in certain patients
Procainamide	Used to control ventricular arrhythmias
Propafenone	Used for the prophylaxis and treatment of ventricular arrhythmias and also for some supraventricular arrhythmias
Quinidine	May be effective in suppressing supraventricular and ventricular arrhythmias

Table 16.5 Details of drugs used to treat supraventricular and ventricular arrhythmias

Drug	Pharmacokinetics	Dose	Adverse effects	Notes
Amiodarone	Slowly absorbed at widely varying rates. Onset of action occurs within 1–3 weeks. It has a long half-life (30–45 days) and effects can be seen months after the drug is withdrawn	Oral: 200 mg three times daily for 1 week, reduced to 200 mg twice daily for 1 week, then maintenance usually 200 mg daily. IV infusion: 5 mg/kg over 20–120 minutes with ECG monitoring	Causes corneal microdeposits on long-term therapy not requiring withdrawal which is reversible on discontinuation (may cause dazzle to night drivers), photosensitisation (sunscreen available), may cause hypothyroidism, or hyperthyroidism, reversible peripheral neuropathy and myopathy, diffuse pulmonary alveolitis and fibrosis, hepatitis	Contraindicated in sinus bradycardia, SA heart block, thyroid dysfunction, pregnancy and breast-feeding. Liver and thyroid function tests are required in long-term therapy. Contains 37% iodine which affects thyroid hormone metabolism
Disopyramide	90% absorbed from GI tract, metabolised in liver, 50% excreted unchanged in urine. Onset of action 30 minutes to 3 hours after oral administration	Oral: 300–800 mg daily in divided doses. Slow IV infusion: 2 mg/kg over at least 5 minutes to a maximum of 150 mg with ECG monitoring, followed immediately by either 200 mg by mouth then 200 mg every 8 hours for 24 hours or 400 micrograms/kg/hour by IV infusion	The negative inotropic effect may cause hypotension and aggravate cardiac failure, and it is important to avoid rapid infusion during the loading dose. Anticholinergic side-effects include dry mouth, blurred vision and urinary retention. May exacerbate glaucoma	Contraindicated in heart block and SA dysfunction (unless pacemaker fitted). Caution in glaucoma, prostatic enlargement, hepatic and renal impairment, pregnancy, the elderly
Flecainide	Well absorbed, reaching peak concentration in 2–3 hours	Oral: 100 mg twice daily to maximum of 400 mg. Slow IV injection: 2 mg/kg over 10–30 minutes – maximum of 150 mg with ECG monitoring	Dizziness and visual disturbances, jaundice, ataxia, peripheral neuropathy, pulmonary fibrosis	Contraindicated in heart failure, long-standing atrial fibrillation, history of MI. Caution in patients with pacemakers, the elderly, hepatic and renal impairment, pregnancy and breast-feeding
Procainamide	90% absorbed from GI tract. 50% is excreted unchanged, the other 50% metabolised including the active metabolite *N*-acetylprocainamide (NAPA), the quantity depending on whether the patient is a fast or slow acetylator. Doses should be reduced in hepatic disease and renal failure	Oral: up to 50 mg/kg daily in divided doses. By slow IV injection: up to 50 mg/minute, 100 mg with ECG monitoring repeated at 5-minute intervals until arrhythmia controlled – maximum 1 g	Cardiac adverse effects include heart failure; nausea, diarrhoea, rashes and fever may occur; lupus erythematosus-like syndrome and agranulocytosis have been noted	Contraindicated in heart failure and hypotension. Caution in the elderly, hepatic and renal impairment, asthma and myasthenia gravis
Propafenone	Rapidly absorbed after oral administration. Extensive hepatic metabolism. Half-life approximately 4–5 hours. Steady concentration attained after 3–4 days. Slow IV injection – works within minutes	Oral: 150–300 mg three times daily after food under hospital supervision with ECG monitoring and blood pressure control	Antimuscarinic side-effects include constipation, blurred vision, dry mouth. May also experience nausea, vomiting, diarrhoea, dizziness, headache, fatigue, postural hypotension, SA and AV block	Contraindicated in uncontrolled congestive heart failure, severe bradycardia, electrolyte imbalance, marked hypotension, myasthenia gravis. Caution in obstructive airways disease due to beta-blockers, hepatic and renal impairment, pacemaker patients, pregnancy
Quinidine	Almost completely absorbed. Onset of action is 30 minutes to 3 hours	Oral: 200 mg test dose to detect hypersensitivity reactions. 200–400 mg three to four times daily	Adverse effects are very common and have limited its usefulness. See under procainamide. In addition	Contraindicated in heart block. Quinidine inhibits renal tubular secretion of digoxin

(*continued*)

Table 16.5 (continued)				
Drug	Pharmacokinetics	Dose	Adverse effects	Notes
			thrombocytopenia and haemolytic anaemia. Also cinchonism with tinnitus, visual disturbances, headache, flushing, confusion, dizziness, vomiting and abdominal pain	and the digoxin dose should be lowered accordingly. Enzyme inducers including rifampicin, phenytoin and phenobarbital increase the metabolism of quinidine, therefore increased dose is required. Should not be used in combination with procainamide, amiodarone or disopyramide because of prolonged effect

Table 16.6 Drugs used in the treatment of ventricular arrhythmias

Drug	Indication	Pharmacokinetics	Dose	Adverse effects	Notes
Bretylium	Given by injection as an anti-arrhythmic in resuscitation	Available only as an injection because GI absorption is erratic. Active within minutes of IV injection in treatment of ventricular tachycardia and ectopy; onset of action takes 20 minutes to 6 hours. Half-life is 5–10 hours. Excreted unchanged by the kidneys over several days	IM injection: 5–10 mg/kg repeated after 6–8 hours if necessary. By slow IV injection: 5–10 mg/kg over 8–10 minutes with ECG and blood pressure monitoring. May be repeated	Severe hypotension, nausea and vomiting	Contraindicated in phaeochromocytoma Adrenaline (epinephrine) or other sympathomimetic amines should not be given
Lidocaine (lignocaine)	First choice in emergency. Effective in suppressing ventricular tachycardia and reducing the risk of ventricular fibrillation following myocardial infarction	Not available in oral form because most of absorbed drug undergoes first-pass metabolism in the liver. Exerts anti-arrhythmic effect in 1–2 minutes after IV administration	By IV injection: 100 mg as a bolus over several minutes followed by infusion of 2–4 mg/minute. Lower doses in congestive heart failure, hepatic failure	Central nervous system disturbances, including confusion, convulsions, drowsiness, paraesthesia	
Mexiletine	Has a similar action to lidocaine (lignocaine) and may be given as slow IV injection if lidocaine is ineffective	Well absorbed from GI tract. Onset of action is 30 minutes to 2 hours	Oral: 400–600 mg followed after 2 hours by 200–250 mg three or four times daily. IV injection: 100–250 mg at 25 mg/minute with ECG monitoring followed by infusion	Adverse cardiovascular and central nervous system effects may limit the dose tolerated. Nausea and vomiting may prevent an effective dose being given by mouth. Side-effects include bradycardia, hypotension, confusion, convulsions	Action antagonised by hypokalaemia; rifampicin accelerates metabolism

- by the Vaughan Williams classification, which classifies drugs into four distinct classes according to their effects on the electrical behaviour of myocardial cells during activity (termed the 'action potential').

To understand the actions of these drugs it is necessary first to examine the cardiac action potential (Fig. 16.3).

The cardiac action potential

Phase 4. Phase 4 is the resting phase in cells normally capable of spontaneous depolarisation (cells in SA node, AV node and His–Purkinje system). There is a voltage difference across the surface membrane of all myocardial cells which is called the resting transmembrane voltage or potential. During the resting phase there

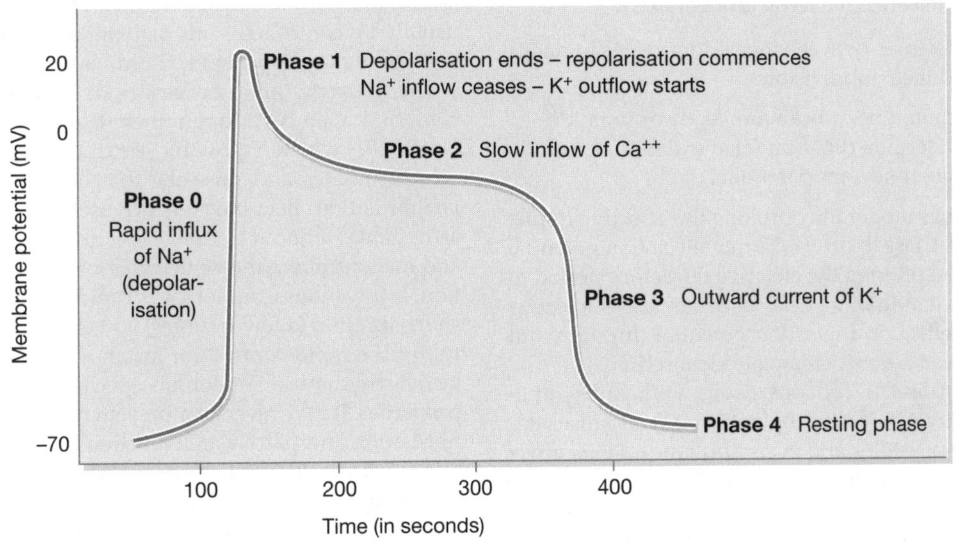

Figure 16.3 Phases of an action potential in the Purkinje fibre cell and the cationic changes which take place.

is a slow drift from the maximum negative potential (around −90 mV) to a potential of about −70 mV. This is due to a small influx of sodium ions into the cell and a small efflux of potassium ions. This depolarisation is spontaneous and continues until it reaches the threshold at which an action potential is initiated automatically (phase 0). Atrial and ventricular cells do not normally exhibit spontaneous depolarisation but remain at rest (diastole) until stimulated by a propagatory impulse.

Phase 0. When the threshold potential is reached and the cell is stimulated, there is a very rapid influx of sodium ions into the cell causing a rapid rise in transmembrane potential (depolarisation) until it reaches a given value (above 120 mV in Purkinje fibres). This inward current of sodium is very intense and very brief.

Phase 1. The potential starts to fall rapidly as repolarisation takes place, until it plateaus.

Phase 2. This phase is known as the plateau phase. There is a slow current of calcium ions into the cell which is balanced by a small outward current of potassium ions. These calcium ions are important to the strength of cardiac contraction, which is discussed under calcium antagonists (p. 192).

Phase 3. Repolarisation continues, marked by an outward flux of potassium ions. As the transmembrane potential falls to its maximum negative value the outward flux is terminated and phase 4 commences with sodium ions entering the cell and potassium ions leaving the cell.

Refractory period

During phases 1 to 3 (repolarisation), depolarisation cannot normally occur. This period is called the refractory period, although when about 50% of repolarisation has occurred a larger than normal stimulus can cause depolarisation.

Vaughan Williams classification of anti-arrhythmic actions

This system of classification categorises drugs by their action on cardiac conduction. A drug may show more than one of the classes of anti-arrhythmic action. Its main function is to define drugs with similar modes of action and to identify possible anti-arrhythmic compounds by their effects on cardiac conduction. The clinical value of this classification is limited and it excludes some anti-arrhythmic agents such as the cardiac glycosides. The four classes are as follows.

Class I. Class I drugs are those with local anaesthetic properties which act as membrane-stabilising agents. Depolarisation of the cardiac cell membrane is depressed by restricting entry of the fast sodium current. This reduces the rate of rise of phase 0 of the action potential and depresses the rate of phase 4 depolarisation. These effects tend to:

- reduce the automatic initiation of the action potential

- reduce the speed of conductivity
- increase the effective refractory period.

Clinical differences between the various drugs in class 1 necessitated their subdivision:

Class Ia: quinidine, procainamide, disopyramide
Class Ib: lidocaine (lignocaine), mexiletine, tocainide
Class Ic: flecainide, propafenone.

Class Ia drugs moderately prolong the effective refractory period. Class Ib drugs shorten the action potential duration and prolong the effective refractory period to a greater extent than do class Ia drugs. Class Ic drugs have little effect on the action potential duration, but increase the His–ventricular conduction time.

Class II. Class II contains drugs with antisympathetic activity. Adrenaline (epinephrine) can cause ventricular extrasystoles and even fibrillation by its effect on the pacemaker potential and the slow inward current, carried by calcium ions, in myocardial cells. Ventricular dysrhythmias following myocardial infarction are due partly to increased sympathetic activity.

The beta-blockers act as competitive antagonists and block receptor sites in the conduction system of the heart. This slows the triggering of the SA node and the conductivity of the AV node and other cells. The beta-blockers also exert a significant negative inotropic effect. By decreasing myocardial oxygen demand, myocardial ischaemia may be reduced. As ischaemia abates, myocardial cells lose their automaticity and this effect suppresses atrial and ventricular ectopy. Examples are propranolol, metoprolol and acebutolol.

Class III. Class III drugs greatly prolong the duration of the action potential and the effective refractory period in both atrial and ventricular tissue. Bretylium and amiodarone are class III drugs.

Class IV. Calcium ions play an essential part in the process of contraction of vascular and myocardial smooth muscle. In the heart this occurs during phase 2 (plateau) of the action potential. The entry of calcium ions into the cells causes fibre shortening and increased myocardial wall tension. The degree of this contraction (or positive inotropic state) is regulated by the amount of calcium ions that reach the contractile proteins. Calcium antagonists block the entry of calcium ions through the slow calcium channels. This blockade greatly increases the effective refractory period of the AV node and slows the conduction rate between atria and ventricles. Verapamil is in class IV.

Management of arrhythmias

Management of an arrhythmia, apart from treatment of the associated heart failure, requires precise diagnosis of the type of arrhythmia and an electrocardiograph is essential. In atrial fibrillation, the ventricular rate can usually be controlled with digoxin. A beta-blocker or verapamil may be added if control is inadequate.

The antiarrhythmic properties of beta-blockers are conferred mainly through their β_1-blocking actions (see p. 181) which oppose the electrophysical effects of catecholamines and raise the threshold for ventricular fibrillation. Beta-blockers are useful in preventing arrhythmias induced by exercise, emotion or anaesthesia and for controlling the ventricular rate in atrial fibrillation. Intravenous esmolol gives rapid beta-blockade of short duration (a few minutes) and is particularly useful for the rapid control, for instance, of perioperative tachyarrhythmias. Sotalol has specific antiarrhythmic properties. It may reverse or prevent recurrence of atrial fibrillation and paroxysmal junction tachycardia associated with the Wolff–Parkinson–White syndrome (see below) and may prevent recurrent life-threatening ventricular arrhythmias. However, sotalol may itself cause serious ventricular arrhythmia, including torsade de pointes, especially in patients with depressed left ventricular function, hypokalaemia, or if given with other drugs that prolong the QT interval. Sotalol should be reserved for patients with serious arrhythmias likely to benefit specifically from its antiarrhythmic actions. In valvular or myocardial disease anticoagulants may be indicated. In atrial flutter the ventricular rate can similarly be controlled by digoxin. Synchronised direct current shock can be utilised where reversion to sinus rhythm is indicated.

The Wolfe–Parkinson–White syndrome

The Wolfe–Parkinson–White syndrome is a congenital abnormality occurring in about 0.2% of the population. It results from an additional conducting system between the atria and the ventricles. It is associated with supraventricular arrhythmias due to re-entry through the additional conducting system.

In treating these arrhythmias it should be remembered that the additional bundle may not respond to drugs in the same way as the normal conducting system. In particular, digoxin and verapamil enhance rather than depress conduction through the additional bundle and are therefore contraindicated. Depending on circumstances amiodarone, disopyramide or flecainide are used.

Paroxysmal supraventricular tachycardia usually remits spontaneously or can be returned to sinus rhythm by reflex vagal stimulation by prompt squatting or respiratory control. If drug treatment is required intravenous adenosine is usually first choice. Digitalisation,

Table 16.7 Features of some beta-blockers

Drug	Feature of selectivity	Dose – oral
Acebutolol	$\beta_1 > \beta_2$	400–1200 mg daily in divided doses
Atenolol	$\beta_1 > \beta_2$	50–100 mg daily
Betaxolol	$\beta_1 > \beta_2$	20–40 mg daily
Bisoprolol	$\beta_1 > \beta_2$	10–20 mg daily
Carvedilol	$\alpha + \beta_1 + \beta_2$	12.5–50 mg daily
Celiprolol	$\beta_1 + \beta_2$	200–400 mg daily
Esmolol	$\beta_1 > \beta_2$	IV only
Labetalol	$\alpha_1 + \beta_1 + \beta_2$	100–800 mg daily in divided doses
Metoprolol	$\beta_1 > \beta_2$	50–300 mg daily in divided doses
Nadolol	$\beta_1 + \beta_2$	40–240 mg daily
Oxprenolol	$\beta_1 + \beta_2$	40–160 mg daily in divided doses
Pindolol	$\beta_1 + \beta_2$	2.5–45 mg daily
Propranolol	$\beta_1 + \beta_2$	80–320 mg daily in divided doses
Sotalol	$\beta_1 + \beta_2$	80–320 mg daily
Timolol	$\beta_1 + \beta_2$	10–60 mg daily

an intravenous beta-blocker, intravenous verapamil or direct current shock may be tried.

Where arrhythmias occur after myocardial infarction, lidocaine (lignocaine) should be given intravenously. Bradycardia, especially if complicated with hypotension, should be treated with intravenous atropine sulphate (0.3–1 mg).

BETA-ADRENOCEPTOR BLOCKING DRUGS

Adrenaline (epinephrine) and noradrenaline (norepinephrine), which are produced by the adrenal glands and at sympathetic nerve endings, exercise their physiological actions via alpha- and beta-adrenoceptors.

Beta-adrenoceptors are widely distributed in the body, being present in the heart, bronchi, blood vessels, eyes, pancreas, liver and gastrointestinal tract. The beta receptors can be divided into two groups:

- β_1 receptors, which predominate in the heart
- β_2 receptors, which are found mainly in the airways and blood vessels.

Stimulation of β_1-adrenoceptors in the heart and coronary arteries will lead to an increase in heart rate, increase in conduction velocity and force of contraction in the heart and vasodilatation of coronary arteries. Excitation of β_2-adrenoceptors will lead to dilatation of peripheral arteries.

Beta-adrenergic blocking agents interfere with catecholamine binding at beta-adrenoceptors. Several beta-blockers (acebutolol, atenolol, betaxolol, bisoprolol and metoprolol) are said to be cardioselective. These agents have the ability to antagonise the action of catecholamines at β_1 receptors at doses smaller than those required to block β_2 receptors. They are not, however, cardiospecific. They have a smaller effect on airways' resistance but are not free of this side-effect. Others block both β_1 and β_2 receptors (i.e. cardiac + bronchial + peripheral blood vessel receptors) and are called non-selective beta-blockers (see Table 16.7). Blocking β_2 receptors causes bronchospasm, which may be of little consequence in normal subjects but in asthmatic patients may make bronchospasm worse and increase dyspnoea. Beta-blockers should be used only in patients with asthma or in those with a history of obstructive airways disease where no alternative treatment is available.

Some beta-blockers (pindolol, oxprenolol, acebutolol and celiprolol) demonstrate various degrees of intrinsic sympathomimetic activity (ISA) which represents the capacity of beta-blockers to stimulate as well as block adrenergic receptors. These drugs cause a slight agonist response at the beta receptor while blocking the effect of endogenous catecholamine. Patients given a drug with ISA experience a smaller reduction in resting heart rate than those receiving a beta-blocker without ISA. They tend to cause less bradycardia and less coldness of the extremities than the other beta-blockers, which is a problem particularly in patients with peripheral vascular disease.

Some beta-blockers are water-soluble and some are lipid-soluble. Lipophilic beta-blockers are able to cross the blood–brain barrier and exert effects on the central nervous system. Nightmares and hallucinations are more of a problem with the lipophilic agents. The most water-soluble are atenolol, celiprolol, nadolol and sotalol. They are less likely to enter the brain and may therefore cause fewer sleep disturbances and nightmares. Water-soluble beta-blockers are excreted by the kidneys and dose reduction may be required in renal impairment.

All beta-blockers slow the heart; the output of blood is reduced and the work done by the heart is thus decreased. They should not therefore be given to patients with heart failure or heart block.

Labetalol is a mixed alpha, and non-selective beta-adrenergic antagonist which reduces peripheral resistance but has little effect on heart rate or cardiac output. Positive hypotension occurs. Labetalol may be useful in hypertension of pregnancy and in patients with renal failure.

Beta-blockers are contraindicated in asthma or obstructive airways disease, second- or third-degree heart block, sinus bradycardia, sick sinus syndrome, severe peripheral arterial disease and uncompensated cardiac failure.

The side-effects of beta-blockers include fatigue, cold extremities, bronchoconstriction, interference with autonomic and metabolic responses to hypoglycaemia, bradycardia, heart block, negative inotropic effect and impotence.

Uses of beta-blockers

Hypertension

Beta-blockers are effective in the treatment of many medical conditions but are most widely used for the treatment of patients with hypertension, in whom they may reduce the long-term morbidity and mortality, and for the prevention of angina. Beta-blockers lower the diastolic blood pressure to less than 95 mm of mercury in about 40–50% of patients with mild to moderate hypertension. The mechanism of hypotensive action of the beta-blockers is not fully understood. Reduction of cardiac output, resetting of baroreceptors, suppression of renin (which is directly responsible for the production of angiotensin, a circulating vasoconstrictor hormone), release of vasodilator prostaglandins, prejunctional beta receptor blockade and a direct action on the central nervous system have all been proposed. It may be due to a combination of several of these factors. Blood pressure can usually be controlled with few side-effects.

Long-term control with a regimen that includes a beta-blocker as first- or second-line therapy (with a thiazide diuretic) reduces mortality and the risk of stroke or of heart attack. These regimens also benefit patients over 60 years with hypertension.

Angina

Beta-blockers, competitive inhibitors of catecholamines, decrease the heart rate, thereby reducing the cardiac workload and increasing the diastolic interval, allowing better coronary perfusion during exercise and reducing the myocardial oxygen demand.

In patients with stable angina, beta-blockers have been shown to be important therapeutic agents as monotherapy or as adjuncts to nitrates. They are particularly useful in the treatment of exertional angina because of their negative inotropic and chronotropic actions. The most commonly prescribed beta-blockers are atenolol, bisoprolol and metoprolol, which are all cardioselective. A sudden withdrawal of a beta-blocker in patients with angina may cause an exacerbation of the symptoms because of an increase in the number of beta receptors available for stimulation when the antagonist is no longer being given. Stopping a beta-blocker should therefore be by gradual withdrawal.

Myocardial infarction

Beta-blockade in the first 24 hours after myocardial infarction, when myocardial damage (e.g. rupture) and risk of serious arrhythmias are greatest, is reliably achieved only by intravenous administration, e.g. metoprolol and atenolol may reduce early mortality after intravenous and subsequent oral administration in acute phase.

- Metoprolol – IV 5 mg over 2 minutes for three doses followed by oral therapy with 50 mg four times daily for 2 days then 100 mg twice daily.
- Atenolol – IV 5 mg over 5 minutes for two doses then oral therapy with 50 mg twice daily for 2 days then 50–100 mg once daily.

Intravenous treatment reduces mortality, reinfarction rate and incidence of cardiac arrest. Follow-on oral treatment with a beta-blocker reduces the risk of reinfarction and death by about 20–25% over 3 years. Where there is pre-existing heart failure, hypotension, bradyarrhythmias or obstructive airways disease this group of drugs is unsuitable.

Other uses of beta-blockers

Beta-blockers (see Table 16.7) are used in preoperative preparation for thyroidectomy 4 days before surgery. Propranolol reverses clinical symptoms of thyrotoxicosis. The thyroid is rendered less vascular, making surgery easier. Beta-blockers are also used:

- to relieve anxiety – patients with palpitations, tremor and tachycardia respond better
- in prophylaxis of migraine (p. 248)
- topically in glaucoma (p. 411).

Pharmacokinetics

Beta-blockers are usually well absorbed from the gastrointestinal tract (atenolol is an exception – about 50%). Acebutolol, labetalol, metoprolol, propranolol and timolol undergo extensive first-pass metabolism in the liver. The duration of action ranges from 4 hours for oral timolol to 24 hours for oral atenolol.

ANTIHYPERTENSIVE DRUGS

Blood pressure

Blood pressure may be defined as the force exerted on the walls of the blood vessels. Arterial blood pressure is the pressure exerted when the heart pumps blood into the already full aorta. The factors determining the blood pressure are:

- cardiac output
- blood volume
- peripheral resistance
- viscosity of the blood
- venous return.

Blood pressure is maintained by sensory receptors found in several of the arteries close to the heart. These baroreceptors convey information to the vasomotor centre in the medulla of the brain in response to changes in the blood pressure. The vasomotor centre in turn transmits impulses via the sympathetic nervous system to the smooth muscle in the walls of the arterioles, which are stimulated to contract. The chemical transmitter between neurone and muscle is noradrenaline (norepinephrine). The arterioles are kept in a state of partial vasoconstriction by the vasomotor centre. If the vasomotor activity increases, the blood vessels will constrict and the blood pressure will rise and vice versa.

Hypertension

Blood pressure changes with emotion, posture, exercise, etc. In such circumstances, the changes are brought about by reflex adjustments, the aim of which is to keep the pressure at the most appropriate level for the body's needs. Physicians have difficulty agreeing what constitutes hypertension. An elevation of the resting blood pressure above the 'normal' for the patient's age, weight and height is a broadly acceptable definition. This would be the result of taking several readings under resting conditions. Some 95% of all cases are described as essential hypertension for which there is no known cause. The remainder of cases are associated with renal disorder, adrenal disorder, coarctation of the aorta or toxaemia of pregnancy. In many instances there are no symptoms. Some cases are picked up on routine examination or when the patient presents with one of the complications of hypertension such as stroke, ischaemic heart disease or renal failure. Malignant hypertension is a rare condition which affects fairly young males. It has a rapid onset and causes severe headache, dizziness, left ventricular failure and papilloedema. The diastolic blood pressure may be as high as 140 mmHg.

In patients with hypertension, controls are not able to maintain the blood pressure at the normal level. This may be due to a number of factors:

- rigidity of blood vessels due to atheroma which inevitably occurs with age
- hormonal changes which alter peripheral resistance or blood volume
- other factors which may set the baroreceptors at the wrong level.

If there is an identified cause for hypertension, this must be treated, e.g. phaeochromocytoma, but this is rare. In the relatively few cases where a cause can be found the hypertension is designated as secondary hypertension.

Hypertension requires to be treated since serious cardiovascular complications may result – such as stroke, heart failure, renal failure or myocardial infarction. Where the cause cannot be removed, high blood pressure is treated with antihypertensive agents. The methods by which these are effective are based on the fact that blood pressure depends on:

- the peripheral vascular resistance
- the output of blood from the heart
- the volume of blood within the circulation.

By decreasing one or more of these it is possible to lower the blood pressure.

Aetiological factors in hypertension

A family history of hypertension is common in patients who present with raised blood pressure. There is also a positive correlation between obesity and blood pressure. It is accepted that a reduction in body weight will reduce blood pressure in hypertensive patients. A high salt and high alcohol intake may elevate blood pressure and these should be corrected.

Antihypertensive therapy

Initiation of antihypertensive therapy is recommended by the British Hypertension Society for patients with a sustained systolic blood pressure ⩾160 mm mercury or a sustained diastolic blood pressure ⩾100 mm of mercury. The aim of antihypertensive treatment is to reduce the blood pressure to within normal limits, thereby reducing the number of subsequent cardiovascular events. Optimum blood pressure treatment targets are systolic blood pressure <140 mm mercury and diastolic blood pressure <85 mm mercury.

Diuretic therapy

Thiazide diuretics (see p. 172) are regarded as first- or second-choice drugs for hypertension. The hypotensive effect of thiazides is not related solely to their promotion of salt and water loss, they also dilate arterioles – leading to reduced resistance. Only low doses are needed for maximal hypotensive effect and increasing the dose merely increases the incidence of adverse effects. A thiazide such as bendroflumethiazide (bendrofluazide) 2.5 mg is inexpensive and allows once-daily dosing. Larger doses can cause more metabolic disturbances without any improvement in blood pressure control. Routine use of low doses minimises adverse effects such as hypokalaemia, hyperuricaemia, glucose intolerance, insulin resistance and elevation of serum cholesterol and calcium. Indapamide is a thiazide-like diuretic. While the incidence of hypokalaemia and hyperuricaemia is the same as with thiazides, indapamide produces no adverse effects on the lipid profile, blood glucose or insulin levels. Indapamide is thought to inhibit progression of left ventricular hypertrophy.

Thiazides are contraindicated in gout, diabetes and hypercalcaemia. Important interactions occur with lithium (lithium toxicity), digoxin (risk of arrhythmia) and non-steroidal anti-inflammatory drugs (hypotensive action reduced).

Loop diuretics have less antihypertensive action than thiazides in uncomplicated patients and are not routinely used for hypertension. They have a valuable role in patients with resistant hypertension, renal impairment, coexistent heart failure and in patients taking the potent vasodilator minoxidil (for further information on diuretics see pp. 172–175).

Beta-adrenoceptor blocking drugs

These are used on their own, or where not effective, in combination with a thiazide diuretic (see p. 172).

Calcium-channel blockers

Calcium-channel blockers have efficacy similar to that of beta-blockers and thiazide diuretics and are normally used if these prove unsuccessful. Within the calcium-channel blocking group of drugs, which includes diltiazem, verapamil, nifedipine, nicardipine and amlodipine, there are important differences (see p. 192).

Angiotensin-converting enzyme inhibitors (ACE inhibitors)

These drugs are commenced at low doses since they may cause a profound fall in blood pressure after the first dose, particularly in patients with renal impairment or receiving diuretic therapy. Diuretic therapy should be ceased 3 days before commencing ACE inhibitor treatment (for further details see pp. 186–189).

A single antihypertensive drug is often not adequate and other antihypertensive drugs are usually added in a stepwise manner until control is achieved. Unless it is necessary to lower the blood pressure urgently, an interval of at least 4 weeks should be allowed to determine response. In uncomplicated mild hypertension (systolic blood pressure <160 mm mercury and diastolic <100 mm mercury) drugs may be substituted rather than added.

Other drugs

Vasodilators (diazoxide, hydralazine, minoxidil) (see Table 16.8), alpha-adrenoceptor blocking drugs (prazosin, terazosin, doxazosin), and centrally acting drugs (methyldopa) are generally reserved for patients whose blood pressure is not controlled by, or who have contraindications to, the drugs already mentioned.

Hypertension in pregnancy

This can be safely treated with methyldopa. Beta-blockers may cause intrauterine growth retardation early in pregnancy but are safe from the third trimester onwards.

Malignant hypertension (accelerated hypertension)

Malignant hypertension (diastolic blood pressure in excess of 140 mm of mercury) requires urgent hospital treatment. Although it is desirable to reduce diastolic blood pressure below 120 mm of mercury within 24 hours this can normally be achieved by oral therapy. If it is lowered too rapidly, cerebral blood flow may fall and brain damage and death can occur from cerebral anoxia, cerebral oedema and cerebral infarction. Normal treatment should be with a beta-blocker (atenolol or labetalol) or a calcium-channel blocker (nifedipine). Only rarely is parenteral treatment necessary, e.g. in patients with acute dissection of aortic aneurysm, hypertensive encephalopathy. Sodium nitroprusside by infusion is the drug of choice.

Table 16.8 Information on vasodilators

Drug	Pharmacokinetics	Dosage	Adverse effects	Notes
Diazoxide	Available only as injection. Metabolised in liver to inactive metabolites. One-third excreted unchanged in kidneys. It acts in a few minutes, its action lasting from 3–12 hours	Rapid IV injection: 1–3 mg/kg to maximum 150 mg. May be repeated	Headache, nausea, tachycardia, hyperglycaemia, sodium and water retention	Caution in pregnancy, ischaemic heart disease and impaired renal function
Hydralazine	Rapidly absorbed from the GI tract. Oral preparations act in 20–30 minutes and much faster by injection	Oral: 25–50 mg twice daily. Slow IV injection: 5–10 mg	Tachycardia, nausea, vomiting, diarrhoea, fluid retention	Contraindicated in systemic lupus erythematosus since at higher doses over longer term it can cause a systemic lupus erythematosus-like syndrome. Caution in coronary disease, pregnancy and breast-feeding
Minoxidil	Well absorbed from GI tract. Onset of action is approximately 30 minutes. Its therapeutic action may last several days	Initially 5 mg daily, increasing by 5–10 mg every 3 days as required. Maximum: 50 mg	Vasodilatation is accompanied by increased cardiac output, tachycardia and sodium and water retention occur. For this reason a beta-blocker and a diuretic (usually furosemide (frusemide) in high dosage) are required. Other side-effects include weight gain and hypertrichosis	Contraindicated in phaeochromocytoma. Caution in angina, pregnancy, after myocardial infarction

Sodium nitroprusside

Mode of action. Sodium nitroprusside has a direct relaxant effect on the smooth muscle of veins and arteries. The resultant peripheral vasodilatation produces a hypotensive effect.

Pharmacokinetics. The half-life of sodium nitroprusside is only a few minutes. Its effects can therefore be accurately controlled when administered by infusion.

Dose. In patients not already receiving antihypertensives, sodium nitroprusside is given at a dose of 0.5–1.5 microgram/kg/minute by infusion in 5% glucose and increased as required to a maximum of 8 micrograms/kg/minute. Patients on current antihypertensive therapy require a lower dose. The infusion should be protected from light.

Adverse effects. The following effects may occur but will reduce on slowing the infusion rate: headache, dizziness, nausea, retching, abdominal pain, perspiration and palpitations.

Vasodilator antihypertensive drugs

Diazoxide, hydralazine and minoxidil are potent drugs, especially when used in combination with a beta-blocker or a thiazide (see Table 16.8). However, they are generally reserved for patients whose blood pressure is not controlled by, or who have contraindications to, the drugs previously described – thiazides, beta-blockers, calcium-channel blockers and ACE inhibitors.

Mode of action. Diazoxide, hydralazine and minoxidil cause peripheral arteriolar dilatation by a direct relaxing effect on vascular smooth muscle. The peripheral dilatation causes a fall in blood pressure. This in turn may cause a resultant reflex tachycardia, negating the fall in blood pressure. This reflex tachycardia can be prevented by administering along with hydralazine or minoxidil a beta-blocker which potentiates their action. For this reason combination therapy is common when these vasodilators are used.

Centrally acting antihypertensive drugs

Methyldopa

Methyldopa is converted in the body to methylnoradrenaline. In the central nervous system this compound stimulates the alpha-adrenergic receptors which results in decreased activity of the sympathetic system. Vascular peripheral tone and arteriolar vasoconstriction are decreased, which lowers standing and supine blood pressures. There is little effect on cardiac output and there is less orthostatic hypotension compared with peripherally acting agents.

Indications. Methyldopa is effective in the treatment of hypertension and is easy to use because the fall in blood pressure is not precipitous. It is no longer widely used because of a high incidence of adverse effects. However, it is safe in asthmatics, in heart failure and in pregnancy.

Pharmacokinetics. Methyldopa is well absorbed from the gastrointestinal tract. The onset of action is immediate when given intravenously and takes 3 to 6 hours after oral administration.

Dose. By mouth, 250 mg two or three times daily increased gradually at intervals of 2 or more days to a maximum of 3 g.

Adverse effects. Central nervous system adverse effects include depression and drowsiness. It may also cause dry mouth, diarrhoea, fluid retention, failure of ejaculation, liver damage, and, rarely, haemolytic anaemia. In patients with severe renal impairment, dosage should be reduced. Methyldopa is contraindicated where there is active liver disease, history of depression and phaeochromocytoma. Where fluid retention is a problem, this can be controlled by a diuretic.

Moxonidine

A second class of binding sites termed imidazoline receptors has also been shown to influence central sympathetic activity. Moxonidine is the first of a new generation of centrally-acting agents which binds selectively and with high affinity to imidazoline 1 receptors. Occupation of the imidazoline binding site by moxonidine leads to reduced peripheral sympathetic activity and a consequent reduction in peripheral resistance of the arterioles, while cardiac output and pulmonary haemodynamics remain generally unaffected.

Pharmacokinetics. Moxonidine is well absorbed from the gastrointestinal tract. Plasma concentration peaks at 1 hour and plasma half-life is around 2 hours. It is excreted largely unchanged in the urine. The dose should be reduced in patients whose glomerular filtration rate is less than 60 mL/min.

Dose. A once-daily dose of 200 micrograms in the morning, increased if necessary after 3 weeks to 400 micrograms daily in one or two divided doses. Maximum 600 micrograms in two divided doses.

Side-effects. Side-effects include dry mouth, headache, fatigue, sedation, dizziness, nausea, sleep disturbances, vasodilatation. Moxonidine is contraindicated in patients with history of angio-oedema, cardiac conduction disorders, bradycardia, life-threatening arrhythmia, severe heart failure, severe coronary artery disease, unstable angina, severe liver disease or renal impairment.

Alpha-adrenoceptor-blocking drugs

Alpha$_1$-adrenoceptor antagonists are effective and well-tolerated drugs that can be used alone or in combination with other groups of drugs in a wide range of hypertensive patients. Alpha-blockers reduce left ventricular hypertrophy. They may be considered in patients who fail to respond to, or have toxicity associated with, diuretics and/or beta-blockers, including hypertensive patients with lipid disorders or diabetes. Prazosin, terazocin and doxazosin are equally effective in reducing blood pressure in older people. They lower elevated blood pressure by reducing peripheral arterial resistance without increasing the heart rate or reducing cardiac output.

The drugs to be considered in Tables 16.9 and 16.10 are doxazosin, indoramin, phenoxybenzamine, phentolamine, prazosin and terazosin.

Angiotensin-converting enzyme inhibitors (ACE inhibitors)

ACE inhibitors act on the renin–angiotensin–aldosterone system (see Fig. 16.4) by inhibiting the angiotensin-converting enzyme (ACE). This system plays an important role in regulating blood pressure, blood volume and electrolyte concentrations. Renin is released from the kidney in response to reduced renal perfusion. It converts angiotensinogen to form angiotensin I. Angiotensin I is then converted in both plasma and tissue to angiotensin II by ACE. Angiotensin II is a potent vasoconstrictor and, in addition, stimulates the release of aldosterone, which promotes water and sodium retention. Both these actions serve to raise blood pressure. ACE inhibitors, by inhibiting the production of angiotensin II, thus effectively lower blood pressure.

ACE also inactivates certain neuropeptides, including bradykinin. ACE inhibitors therefore increase levels of bradykinin, which may play an important role in preventing left ventricular hypertrophy (LVH). Bradykinin

Table 16.9 Alpha-adrenoceptor blocking drugs: mode of action and indications

Drug	Mode of action	Indications
Doxazosin	As for prazosin	Hypertension usually in conjunction with a thiazide or beta-blocker
Indoramin	As for prazosin	Hypertension usually in conjunction with a thiazide or beta-blocker, benign prostatic hyperplasia
Phenoxybenzamine	As for phentolamine	Used with beta-blockers for short-term management of severe hypertensive episodes associated with phaeochromocytoma. It is also used in the management of severe shock unresponsive to conventional therapy
Phentolamine	Acts directly on both α_1- and α_2-adrenoceptors, blocking the pharmacological action of noradrenaline (norepinephrine) – producing vasodilatation by reducing peripheral resistance. Its action is not selective on α_1 receptors, and reflex tachycardia occurs	Hypertensive crisis due to phaeochromocytoma
Prazosin	Selectively blocks α_1 receptors, interfering with sympathetic stimulation and directly relaxing arteriolar smooth muscle. This interference reduces peripheral vascular resistance and produces vasodilatation without causing tachycardia or reducing cardiac output	Hypertension, congestive heart failure, Raynaud's syndrome, benign prostatic hyperplasia
Terazosin	As for prazosin	Mild to moderate hypertension, benign prostatic hyperplasia

Table 16.10 Alpha-adrenoceptor blocking drugs: dose and adverse effects

Drug	Dose	Adverse effects	Notes
Doxazosin	Oral: 1 mg daily increased after 1–2 weeks to 2 mg daily. Maximum: 16 mg daily	Postural hypotension, dizziness, headache, fatigue, oedema	
Indoramin	Hypertension, oral: usually in conjunction with a thiazide diuretic or a beta-blocker – initially 25 mg twice daily increased by 25–50 mg daily at intervals of 2 weeks; maximum daily dose 200 mg in two to three divided doses	Drowsiness, dizziness, depression, dry mouth, weight gain, extrapyramidal effects, failure of ejaculation	Avoid alcohol (enhances absorption). Caution in Parkinson's disease, epilepsy, history of depression, hepatic or renal impairment
Phenoxybenzamine	Oral – phaeochromocytoma: 10 mg daily increased by 10 mg daily – usual dose 1–2 mg/kg daily in two divided doses	Postural hypotension, dizziness, compensatory tachycardia, lassitude, nasal congestion, inhibition of ejaculation	Caution in renal impairment, pregnancy, elderly, heart failure, ischaemic heart disease
Phentolamine	IV injection: 2–5 mg, repeated if necessary	Hypotension, tachycardia, dizziness, nausea, diarrhoea, nasal congestion	Monitor blood pressure and heart rate
Prazosin	Hypertension, oral: 500 micrograms two to three times daily, increased to 1 mg two to three times daily after 3–7 days, further increased to a maximum 20 mg daily	Dizziness and loss of consciousness may occur following the first dose because of profound hypotension. The initial dose should be taken in bed. Other common effects include drowsiness, weakness, headache, urinary frequency	Reduce initial dose in renal impairment
Terazosin	Oral: 1 mg at bedtime, dose doubled after 7 days if necessary, usual maintenance dose 2–10 mg daily	Dizziness, lack of energy, peripheral oedema, urinary frequency. Initial dose taken at bedtime as for prazosin	

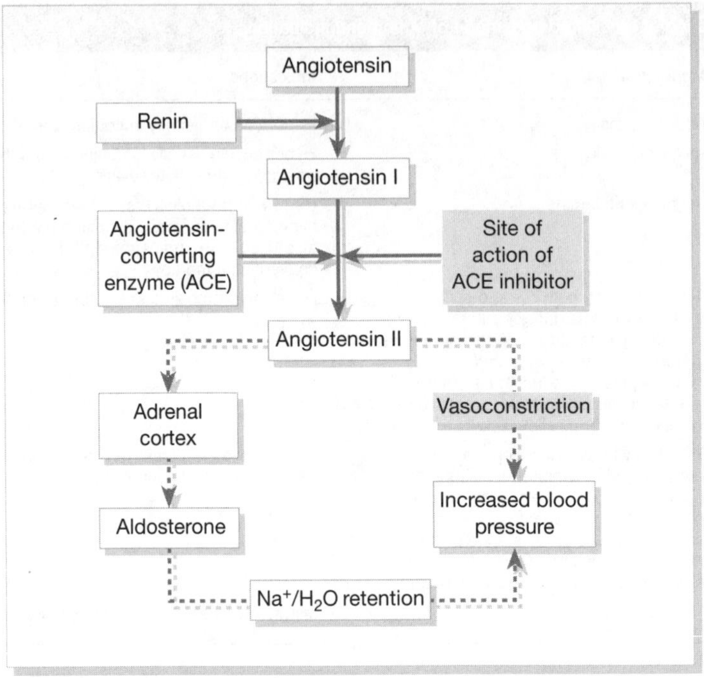

Figure 16.4 Sites of action of ACE inhibitors.

is also a vasodilator and may have a key role in the cardioprotective actions of ACE inhibitors. In the kidney they reduce proteinuria by local inhibition on the post-glomerular efferent arteriole. This causes greater dilatation of the efferent than the afferent arteriole, reducing the intraglomerular pressure and thereby reducing proteinuria. This forms the basis of ACE inhibitors as the antihypertensives of choice in diabetics, thus protecting the kidney from further damage. These drugs are now being increasingly used to protect the kidney in non-diabetic kidney disease, except in polycystic disease.

Indications. ACE inhibitors are used to control hypertension, particularly when thiazides and beta-blockers are contraindicated or ineffective. They are particularly indicated for hypertension in insulin-dependent diabetics with nephropathy and possibly for hypertension in all diabetics. Since, in some patients, all cause a very rapid fall in blood pressure, diuretic therapy should be stopped for several days before commencing ACE inhibitors in order to avoid an additive effect. This is termed first-dose hypotension, and treatment should be commenced at low dose, being taken at bedtime.

ACE inhibitors are also used in the treatment of heart failure, either as an adjunct to diuretics or in cases where there is no response to diuretics. They may also be used, where appropriate, with digoxin. Dilatation of the arterioles reduces the load on the heart and improves its function. Potassium-sparing diuretics or potassium supplements should not be given concomitantly with ACE inhibitors as dangerous hyperkalaemia may result.

Indications and dosages of ACE inhibitors are given in Table 16.11.

Pharmacokinetics. The ACE inhibitor should be started at a very low dose (e.g. captopril 6.25 mg) with the patient recumbent and under close medical supervision with facilities to treat profound hypotension. In these circumstances, and in other special risk groups, therapy should be commenced in hospital.

Following myocardial infarction, compensatory changes occur in the heart which lead to ventricular hypertrophy and ultimately heart failure. ACE inhibitors given post-myocardial infarction can reduce these compensatory changes.

Side-effects. ACE inhibitors are generally well tolerated. Dry cough caused by the inhibition of bradykinin breakdown is a feature of ACE inhibitor therapy in up to 15% of patients. This is unresponsive to antitussives and can be severe enough to cause patients to discontinue therapy.

Hypotension, which may be profound, can occur after the first dose of an ACE inhibitor. Patients most at risk include those with congestive cardiac failure (CCF), volume depletion and high-renin hypertension. The

Table 16.11 Indications and dosages for ACE inhibitors

Drug	Dose	Indications		
		Hypertension	Heart failure	Post-MI
Captopril	Hypertension 6.25–50 mg twice daily Heart failure (adjunct) 6.25–150 mg two to three times daily Diabetic neuropathy 75–100 mg daily in divided doses	Yes	Yes	Yes
Cilazapril	Hypertension 1–5 mg daily Heart failure (adjunct) 500 micrograms–2.5 mg daily	Yes	Yes	No
Enalapril	Hypertension 2.5–40 mg once daily Heart failure (adjunct) 2.5–20 mg in one or two divided doses	Yes	Yes	No
Fosinopril	Hypertension and heart failure (adjunct) 10–40 mg daily	Yes	Yes	No
Imidapril	Hypertension 2.5–20 mg daily	Yes	No	No
Lisinopril	Hypertension 2.5–40 mg daily Heart failure (adjunct) 2.5–20 mg daily	Yes	Yes	Yes
Moexipril	Hypertension 3.75–30 mg daily	Yes	No	No
Perindopril	Hypertension 2–8 mg daily Heart failure (adjunct) 2–4 mg daily	Yes	Yes	No
Quinapril	Hypertension 2.5–80 mg in one or two divided doses Heart failure (adjunct) 2.5–40 mg in one or two daily doses	Yes	Yes	No
Ramipril	Hypertension 1.25–10 mg daily Heart failure (adjunct) 1.25–10 mg in one or two divided doses	Yes	Yes	Yes
Trandolapril	Hypertension and post-MI 500 micrograms–4 mg daily	Yes	No	Yes

risk may be minimised by stopping or reducing existing diuretic therapy and administering a low test dose of an ACE inhibitor with a short half-life. ACE inhibitors have produced acute renal failure in patients with bilateral renal artery stenosis and atherosis of the artery supplying a single functioning kidney, because of loss of perfusion pressure. ACE inhibitors are contraindicated in such patients. Hyponatraemia, high-dose diuretic therapy and severe CCF are other predisposing factors to worsening renal function. Haematological side-effects may occur, in particular when ACE inhibitors are administered with other drugs causing blood dyscrasias; these side-effects are generally reversible. ACE inhibitors may have a lesser antihypertensive response in Afro-Caribbean patients.

A maculopapular or pruritic rash occurring early on in therapy may be a feature, though this is often self-limiting. Rarely, photosensitivity may occur. Similarly, taste disturbance (characterised by a metallic taste) or taste suppression may arise within the first 1–3 months but is also self-limiting. Hyperkalaemia may occur due to renal potassium retention and may become clinically significant in patients with renal impairment or those taking potassium-sparing diuretics or potassium supplements. Angio-oedema involving the face and lips, and more dangerously the larynx, may rarely occur.

Contraindications. ACE inhibitors are best avoided in patients with known or suspected renovascular disease, including patients with symptomatic peripheral vascular disease or severe generalised atherosclerosis. Bilateral renal artery stenosis or arterial stenosis to a single kidney are contraindications. ACE inhibitors should not be used in aortic stenosis or outflow tract obstruction.

All ACE inhibitors are contraindicated in any trimester of pregnancy as they may adversely affect fetal growth, neonatal blood pressure control and renal function.

Angiotensin-II receptor antagonists

Mode of action. There are two classes of angiotensin II receptors termed AT_1 and AT_2. The AT_1 receptor appears to be responsible for the known effects of angiotensin II. AT_1 receptors are found mainly in the heart and blood vessels, the kidney, adrenal cortex, lung and brain. The exact role of AT_2 receptors is unclear.

Among the functions of these receptors are vasoconstriction, promotion of aldosterone release and sodium retention. Antagonism, or blockade, of these receptors therefore leads to an effective blood pressure lowering response.

Angiotensin II antagonists are licensed for use only in hypertension and have been shown to be effective antihypertensive agents.

Side-effects. Unlike ACE inhibitors, the angiotensin-II receptor antagonists do not inhibit the breakdown of bradykinin and other kinins. As a result they do not appear to cause the persistent dry cough commonly occurring in ACE inhibitor therapy. They are therefore a useful alternative for patients who have to discontinue an ACE inhibitor because of persistent cough. Side-effects are usually mild and transient in nature. Hypotension, hyperkalaemia, gastrointestinal disturbances, dizziness and myalgia have been reported.

Cautions. Angiotensin-II receptor antagonists should be used with caution in renal artery stenosis. Plasma potassium monitoring is advised, particularly in the elderly and in patients with renal impairment. These drugs should be avoided in pregnancy. (See Table 16.12 for doses.)

NITRATES

The nitrates are used in the prophylaxis and treatment of angina pectoris and also to treat left ventricular failure. Beta-blockers and calcium-channel blockers are widely used to treat angina; however, short-acting nitrates retain an important role both for prophylactic use before exertion and for chest pain occurring during exercise.

Mode of action. Nitrates have several effects:

- dilatation of vessels in the venous system decreases venous return and thus the preload to the heart; the reduced preload prevents the left ventricle from overfilling and reduces the symptoms of cardiac failure
- dilatation of arterioles lowers peripheral resistance and left ventricular pressure, reducing myocardial work and oxygen demand
- dilatation of coronary arteries increases blood supply (and therefore oxygen supply) to the myocardium.

The mode of action of nitrates to produce these effects is as follows. Mononitrates enter the walls of veins and arteries, combine with sulphydryl groups and form the vasodilating substance nitric oxide. (The nitric oxide activates guanylate cyclase to produce cyclic guanosine monophosphate which causes relaxation of vascular smooth muscle with dilatation of veins and arterioles.)

Table 16.12 Dosages for angiotension-II receptor antagonists

Drug	Dose
Candesartan	2–16 mg once daily
Eprosartan	300–800 mg once daily
Irbesartan	75–300 mg once daily
Losartan	25–100 mg once daily
Telmisartan	40–80 mg once daily
Valsartan	40–160 mg once daily

Sublingual glyceryl trinitrate

Glyceryl trinitrate is used as soon as an attack of angina occurs or may also be used prophylactically before physical activity. It undergoes extensive first-pass metabolism when taken orally but the sublingual administration bypasses the hepatic circulation. The tablets are placed under the tongue and allowed to dissolve. A burning or tingling sensation in the mouth is commonly experienced. Rapid symptomatic relief of angina is normally obtained within a minute but the effect lasts for only 20–30 minutes. Initially one tablet should be used, but if no relief is obtained a second and then a third may be taken at 5-minute intervals. If no relief is obtained after three tablets the patient should seek medical attention.

Patients should be advised that when they get chest pain and need to take a glyceryl trinitrate tablet they should sit down. The purpose of this is twofold: first, sitting down may in itself relieve the angina symptoms, and second, by sitting, any dizziness caused by the glyceryl trinitrate will be minimised. Patients should be warned of the possible side-effects to expect – such as headache, facial flushing, dizziness, nausea and light-headedness. These effects can be minimised by spitting out or swallowing any tablet remaining when the pain has subsided. The side-effects usually subside after a few weeks of regular glyceryl trinitrate use.

Patients should be advised to store the tablets in a cool dry place in the original container with the original cap. Any tablets left 8 weeks after first opening the bottle should be discarded and replaced with a fresh supply. Some patients prefer using glyceryl trinitrate spray as it offers more convenience in terms of longer expiry and easier storage but it is more expensive. The tablets are available in 300, 500 and 600 microgram strengths. An aerosol spray provides an effective alternative to tablets.

Buccal nitrate

Buccal nitrate tablets consist of glyceryl trinitrate impregnated in an inert polymer matrix, allowing slow diffusion across the buccal mucosa. The tablet is placed under the top lip without chewing, where a gel-like coating forms around the tablet. This allows adherence to the buccal mucosa with the release of drug over 3–5 hours.

Oral preparations

Higher doses of organic nitrates are used to overcome the effect of first-pass metabolism, and high doses of oral glyceryl trinitrate in a sustained-release form can be effective.

Transdermal preparations

Several transdermal preparations, either as patches or ointment, have been developed for prophylaxis of angina. They bypass first-pass metabolism. Using the patches, therapeutic blood levels are achieved within an hour and last up to 24 hours. The patches should be applied to a clean, dry, non-hairy part of the skin (extremities should be avoided). Absorption depends on site of application and blood flow. Skin irritation and variable absorption may limit their use. If tolerance is suspected during the use of transdermal patches, they should be left off for several consecutive hours in 24 hours (during a period of time when the patient is least likely to develop chest pain) in order to have a nitrate-free interval.

Intravenous nitrates

Glyceryl trinitrate or isosorbide mononitrate may be tried by intravenous injection when the sublingual form is ineffective in patients with chest pain due to myocardial infarction or severe ischaemia. Intravenous injections are also useful in the treatment of acute left ventricular failure. It may not always be possible to proceed to doses which are high enough to relieve symptoms, because of adverse effects such as headache or hypotension. In the longer term the infusion rate may need increasing owing to the development of tolerance, since a continuous infusion of glyceryl trinitrate does not permit a nitrate-free period and tolerance may develop within 24–48 hours of commencing the infusion.

Isosorbide mononitrate and isosorbide dinitrate

Isosorbide mononitrate and isosorbide dinitrate are effective when taken orally, and the mononitrate is less readily metabolised than glyceryl trinitrate in the liver. Isosorbide dinitrate is active sublingually and orally but has a short half-life (0.5–1 hour). It undergoes extensive first-pass metabolism with the main active metabolite being isosorbide mononitrate. No matter which long-acting nitrate preparation is used, the dose has to be titrated to attain the desired response or until the dose is limited by side-effects such as headache. The dose varies greatly between patients (see Tables 16.13 and 16.14 for further information).

Table 16.13 Nitrate information

Drug	Dose	Adverse effects	Notes
Glyceryl trinitrate	Sublingually: 0.3–1 mg repeated as required. Oral: 2.6–12.8 mg as modified-release tablets two to three times daily. Severe angina: 10 mg three times daily. IV infusion: 10–200 micrograms per minute. Spray: 1–2 doses under tongue. Patches: 5 mg, 10 mg and 15 mg patches are available	Throbbing headache, flushing, dizziness, postural hypotension, tachycardia	Glyceryl trinitrate tablets should be supplied in glass containers containing no cotton wool wadding. They should be discarded 8 weeks after first opening the container. Contraindicated where marked anaemia, closed-angle glaucoma, cerebral haemorrhage. Caution in hypotensive conditions
Isosorbide dinitrate	Sublingually: 5–10 mg. Oral: daily in divided doses. Angina: 30–120 mg. Left ventricular failure: 40–160 mg. IV infusion: 2–10 mg/hour	As for glyceryl trinitrate	Contraindications and cautions as for glyceryl trinitrate
Isosorbide mononitrate	Initially 20 mg two to three times daily (half this in those who have not received nitrates previously). Up to 120 mg daily in divided doses where required	As for isosorbide dinitrate	As for isosorbide dinitrate

Nitrate tolerance

The release of the vasodilating substance nitric oxide depends on the presence of sulphydryl groups. Continuous 24-hour nitrate therapy leads to the depletion of sulphydryl groups preventing further release of nitric oxide and the development of tolerance. Development of tolerance can be avoided by allowing the plasma nitrate concentration to fall at some period during the 24 hours. A nitrate-free gap of several consecutive hours in each 24-hour period is necessary for the regeneration of sulphydryl groups. This can be achieved by removing glyceryl trinitrate patches for a period of 6 hours. A dosage schedule in which an oral nitrate is taken three times daily, but with the last dose at the time of the evening meal, allows an appropriate interval to counter the development of tolerance. Sustained-release nitrate preparations provide a nitrate-free interval if given once daily.

Table 16.14 Onset and duration of action of nitrates

	Onset of action (min)	Duration of action
Sublingual glyceryl trinitrate	2–5	10–30 minutes
Buccal glyceryl trinitrate	2–5	30–300 minutes
Glyceryl trinitrate ointment	15–60	3–8 hours
Glyceryl trinitrate patch	30–60	18–24 hours
Oral isosorbide dinitrate	15–45	2–6 hours
Oral isosorbide mononitrate	60	5 hours

CALCIUM-CHANNEL BLOCKERS

Mode of action. Calcium ions play an important role in the maintenance of vascular smooth muscle tone. Calcium-channel blockers inhibit the influx of calcium ions into the muscle cells in the arterial walls resulting in relaxation of the muscle and dilatation of the artery. As a result, coronary or systemic vascular tone may be diminished and calcium-channel blockers are used to lower blood pressure in hypertension and to dilate coronary arteries in angina. (In addition, verapamil slows conduction in the AV node and is used to treat cardiac arrhythmias.)

Although their actions are similar, the balance of their effects on the myocardium, on conducting tissue and on blood vessels varies and so there is variation between the drugs in this class. They are all given orally and broken down by the liver (see Table 16.15).

The smooth muscle relaxant effect of nimodipine acts preferentially on cerebral arteries. Its use is confined to the prevention of vascular spasm following subarachnoid haemorrhage.

Side-effects. Headache, flushing and ankle oedema can occur because of vasodilatation but become less of a problem after a few days. Constipation may be a problem with verapamil. Great care is necessary in patients who have heart failure as several calcium-channel blockers may further depress cardiac function and cause clinically significant deterioration.

POTASSIUM-CHANNEL ACTIVATORS

Mode of action. Nicorandil combines the properties of an organic nitrate with those of a potassium-channel opener, thereby causing dilatation of coronary arteries and arterioles and also large veins (see Fig. 16.5).

Nicorandil is a nitrate derivative of nicotinamide. Similar to other organic nitrates, it relaxes vascular smooth muscle, particularly on the venous side, reducing the preload (ventricular filling and myocardial work). In addition to dilatation of coronary arteries,

Table 16.15 Calcium-channel blockers

Drug	Hypertension	Angina	Dose
Amlodipine	✓	✓	5–10 mg once daily
Diltiazem	✓	✓	Angina 60–360 mg three times daily Longer-acting formulations used in hypertension
Felodipine	✓	✓	Angina 5–10 mg once daily Hypertension 2.5–20 mg once daily
Isradipine		✓	1.25–10 mg twice daily
Lacidipine	✓		2–6 mg daily
Lercanidipine	✓		10–20 mg daily
Nicardipine	✓	✓	20–30 mg three times daily
Nifedipine	✓	✓	Varies according to which of the many available preparations are used
Nisoldipine	✓	✓	10–40 mg daily
Verapamil	✓	✓	Angina 80–120 mg three times daily Hypertension 240–480 mg daily in two to three divided doses

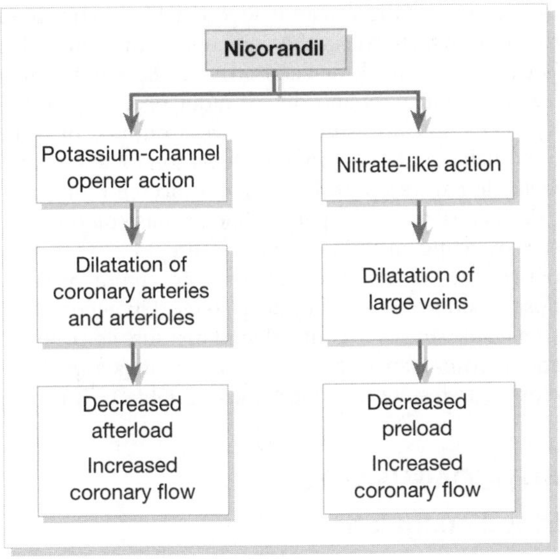

Figure 16.5 Actions of nicorandil.

nicorandil activates ATP-dependent potassium channels and increases the efflux of potassium ions. This hyperpolarises the cell membrane, inhibits calcium entry and causes arterial vasodilatation (similar to calcium blockers).

The commonest side-effect of nicorandil is headache (especially in initiation, usually transitory).

Pharmacokinetics. Pharmacokinetically, nicorandil is rapidly and almost completely absorbed into the circulation with little or no first-pass metabolism in the liver. Peak plasma effects are reached after 20–60 minutes and steady-state concentrations are reached in 5 days following a twice-daily dosing regimen. Nicorandil has a half-life of 1 hour and is mainly metabolised through the liver and excreted via the kidneys.

Dose. Initially 10 mg twice daily (halved if susceptible to headache); usual dose 10–20 mg twice daily; up to 30 mg twice daily may be used.

Side-effects. The commonest side-effect of nicorandil is headache (especially on initiation, usually transitory). Other adverse effects may include nausea, vomiting, malaise, dizziness, palpitations and fatigue. Continuous treatment may lead to the development of tolerance to the organic nitrate component of nicorandil but the drug's efficacy tends to be maintained owing to the potassium-channel opening effect.

PERIPHERAL VASODILATORS

The blood supply to the limb may be diminished by disease or spasm of the peripheral arteries. This leads to an inadequate oxygen supply to the muscle and thus pain in the muscle on walking (intermittent claudication). The cause of this is occlusion of the vessels either by spasm or sclerotic plaques. Vasodilators may increase blood flow at rest but have not been shown to be of benefit during exercise.

Since most vasodilators dilate the blood vessels to the skin rather than those to the muscle, they are more useful in the treatment of Raynaud's syndrome where spasm is a major factor in poor circulation. It is important that non-drug measures be carried out, e.g. stopping smoking, reducing weight and fat intake, increasing exercise to improve muscle efficiency and prevent build-up of metabolites, avoidance of exposure to the cold.

Many of these drugs have unpleasant side-effects such as gastrointestinal disturbances, headache, dizziness. They may adversely affect patients suffering from angina, recent myocardial infarction (by diverting blood from ischaemic areas), those taking antihypertensives (by potentiating their effects) and diabetics (may potentiate insulin and oral hypoglycaemics). Examples of drugs in this class include cinnarizine, nicotinic acid derivatives, pentoxifylline (oxpentifylline), moxisylyte (thymoxamine) and naftidrofuryl oxalate (also a cerebral vasodilator).

SYMPATHOMIMETICS

Inotropic and vasoconstrictor sympathomimetics are discussed in this section.

Inotropic sympathomimetics

The properties of the sympathomimetics vary according to whether they act on alpha- or on beta-adrenergic receptors. Adrenaline (epinephrine) acts on both alpha and beta receptors:

- alpha effect – vasoconstriction
- β_1 effect – increase in heart rate and contractility
- β_2 effect – peripheral vasodilatation.

Although a powerful sympathomimetic agent, adrenaline (epinephrine) is used less frequently as more selective drugs are available. It is of value in anaphylaxis and bronchospasm and is the first drug given in cardiac arrest. In the latter indication it has a direct myocardial stimulatory effect, improving the quality of ventricular contraction and improving cardiac output. Adrenaline (epinephrine) 1 in 10 000 (1 mg per 10 mL) is recommended in a dose of 10 mL by central intravenous injection.

Dopamine is a naturally occurring substance which is changed to noradrenaline (norepinephrine) in the body. However, dopamine has pharmacological actions of its own:

- β_1 effect: potent inotropic action, i.e. it increases the force of contraction more than the rate of the heart
- stimulates alpha receptors in the peripheral vascular system causing vasoconstriction at higher doses
- stimulates dopamine receptors in the mesenteric, coronary, intracerebral and renal vascular systems; this causes dilatation, and in the renal system, blood flow and urinary output are increased, which is useful in shock where there is a decline in renal function – this effect occurring at low dosage
- causes release of noradrenaline (norepinephrine) from sympathetic nerves.

Dopamine is used in cardiogenic shock in infarction or cardiac surgery. It is administered by intravenous infusion (2.5–5 micrograms/kg/minute), the dose being adjusted according to response.

Its use requires considerable care, as higher doses lead to vasoconstriction and may exacerbate heart failure. Once the condition is under control the drug should be withdrawn slowly.

Dobutamine has a more selective action than dopamine, acting mainly on the beta-adrenoceptors, and it does not cause release of noradrenaline (norepinephrine). It produces an increase in the force of contraction of the heart and at high doses causes peripheral vasodilatation. For the latter reason it is not appropriate in the treatment of shock where there is marked hypotension. However, it is preferable to dopamine if blood pressure is normal.

Dopexamine is indicated as inotropic support and vasodilator in exacerbations of chronic heart failure and in heart failure associated with cardiac surgery. It is a synthetic catecholamine, structurally related to dopamine with marked intrinsic agonist activity at β_2-adrenoceptors and lesser activity at β_1-adrenoceptors. Its use in critically ill patients is often aimed at improving vital organ perfusion, specifically gastrointestinal tract, renal, hepatic and splanchnic blood flow, thus preventing the translocation of endotoxins and microorganisms.

Isoprenaline is less selective and increases both heart rate and contractility. It is now used only as emergency treatment of heart block or severe bradycardia.

Vasoconstrictor sympathomimetics

Although some people have a naturally low blood pressure and come to no harm, when the blood pressure is unusually low there is an inadequate blood supply to the brain which causes the person to faint. Where this is caused by shock of haemorrhage the patient may lose consciousness and die. In older people, postural hypotension can result from rising from bed or chair too quickly and may provide the reason for some falls. Delay in baroreceptor response may account for this.

Vasoconstrictor sympathomimetics raise blood pressure by acting on alpha-adrenergic receptors to constrict peripheral vessels. They are used in emergencies to raise blood pressure. They are also used in general and spinal anaesthesia to control blood pressure since spinal and epidural anaesthesia may result in sympathetic block with resultant hypotension (see Table 16.16).

ANTICOAGULANTS

Blood coagulation

Platelets, disc-shaped cells 2–3 μm in diameter, are formed in the bone marrow under the control of a regulator called thrombopoietin. Aggregation of platelets occurs in response to blood-vessel injury and the platelets plug the disrupted vessel wall. Platelet aggregates are reinforced by precipitation of the insoluble protein called fibrin from soluble precursors in the plasma. Erythrocytes then become enmeshed within this fibrin framework. The formation of fibrin depends on the activation of the clotting cascade along extrinsic and intrinsic pathways (Fig. 16.6).

Exposure of collagen in damaged blood vessels initiates the action of factor XII and this leads to activation of the intrinsic pathway. The extrinsic part of the cascade is stimulated by tissue thromboplastin released from damaged tissue which activates factor VII. Once triggered the coagulation process accelerates. Platelet aggregation leads to release of various mediators including phospholipid factor III, which is a major accelerating influence upon blood coagulation. Thrombin generation also acts as a further stimulus to platelet aggregation. Thrombin (IIa) stimulates the conversion of fibrinogen to fibrin in the presence of calcium ions. The initial fibrin clot is soluble and is converted to an insoluble polymer when factor XIII is activated by thrombin and calcium. The initial conversion of fibrinogen to fibrin is rapid; the conversion to the polymer is slow and complete cross-linking takes several hours.

Eventually the process terminates because of the action of physiological inhibitors of coagulation factors (e.g. antithrombin) as well as through the inactivation of factors V and VII by high concentrations of thrombin. Phagocytosis facilitates the removal of precipitated fibrin complexes. Fibrin thrombus undergoes enzymatic

Table 16.16 Vasoconstrictor sympathomimetics

Drug	Receptor activity	Action	Use	Dose	Adverse effects	Notes
Ephedrine	Alpha	Constricts peripheral vessels	Hypotension in anaesthesia with associated bradycardia	Reversal of hypotension from spinal or epidural anaesthesia by slow IV injection 3–6 mg repeated every 3–4 minutes to maximum 30 mg	Tachycardia, anxiety, restlessness, insomnia, tremor, arrhythmias, dry mouth, cold extremities	Caution in hyperthyroidism, diabetes mellitus, ischaemic heart disease, hypertension, elderly. May cause acute retention in prostatic hypertrophy
	Beta	Accelerates the heart				
Metaraminol	Alpha greater than beta	Mainly constriction of peripheral vessels	Acute hypotension	By IV infusion: 15–100 mg adjusted according to response	Tachycardia, arrhythmias, reduced renal blood flow	Extravasation at injection site may cause necrosis Contraindicated in myocardial infarction and pregnancy
Methoxamine	Alpha	Increased peripheral resistance due to vasoconstriction; no direct action on heart	Hypotension in anaesthesia; when the hypotension occurs in association with tachycardia methoxamine is the drug of choice	IM injection: 5–20 mg Slow IV injection: 5–10 mg	Headache, hypertension, bradycardia	Caution in hyperthyroidism, pregnancy
Noradrenaline (norepinephrine)	Alpha greater than β_1	Vasoconstriction	Acute hypotension, cardiac arrest	Acute hypotension, by IV infusion, via central venous catheter of a solution of 80 micrograms/mL at an initial rate of 0.16–0.33 mL per minute, adjusted according to response. Rapid IV or intracardiac injection: 0.5–0.75 mL of a solution of noradrenaline acid tartrate 200 micrograms/mL	Headache, palpitations, bradycardia	Caution in coronary, mesenteric or peripheral vascular thrombosis, following myocardial infarction, Prinzmetal's variant angina, thyroid disease, diabetes mellitus
Phenylephrine	Alpha, beta (weak)	Vasoconstriction	Acute hypotension	SC or IM injection: 2–5 mg. Slow IV injection: 100–500 micrograms. IV infusion: initial rate up to 180 micrograms/minute reduced to 30–60 micrograms/minute according to response	Hypertension with headache, palpitations, vomiting, tingling and coolness of skin, tachycardia or reflex bradycardia	Contraindicated in hypertension, hyperthyroidism, myocardial infarction and pregnancy. Extravasation at injection site may cause necrosis

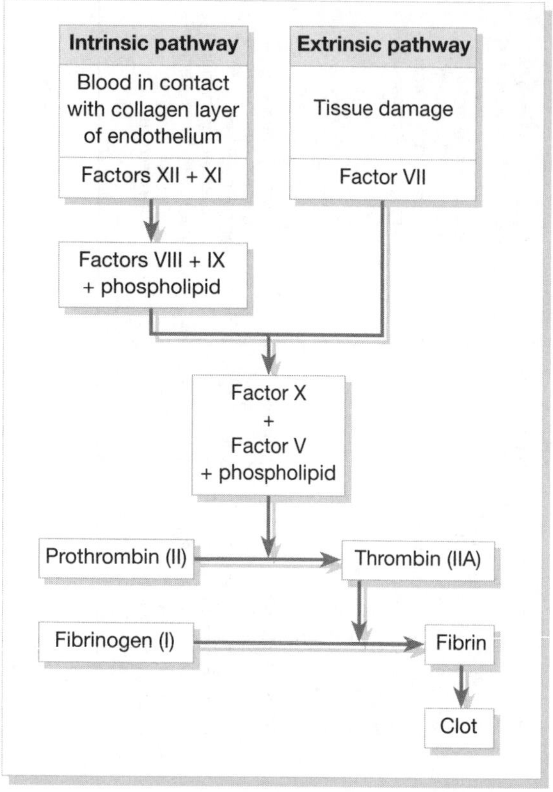

Figure 16.6 Blood coagulation system.

digestion to soluble polypeptides by the process of fibrinolysis. The proteolytic enzyme involved is called plasmin.

Plasminogen is incorporated in the clot and is converted to plasmin when the activators diffuse into the clot (Fig. 16.7). In addition to converting fibrin clot to soluble fragments, plasmin acts on fibrinogen, prothrombin, and factors V and VIII, rendering them ineffective in the coagulation system, thus preventing excessive coagulation.

Types of anticoagulant

Parenteral anticoagulants

Mode of action. Heparin promotes the action of antithrombin III which, in turn, inhibits factor X at low (prophylactic) doses, and factors IX and XI in anticoagulant doses. The outcome is inhibition of the conversion of prothrombin to thrombin and this prevents the conversion of fibrinogen to fibrin. This results in the prolongation of clotting time.

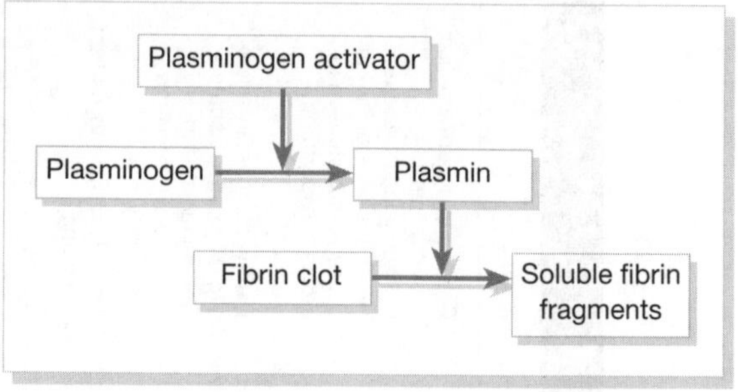

Figure 16.7 Action of plasmin in fibrinolysis.

Indications. Heparin is used as an anticoagulant in the treatment of deep-vein thrombosis (DVT) and pulmonary embolism or in the prevention of DVT.

Pharmacokinetics. Heparin is not well absorbed from the gastrointestinal tract so it must be administered parenterally. The intravenous route is preferred for high-dose treatment of acute thrombotic episodes, while the subcutaneous route is preferred for low-dose prophylactic therapy. The intramuscular route should be avoided because of the danger of local bleeding. With intravenous administration, the onset of action of heparin is almost immediate, and peak concentration levels occur within minutes. The patient's clotting time will return to normal within 2–6 hours after administration of an intravenous bolus. With subcutaneous administration, onset is delayed for about 2 hours. The serum half-life of heparin is dose-related, the duration of action being extended with higher doses.

The enzyme heparinase metabolises heparin in the liver. Half-life, approximately 1–1.5 hours, is dose-related. The anticoagulant effect is measured by the activated partial thromboplastin time (APTT) test and the partial thromboplastin time. Dosage is adjusted daily with laboratory monitoring and adjustment according to the APTT.

Dose. Treatment of deep-vein thrombosis and pulmonary embolism by intravenous injection, loading dose of 5000 units (10 000 units in severe pulmonary embolism) followed by continuous infusion of 15–25 units/kg/hour or by subcutaneous injection of 15 000 units every 12 hours (laboratory monitoring essential – preferably on a daily basis).

By subcutaneous injection, prophylaxis of deep-vein thrombosis, 5000 units 2 hours before surgery then every 8–12 hours for 7 days or until the patient is ambulant.

Side-effects. Haemorrhage, thrombocytopenia, hypersensitivity reactions, osteoporosis after prolonged use.

Contraindicated in haemophilia and other haemorrhagic disorders, thrombocytopenia, peptic ulcer, cerebral aneurysm, severe hypertension, severe liver disease.

Low-molecular-weight heparin. Low-molecular-weight heparins are used for prophylaxis of deep-vein thrombosis by subcutaneous injection, particularly in high-risk orthopaedic surgery. A number of similar drugs are available (certoparin, dalteparin, enoxaparin, reviparin and tinzaparin), the timing of the first dose varying from 12 hours before surgery to 1–2 hours before surgery. The regimen is continued daily for 7–10 days or until the patient is ambulant. Some low-molecular-weight heparins are also used in the treatment of deep-vein thrombosis, unstable coronary artery disease and for the prevention of clotting in extracorporeal circuits.

Heparin flushes are used to maintain the patency of cannulae intended to be in place for longer than 48 hours. They are available as solutions of 10 units per mL and 100 units per mL. For under 48 hours, sodium chloride injection 0.9% is effective.

Bleeding due to overdosage may occur with heparin. As with all anticoagulants, this often first appears as haematuria but may develop from any site. Protamine sulphate is a strong base that neutralises acidic heparin by binding with it to form a stable compound with no anticoagulant effect. 1 mg of protamine sulphate will neutralise approximately 100 units of heparin. The dose to be given should be carefully calculated bearing in mind the short half-life of heparin. The maximum dose is 50 mg. Protamine sulphate is given slowly by intravenous injection. Rapid injection can cause complications such as dyspnoea, flushing, bradycardia and hypotension. If used in excess, protamine has an anticoagulant effect. It is derived from fish sperm, and hypersensitivity reactions may occur in patients with allergies to fish.

Low-molecular-weight heparin has a longer half-life than heparin, which facilitates once-daily dosing. The standard prophylactic regimen does not require monitoring.

Oral anticoagulants

There are three substances in the coumarin group, warfarin, acenocoumarol (nicoumalone) and phenindione. The drug of choice is warfarin, the others being seldom used.

Mode of action. Warfarin is effective by mouth. It antagonises the synthesis of vitamin K-dependent clotting factors in the liver, including prothrombin and factors VII, IX and X. The resulting therapeutic anticoagulant effect does not occur until the already circulating clotting factors are depleted. This takes from several hours for factor VII to 2–3 days for prothrombin. It therefore takes several days before the anticoagulant effect develops, and heparin is used until warfarin is effective. Liver disease, in which synthesis of clotting factors is defective, potentiates warfarin.

Indications. Warfarin is indicated for:

- prophylaxis and treatment of venous thrombosis and pulmonary embolism
- prophylaxis of embolisation in rheumatic heart disease and atrial fibrillation
- prophylaxis after insertion of a prosthetic heart valve to prevent emboli developing on the valves.

Pharmacokinetics. Warfarin is absorbed rapidly and almost completely after oral administration; it is highly protein-bound, although binding and half-life may vary considerably between patients. Dosage must therefore be individualised. The anticoagulant effect must be carefully monitored when other drugs which alter protein binding or metabolism are introduced or withdrawn.

Dose. Whenever possible, the baseline prothrombin should be determined before the initial dose is given. An initial adult dose of 10 mg is given once daily for 2 days with daily measurements of International Normalised Ratio (INR) for prothrombin time and adjustments as required. The daily maintenance dose (usually between 3 and 6 mg) is adjusted to provide a target INR.

Recommended target INR values:

- *INR 2–2.5* – prophylaxis of deep-vein thrombosis, including surgery on high-risk patients
- *INR 2.5* – treatment of deep-vein thrombosis and pulmonary embolism, atrial fibrillation, mural thrombus following myocardial infarction and rheumatic mitral valve disease
- *INR 3.5* – recurrent deep-vein thrombosis, pulmonary embolism and mechanical prosthetic heart valves.

Adverse reactions. The main adverse reaction of all oral anticoagulants is haemorrhage. The level of INR at which bleeding occurs varies from patient to patient. However, an INR of 8 or over is considered dangerously high and usually necessitates the administration of plasma and possibly blood if haemorrhage has already occurred. Phytomenadione (vitamin K) 5 mg by slow intravenous injection will counteract the effects of warfarin but it is not ideal since it takes up to 6 hours to act and will render the patient resistant to anticoagulants for several weeks. Where the INR is raised but to a lesser extent (4.5–7 without haemorrhage) it may be sufficient to withdraw warfarin for 1 or 2 days and then review. Anticoagulant treatment cards are supplied by the pharmacist and must be carried by the patient.

Warfarin is contraindicated in pregnancy since it is teratogenic. It is also contraindicated in peptic ulcer, severe hypertension and bacterial endocarditis.

Interactions. Drug interactions occur commonly with warfarin for a number of reasons, for example:

- protein-binding displacement – warfarin is highly bound and is displaced, e.g. by salicylates and sulphonamides, which enhances its action
- inhibition of metabolism increases its effect, e.g. metronidazole, cimetidine
- induction of metabolism by drugs which induce microsomal enzymes (including phenytoin, rifampicin, carbamazepine) reduces the effect of warfarin.

Antiplatelet drugs

Arterial thrombosis, such as occurs in coronary thrombosis and strokes, is partly due to an aggregation of platelets which ultimately form plugs in blood vessels. By decreasing platelet aggregation, thrombus formation on the arterial side of the circulation is inhibited (anticoagulants have little effect on arterial thrombus and antiplatelet drugs have little effect in venous thromboembolism). Dipyridamole is used orally as an adjunct to warfarin for prophylaxis of thromboembolism associated with prosthetic heart valves. The dose is 300–600 mg daily in three to four divided doses before food. The most common adverse effects are headache and diarrhoea. Peripheral vasodilatation may result in facial flushing and hypotension.

Aspirin is used in the prophylaxis of cerebrovascular disease or myocardial infarction; 75–300 mg is given daily. Low-dose aspirin (75 mg daily) is given following bypass surgery. Adverse reactions include gastrointestinal bleeding and bronchospasm. It is contraindicated in children under 16 and in breast-feeding because of the risk of Reye's syndrome. Clopidogrel and ticlopidine are licensed for the prevention of atherosclerotic events in patients with a history of symptomatic ischaemic disease.

Fibrinolytic drugs

Fibrinolytic drugs act as thrombolytics by activating plasminogen to form plasmin which degrades fibrin and breaks up thrombi. Streptokinase, alteplase (recombinant human tissue type plasminogen activator) reteplase and tenecteplase are used for the treatment of myocardial infarction. Alteplase, reteplase and streptokinase need to be given within 12 hours of a myocardial infarction, ideally within 1 hour; use after 12 hours requires specialist advice. Tenecteplase should be given within 6 hours of a myocardial infarction. Streptokinase remains the drug of choice, although antibodies appear after 4 days and streptokinase should not therefore be used again after this time. Streptokinase is, in addition, indicated for deep-vein thrombosis, pulmonary embolism, acute arterial thromboembolism and thrombosed arteriovenous shunts.

The potential for benefit in myocardial infarction lessens as the delay from onset of major symptoms increases, the value of treatment within the first 12 hours being well established. An alternative to streptokinase should be used in patients who have received therapy in the previous 12 months or where an allergic action has occurred.

Streptokinase is an enzyme made by haemolytic streptococci. The initial dose is 250 000 units by intravenous infusion over 30 minutes in 0.9% sodium chloride. The maintenance dose is 100 000 units every hour for 24–72 hours.

The most common adverse effects are nausea, vomiting and bleeding.

Antifibrinolytic drugs and haemostatics

Tranexamic acid has the opposite effect to streptokinase by inhibition of plasminogen activation and fibrinolysis. It is useful in stemming haemorrhage in dental extraction or prostatectomy and in streptokinase overdose.

Aprotinin inhibits the action of plasmin. It is indicated for blood conservation in open-heart surgery. A loading dose is given after induction of anaesthesia and maintained by intravenous infusion until the end of the operation.

LIPID-LOWERING DRUGS

Cardiovascular disease is the most common cause of mortality in the UK. One in four men and one in five women die from coronary heart disease (CHD). Lowering the concentration of low-density lipoprotein (LDL) cholesterol and raising high-density lipoprotein (HDL) cholesterol reduces the progression of coronary atherosclerosis. Lowering total cholesterol by 20–25% (or lowering LDL cholesterol by about 30%) is effective in lowering the risk of atheroma and coronary thrombosis.

Lipoproteins are substances which are composed of fats and proteins and are produced by the liver. The concentration of blood lipoproteins is determined partly by the dietary intake of fats and partly by metabolic processes within the body. There are several ways of lowering lipoprotein levels. These are by decreasing the intake of fats, reducing absorption or reducing the synthesis of these.

A decrease in the total fat intake and the proportion of saturated (animal) fat to unsaturated (fish and vegetable) fat will reduce plasma cholesterol but requires

Table 16.17 Lipid-lowering drugs

Drug	Dose
Atorvastatin	10–80 mg daily
Fluvastatin	20–80 mg daily
Pravastatin	10–40 mg daily
Simvastatin	10–80 mg daily

adherence to a strict diet. Oxidised LDL is highly atherogenic but naturally occurring antioxidants are present in fruit and vegetables and may be protective against CHD. At least five portions of fruit and vegetables daily is recommended.

Anion-exchange resins are used in the management of hypercholesterolaemia. Colestyramine and colestipol are examples. They bind to bile acids in the gut preventing their absorption. This promotes the conversion of cholesterol in the liver to bile acids, effectively reducing LDL cholesterol. However, they may cause abdominal discomfort and diarrhoea.

Fibrates such as bezafibrate, fenofibrate and gemfibrozil lower blood cholesterol and triglycerides and have been shown to reduce the risk of CHD. Their side-effects include nausea, gastric pain, headache, fatigue and rashes.

Statins are the drugs of first choice for treating hypercholesterolaemia. They block the synthesis of cholesterol in the liver, resulting in a lower blood level. For primary and secondary prevention of CHD, statin treatment should be adjusted to achieve a target total cholesterol concentration of less than 5 mmol/litre. Liver function tests should be carried out before and within 1–3 months of starting treatment and thereafter at intervals of 6 months for 1 year.

The statins are well tolerated and side-effects are generally mild and transient. They include headache and gastrointestinal effects. They are taken at night since cholesterol synthesis is greatest at this time (see Table 16.17).

ISCHAEMIC HEART DISEASE

Ischaemia arises when the normally smooth endothelial surface of one or more of the coronary arteries becomes roughened. Narrowing occurs as a result of deposits (atheroma) which partly occlude the artery. Atheroma starts at an early age and consists of abnormal plaques of fatty compounds which develop in the muscular layer of an artery. As they grow they project into the lumen of the artery, thus reducing blood flow. The resulting reduction in blood flow leads to a reduction of oxygenated blood supply to the myocardium.

Angina pectoris

Angina pectoris is the clinical sign of transient myocardial ischaemia. It occurs when the metabolic demands of the heart for oxygen exceed the ability of diseased coronary arteries to supply adequate blood flow to the myocardium (physical exercise, anaemia). Angina is one of the principal symptoms of coronary heart disease. It is characterised by tightness of the chest which may or may not radiate to the jaw, down one or both arms or through into the back. The pain tends to occur during exertion and is of an alarming nature.

Chronic stable angina is by far the commonest form, and is characterised by brief (10-minute) episodes of pain closely related to precipitants which increase cardiac output, such as exertion, emotion and, less commonly, heavy meals. The treatments used have little or no effect on the obstructed coronary artery itself but prevent angina by reducing or limiting the work of the heart. As its name suggests, this form of angina often follows a stable pattern for many years but may be complicated by myocardial infarction, unstable angina or sudden death.

Unstable angina presents as a worsening pattern of pre-existing angina, or with episodes of pain which are prolonged (30 minutes or longer) or which occur spontaneously. It is caused by a non-occlusive thrombus forming on an atherosclerotic plaque which has developed a fissure or had a haemorrhage into its substance. Unstable angina is a threatening condition because it confers a high risk of myocardial infarction or sudden death within weeks or months.

Management of stable angina

All patients with angina who smoke should be advised to stop. Diet should be modified in line with healthy eating advice

- increase fruit and vegetable consumption to five portions per day
- increase consumption of oil-rich fish to three portions per week
- decrease total fat consumption
- increase starchy food intake and reduce sugary food intake.

All patients with angina should have their cholesterol level measured. Appropriate dietary measures should be recommended. If required, drug therapy (see p. 198) should be initiated to reduce total cholesterol to <5 mmol/litre.

Patients should be encouraged to increase exercise levels within limits set by their disease state. Alcohol consumption should be limited to three units per day for men and two for women.

Patients with stable angina should be treated with aspirin 75 mg per day. In the event of true aspirin intolerance or allergy, clopidogrel 75 mg daily should be considered.

All patients with symptomatic coronary heart disease should be prescribed sublingual glyceryl trinitrate (GTN) and should be educated to its use for short-term symptom control.

Patients who require regular symptomatic treatment should be treated initially with a beta-blocker and warned not to stop the treatment suddenly.

Patients intolerant of beta-blockers and who show no left-sided ventricular systolic dysfunction should be treated with one of the following (see pp. 190–192):

- a rate-limiting calcium-channel blocker
- a long-acting dihydropyridine
- a nitrate
- a potassium-channel-opening agent

If symptoms are not controlled in patients taking beta-blockers, isosorbide mononitrate, a long-acting dihydropyridine (e.g. felodipine) or diltiazem can be added.

Myocardial infarction (MI)

In western countries heart attacks are responsible for 30–50% of all deaths. The incidence increases with age and is greater in men. Factors which may contribute to the development of myocardial infarction include:

- family history of coronary heart disease
- stress
- cigarette smoking
- lack of exercise
- hypertension
- raised serum cholesterol
- obesity
- oral contraceptives
- diet rich in saturated fats and cholesterol.

Myocardial infarction occurs when there is a prolonged reduction in the oxygen supply to a region of myocardium (heart muscle). Tissue death follows and the area is said to be infarcted. This occurs primarily in patients with coronary artery disease where there is significant narrowing of one or more of the three major coronary arteries. As a result of turbulent blood flow at the site of the atheroma, platelets aggregate to form thrombi and blockage of the coronary artery occurs.

Typically, the symptom of myocardial infarction is severe chest pain which is sudden in onset and prolonged. The pain is characteristically tight or 'band like' and may radiate to the jaw, shoulders, neck, back or arms. It is often associated with breathlessness, anxiety, weakness, sweating, nausea and vomiting.

The diagnosis is made primarily on the individual's history supported by evidence from an electrocardiogram and biochemical tests. As infarcted myocardium breaks down, enzymes are liberated into the bloodstream and these can be measured. The three enzymes most frequently assayed are creatine kinase, lactate dehydrogenase and aspartate aminotransferase. Each enzyme has a particular time course for release from damaged myocardial cells during MI.

The most common causes of sudden death following an MI are ventricular fibrillation, heart block (blockage of electrical conduction in the heart) or asystole (total absence of heart beat).

Pharmacological intervention following MI

Patients with suspected myocardial infarction are best transferred to hospital, particularly because the risk of early cardiac arrest makes it crucial to ensure rapid access to a defibrillator. Also, patients should be in a position to receive reperfusion therapy as soon as infarction is confirmed by prompt clinical and ECG assessment.

The patient should have an intravenous cannula inserted and, to relieve pain and distress, should be given intravenous injections of diamorphine (2.5–5 mg) and an anti-emetic (e.g. metoclopramide 10 mg), with further doses if pain persists. Injections should not be given intramuscularly because this delays pain relief, can increase serum creatine kinase (CK) levels and could lead to intramuscular bleeding with thrombolytic therapy. The patient should be given aspirin, unless there is a clear contraindication. 300 mg of aspirin should be given at the onset of MI. This reduces the risk of death by about 25%. Aspirin irreversibly inhibits cyclooxygenase, the main enzyme involved in the synthesis of prostaglandins and ultimately thomboxane, thereby blocking this pathway of platelet aggregation. Aspirin should be continued indefinitely at a dose of 75–150 mg daily. Clopidogrel should be considered for patients in whom aspirin is contraindicated.

Thrombolysis (see p. 198), in addition to aspirin, can further reduce the risk of death by 20–25% with the largest benefit seen when given early. Ideally, thrombolytic therapy should be started within 1 hour of onset of symptoms.

Beta-blocker therapy should be considered for patients following MI unless there are contraindications. Beta-blockers reduce myocardial ischaemia by lowering blood pressure and heart rate. They could also

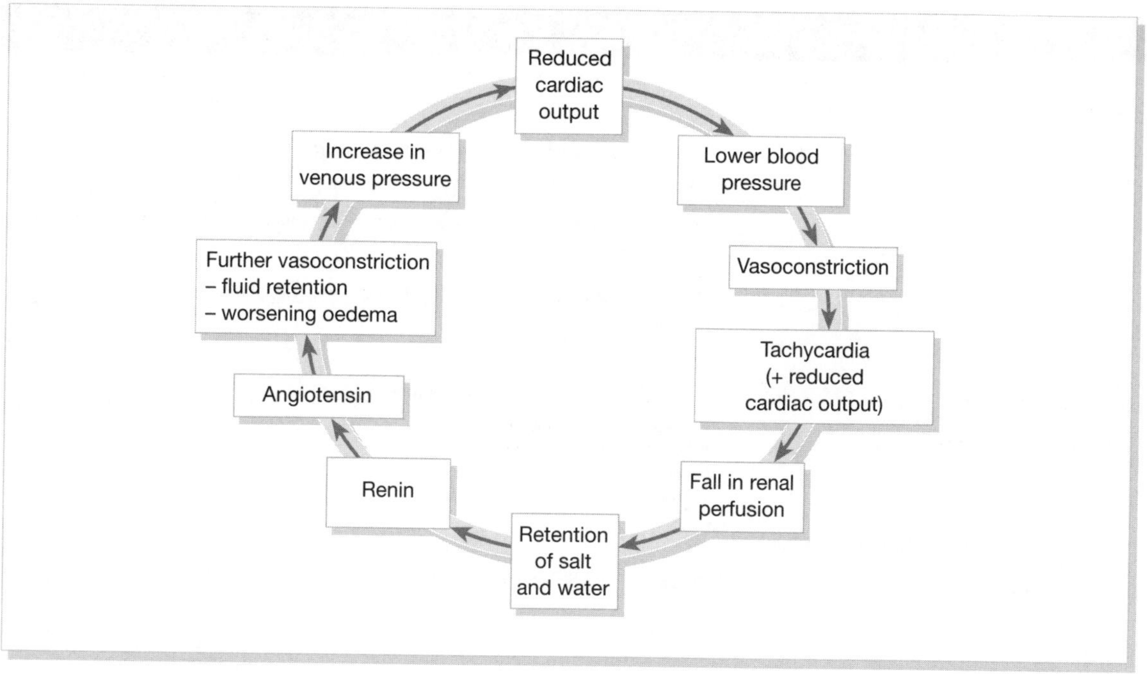

Figure 16.8 Cycle of heart failure.

block arrhythmogenic effects of catecholamines released in acute myocardial infarction. Beta-blockers have been shown to prolong life following MI by reducing the risk of reinfarction and both supraventricular and ventricular arrhythmias.

Beta-blockade added to angiotensin-converting enzyme (ACE) inhibitor therapy (see p. 186) can also reduce mortality and progression to severe heart failure. Serum cholesterol and LDL cholesterol are major risk factors for recurrent cardiac events in patients following MI. Statins (see p. 199) are the drugs of choice for lipid-lowering for secondary prevention of CHD following MI.

Cardiac failure (heart failure)

The volume of blood passing through the heart per minute is known as the cardiac output. This output varies considerably depending on the needs of the body, being low at rest and rising with exercise. The healthy heart has a great functional reserve and can cope with the demands for increased output which occur from time to time. In cardiac failure the cardiac output is reduced (Fig. 16.8). At first this may be apparent only on exercise, but as the condition progresses it may be insufficient for the needs of the body even at rest. As a result, the tissues and organs receive an inadequate blood supply and therefore insufficient oxygen and nutrients.

Drug therapy can control the symptoms of cardiac failure, but the natural course of the condition is often one of progressive deterioration. Cardiac failure is common, affecting 1–2% of the population, and is becoming more prevalent as older people form a larger part of the population.

Types and causes of heart failure

Heart failure is not a diagnosis in itself, rather a 'state' that patients can move into and out of. For example, in otherwise healthy people, a profound anaemia, hyperthyroidism or an overwhelming infection may precipitate heart failure. As these conditions are treated, so the failure will improve. For many patients, however, heart failure exists to a greater or lesser extent as the result of a specific condition and this will dictate which part of the heart's pumping mechanism is failing and therefore which features present. Table 16.18 summarises the types of heart failure, what causes them to develop, and the resulting clinical features. This is based on the kidneys helping to regulate blood pressure through the renin–angiotensin system (see p. 186).

Management of heart failure

The aims of management in heart failure are to decrease symptoms, limit progression and prolong survival.

Table 16.18 Types of heart failure

Causes	Clinical features
Left heart failure Hypertension Aortic valve disease Coronary artery disease	Those associated with increased venous pressure: • dyspnoea (in acute pulmonary oedema, the patient will also be acutely anxious, sweating, pale and very ill-looking) • cough (this may or may not be accompanied by sputum; sputum is generally copious, frothy and tinged with blood) • cyanosis Those associated with low cardiac output and poor peripheral perfusion: • tiredness • weakness
Right heart failure Chronic lung disease (e.g. chronic bronchitis) Pulmonary valve disease Congenital defects	These are predominantly the result of increased venous pressure: • raised jugular venous pressure • hepatomegaly, jaundice • anorexia, nausea, vomiting • constipation • peripheral oedema
Biventricular failure (congestive cardiac failure) (Fig. 16.8) Left heart failure	Those associated with left heart failure: • dyspnoea • cough • cyanosis Those associated with increased venous pressure: • raised jugular venous pressure • hepatomegaly, jaundice • constipation • peripheral oedema Those associated with insufficient cardiac output: • mental confusion, Cheyne–Stokes respirations • oliguria, proteinuria • fatigue

Related aims include improving the potential for activity and quality of life.

Non-pharmaceutical measures

Non-pharmaceutical measures include dietary advice. Since sodium and fluid retention are hallmarks of heart failure, sodium restriction is indicated: salt-rich foods and the addition of salt in cooking or at table should be avoided.

Reducing obesity will reduce the work of the heart, help lower blood pressure and improve the lipid profile. However, stepped changes towards a modest target will have greater success than aiming for large weight loss. In addition, heart failure patients may suffer from malnutrition and muscle wasting. Therefore, dietary interventions may require the contribution of a dietician.

Alcohol is absolutely contraindicated in those with alcohol-induced cardiomyopathy. In other patients with heart failure it should be restricted to small quantities (e.g. one or two units a day). Smoking is harmful and should be stopped if the patient will cooperate.

Rest is an essential element of the management of acute heart failure; however, there is a large body of evidence to suggest that appropriate exercise is beneficial for patients with chronic heart failure.

Drug management

The use of ACE inhibitors (see p. 186) is central to the management of heart failure. ACE inhibitors reduce symptoms, mortality rates, hospital admissions and the risk of developing myocardial infarction in patients with mild to severe heart failure.

All patients with signs of sodium and water retention should be considered for treatment with diuretics to reduce breathlessness and oedema and improve exercise tolerance. Thiazide diuretics are effective in patients with normal renal function and mild heart failure. Loop diuretics are more effective in older people, in patients with impaired mental function and where heart failure is severe. Digoxin (see p. 171) has long been used to relieve symptoms, increase exercise tolerance and reduce the need for hospital admission due to acute exacerbations in patients with heart failure. It tends to be reserved for patients with atrial fibrillation or those with moderate to severe heart failure who remain symptomatic despite treatment with a diuretic, an ACE inhibitor and a beta-blocker.

In general, because of their negative inotropic effects, beta-blockers can cause worsening of heart failure. However, beta-blockers can reduce mortality when small, carefully titrated doses are added to conventional therapy in patients with stable mild to moderate heart failure. Carvedilol and bisoprolol are both licensed for use in selected patients with heart failure.

While aldosterone is indirectly suppressed by ACE inhibitors, this may be incomplete and transient in some patients. Spironolactone (see p. 174) is a potassium-sparing diuretic but unlike triamterene and amiloride is a direct antagonist of aldosterone. Spironolactone is associated with improved survival and morbidity when added to ACE inhibitor and diuretic therapy.

The use of hydralazine and isosorbide dinitrate combination in heart failure is now reserved for those patients in whom ACE inhibitors or beta-blockers are contraindicated.

STROKE

Stroke is a common condition and, for those who survive, a source of functional disability to varying degrees. The two types of stroke are haemorrhagic stroke and ischaemic stroke.

Some patients experience a minor episode known as a transient ischaemic attack (TIA) which lasts for a few minutes or hours; for others, the event is catastrophic, resulting in death or severe disability.

Stroke usually occurs without warning. Occasionally, there may be preceding headache, especially with intracerebral or subarachnoid haemorrhage. Neurological symptoms most often develop within a few minutes, although they can develop in an irregular manner over several hours. Classically, haemorrhage develops rapidly and is associated with headache, vomiting and sometimes clouding of consciousness.

The symptoms that a patient presents with will depend upon which part of the brain has been damaged. No one patient is likely to be the same as any other, making predictions as to the likely outcome of the stroke almost impossible to make with any degree of certainty. The basic organisation of the brain differs from one person to the next and there are differences in the degree to which certain functions are represented in both cerebral hemispheres. This means that if one hemisphere is affected by the stroke, some people will carry on regardless because the other side of the brain can compensate, although others will be severely affected. There are also differences in the ability of individual brains to compensate for localised damage.

The major risk factor for stroke is hypertension. Smoking increases the risk of stroke by around 50%. Cholesterol lowering using statins reduces the stroke risk by around 25%.

Management of stroke

- All patients should have their blood pressure checked, and hypertension persisting for over 1 month should be treated.
- All patients, not on anticoagulation, should be taking aspirin (75–300 mg) daily or low-dose aspirin and dipyridamole modified-release (MR). Where patients are aspirin intolerant, clopidogrel 75 mg daily or dipyridamole MR 200 mg twice daily should be used.
- Anticoagulation should be started in every patient with atrial fibrillation unless contraindicated.
- Anticoagulation should not be started until brain imaging has excluded haemorrhage and 12 days have passed from the onset of an acute ischaemic stroke.
- Anticoagulation should not be used after transient ischaemic attacks or minor strokes unless cardiac embolism is suspected.
- Therapy with a statin should be considered for patients with a history of myocardial infarction and a cholesterol above 5 mmol/litre following stroke.

FURTHER READING

[Anonymous] 2000 Heart failure drugs: What's new? Drug and Therapeutics Bulletin 38(4):25–27

[Anonymous] 2000 Tackling myocardial infarction. Drug and Therapeutics Bulletin 38(3):17–22

[Anonymous] 2001 Statin therapy – What now? Drug and Therapeutics Bulletin 39(3):17–24

ASHP Report 2000 ASHP therapeutic position statement on optimising treatment of hypertension. American Journal of Health-System Pharmacists 57:162–172

Lip G Y H, Kamath S 2000 Antiarrhythmic agents. Pharmaceutical Journal 264:659–663

McAnaw J, Hudson S, McGlynn S et al 1999 Chronic heart failure. Pharmaceutical Journal 262:502–509

Oates C, Lawrence R A, Petty D 2002 Current thinking in heart failure management. Pharmacy in Practice 12(2):74–82

Ramsay L E, Williams B, Johnston G D et al 1999 Guidelines for management of hypertension: a report of the third working party of the British Hypertension Society. Journal of Human Hypertension 13:569–592

Sani M, Lacey J, Rudd A 2002 The management of stroke. Hospital Pharmacist 9:37–41

Scottish Intercollegiate Guidelines Network (SIGN) 1997 Management of patients with stroke. SIGN, Edinburgh

Scottish Intercollegiate Guidelines Network (SIGN) 1999 Antithrombotic therapy. SIGN, Edinburgh

Scottish Intercollegiate Guidelines Network (SIGN) 1999 Diagnosis and treatment of heart failure due to left ventricular systolic dysfunction. SIGN, Edinburgh

Scottish Intercollegiate Guidelines Network (SIGN) 1999 Lipids and the primary prevention of coronary heart disease. SIGN, Edinburgh

Scottish Intercollegiate Guidelines Network (SIGN) 2000 Secondary prevention of coronary heart disease following myocardial infarction. SIGN, Edinburgh

Scottish Intercollegiate Guidelines Network (SIGN) 2001 Hypertension in older people. SIGN, Edinburgh

Scottish Intercollegiate Guidelines Network (SIGN) 2001 Management of stable angina – a national clinical guideline. SIGN, Edinburgh

Smith A J, Wehner J S, Manley H J et al 2001 Current role of beta-adrenergic blockers in the treatment of chronic congestive heart failure. American Journal of Health-System Pharmacists 58:140–145

Spencer C, Lip G 1999 Antihypertensive drugs. Pharmaceutical Journal 263:351–354

Spencer C, Lip G 1999 Management of the hypertensive patient. Pharmaceutical Journal 263:383–386

Topol A, Bijarboneh A, Bakhai A et al 2001 Myocardial infarction and angina – current drug therapy. Hospital Pharmacist 8:125–132

CHAPTER CONTENTS

17

Drug treatment of respiratory disorders

ANATOMY AND PHYSIOLOGY

The organs of the respiratory system comprise the nose, pharynx, larynx, trachea, bronchi, bronchioles, alveoli and lungs (Fig. 17.1).

The main functions of respiration are to take in oxygen and to give off carbon dioxide. In health the respiratory epithelium is protected by a mucous blanket of secretions, and ciliary activity ensures that the airways remain clear to allow the transport of gases between the alveoli and the atmosphere. The commonest disorders of the respiratory system are the result of:

- upper respiratory tract infection
- inhaled irritants
- allergens
- intrinsic causes.

Changes to mucus production and cilia lead to cough, while narrowing of the airways produces dyspnoea and, in some cases, wheezing. Depending on the body's capacity to compensate for diminished oxygen intake the patient may or may not become cyanosed. Drug treatment is directed primarily towards getting the airways to function normally. A variety of pulmonary function tests assists the doctor in both making a diagnosis and selecting the appropriate drug therapy.

ASTHMA

The characteristic symptom of asthma is wheezing resulting from narrowing of the bronchi and bronchioles. Asthma can be divided into two broad types:

- early onset, which occurs in childhood or adolescence, is allergy-related and occurs in patients who develop allergic disorders such as eczema or hay fever; there is a strong familial tendency
- late onset, which affects older people, has no allergic cause and is often referred to as intrinsic asthma.

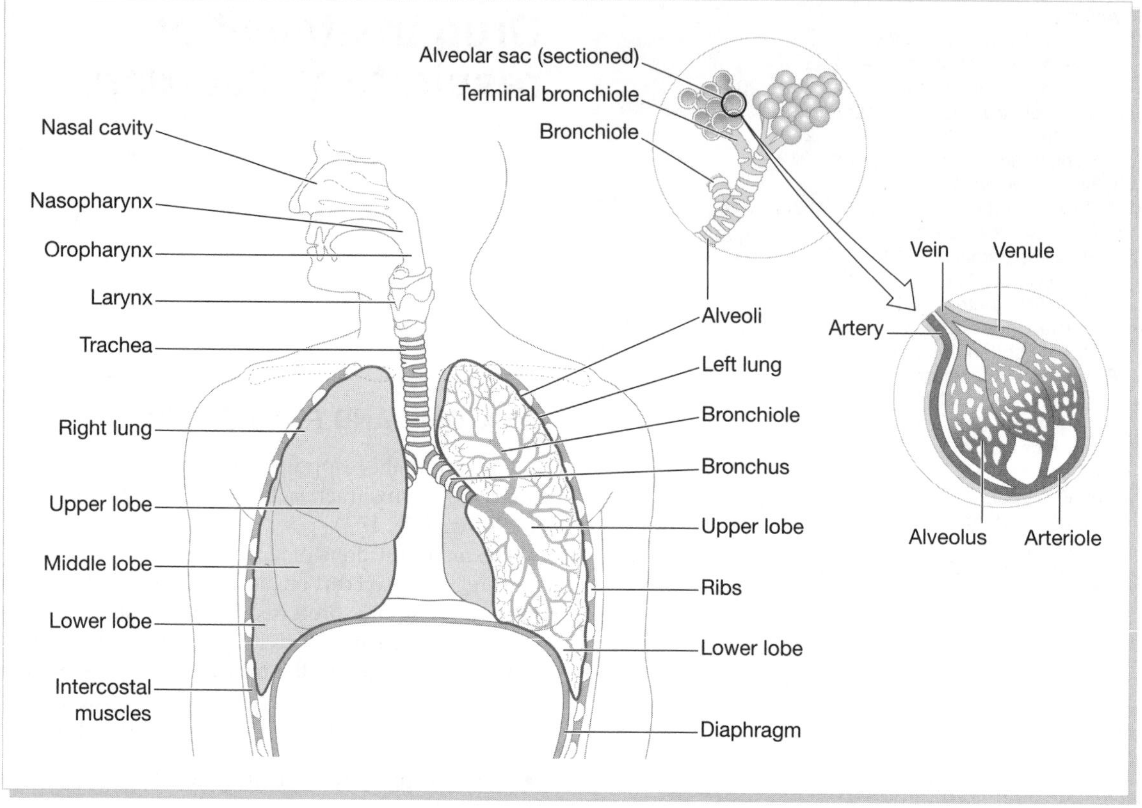

Figure 17.1 The lungs and an alveolus.

Various factors can aggravate both types, and these include dust, tobacco smoke, environmental pollution, rapid changes in humidity or temperature, respiratory tract infection, exercise and stress.

While allergic asthma often resolves after a few years, intrinsic asthma rarely does. Severe acute asthma is a medical emergency clinically recognised by severe wheeze, inability to speak sentences without pausing for breath and a pulse rate over 110 per minute in the adult.

Allergic conditions

Allergic conditions vary from mild forms of hay fever, skin rashes and eczema to more severe forms such as asthma and anaphylactic shock. Allergens which provoke this response in certain individuals include pollen, animal hair, dust, components of various foods, such as fish and eggs, some food dyes, notably tartrazine, drugs, feathers, etc.

Initial exposure to an allergen inhaled or ingested into the body stimulates the production and release of IgE from lymph nodes in atopic individuals. The IgE becomes fixed to mast cells (to produce sensitised mast cells) which, on a second exposure to the allergen, causes release of inflammatory mediators, histamine and serotonin.

Histamine is a major factor in allergic and anaphylactic reactions; it causes:

- contraction of smooth muscle in the bronchial tract
- a short-lasting fall in blood pressure owing to dilatation of the arterioles
- increased permeability of the capillaries, leading to formation of weals and blisters (all actions on H_1-receptors)
- increased secretion of exocrine glands, e.g. acid in stomach (H_2-receptors).

Drug treatment of asthma

Drugs are given either regularly to prevent an attack of asthma or intermittently to relieve one. The asthma attack is due to narrowing of the bronchi and bronchioles by:

- spasm of the circular muscle in the bronchial wall
- inflammation with oedema of the bronchial mucosa.

Drugs used in the management of asthma include:

- β_2 agonists
- antimuscarinic bronchodilators
- theophylline
- corticosteroids
- cromones
- leukotriene receptor antagonists.

Administration of drugs for asthma

Inhalation delivers the drug directly to the airways, requiring a smaller dose than with the oral route resulting in reduced side-effects. Various devices are available for delivering a measured dose (see p. 212). The use of a spacer device may improve drug delivery. Solutions for nebulisation are available for use in acute severe asthma. They are administered over a period of 5–10 minutes from a nebuliser (see p. 214).

Oral preparations are taken when administration by inhalation is not possible. Systemic side-effects occur more frequently when a drug is given orally rather than by inhalation because of the higher dose required orally. Drugs given by mouth for the treatment of asthma include β_2 agonists, corticosteroids, theophylline and leukotriene receptor antagonists.

In acute severe asthma, drugs such as β_2 agonists, corticosteroids and aminophylline may be given by injection when administration by nebulisation is inadequate or inappropriate.

Selective β_2 agonists

Mild to moderate symptoms of asthma respond rapidly to the inhalation of a selective short-acting β_2 agonist such as salbutamol or terbutaline. They are indicated in step 1 of the British Thoracic Society guidelines (BTS et al 1997) (see Table 17.1). If β_2 agonist inhalation is required more often than once daily, prophylactic treatment should be considered.

Salmeterol and formoterol are longer-acting β_2 agonists which are administered by inhalation. They are not suitable for relief of an acute asthma attack and are administered as a preventive. β_2 agonists are highly effective at preventing bronchoconstriction when used shortly before exercise or exposure to known allergens. The longer-acting β_2 agonists are included in step 3 (Table 17.1) for regular, twice-daily use as second-line controlling treatment in conjunction with a low dose of inhaled corticosteroid. Dosages of β_2 agonists are shown in Table 17.2.

Mode of action. β_2 agonists act by directly stimulating β_2 receptors in the smooth muscle of the airways producing bronchodilatation. They also stabilise mast cells, preventing release of inflammatory mediators and histamine on exposure to allergens.

Side-effects. Only small doses of β_2 agonists are required by the inhalation route. In this way side-effects are minimised. Side-effects may occur with the much higher doses required by the oral route and include fine tremor in the hands or headaches.

Antimuscarinic bronchodilators

In patients who already require high-dose inhaled corticosteroids, ipratropium or oxitropium may be used by inhalation in the management of chronic asthma. Ipratropium by nebulisation may be added to other standard treatment in life-threatening asthma or where acute asthma fails to improve with standard therapy (see step 4, Table 17.1).

Antimuscarinic bronchodilators are regarded as being more effective in relieving bronchoconstriction associated with chronic obstructive pulmonary disease (see pp. 210–212) than in relieving asthma. The aerosol inhalation of ipratropium has a maximum effect 30–60 minutes after use, with a duration of action of 3–6 hours. Oxitropium has a similar action.

Theophylline

Theophylline is a bronchodilator used for reversible airways obstruction. It may have an additive effect when used in conjunction with small doses of β_2 agonists. The bronchodilatory effect of theophylline has been used for many years in the management of patients with persistent symptoms. Theophylline is indicated in step 4 of the BTS guidelines (Table 17.1) as an additional bronchodilator to β_2-receptor agonists in patients taking high-dose (800–2000 micrograms daily) inhaled corticosteroids whose asthma is still uncontrolled. In patients unable to tolerate high-dose inhaled corticosteroids, theophylline may be prescribed as additional therapy to standard-dose inhaled corticosteroids (step 3 of the BTS guidelines). Patients who suffer from nocturnal asthma may benefit from slow-release preparations of theophylline as these can provide therapeutic plasma concentrations overnight.

Mode of action. Theophylline inhibits the enzyme phosphodiesterase in bronchial muscle causing it to

Table 17.1 Management of chronic asthma in adults or children

	Treatment	Notes
Step 1	Occasional use of relief bronchodilators	Inhaled short-acting beta agonists 'as required' for symptom relief are acceptable If they are needed more than once daily move to step 2 Before altering a treatment step ensure that the patient is having the treatment and has a good inhaler technique Address any fears
Step 2	Regular inhaled anti-inflammatory agents	Inhaled short-acting beta agonists are required plus either beclometasone or budesonide 100–400 micrograms twice daily or fluticasone 50–200 micrograms twice daily or use cromoglicate or nedocromil, but if control is not achieved change to inhaled corticosteroids
Step 3	High-dose inhaled corticosteroids or standard-dose inhaled corticosteroids plus long-acting inhaled β_2 agonist bronchodilator	Inhaled short-acting beta agonists as required plus either beclometasone or budesonide increased to 800–2000 micrograms daily or fluticasone 400–1000 micrograms daily via a large volume spacer or beclometasone or budesonide 100–400 micrograms twice daily or fluticasone 50–200 micrograms twice daily plus salmeterol 50 micrograms twice daily. In a very small number of patients who experience side-effects with high-dose inhaled corticosteroids, either the long-acting inhaled beta agonist option is used or a sustained-release theophylline may be added to step 2 medication. Cromoglicate or nedocromil may also be tried
Step 4	High-dose inhaled corticosteroids and regular bronchodilators	Inhaled short-acting beta agonists as required with inhaled beclometasone or budesonide 800–2000 micrograms daily or fluticasone 400–1000 micrograms daily via a large volume spacer plus a sequential therapeutic trial of one or more of: • inhaled long-acting β_2 agonist • modified-release theophylline • inhaled ipratropium or in adults oxitropium • long-acting beta agonist tablets • high-dose inhaled bronchodilators • cromoglicate or nedocromil
Step 5	Addition of regular corticosteroid tablets	Inhaled short-acting beta-agonists as required with inhaled beclometasone or budesonide 800–2000 micrograms daily or fluticasone 400–1000 micrograms daily via a large volume spacer and one or more of the long-acting bronchodilators plus regular prednisolone tablets in a single daily dose
Stepping down		Review treatment every 3–6 months. If control is achieved, a stepwise reduction in treatment may be possible. In patients whose treatment was recently started at step 4 or 5, or included corticosteroid tablets for gaining control of asthma, this reduction may take place after a short interval. In other patients with chronic asthma, a 3- to 6-month period of stability should be shown before slow stepwise reduction is undertaken

The British Thoracic Society guidelines on asthma management (BTS et al 1997).

relax and thus relieve bronchospasm. Theophylline may also have an anti-inflammatory effect and may therefore be of benefit when used in combination with inhaled corticosteroids, providing an alternative to increasing the dosage of corticosteroids in suitable patients.

Dose. Theophylline has a narrow margin between the therapeutic and the toxic dose. In most patients a plasma theophylline concentration of 10–20 mg/litre is usually required for satisfactory bronchodilatation. A dose of theophylline of 125–250 mg three to four times daily is given after food. However, theophylline modified-release preparations are usually able to produce adequate plasma concentrations for up to 12 hours. When given as a single dose at night they have a useful role in controlling nocturnal asthma and early morning wheezing.

Table 17.2 β_2 agonists

Drug	Dose
Formoterol	Dry powder for inhalation: 12–24 micrograms twice daily
	By turbohaler: 6–24 micrograms twice daily
Salbutamol	Aerosol inhalation for persistent symptoms: 100–200 micrograms three to four times daily: for prophylaxis in exercise-induced bronchospasm: 100–200 micrograms (1–2 puffs)
	Inhalation of powder: 200–400 micrograms for persistent attacks three to four times daily; for prophylaxis of exercise-induced asthma: 100–200 micrograms
	Inhalation of nebulised solutions: 2.5–5 mg up to four times daily
	Oral: 2–8 mg three to four times daily
Salmeterol	By inhalation: 50–100 micrograms twice daily
Terbutaline	Aerosol inhalation: 250–500 micrograms up to three to four times daily for persistent symptoms
	Inhalation of powder: 500 micrograms up to four times daily
	Inhalation of nebulised solution: 5–10 mg two to four times daily
	Oral: 2.5–5 mg three times daily

Theophylline is given by injection as aminophylline, a mixture of theophylline with ethylenediamine, which is 20 times more soluble than theophylline alone. Aminophylline must be given by *very slow* intravenous injection (over at least 20 minutes); it is too irritant for intramuscular use.

Intravenous aminophylline has a role in the treatment of severe attacks of asthma that do not respond rapidly to a nebulised β_2 agonist. Measurement of plasma theophylline concentration may be helpful and is essential if aminophylline is to be given to patients who have been taking oral theophylline preparations, because serious side-effects such as convulsions and arrhythmias can occasionally precede other symptoms of toxicity.

Side-effects. Side-effects can occur within the 10–20 mg/litre plasma theophylline concentration but their frequency and severity increase at concentrations above 20 mg/litre. These include palpitations, tachycardia, arrhythmias, convulsions and headache.

Metabolism/drug interactions. Theophylline is metabolised in the liver; there is considerable variation in its half-life particularly in smokers, in patients with hepatic impairment or heart failure, or if certain drugs are taken concurrently. The half-life is *increased* in heart failure, cirrhosis, viral infections, in the elderly and by drugs such as cimetidine, ciprofloxacin, furosemide (frusemide), calcium-channel blockers, erythromycin, fluvoxamine and oral contraceptives. The half-life is *decreased* in smokers and in chronic alcoholism and by drugs such as phenytoin, carbamazepine, rifampicin and barbiturates.

These differences in half-life are important because theophylline has a narrow margin between the therapeutic and toxic dose and will necessitate a reduction or an increase in dosage in order to maintain the plasma level between 10–20 mg/litre.

Corticosteroids

Inhaled corticosteroids

Inhaled steroids are the mainstay of preventive therapy in asthma. Inhaled steroids are best started at high dose and reduced as control is achieved. High-dose steroids via metered-dose inhalers should be taken through large-volume spacers (see p. 212). Dry powder inhalers may be more effective in some patients.

Mode of action. Inhaled corticosteroids act by inhibiting a variety of inflammatory agents, reducing inflammatory aspects of asthma and decreasing bronchospasm.

Inhaled corticosteroids are recommended for prophylactic treatment of asthma when patients are using a β_2 agonist more than once daily (see Table 17.1). Corticosteroid inhalers must be used regularly to obtain maximum benefit; alleviation of symptoms usually occurs 3–7 days after initiation. Beclometasone dipropionate, budesonide and fluticasone propionate appear to be equally effective. Doses for chlorofluorocarbon (CFC)-free corticosteroid inhalers may be different from those that contain CFCs.

CFC-free inhalers. Chlorofluorocarbon (CFC) propellants in prescribed inhalers are being replaced by hydrofluoroalkane (HFA) propellants. Patients receiving CFC-free inhalers should be counselled that the new inhaler may taste different and reassured of its efficacy. If the inhaled corticosteroid causes coughing, the use of a β_2 agonist beforehand may help. If a patient is using a β_2 agonist inhaler and a corticosteroid inhaler concurrently, the β_2 agonist should be inhaled first, as the resulting bronchorelaxation will result in a more effective dose of corticosteroid.

Patients who have been taking long-term oral corticosteroids can often be transferred to an inhaled corticosteroid but the transfer must be slow, with gradual reduction in the dose of oral corticosteroid and at a time when the asthma is well controlled. High-dose inhalers are available for patients who respond only partially to standard-dose inhalers.

Systemic therapy may be necessary during episodes of infection or if asthma is worsening, when higher doses are needed and access of inhaled drug to small airways may be reduced.

Side-effects of inhaled corticosteroids. Because of the much smaller dose administered, inhaled corticosteroids have considerably fewer systemic effects than oral corticosteroids, but adverse effects have been reported, including a small increased risk of glaucoma with prolonged high doses of inhaled corticosteroids; cataracts have also been reported with inhaled corticosteroids. Higher doses of inhaled corticosteroids may induce adrenal suppression and patients on high doses should be given a steroid card.

Bone mineral density is reduced following long-term inhalation of higher doses of corticosteroids and this may predispose patients to osteoporosis.

Patients on inhaled steroids should wash out the mouth and teeth after treatment to reduce the occurrence of fungal infection.

Oral corticosteroids

Acute attacks of asthma should be treated with short courses of oral corticosteroids starting with a high dose, e.g. prednisolone 30–60 mg (30–40 mg usually adequate) daily for a few days. Patients whose asthma has deteriorated rapidly usually respond quickly to corticosteroids. The dose can usually be stopped abruptly in a mild exacerbation of asthma.

Cromones

The cromones consist of sodium cromoglicate and nedocromil sodium, which are indicated for use in step 2 of the BTS guidelines (Table 17.1) as an alternative to low-dose inhaled steroids in patients whose asthma is uncontrolled by occasional β_2-receptor agonist use. The cromones improve symptom control in mild to moderate asthmatics, but are less effective than corticosteroids and have therefore been superseded by inhaled steroids and their use in practice has declined. Cromones can also be used as additional therapy at steps 3 and 4 of the BTS guidelines but in clinical practice are rarely used as add-on therapy.

Mode of action. Cromones inhibit the release of substances from mast cells responsible for bronchospasm by causing mast cell stabilisation and are therefore referred to as mast cell stabilisers. They have also been shown to have an inhibitory effect on several inflammatory cells such as eosinophils, neutrophils and macrophages. Both cromoglicate and nedocromil reduce allergen-induced early and late phase responses to immunological stimuli and inhibit bronchospasm during and after exercise and exposure to cold or dry air. They tend to be more effective in patients with mild atopic asthma, in particular children with exercise- or allergen-induced asthma.

Because of their short duration of action and four-times-daily dosing, compliance with therapy can be a problem. However, cromones are well tolerated and rarely cause adverse effects.

Leukotriene receptor antagonists

Cysteinyl leukotrienes cause potent stimulation of bronchial smooth muscle, release of eosinophils and production of secretions in the airways. Leukotriene receptor antagonists block these effects relieving smooth muscle bronchoconstriction and preventing inflammation.

Montelukast and zafirlukast are indicated for the prophylaxis of asthma. They are also useful in preventing exercise-induced asthma and aspirin-sensitive asthma.

Dose. Montelukast – 10 mg daily at bedtime; zafirlukast – 20 mg twice daily.

Side-effects. Appear to be mild but include gastrointestinal disturbances.

CHRONIC OBSTRUCTIVE PULMONARY DISEASE

Chronic obstructive pulmonary disease (COPD) is defined in the BTS guidelines for the management of chronic obstructive pulmonary disease (COPD Guidelines Group of the Standards of Care Committee of the BTS 1997) as a chronic, slowly progressive, largely irreversible disorder characterised by air flow obstruction that does not change markedly over several months. COPD encompasses:

- emphysema
- chronic bronchitis
- chronic obstructive airways disease.

COPD is largely a disease of smokers and the risk of developing COPD increases with increased tobacco exposure, although other factors may contribute.

Emphysema results from destruction of the walls of the alveoli resulting in a reduction of the surface area available for the diffusion of gases.

Chronic bronchitis is associated with prolonged exposure to non-specific bronchial irritants and accompanied by hypersecretion of mucus and by structural changes in the bronchi.

Chronic obstructive airways disease is characterised by an increased resistance to air flow during forced expiration.

Size of the problem

Chronic obstructive pulmonary disease is a major cause of morbidity and is the fifth major cause of death in the UK (Calverly & Bellamy 2000). Stopping smoking is the single most important way of affecting outcome in patients at all stages of COPD. Patients who continue to smoke are certain to lose FEV_1 (forced expiratory volume produced in the first second) at an accelerated rate (see Table 17.3). Stopping smoking is just as important in severe COPD as at earlier stages of the disease. Although lost function cannot be restored, those who stop smoking will deteriorate more slowly. The degree of exposure to cigarette smoking is usually measured in 'pack years', with each year classed as being equivalent to 7305 cigarettes or an average of a pack of 20 cigarettes a day.

Clinical features

The symptoms and signs vary with the severity of the disease (see Table 17.3).

Treatment options for COPD

Non-pharmacological

- Smoking cessation
- Exercise, where possible
- Diet (to deal with obesity or poor nutrition)
- Vaccination against influenza (recommended, especially for moderate to severe disease).

Table 17.3 Signs and symptoms of COPD relating to severity

Category of COPD	FEV_1	Symptoms and signs
Mild	60–80	No abnormal signs Smokers cough Little or no breathlessness
Moderate	40–59	Breathlessness (±wheeze) on moderate exertion Cough (±sputum) Variable abnormal signs (general reduction in breath sounds, presence of wheeze)
Severe	<40	Wheeze and cough often prominent Lung overinflation usual; cyanosis, peripheral oedema and polycythaemia in advanced disease, especially during exacerbation

Pharmacological

- Bronchodilators:
  - β agonists
  - antimuscarinic
- Corticosteroids
- Long-term oxygen therapy (for patients with more advanced disease who are chronically hypoxaemic).

As with the initial diagnosis of COPD, spirometry plays a key role in individualising treatment to a patient's response.

Short-acting β_2 agonists

Short-acting inhaled β_2 agonists (e.g. salbutamol, terbutaline) are the most commonly used bronchodilators. They are best used as required for symptom relief.

Antimuscarinic bronchodilators

Inhaled antimuscarinic bronchodilators (i.e. ipratropium bromide and oxitropium bromide) are at least as effective as short-acting inhaled β_2 agonists in the short term at relieving symptoms and improving lung function. They differ, however, in having a slower onset of action and a more sustained bronchodilatory effect. Regular use of an antimuscarinic bronchodilator alone is therefore recommended in patients with stable COPD who remain symptomatic despite using a short-acting β agonist 'as required'.

Mode of action. Antimuscarinics are specific antagonists to muscarinic receptors. They inhibit muscarinic-induced bronchoconstriction.

Dose. The dosages of antimuscarinics are given in Table 17.4.

The aerosol inhalation of ipratropium has a maximum effect 30–60 minutes after use with a duration of action of 3–6 hours. A more recently introduced antimuscarinic is tiotropium. It has a similar mode of

Table 17.4 Dosages of antimuscarinics

Drug	Dose
Ipratropium	Aerosol inhalation: 20–80 micrograms three to four times daily Inhalation of powder: 40 micrograms three to four times daily Inhalation of nebulised solution: 100–500 micrograms up to four times daily
Oxitropium	Aerosol inhalation: 200 micrograms two to three times daily

action to ipratropium but has a longer duration of action necessitating only once-daily dosing with a dry breath-activated powder inhaler.

Side-effects. Dry mouth can be experienced.

Long-acting β_2 agonists

These are as effective as ipratropium in terms of reducing breathlessness and increasing FEV.

Corticosteroids

There is no evidence of benefit on lung function from corticosteroids. However, they may reduce the occurrence of exacerbations.

ADMINISTRATION OF INHALED DRUGS

The fact that drugs can be introduced directly into the pulmonary system is highly advantageous. Not only is their absorption through the lungs rapid but also high concentrations of drugs can be obtained in the bronchial mucosa and smooth muscle with minimal systemic side-effects. Inhaled drugs are available in the form of a spray (wet), a powder (dry) or a gas. Some drugs are inhaled via the mouth, some via the nose and some through both mouth and nose. The appliances used include the hand-held inhaler, with or without any additional device; nebuliser; face mask and nasal cannulae.

INHALER DEVICES

Pressurised metered-dose inhalers

How they work

Most commonly, drugs are delivered to the lungs as sprays from pressurised aerosol dispensers (aerosol inhalers). The drug and an inert propellant, such as freon, are maintained under pressure in a small canister. When the valve is activated, a measured quantity of propellant carrying the drug is released through the mouthpiece. CFC-free inhalers are being developed as part of the wider approach to prevent damage to the ozone layer.

Administration

Maximum benefit is obtained by the patient only when the proper technique of inhalation is used. It has been estimated that 30% of adults and 80% of children have difficulties with aerosol inhalers (Hilton et al 1986). The problems include coordinating activation and inhalation, too rapid inspiration and too short breath-holding after inspiration (Price 1997). Difficulties arise because: (i) patients are not always adequately taught to use the devices prescribed; (ii) the technique is difficult for some patients to master; (iii) patients who are competent often develop poor technique, and need reassessment and education.

Inhaler technique

Counselling the patient on proper technique is vitally important, with periodic checks to ensure that efficiency is being maintained. Instruction in inhaler technique takes time. Oral instruction should be backed up by demonstration using a placebo inhaler, and written guidelines.

First, the cover should be removed from the mouthpiece and the inhaler shaken vigorously. With the inhaler held upright, the patient breathes out gently and then places the mouthpiece in the mouth and closes the lips around it. The patient should breathe in through the mouth, press the canister to release the medication and continue to breathe in steadily and deeply. The breath is held while the inhaler is removed from the mouth and should continue to be held for as long as is comfortable. The patient should breathe out slowly. If a second puff is to be taken, the inhaler should be kept upright and, after a pause of 0.5–1 minute, the procedure is repeated. On completion, the cover is replaced. People lacking the necessary power to depress the canister may find it easier to use both hands.

The dose delivered from the inhaler can be seen as a fine mist. If any can be seen escaping from the mouth or nose, the inhaler is not being used correctly. In patients with an ideal technique only about 12% of the dose enters the lungs (Fig. 17.2). Although this is only a tiny fraction of the oral dose it is enough to be effective. The remainder of the dose lands on the tongue or the back of the throat and is swallowed, but in such a small quantity that it has no systemic effect.

Spacer devices

In certain situations, spacer devices are particularly useful. For example:

- patients with poor inhalation technique
- patients requiring higher doses
- children
- patients susceptible to candidiasis with inhaled corticosteroids.

A spacer device attached to the inhaler improves the dose delivery to 15%. Spacer devices provide a space

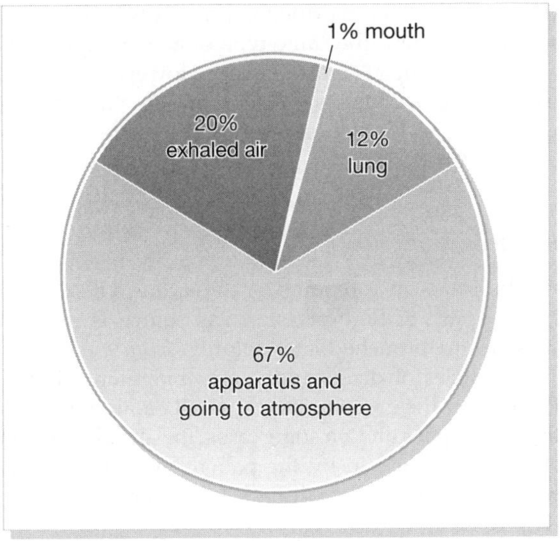

Figure 17.2 Destinations of an inhaled 'dose'.

between the inhaler and the mouth, so allowing for a reduction in the velocity of the aerosol. There is thus less impaction of particles on the oropharynx and this, together with the greater time for evaporation of the propellant, results in a larger proportion of particles reaching the lungs. In utilising a spacer device, coordination of inspiration and actuation of the aerosol is less important. It is important, however, that the patient inhales as soon as possible after actuation because the aerosolised drug is short-lived. Spacing devices range in size from the Bricanyl Spacer, a foldaway extended mouthpiece, to larger devices with a one-way valve. The latter include the Nebuhaler and the Volumatic.

Nebuhaler and Volumatic. The Nebuhaler, a plastic cone of 750 mL capacity, increases efficiency to about 20% (Fig. 17.3). A pressurised aerosol is fitted at one end, and the patient breathes in through a one-way valve at the other. On expiration, the valve returns to the closed position and a hole in the mouthpiece allows the escape of gas which prevents re-breathing and build-up of carbon dioxide. The Nebuhaler is designed in a cone shape to minimise deposition of bronchodilator on the walls, and the patient can inhale when ready. There is no need to coordinate firing of the canister with inhalation.

The Volumatic is similar to the Nebuhaler and serves the same purpose. Each is designed for use with different aerosol medications.

Spacer device care. Large-volume spacer devices should be washed, rinsed and allowed to dry naturally on a weekly basis. An electrostatic charge may be set

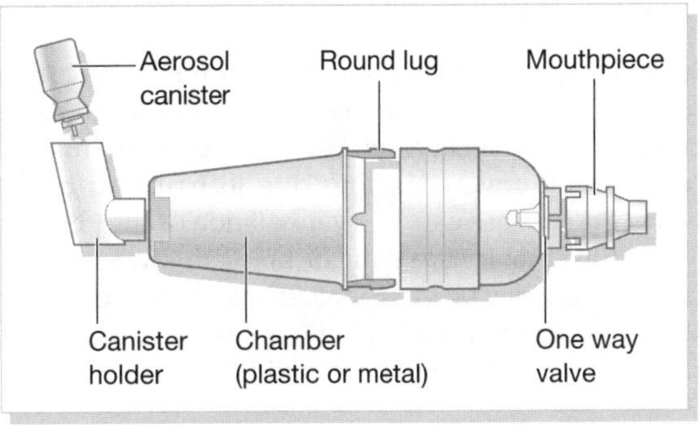

Figure 17.3 The Nebuhaler.

up by wiping with a cloth or paper which could interfere with delivery of the drug. The spacer device should be replaced after 6–12 months.

Breath-actuated inhaler

For those who cannot coordinate aerosol inhalation, several alternative methods of administration are available. The breath-actuated inhaler, when used correctly, is automatically activated by breathing in, and a click is heard so that the patient knows that medication is being received. Examples include the Rotahaler and Spinhaler (see below).

Adaptive aerosol delivery

This hand-held system monitors each patient's breathing pattern, adapts accordingly and then delivers a precise pre-set dose of drug on inspiration only. It is believed to be an advance on nebuliser therapy as it overcomes difficulties with poorly defined drug dose and wastage of the drug into the atmosphere.

Dry powder inhalers

Examples of dry powder inhalers include the Rotahaler – salbutamol or beclometasone dipropionate and the Spinhaler – sodium cromoglicate.

How they work

Gelatin capsules (e.g. Rotacaps) containing the active drug, diluted with a suitable inert powder such as lactose, are placed in this small hand-held device which is twisted to break the capsule. With the mouth placed on the mouthpiece, the patient inhales through the device, causing drug particles to be entrained and drawn into the respiratory system. No coordination of hand movement and breathing is required.

Administration

It should be remembered that twice as much drug from a dry powder inhaler is needed for the same effect compared with an aerosol. Some dry powder inhalers occasionally cause coughing due to irritation of the throat and trachea caused by inhalation of the powder.

For the chronic asthmatic or bronchitic who is very breathless, a dry powder inhaler may be easier to use than a pressurised aerosol but it is particularly in these patients that wet nebulisers should be considered.

Patient education

Compliance is more likely to be achieved if the patient is well informed. The patient should know:

- how to use and care for the inhaler
- the dose to be taken
- the time interval
- the maximum number of inhalations which should be taken in 24 hours.

With the exception of the Nebuhaler and Volumatic, aerosol inhalers are easily carried in the pocket or handbag, helping the patient to be independent. Nurses supervising patients using this type of device should discreetly observe their inhaling technique but avoid giving any impression of hurrying them in the process. Patients need to concentrate on what they are doing at this time and so cannot engage in conversation.

More cooperation can be achieved if the patient is informed about the disease, the purpose of the therapy, how to recognise deterioration in the condition and what to do if deterioration is suspected.

It is the responsibility of doctors, nurses and pharmacists to promote understanding of the technique involved by teaching, demonstrating and checking the patient's performance at intervals. On this basis, alterations in the choice of device may be made so that the patient derives maximum benefit.

Nebulisers

For the treatment of acute breathlessness and wheeze in patients with air flow obstruction, e.g. chronic obstructive airways disease (COAD), and asthma, the method of choice for administering bronchodilator drugs is by inhalation via a mini-nebuliser. This route is particularly useful for patients in respiratory distress or who are unable to inhale properly (Lund 1994). The aim of nebuliser therapy is to deliver a therapeutic dose of the desired drug as an aerosol in the form of respirable particles within a fairly short period of time, usually 5–10 minutes (Muers & Corris 1997). Nebuliser solutions contain the same type of active ingredients as those used in an aerosol inhaler. However, the doses used are up to 25 times greater than those in inhalers, which is why the nebuliser is used in states of acute bronchoconstriction.

How they work

A nebuliser is an apparatus for converting a liquid into a fine spray. A high-pressure gas source is used to suck up the bronchodilator solution from a reservoir. The particles of drug produced impinge on a baffle. Particles of the correct size, i.e. small enough to reach the bronchioles and, in some cases, the alveoli, pass on and are breathed in by the patient via a face mask, while larger particles fall back to be nebulised again (Fig. 17.4).

Because a nebuliser has a 'dead space', a quantity of respirator solution has to be nebulised to fill this space before the particles start to leave the nebuliser and achieve a therapeutic effect. Depending on the design of the nebuliser this volume of solution may be 1–2 mL, and for the nebuliser to function efficiently (i.e. 80% of

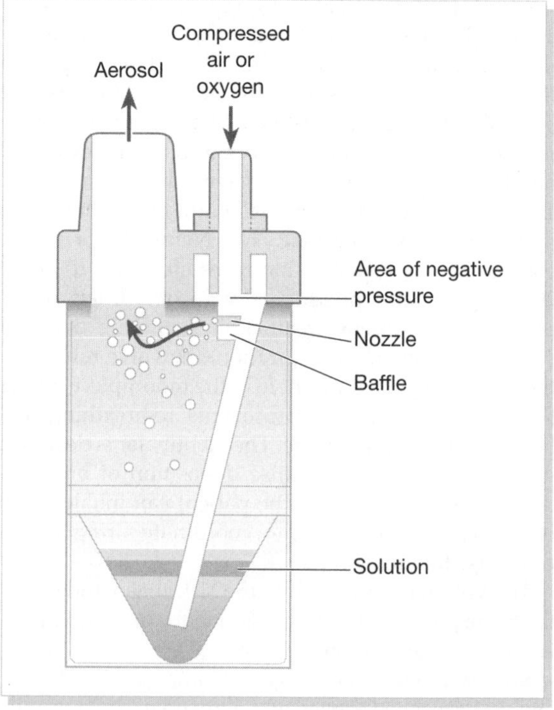

Figure 17.4 Wet nebuliser – in detail.

the drug to reach the patient) it must have a starting volume of fluid of not less than 4 mL. In order to achieve this volume, sufficient diluent must be added to the bronchodilator solution(s). Sterile 0.9% w/v sodium chloride is chosen since it is isotonic, non-irritant and compatible with commercially available bronchodilator solutions; 25 mL sachets of 0.9% w/v sodium chloride solution are available for this purpose. Water would result in hypotonic solutions which may cause bronchoconstriction.

An increasing number of drugs are given by this route – with the result that more than one agent may be required for the treatment of any patient at one time. The question of stability of drug admixtures in this situation may therefore arise. Drugs can be mixed where there is evidence of compatibility as stated in the relevant data sheet (Harriman & Purcell 1996); otherwise, as a general principle, drugs should not be mixed.

Typical drug regimens

For administration via a wet nebuliser: (i) β_2-adrenoceptor stimulant respirator solution made up to 4 mL with 0.9% sodium chloride solution, *or* (ii) anticholinergic bronchodilator solution made up to 4 mL with 0.9% sodium chloride solution, *or* (iii) a combination of β_2-adrenoceptor stimulant and anticholinergic bronchodilator solutions.

It is common practice in patients receiving a combination of β_2-adrenoceptor stimulant and anticholinergic bronchodilator solutions for the drugs to be mixed in the same nebuliser and administered concurrently. Other combinations of drugs should not be mixed without consulting the pharmacy.

Nebulised drugs are normally administered 4-hourly. In severe cases of airways obstruction, however, provided pulmonary function tests show reversibility of the obstruction to be possible, the frequency may be increased to 2-hourly or even hourly. Where the obstruction is irreversible artificial ventilation must be begun.

The carrier gas

The carrier gas used may be either compressed air or oxygen. The choice of air or oxygen, however, depends on each individual patient's clinical status.

Oxygen. Oxygen must not be used for patients with chronic obstructive airways disease and carbon dioxide retention. In such cases, air must be used. Oxygen may be used for asthmatics and some patients with chronic obstructive airways disease but must be prescribed indicating the flow rate in litres per minute as well as the percentage of oxygen to be used. Where the prescribed driving gas is oxygen, a piped supply should be used wherever possible. Patients receiving controlled oxygen should have the prescribed flow rate re-established following nebulisation.

Air. Air is supplied via a portable air compressor or a medical air cylinder. It should be used for patients with chronic bronchitis and evidence of carbon dioxide retention. The use of air in patients with respiratory failure without carbon dioxide retention will aggravate their hypoxia.

Administration

Patients who are to receive nebulised drugs should preferably be in the sitting position, either in bed or in a chair. A gentle approach by the nurse can encourage the patient to relax. The patient should be advised to breathe through the mouth.

Face masks should be tight fitting. Mouthpieces rather than face masks should be considered in elderly patients susceptible to glaucoma and those using high doses of anticholinergic drugs. They should also be used for nebulised steroids to prevent deposition on the face.

As with the administration of any medicine, the patient is identified, the prescription carefully read and the expiry date on the respiratory solution checked. Where a multidose bottle is being used, it must be discarded 1 month after opening. The nurse should therefore record the date opened on any container used.

Sachets of 0.9% sodium chloride solution used to give the necessary volume to the bronchodilator solution may be used for more than one patient during a medicine round but must be discarded immediately thereafter.

The required amount of each solution used is drawn up using a sterile syringe and needle to avoid bacterial contamination. However, as there is no patient contact there is no need to change the syringe and needle when drawing up the same drug for use in a number of patients.

To produce particles of the correct size, a minimum flow rate of 6 litres per minute is required. This flow rate will deliver at least 65% of the droplets in a size which enables drug penetration into the distal airways. During nebulisation, it is helpful to tap the nebuliser periodically so that large droplets may be shaken down and to ensure maximum delivery of the drug. Optimal nebulisation of 4 mL takes approximately 10 minutes. A proportion of respirator solution (approximately 0.5 mL) will remain in the nebuliser chamber.

Nebuliser care

After each use, the nebuliser chamber and mask should be washed in hot, soapy water, rinsed thoroughly and dried using a paper towel to reduce the risk of bacterial contamination and prevent a build-up of crystallised drug in the nebuliser. The inner tubing should be washed once a week in hot soapy water and dried by attaching it to the gas supply for about 3–4 minutes. If the patient has a chest infection, then nebuliser, tubing and mask should be changed every week.

Portable nebulisers

A portable nebuliser unit is designed to allow greater mobility and independence, and is therefore suitable for use by patients at home. The unit consists of an electrically driven compressor which provides clean breathable air; nebuliser; mask; mouthpiece; supply tube; and filters. In addition, a 12 volt connection cable and adaptor are available for operating the unit from a car, boat or caravan.

Peak flow meters

Peak flow meters are used in helping to diagnose air flow obstruction, as in chronic obstructive airways disease and asthma, and in measuring the effectiveness of treatment prescribed for the individual patient.

Peak flow or the peak expiratory flow rate (PEFR) is the maximum flow of air achievable while breathing out as hard as possible. It is an indication of how wide the airways are at the time the measurement is taken. The speed of air passing through the meter is measured in litres per minute and will vary according to sex, age and height (Table 17.5). Peak flow readings are usually higher in men than in women. Peak flow varies throughout the day, and the morning reading is often lower than that of the evening. It is the difference between these two readings that is important. When asthma is out of control, great swings occur with the morning readings being much lower and the evening readings much higher than normal.

Types of peak flow meter

The Mini-Wright and the Vitalograph peak flow meter are available on prescription. The use of peak flow meters is the same whichever type is used. The marker is first set to zero. Those able to stand to use the meter are advised to do so. Patients may be taught how to make an accurate recording of peak flow. Some patients may be instructed as to what action to take in the event of a low reading. Readings should be taken at the same time every morning and evening, and a careful record kept to show to the doctor at the outpatient clinic.

ANTIHISTAMINES

Antihistamines compete with histamine and block its action at histamine receptor sites. They do not reverse histamine effects once established. Some antihistamines have anti-emetic properties.

Usage

Antihistamines are used in the treatment of allergic skin rashes, nasal allergy (particularly the seasonal type,

Table 17.5 Table of predicted peak flow (litres/min)*

Height	Age									
	25	30	35	40	45	50	55	60	65	70
Males										
5′3″ (160 cm)	572	560	548	536	524	512	500	488	476	464
5′6″ (167 cm)	597	584	572	559	547	534	522	509	496	484
5′9″ (175 cm)	625	612	599	586	573	560	547	533	520	507
6′0″ (183 cm)	654	640	626	613	599	585	572	558	544	530
6′3″ (191 cm)	679	665	650	636	622	608	593	579	565	551
Females										
4′9″ (144 cm)	377	366	356	345	335	324	314	303	293	282
5′0″ (152 cm)	403	392	382	371	361	350	340	329	319	308
5′3″ (160 cm)	433	422	412	401	391	380	370	359	349	338
5′6″ (167 cm)	459	448	438	427	417	406	396	385	375	364
5′9″ (175 cm)	489	478	468	457	447	436	426	415	405	394

Standard deviation: 60 min. Negligible ethnic variation.
*A severe asthmatic attack is recognised when the peak expiratory flow is less than 40% of the predicted peak flow. (Figures produced by the National Asthma Campaign.)

e.g. hay fever), pruritus, insect bites and stings, drug allergies and anaphylactic shock (see pp. 136–137) and for the prevention of urticaria and motion sickness.

Drugs used in this group

Non-sedating antihistamines such as acrivastine, cetirizine, desloratidine, fexofenadine, levocetirizine, loratidine, mizolastine and terfenadine cause less sedation than the older antihistamines because they penetrate the blood–brain barrier only to a slight extent. All older antihistamines cause sedation. These include alimemazine, azatidine, brompheniramine, clemastine, chlorphenamine (chlorpheniramine), hydroxyzine and promethazine.

Formulation and dosage. Most antihistamines are available only in the oral form. Following oral administration, symptomatic relief of allergic reactions and side-effects may begin within 15–30 minutes, lasting for 3–6 hours.

Chlorphenamine (chlorpheniramine) and promethazine are also available as injections to treat severe conditions. Chlorphenamine can be administered by subcutaneous or intramuscular injection (10–20 mg) or by slow intravenous injection (10–20 mg) over 1 minute.

Side-effects. Influence on the central nervous system, namely, drowsiness, headaches and dulling of mental alertness. In newer antihistamines, greatly reduced sedative and psychomotor impairment effects. Antimuscarinic effects such as urinary retention, dry mouth, blurred vision and gastrointestinal disturbances.

Interactions. Antihistamines may enhance sedative effects of central nervous system depressants such as alcohol, analgesics, sedatives and antipsychotics. The newer antihistamines do not seem to potentiate the effect of alcohol.

Caution. Sedating antihistamines have significant antimuscarinic activity and should be used with caution in prostatic hypertrophy, urinary retention and glaucoma. Caution may be required in epilepsy and hepatic disease.

Important point. Patients should be advised to take antihistamines with or after food to avoid gastric disturbances.

RESPIRATORY SURFACTANTS

Improved neonatal healthcare and the development of mechanical ventilation techniques have markedly reduced infant mortality from respiratory distress syndrome. Replacement therapy with colfosceril palmitate can further reduce the morbidity and mortality associated with this condition. Used either prophylactically in infants at risk of developing respiratory distress syndrome or as rescue therapy in infants with the established condition, colfosceril palmitate, beractant or poractant alfa improve the clinical outcome in infants weighing 700 g or more at birth.

Neonatal respiratory distress syndrome is a condition caused by pulmonary immaturity affecting approximately 10% of infants born at less than 37 weeks' gestation. It is characterised by tachypnoea, expiratory grunting and cyanosis. The primary pathogenic feature is a deficiency of endogenous lung surfactant. Surfactant is necessary to lower surface tension forces at the air—alveolar interface in order to prevent the alveoli collapsing during expiration. In the absence of surfactant the infant tires, and progressive pulmonary failure develops.

Administration. Pulmonary surfactants are given by endotracheal tube and may be repeated. Continuous monitoring of heart rate and arterial oxygenation is required to avoid hyperoxaemia due to a rapid improvement in arterial oxygen concentration.

Side-effects. The incidence of pulmonary haemorrhage may be increased. Obstruction of the endotracheal tube may occur due to mucous secretions.

OXYGEN

Oxygen, which comprises approximately 21% of air, is essential to all forms of animal life.

Tissue hypoxia results from failure of any one or a combination of the following:

- adequate ventilation
- gas exchange
- circulatory distribution.

Arterial blood gas analysis provides accurate information on pH, partial pressure of oxygen, oxygen saturation and partial pressure of carbon dioxide.

Medical uses of oxygen include maintaining tissue oxygenation during anaesthesia; treatment of diseases including chronic lung disease, myocardial infarction, and pulmonary embolism; treatment of cardiopulmonary arrest; and the treatment of newborn babies with respiratory distress.

Administration of oxygen

Medical grade oxygen is regarded as a drug. It should therefore normally be prescribed by a doctor on the patient's prescription sheet, stating: the word 'oxygen'; the type of appliance to be used (i.e. mask, nasal cannulae), and, in the case of a mask, the appropriate percentage of oxygen, the flow rate of oxygen (i.e. litres per minute) and the duration of administration.

Oxygen may be delivered to the patient using either a variable oxygen delivery system or a fixed oxygen delivery system. These terms refer to the rates of oxygen delivered by the equipment.

Variable oxygen delivery systems, which include nasal cannulae and face masks, deliver oxygen at flow rates that supplement the oxygen concentration in room air. The range can vary from as low as 21% to as high as 90%. The exact concentration, however, depends on the flow rate of oxygen and the patient's rate and depth of breathing. Variable-delivery systems are commonly used postoperatively, and in pulmonary oedema and pulmonary embolus.

Fixed oxygen delivery systems, which include masks and nebulisers incorporating the Venturi principle, provide the person's total inspiratory needs, and can deliver a precise and accurate concentration of oxygen which is not significantly affected by the rate and depth of the patient's breathing, and is largely independent of the oxygen flow rate. It is essential that patients with chronic obstructive pulmonary disease who require oxygen receive a fixed concentration such as 24 or 28%.

In health, there are two drives for breathing. The predominant drive is the presence of carbon dioxide; the less important one is lack of oxygen. In chronic obstructive pulmonary disease, the sensitivity to carbon dioxide may be lost, in which case the hypoxic drive predominates. If the patient then receives high concentrations of oxygen, the hypoxic drive will also disappear, leaving the patient respiratorily depressed and likely to develop carbon dioxide narcosis resulting in loss of consciousness.

As well as ensuring the patient receives the correct percentage of oxygen at the correct flow rate, it is important to note how long the oxygen should be given. The administration of high concentrations of oxygen (>60%) for more than 48 hours may damage the alveolar membrane of the lungs.

Oxygen may be administered on a nurse's own initiative only in a life-threatening situation, because in an inappropriate concentration it has potentially harmful effects in some patients.

Devices for the administration of oxygen

Face mask. This is the commonest method for administering oxygen. Face masks are designed to deliver different concentrations of oxygen according to the flow system involved. The main ones are:

- *high flow* masks which accurately deliver *low concentrations* of oxygen (24–35%) used in chronic obstructive pulmonary disease
- *low flow* masks achieving *high concentrations* of oxygen (up to 60%) used in pulmonary oedema and pulmonary embolus.

A variety of masks are available which are lightweight, efficient, and, for most patients, comfortable, and which allow for observation of lip colour. Care must be taken to ensure that the mask fits snugly and that its position is maintained for effective delivery. Redness and sores can result from pressure and chafing from the mask over the bridge of the nose and from the elastic strap over the temporal region and above the ears. When discomfort persists after adjusting the tension of the elastic, this may be relieved by inserting a neat layer of cotton wool between the appliance and the skin. In the course of time, the mask can become moist and sticky, and patients appreciate having it removed for a few moments to allow the face and the mask to be wiped clean and dry. Unless it is delivered at a flow rate of more than 4 litres/minute, oxygen taken through a mask or nasal cannulae does not require to be humidified as the air with which it mixes on inspiration contains sufficient water vapour.

Nasal cannulae. These have an advantage over face masks in that they do not interfere to the same extent with feeding and communication. In addition, those patients who experience feelings of claustrophobia with a mask may find nasal cannulae acceptable. Before inserting nasal cannulae the patient is asked to blow the nose, or else the nostrils are cleaned with moist cotton-tipped applicators.

Oxygen tent/hood. These are used in paediatric wards because very young children do not tolerate oxygen masks. A nurse can do much to help a child overcome feelings of isolation by staying close by and making physical contact with the child through the appropriate openings in the apparatus.

Safety

Oxygen administration is a potentially dangerous procedure and every precaution must be taken to ensure that standards of safety are maintained.

Although in most hospitals oxygen is piped to the bedside or operating theatre, portable cylinders still have to be used, for example on patient trolleys and during emergencies outside the ward. All nurses must therefore be able to identify a cylinder of oxygen correctly, i.e. black with a white shoulder and marked with the word **OXYGEN**. Since the oxygen in cylinders is in compressed form, removal of valves or flow meters should be carried out only by those trained to do so and in accordance with local policy. This noisy procedure should take place outside patient areas. At all times cylinders should be supported in a stand so that they cannot be knocked over, and they should be stored away from direct heat to prevent explosion. Nurses require to anticipate when a replacement cylinder will be needed, taking into account that there will be a rapid decrease in pressure as the gauge reaches the empty mark. Sufficient time also needs to be allowed for a new supply to be delivered to the ward.

Emergency equipment should be checked daily!

Precautions

Since oxygen supports combustion and can convert a spark into a flame, precautions must be taken in the immediate area of its use. The patient involved, the surrounding patients and any visitors should have these precautions explained to them. Printed warnings should be in evidence. Items likely to be a danger should be removed – for example, matches and cigarette lighters, electric shavers and battery-operated or friction toys. Care should be exercised when bedmaking and combing hair to reduce risk of sparks created by static electricity.

Observations

Periodic observations must be made by the nurse as long as the patient is receiving oxygen. A check should be made of the patient's condition, generally, and respirations, specifically. It is important to recognise whether the oxygen is benefiting the patient. Acute hypoxaemia produces alterations to rate and depth of respiration; bounding pulse; high blood pressure; cyanosis; restlessness; and confusion. Pulse oximetry provides non-invasive continuous monitoring of the state of oxygenation.

Other observations include the flow of oxygen; the volume of oxygen remaining in the cylinder; and the general environment to ensure that safety is being maintained. When working with patients receiving oxygen, care should be taken to prevent obstruction of the oxygen tubing by, for example, a cot side, backrest or the patients themselves.

Effects of oxygen therapy

To counteract the drying effect of oxygen, patients should be assisted and encouraged to increase their fluid intake. For the same reason, the frequency of oral and nasal hygiene should be increased. Since flammable materials such as oils are unsafe to use in the presence of oxygen, water-soluble lubricants such as glycerin should be used for soothing the lips or nasal mucosa. Soft paraffin is ill-advised.

Oxygen therapy at home

Patients with chronic obstructive pulmonary disease may require to have oxygen therapy continued on their discharge from hospital. Time must be spent with the patient and, if possible, a member of her family, giving clear instructions on the safe and effective use of oxygen. The community nursing service should be informed so that a domiciliary visit may be arranged.

Cylinders for home use in the UK contain 1360 litres of oxygen providing 11 hours of treatment at a flow rate of 2 litres/minute. Portable cylinders containing 300 litres are also available but last for only 2 hours at a flow rate of 2 litres/minute.

A register is maintained of community pharmacists who stock oxygen cylinders and administration sets. These are supplied on prescription to patients who require to use oxygen or to have it on standby.

An oxygen concentrator for domiciliary use may be supplied for those patients who would otherwise require many cylinders. This device, which is powered by electricity, draws in air from the atmosphere and then filters out unwanted gases to produce oxygen in a concentrated form. In England and Wales, concentrators are prescribable on the NHS. In Scotland, arrangements for the provision of a concentrator may be made only by a respiratory consultant through the Common Services Agency (British National Formulary, 1997). The concentrator is an economical method of supplying oxygen. A back-up cylinder should also be available, however, for use in the event of a power cut.

Clearly, education of the patient and family in the safe use of oxygen in the home is an important aspect of the work of community nurse, doctor and pharmacist. In some districts, supervision of patients at home is undertaken by a respiratory nurse.

MUCOLYTICS

Mucolytics such as carbocisteine are used to ease expectoration by reducing sputum viscosity in chronic asthma and bronchitis. Their therapeutic value, however, is doubtful. Steam inhalation is beneficial in some cases.

INHALATIONS

Decongestants such as steam and menthol may be helpful when breathed in from a Nelson-type inhaler.

COUGH PREPARATIONS

Cough suppressants

The cough reflex is important in maintaining an open airway. A productive cough expels secretions and foreign material and should not be suppressed.

Cough suppressants act directly on the medullary mechanism in the brain, suppressing the cough reflex.

Usage. The effectiveness of cough suppressants is dubious. Therefore they are only occasionally useful in the treatment of:

- a dry, hacking, non-productive cough which disturbs sleep (codeine, dextromethorphan and pholcodine)
- an extremely distressing cough associated with lung cancer; in this case the most powerful narcotics are used.

Side-effects and contraindications. All cough suppressants tend to cause constipation. Large doses cause respiratory depression and are contraindicated in patients suffering from asthma.

Important point. Cough suppressants are not recommended for children under the age of 1 year, and only occasionally in older children.

Expectorants

Theoretically, expectorants liquefy mucus and facilitate its removal from the lungs through coughing but there is no scientific basis for this.

Demulcents

Demulcent cough preparations contain soothing, moistening substances such as syrup or glycerol. Some patients find this useful in relieving a dry irritating cough. A demulcent such as simple linctus may be helpful.

NASAL DECONGESTANTS

Local nasal decongestants cause vasoconstriction and reduce congestion and oedema of the nasal mucosa.

Systemic decongestants also cause bronchodilatation.

Preparations. Local preparations such as nasal drops and sprays contain, for example, ephedrine, xylometazoline.

Systemic preparations contain mixtures of paracetamol, antihistamines, and nasal decongestants such as pseudoephedrine. These preparations are of doubtful therapeutic value.

Side-effects. Local decongestants are subject to tolerance and rebound vasodilatation, and cause damage to the nasal mucosa and cilia. They are not generally effective for more than a few days and therefore have limited usefulness.

The sympathomimetic (e.g. pseudoephedrine) component in systemic preparations may cause tachycardia and a rise in blood pressure.

The antihistamine component may cause drowsiness and affect the ability to drive or operate machinery.

Caution. Systemic nasal decongestants should be avoided in patients with hypertension, hyperthyroidism, coronary heart disease, diabetes (interfere with blood sugar control) and in patients taking monoamine-oxidase inhibitors (MAOIs).

REFERENCES

British Thoracic Society (BTS), National Asthma Campaign, Royal College of Physicians of London in association with the General Practitioner in Asthma Group, British Association of Accident and Emergency Medicine, British Paediatric Respiratory Society and Royal College of Paediatrics and Child Health 1997 The British Guidelines on Asthma Management 1995. Review and Position Statement. Thorax 52(suppl 1):S1–S21

Calverly P, Bellamy D 2000 The challenge of providing better care for patients with chronic obstructive airways disease: the poor relation of airways obstruction? Thorax 55:78–82

COPD Guidelines Group of the Standards of Care Committee of the BTS 1997 BTS Guidelines for the Management of Chronic Obstructive Pulmonary Disease. Thorax 52(suppl 5):S1–S28

Harriman A-M and Purcell N 1996 Can we mix nebuliser solutions? Pharmacy in Practice 6(9):347–348

Hilton S, Sibbald B, Ross Anderson 1986 Controlled evaluation of the effects of patient education on asthma morbidity in general practice. Lancet i:26–29

Lund W (ed) 1994 Inhalational products. British pharmaceutical codex. Pharmaceutical Press, London

Muers M F, Corris P A (eds) 1997 Current best practice for nebuliser treatment. Thorax 52(suppl 2): S1–S3

Price D 1997 Improving compliance with asthma therapy. Update 7(May):619–624

FURTHER READING

[Anonymous] 2000 Inhaler devices for asthma. Drug and Therapeutics Bulletin 38(2):9–14

[Anonymous] 2001 Managing stable chronic obstructive pulmonary disease. Drug and Therapeutics Bulletin 39(11):81–85

Barnes P 2000 COPD: therapeutic prospects for future management. Future Prescriber (6):6–9

Hassan M, Topol A, Oldfield W et al 2001 Current drug treatment of asthma. Hospital Pharmacist 8:241–247

Lipwork B J 1999 Modern drug treatment of chronic asthma. British Medical Journal 318:380–384

Robinson D 2001 Current treatments for asthma in primary care. Prescriber 12(17):46–55

Scottish Intercollegiate Guidelines Network (SIGN) 1999 Emergency management of acute asthma. SIGN, Edinburgh

Scottish Intercollegiate Guidelines Network (SIGN) 1998 Primary care management of asthma. SIGN, Edinburgh

CHAPTER CONTENTS

18

Drugs acting on the central nervous system

ANATOMY AND PHYSIOLOGY

The central nervous system comprises the brain, spinal cord and peripheral nerves. There is a vast number of nerves, each consisting of a nerve cell otherwise termed a neurone and its processes, axons and dendrites. The neurones conduct nerve impulses which are akin to tiny electrical charges. Axons, which are usually longer than dendrites, carry nerve impulses away from the cell. Large axons are surrounded by a myelin sheath. Dendrites are nerve fibres which carry impulses towards nerve cells. They form synapses with dendrites of other neurones or terminate in specialised sensory receptors such as those in the skin (Fig. 18.1).

Synapse and chemical transmitters

A synapse is where nerve impulses are transmitted from one neurone, called the presynaptic neurone, to another neurone, called the postsynaptic neurone. The space between them is the synaptic cleft. Chemical transmitters carry nerve impulses across the synaptic cleft (Fig. 18.2). Noradrenaline (norepinephrine), gamma-aminobutyric acid (GABA), acetylcholine, dopamine and 5-hydroxytryptamine (serotonin) are examples of chemicals which act as transmitters. The endings of autonomic nerves supplying smooth muscle and glands release a transmitter substance which stimulates or depresses the activity of the structure.

The brain

The parts comprising the brain are the:

- cerebrum
- midbrain } brain stem
- pons varolii } brain stem
- medulla oblongata } brain stem
- cerebellum.

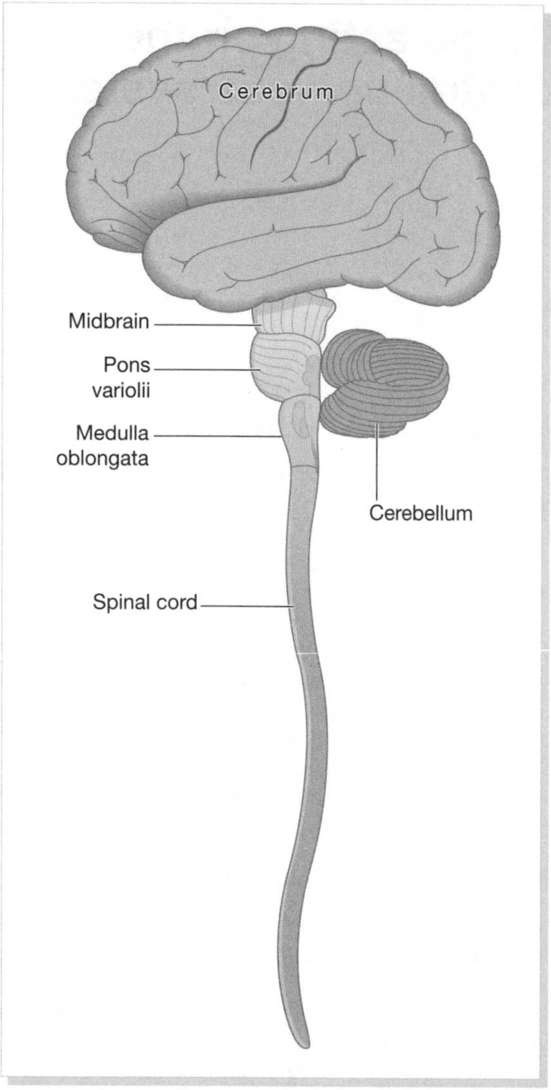

Figure 18.1 The brain. (From Waugh A, Grant A 2001 Ross and Wilson Anatomy and physiology in health and illness, 9th edn. Churchill Livingstone, Edinburgh.)

The peripheral part of the cerebrum is composed of nerve cells or grey matter forming the cerebral cortex, and the deeper layers consist of nerve fibres or white matter. The types of activity associated with the cerebral cortex are:

- mental activities – memory, reasoning, learning
- sensory perception – pain, temperature, touch, sight, hearing, taste, smell
- control of voluntary muscle contraction.

The midbrain consists of nerve cells and fibres connecting the cerebrum with lower parts of the brain and

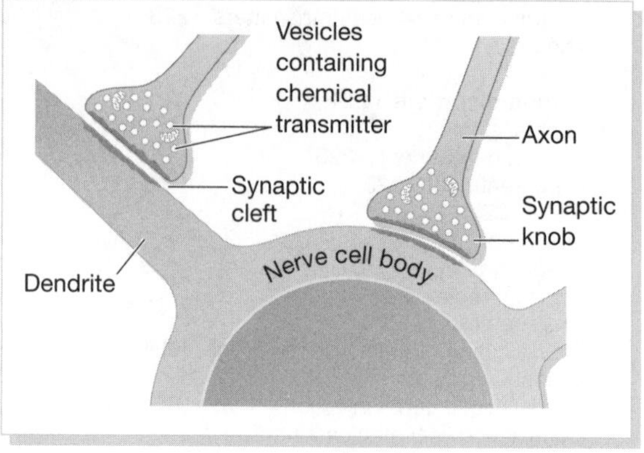

Figure 18.2 Synaptic cleft. (From Waugh A, Grant A 2001 Ross and Wilson Anatomy and physiology in health and illness, 9th edn. Churchill Livingstone, Edinburgh.)

Table 18.1 The vital centres of the brain

Centre	Effect of stimulation
Cardiac centre	Sympathetic stimulation increases the rate and force of the heartbeat; parasympathetic stimulation has the opposite effect
Respiratory centre	Controls rate and depth of respiration
Vasomotor centre	Controls diameter of blood vessels; the vasomotor centre may be stimulated by baroreceptors, body temperature, emotion
Reflex centre	Irritating substances in the stomach or respiratory tract cause nerve impulses to pass to the medulla oblongata which initiate reflex actions such as vomiting, coughing or sneezing

with the spinal cord. The medulla oblongata extends from the pons varolii and is continuous with the spinal cord. The vital centres, comprising groups of cells associated with the autonomic reflex activity, lie within the medulla oblongata; they are listed in Table 18.1.

The cerebellum coordinates voluntary muscle movement, posture and balance. The sensory input is derived from the muscles, joints, eyes and ears. Damage to the cerebellum results in uncoordinated muscular movement such as staggering gait.

COMMON DISORDERS

INSOMNIA

Normal sleep is of two kinds:

- slow wave sleep (SWS)
  - heart rate, blood pressure, respiration are steady or in decline

- muscles are relaxed
- growth hormone secretion is maximal
- rapid eye movement (REM)
  - heart rate, blood pressure, respiration fluctuate
  - cerebral blood flow increases above that during wakefulness
  - skeletal muscles are profoundly relaxed though body movements are more pronounced (dreaming sleep).

A 'normal night' consists of a sleep latency period which varies from person to person (the 'dropping off' stage) followed by SWS sleep for about 1 hour, REM sleep for about 20 minutes, SWS for approximately 90 minutes, REM sleep for about 20 minutes and the rest of the night alternating between SWS and REM sleep until wakefulness. Both kinds of sleep appear necessary for normal health.

Insomnia affects most of us at some time in our lives. For the majority it is transient but for some people insomnia becomes a chronic problem. Many people who sleep badly complain of tiredness during the day and mood disturbance. Insomnia may be characterised by:

- difficulty in falling asleep
- difficulty in staying asleep
- short unrefreshing sleep.

However, individual requirements differ, some people finding that only 4–6 hours is adequate whereas others require 8 or 9 hours to feel refreshed the following day. In general, the elderly require less sleep than the young.

Hypnotics are often prescribed without adequate clinical evaluation to recognise underlying emotional or physical causes that may respond to specific psychotherapy or pharmacotherapy.

Where insomnia is caused by the following symptoms, treatment of these primary symptoms may relieve the problem: pain; dyspnoea; cough; frequency of micturition; excitatory drugs, e.g. caffeine; pruritus.

Insomnia is a common feature of psychiatric illness, particularly in anxiety states and depressive illness. Difficulty in getting to sleep is found in both depression and anxiety, and early morning awakening is common in depression. Choosing a medication to treat the illness with a secondary hypnotic activity can assist in alleviating the insomnia. For example, in depressed patients with early wakening a sedative antidepressant, e.g. trazodone, may be sufficient.

Certain drugs may produce insomnia, particularly the methylxanthines (theophylline and caffeine), the amfetamines and selegiline. Sleep disturbance is likely to be experienced in the early stages of treatment, and medication may need to be reviewed if problems persist.

Three main types of insomnia have been identified according to their duration:

- Transient insomnia. This may occur in those who normally sleep well, owing to factors such as jet lag, shift work or acute stress, and lasts for only a few days. Only one or two doses of a hypnotic should be given.
- Short-term insomnia. This is usually related to an emotional problem such as bereavement, problems at work or with marital relations. A hypnotic should not be given for more than 2 weeks, omitting doses when not required.
- Long-term (chronic) insomnia. This can have many causes. Prescription of hypnotics in long-term insomnia is rarely beneficial.

Non-drug treatment

A regular bedtime routine helps to induce sleep. Warm, milky drinks (not tea or coffee) can help. Relaxation exercises or relaxing with a book may be beneficial. An equable environmental temperature will be conducive to sleep.

Drug treatment

Hypnotics and anxiolytics

Hypnotic drugs are thought to inhibit excitatory pathways in the brain. Benzodiazepines facilitate transmission of gamma-aminobutyric acid (GABA), an inhibitory neurotransmitter.

Benzodiazepines

Benzodiazepines reduce the latent period and prolong the duration of sleep. Approximately 25% of total normal sleep time is REM sleep. This can be reduced by as much as 75% by the administration of benzodiazepines. When the benzodiazepine is stopped, there is a rebound increase in REM sleep as if the body required to recover what has been lost. Nightmares occur with severe rebound, and it is at this point that many people resort to restarting the medication. The rebound increase in REM sleep does revert to normal over a period of weeks after ceasing medication, but it is a major factor in the development of dependence on this group of drugs.

Benzodiazepines that are promoted for use as hypnotics may be divided into those with a short or longer duration of action. Shorter-acting benzodiazepines (temazepam and lormetazepam – half-lives of 6–15 hours) are indicated for patients for whom residual effects are undesirable and they are generally preferred when insomnia is not accompanied by daytime anxiety. They are also the most suitable benzodiazepine hypnotics for elderly people, although caution is still required. It should be noted that half-lives of benzodiazepines may be greatly extended in the elderly where hepatic and renal function are known to deteriorate with age. The dosage should therefore be reduced accordingly. Benzodiazepines such as nitrazepam and diazepam which have long half-lives, should be avoided, particularly in the elderly; the same is true where the metabolites of benzodiazepines have long half-lives. Benzodiazepines have hangover effects such as drowsiness and light-headedness the following day, confusion and ataxia, particularly in older people.

Interactions. Alcohol and benzodiazepines taken concomitantly may result in greater impairment of psychomotor function than either agent alone. The usual effect of the combination of alcohol and benzodiazepines is an increase in the sedative effects of the benzodiazepine.

Dependence. Dependence on benzodiazepines does occur and is now regarded as a serious problem, particularly with longer-term treatment and in patients with some types of personality disorder. Patients taking these drugs, even in therapeutic doses, may develop a physical withdrawal syndrome. The main symptom of this is anxiety, which usually subsides in 2–4 weeks, but sometimes lasts longer, although many patients would have been prone to anxiety prior to treatment. In addition, depression, nausea, depersonalisation and perceptual changes such as intolerance of loud noises, bright lights or touch may occur. Insomnia may also be expected but the symptoms are variable. Occasionally, epileptic seizures, confusion and visual hallucinations may occur.

Stopping treatment with short-acting benzodiazepines leads to withdrawal symptoms within about 2–3 days, whereas with longer-acting drugs there may be a delay of 7 days. Patients being weaned from benzodiazepines need close supervision and support, and the drugs should be withdrawn slowly over weeks or even months.

Benzodiazepine withdrawal. The benzodiazepine is substituted with an equivalent dose of diazepam, e.g. diazepam 10 mg is equivalent to temazepam 20 mg or nitrazepam 10 mg. Diazepam is used because of its long half-life. The withdrawal symptoms from diazepam appear to be less severe with little associated craving. However, there may be a problem with daytime sedation.

Once substitution has been achieved a gradual reduction of the diazepam dosage should follow. Diazepam is available in 2 mg, 5 mg and 10 mg tablets, all of which can be halved, and in an oral solution of 2 mg in 5 mL and 5 mg in 5 mL. Stepwise reductions in dosage should be made weekly, fortnightly or even monthly, depending on the patient's response. These reductions can be in steps of 1 mg, 2 mg or 2.5 mg fortnightly. If withdrawal symptoms occur the dose is maintained until symptoms improve. As the dose is reduced small reductions are made as it is better to reduce too slowly than too quickly.

Once the patient is at a dosage of 0.5 mg daily, the dose interval can be increased to every 2 or 3 days. Many long-term benzodiazepine users can successfully withdraw without experiencing significant withdrawal symptoms. A number of patients may find it extremely difficult to withdraw completely.

Chloral and derivatives

Drugs such as chloral hydrate and cloral (chloral) betaine have been used as hypnotics for a long time, particularly for elderly patients. Gastric irritation has been reported, the incidence being higher with chloral hydrate than with triclofos sodium.

Chloral hydrate can displace anticoagulants such as warfarin from plasma protein-binding sites, and may produce excessive prolongation of prothrombin time and a risk of haemorrhage in anticoagulated patients. Chloral derivatives should therefore be avoided in those patients. Use of chloral derivatives can also lead to dependence. There is no convincing evidence that they are particularly useful in the elderly and their role as hypnotics is now very limited.

Clomethiazole (chlormethiazole)

Clomethiazole has both hypnotic and anticonvulsant properties. It may be a useful hypnotic for elderly patients because of its freedom from hangover but, as with all hypnotics, routine administration is undesirable and dependence occurs. It is indicated as a hypnotic only in the elderly.

Pharmacokinetics. It is rapidly absorbed by mouth, taking around 20 minutes to reach peak concentration. Following extensive metabolism, probably in the liver, it is rapidly excreted and has a half-life of between 3 and 5 hours.

Dose. One or two capsules (or 5–10 mL syrup) at bedtime. Clomethiazole capsules each contain 192 mg of clomethiazole base, and the syrup contains 250 mg of clomethiazole edisilate in 5 mL.

Side-effects. Nasal and conjunctival irritation may be troublesome. Other side-effects include headache, gastrointestinal disturbance and increased bronchial secretion.

Antihistamines

Antihistamines are commonly prescribed as hypnotics and sedatives in paediatric practice. Caution should be exercised as these drugs can produce a paradoxical hyper-excitability in children. In general, hypnotics should not be used for children except for occasional use in night terrors and sleep-walking. Promethazine is occasionally used short-term in children.

Zolpidem and zopiclone

Although neither is a benzodiazepine, both act on the same receptors as benzodiazepines. Both have a short duration of action with little or no hangover effect but, as with other hypnotics, they should not be used for long-term treatment. Both are relatively expensive and offer little or no advantage over the short-acting benzodiazepines in terms of efficacy. The side-effect profiles, contraindications and precautions which must be observed with these drugs also differ little from those of established treatments.

Mode of action. Both drugs bind to the benzodiazepine receptor complex, of which there are three sub-types. They have a greater affinity for type 1 receptors.

Pharmacokinetics. They are rapidly absorbed. Zolpidem and zopiclone have a rapid onset of action so that sleep is induced in about 30 minutes. The elimination half-life is 2.5 hours in young adults and 3 hours in the elderly. They preserve normal sleep patterns and appear to be effective agents in inducing and maintaining sleep without adverse effects on daytime alertness or memory function.

Zopiclone has a half-life of 5 hours in young adults and 8 hours in the elderly. Zopiclone has been found to alter normal sleep patterns, but to a lesser extent than the benzodiazepines. A dose of 7.5 mg delays the onset of the first period of REM sleep, but does not consistently affect the overall duration of REM sleep. Both drugs should be avoided in severe hepatic and renal impairment.

Dose

- zolpidem – 10 mg at bedtime (elderly 5 mg)
- zopiclone – 7.5 mg at bedtime (elderly 3.75 mg).

Side-effects

- zolpidem – gastrointestinal disturbance, headache, daytime drowsiness, memory disturbances, ataxia, confusion and nightmares
- zopiclone – gastrointestinal disturbance, bitter or metallic taste, dry mouth, irritability, confusion, headache and dizziness.

The Committee on the Safety of Medicines advises that zopiclone has the same potential for dependence as the benzodiazepines and its use should therefore be subject to the same cautions.

Table 18.2 indicates the half-lives and dosages of commonly used hypnotics.

Table 18.2 Half-lives and dosages of commonly used hypnotics*

Drug	Elimination half-life (hours)	Hypnotic dose
Benzodiazepines		
Loprazolam	6–12	0.5–2 mg
Lormetazepam	10–12	0.5–1.5 mg
Nitrazepam	15–38	5–10 mg
Temazepam	8–15	10–30 mg
Non-benzodiazepines		
Zolpidem	2½–3	5–10 mg
Zopiclone	5–8	3.75–7.5 mg
Chloral hydrate	(8)	0.5–1 g
Clomethiazole	4	192–384 mg
Antihistamines		
Promethazine	12	50 mg

* The figure in brackets is the half-life of pharmacologically active metabolites. Doses are adult doses. Dosage should be reduced in older people.

Summary

The ideal hypnotic does not exist and hypnotics should be reserved for people whose insomnia is debilitating. They should be prescribed for short courses and only when all underlying causes of insomnia have been investigated and treated.

ANXIETY

Anxiety is a normal reaction we all experience when faced with major events in our lives such as moving house, attending interviews, etc. It becomes a medical problem only when it is excessive or inappropriate. It can then be described as anxiety neurosis.

Anxiety neurosis is twice as common in women as in men; it is most prevalent in young women. The patient may describe a sensation of fear or dread, varying from mild to an overwhelming feeling of terror, the latter leading to panic attacks.

Physical symptoms include tremor, tensing of muscles, perspiration (particularly of the hands and forehead), hypertension, palpitations, gastrointestinal disturbances (such as frequency of defecation), back pain, chest pain, dizziness and dyspnoea. These symptoms are very marked in panic attacks.

Treatment

Treatment of anxiety neurosis includes psychotherapy (relaxation, behavioural and reassurance techniques), as well as drug therapy. The decision whether to use psychotherapy, drug therapy or a combination of both is determined by the practitioner.

Drug treatment relies mainly on the use of anxiolytics such as benzodiazepines and buspirone but β-blockers, antidepressants with a sedative action (such as clomipramine) and antipsychotics (such as zuclopenthixol) have also been used, with varying degrees of success.

Benzodiazepines

Benzodiazepines are anxiolytic, sedative and, in large doses, hypnotic. They also show muscle relaxant and anticonvulsant properties.

Mode of action. Benzodiazepines potentiate the effects of gamma-aminobutyric acid (GABA), the major inhibitory transmitter in the brain, by binding with the receptor complex.

Pharmacokinetics. Compounds with a high potency at the receptor site and with a long half-life are best suited for use in anxiety as they are less likely to cause withdrawal problems. For this reason, diazepam is suitable with a half-life of 14–17 hours and active metabolites. It is rapidly absorbed and quick-acting.

Chlordiazepoxide is also a long-acting benzodiazepine and this type is most useful when a sustained action is required. Short-acting benzodiazepines (lorazepam, oxazepam) are used in intermittent anxiety such as episodes of panic, phobic disorders and acute stressful situations (e.g. public speaking) when a briefer action is required.

Table 18.3 gives dose ranges of benzodiazepines.

Reduced doses should be used in the elderly and in hepatic impairment.

Side-effects. Benzodiazepines are generally well tolerated. However, sedation, ataxia, confusion, amnesia and dependence may occur.

Beta-blockers (see p. 181)

Beta-blockers (e.g. propranolol, oxprenolol) do not affect psychological symptoms such as fear, worry and tension. They do, however, reduce autonomic symptoms such as palpitations and tremor.

Table 18.3 Dose ranges of benzodiazepines

Drug	Dose
Chlordiazepoxide	10 mg three times daily increased if necessary to 60–100 mg daily in divided doses
Diazepam	2 mg three times daily increased if necessary to 15–30 mg daily in divided doses
Lorazepam	1–4 mg daily in divided doses
Oxazepam	15–30 mg three or four times daily

Buspirone

Buspirone has anxiolytic effects but lacks sedative, anticonvulsant and muscle-relaxant properties.

Pharmacokinetics. Buspirone is rapidly absorbed and undergoes considerable first-pass metabolism. It is eliminated by the liver and has a half-life of 2–11 hours. Its anxiolytic effect occurs after 2 weeks of continuous therapy.

Dose. Initially, 5 mg two or three times daily, increased as necessary every 2–3 days; usual range 15–30 mg daily in divided doses; maximum 45 mg daily.

Side-effects. Common side-effects include drowsiness, dizziness, headache, light-headedness, excitement and nausea which occur most commonly at the beginning of treatment. No withdrawal symptoms have been reported on stopping treatment after 6 weeks to 6 months, and there is no evidence of tolerance. Buspirone does not appear to have an additive effect with alcohol. Diazepam remains the drug of choice for anxiety neurosis.

PSYCHOSES

Antipsychotic drugs, also known as neuroleptics, are used in the symptomatic treatment of psychoses, including schizophrenia and the manic phase of manic depressive illness. Antipsychotics can also be used to calm mentally retarded children and agitated elderly patients.

Schizophrenia

Schizophrenia is a severe mental illness affecting 1% of the population at some time in life. It can have a profound effect on a person's reasoning and thought processes, emotions and behaviour. Most people with schizophrenia are unable to hold down a job, have few friends and find it difficult to interact socially.

Schizophrenia can develop at any age but most commonly manifests itself in the late teens or early twenties. It affects both sexes equally, but women have a slightly later average age of onset. About 250 000 people are suffering from schizophrenia in Britain today, and each year about 35 000 patients with the condition are admitted to hospital. It involves the most basic attributes that give people a sense of individuality, uniqueness and direction in life. It causes a disintegration of the personality with a wide range of symptoms and abnormal behaviour. These include delusions, often of persecution, hallucinations, usually of accusatory or abusive voices, incoherence of speech and thought, abnormal movements and a flattened affect. Hallucinations can, however, involve all senses including olfactory, tactile and taste. During the illness, functioning at work, family life, social relations and self-care may deteriorate markedly. The symptoms are divided into:

- positive symptoms such as hallucinations, delusions and thought disorders
- negative symptoms, including marked social isolation or withdrawal, lack of volition, poverty of speech, anhedonia, failure in role functioning as wage-earner or home-maker and marked lack of interests, motivation and energy. Some patients are predominantly disorganised in their behaviour and others mainly paranoid. The negative symptoms are often more prominent during the later stages of the illness, hampering rehabilitation and discharge into the community.

The disease frequently creates heavy burdens for the sufferer, often throughout the person's adult life. Furthermore, there is likely to be considerable impact on the patient's family and on society. The course of the illness varies. About 25% of people who present recover fully within a few months; another 50% recover, but suffer recurring episodes of illness throughout their life. The remaining 25% are permanently disabled and provide the bulk of management problems and require constant intensive treatment. Table 18.4 provides prognostic indicators.

Drug treatment

The aim is to treat both positive and negative symptoms and to increase social functioning. Consent must be obtained for treatment unless there is a risk of significant harm to the patient or others by virtue of non-treatment of the illness, at which point the mental health legislation may require to be invoked to enable the patient to receive the appropriate treatment. Compulsory admission to hospital for treatment can be applied for under the terms of the relevant sections of the Mental Health Act (1983) if there is a significant risk of patients harming themselves or others as a result of their mental illness.

Detention can be for 24 hours (for assessment), then for 28 days followed by a 12-month detention. The detention may be at the request of the patient's next of kin (including common law spouse) or general practitioner and must have the approval of a mental health officer (usually a social worker). The patient has the right of appeal in law to the 28-day and 12-month detention orders. Patients can have medication administered against their will for the first 3 months only.

After the first 3 months of detention, formal consent to treatment is required. This may be given by the patients themselves or, where they are either considered to be incapable of giving consent or are refusing treatment, by a second-opinion psychiatrist appointed for the purpose by the Mental Welfare Commission. In either case, the agreed treatment must be listed on the appropriate form, a copy of which must be sent to the Mental Welfare Commission.

The choice of drug treatment should be discussed with the multidisciplinary team. The choice of antipsychotic drug and the route of administration will depend on the individual circumstances of the patient. The dose will require to be titrated against clinical symptoms and side-effects. Counselling and discussion with the patient of anticipated effects and side-effects will create a better understanding, resulting in improved compliance and an increased likelihood of a positive outcome.

Mechanism of action of antipsychotic drugs. The mechanism of action is complex and many details remain to be established. However, psychotic symptoms result from overactivity of the dopaminergic system. Antipsychotic drugs are believed to act by blocking dopamine receptors, especially D_2-dopaminergic receptors in the brain and, in this way, counterbalance the overactive dopaminergic system. While this will result in an antipsychotic effect, depending on the ability of the drugs to block the dopamine receptors, there may be extrapyramidal side-effects and parkinsonian symptoms.

The antipsychotics may block other central neurotransmitter pathways and this may be clinically relevant.

- Cholinergic blockade is associated with dry mouth, blurred vision, constipation and urinary retention. Antipsychotic drugs with a significant anticholinergic effect should not therefore be administered to patients with angle-closure glaucoma or prostatism.

Table 18.4 Prognostic indicators in schizophrenia

Good	Bad
No family history	Family history
Good pre-morbid personality	Shy, solitary
Functions well in work environment	Poor work record
Precipitating cause	No precipitating cause
Acute onset	Gradual onset
Prompt treatment	Delayed treatment

- Alpha-adrenergic blockade is associated with postural hypotension, particularly in the elderly.
- Histamine receptor blockade is associated with sedation – which may be desirable in some patients but not in others.

Pharmacokinetics. Oral antipsychotics generally show unpredictable absorption. Drug availability may be increased four to 10 times on intramuscular administration. Most antipsychotics have long elimination half-lives of about 20–40 hours, which allow once-a-day dosage after stabilisation of the patient's condition. Older patients have a reduced capacity to metabolise and eliminate these drugs.

Administration of medication. The dose of antipsychotic drugs must be individualised for each patient with respect to severity of illness, drug potency, route of administration, age, weight and liver function. A key factor is to ensure that the dose of medication is kept as low as possible. Treatment is usually initiated at low dose and increased gradually until symptom control is achieved or until side-effects limit further increases. Very large doses rarely improve response and usually increase the burden of side-effects. Because of slower metabolism and elimination rate, older people require much smaller doses.

Three main factors influence the choice of antipsychotic medication:

- previous good response to an individual drug would point to use of the same drug on a subsequent occasion, and vice versa
- severity of the illness and the predominant symptoms
- side-effect profile.

Side-effects. Antipsychotics have a wide range of side-effects, the severity varying between different groups and between individual drugs. These are grouped as follows:

Behavioural

- depression
- anxiety
- agitation.

Autonomic nervous system (anticholinergic)

- dry mouth
- blurred vision
- nasal congestion
- hypotension
- urinary hesitancy.

Particular care is required in older people because of the possibility of precipitating urinary retention or adversely affecting glaucoma. Postural hypotension associated with alpha-adrenergic blockade may also be troublesome in the elderly.

Metabolic/endocrine

- weight gain
- hyperprolactinaemia
- galactorrhoea
- gynaecomastia
- amenorrhoea
- hypo/hyperthermia.

Neuroendocrine effects, which include gynaecomastia, galactorrhoea and amenorrhoea, occur less frequently. They are a consequence of a rise in prolactin (hyperprolactinaemia) following dopamine blockade of the pituitary gland.

Allergic/toxic effects

- cardiac arrhythmias
- neuroleptic malignant syndrome
- jaundice (chlorpromazine)
- dermatitis
- photosensitivity
- pigmentation of lens (thioridazine)
- blood dyscrasias.

All antipsychotic medications have the potential to cause blood dyscrasias. Clozapine has a much greater potential to cause agranulocytosis. Neuroleptic malignant syndrome is thought to occur in 0.5% of newly treated patients and to be greatly underdiagnosed. It is a potentially life-threatening complication of neuroleptic treatment. The main symptoms are hyperthermia, fluctuating consciousness, muscular rigidity, autonomic disturbance and extrapyramidal symptoms. The risk is greater the higher the starting dose of antipsychotic and the more rapidly it is increased. Antipsychotic symptomatic treatment should be stopped while the drug washes out. Intensive medical treatment is required where bromocriptine (a dopaminergic agonist) and dantrolene (a skeletal muscle relaxant) are usually administered.

Central nervous system

- sedation
- reduced convulsive threshold
- extrapyramidal side-effects.

Sedation may be useful where a patient is agitated. Antipsychotics lower the seizure threshold in a dose-dependent manner. The more potent, less sedative drugs tend to carry a greater risk than the less potent, more sedative drugs. Clozapine carries the greatest risk.

Extrapyramidal side-effects. Extrapyramidal reactions are well-recognised complications of antipsychotic medication. Clinical features are acute dystonia, akathisia, tardive dyskinesia and parkinsonism.

Acute dystonia

Acute dystonias most commonly affect children and young adults. These frightening and sometimes painful conditions affect mainly the muscles of the face, jaw, neck and trunk. Typically, patients present with torticollis, facial grimacing and oculogyric spasm. Dystonias usually occur within 1–2 days of starting antipsychotic treatment, but may also develop on drug withdrawal. Occasionally, persistent dystonias develop during prolonged treatment with antipsychotic drugs. Acute and sub-acute reactions will often improve or resolve rapidly on drug withdrawal. Where this is not possible, reducing the dose of the drug or switching to another drug may improve symptoms. Acute dystonic reactions are treated with an anticholinergic drug (e.g. procyclidine) given parenterally and continued by mouth, or with a benzodiazepine (e.g. diazepam).

Akathisia

This is characterised by restlessness and unease which may be intense and distressing. Patients typically describe an inability to keep their legs still and feel a compulsion to move about. Akathisia usually occurs soon after starting drug therapy or after a rapid increase in dose. Persistent akathisia can develop in patients on long-term treatment with antipsychotics. Acute akathisia only rarely responds to treatment with anticholinergic drugs and these may exacerbate the problem, but a low dose of a beta-blocker or benzodiazepine may be helpful.

Tardive dyskinesia

This is most commonly seen in patients on chronic antipsychotic medication. It develops after months or years of treatment and is characterised by abnormal involuntary movements of the face (e.g. lip smacking, lateral jaw movements, fly-catching movements of the tongue) or trunk (e.g. rocking). Increasing age appears to be a risk factor. Withdrawal of long-term antipsychotics may unmask tardive dyskinesia. Symptoms may persist for an indefinite period after the drug has been discontinued. Concomitant administration of anticholinergic drugs can worsen tardive dyskinesia and these should be stopped if this can be done without precipitating severe parkinsonism. There is, however, no convincing evidence to support the idea that long-term anticholinergics increase the risk of tardive dyskinesia. In severe cases, a specific antidyskinetic drug may be indicated – e.g. tetrabenazine may be worth trying. Benzodiazepines, baclofen and valproate have also been used with some success.

Parkinsonism

This is the commonest extrapyramidal effect characterised by lack (akinesia) or slowness (bradykinesia) of movement, muscle rigidity and tremor. The patient has an expressionless face, speaks monotonously, develops a coarse tremor of the hands and can have difficulty in swallowing. It closely resembles the idiopathic form of the disease. Symptoms usually develop within days or weeks of starting antipsychotic treatment or after a recent increase in dose. Elderly patients are particularly susceptible to iatrogenic parkinsonism, especially those with dementia. The condition responds to lowering the dose of antipsychotic or treatment with an anticholinergic drug (e.g. procyclidine or orphenadrine).

Drugs associated with extrapyramidal reactions (Table 18.5)

Extrapyramidal reactions are associated with dopamine receptor antagonists which include antipsychotic and anti-emetic drugs. High potency (relatively high dopamine D_2 activity and low anticholinergic activity) and depot antipsychotics have been particularly implicated. Tricyclic antidepressants and selective serotonin reuptake inhibitors have also caused acute reactions. Other drugs occasionally reported to produce extrapyramidal reactions include anticonvulsants (carbamazepine) and methyldopa.

Classification of antipsychotic drugs

The phenothiazine group comprises a large proportion of the antipsychotics. This group can be divided into

Table 18.5 Some drugs associated with extrapyramidal reactions

Drug group	Example
Antipsychotics	Chlorpromazine Flupentixol Fluphenazine Haloperidol Risperidone Trifluoperazine
Anti-emetics	Metoclopramide Prochlorperazine
Antidepressants	Tricyclics, e.g. amitriptyline
SSRIs	Paroxetine

Table 18.6 Adverse effects of phenothiazines

Group	Adverse effects		
	Sedative	Antimuscarinic	Extrapyramidal
Group 1 (aliphatic phenothiazines) Chlorpromazine Levomepromazine (methotrimeprazine)* Promazine*	Pronounced	Moderate	Moderate
Group 2 (piperidine phenothiazines) Pericyazine* Pipotiazine	Moderate	Pronounced	Low
Group 3 (piperazine phenothiazines) Fluphenazine Perphenazine* Trifluoperazine	Low	Low	Pronounced

* Little or no antipsychotic action.

three sub-groups with respect to the chemical side-chain of the molecule. By altering the side-chain, new molecules were formed but this influenced the side-effect profile with particular regard to sedative effects, antimuscarinic effects and extrapyramidal side-effects (Table 18.6).

Aliphatic phenothiazines (group 1)

The first antipsychotic to be introduced was chlorpromazine in 1952. It is used for a wide range of indications, including control of disturbed behaviour and psychotic symptoms, and control and maintenance of schizophrenia and other psychoses. Chlorpromazine is also used to treat nausea, vomiting and intractable hiccup. Photosensitisation is more common with chlorpromazine than with other antipsychotics. Promazine is indicated for agitation, restlessness and anxiety, especially in the elderly. It is not sufficiently active by mouth to be used as an antipsychotic drug.

Piperidine phenothiazines (group 2)

Pericyazine can be used for the control of disturbed behaviour, schizophrenia and other psychoses. Pipotiazine is available only as an intramuscular injection. It is fairly sedative with a relatively low potential for causing extrapyramidal reactions as it has pronounced anticholinergic activity.

Piperazine phenothiazines (group 3)

Fluphenazine is used as a depot formulation. Trifluoperazine is commonly used in paranoia, but its use is limited by the high incidence of extrapyramidal side-effects.

Box 18.1 **The non-phenothiazine antipsychotic drugs**

Butyrophenones
Benperidol, haloperidol
Diphenylbutylpiperidines
Pimozide
Thioxanthenes
Flupentixol, zuclopenthixol

Non-phenothiazines (Box 18.1)

The non-phenothiazines tend to have adverse effects similar to those of the phenothiazines group 3 (piperazine phenothiazines), i.e. they are generally characterised by fewer sedative and fewer antimuscarinic effects, but more pronounced extrapyramidal effects.

Butyrophenones

Benperidol is used for the control of deviant antisocial sexual behaviour resulting from mental illness. However, its value has not been established. Haloperidol is a widely used antipsychotic and is possibly the drug of choice for acute mania. It is less sedating than chlorpromazine but has more pronounced extrapyramidal side-effects.

Diphenylbutylpiperidines

These are long-acting antipsychotics. Pimozide is long-acting, less sedating than chlorpromazine. An electrocardiogram (ECG) is required prior to commencing treatment and at regular intervals if doses greater than 16 mg daily are being prescribed.

Table 18.7 Antipsychotics – type and dosage

Drug type	Drug	Oral dose
Butyrophenones	Benperidol	0.25–1.5 mg daily in divided doses
	Haloperidol	Initially 1.5–3 mg two to three times daily or 3–5 mg two to three times daily in severely affected or resistant patients; in resistant schizophrenia up to 100 mg daily
Diphenylbutylpiperidine	Pimozide	2–20 mg daily
Phenothiazines	Chlorpromazine	Initially 25 mg three times daily; usual maintenance dose 75–300 mg daily; maximum dose 1 g daily
	Levomepromazine (methotrimeprazine)	Initially 25–50 mg daily in divided doses, increased as necessary to 1 g daily
	Promazine	100–200 mg four times daily; agitation and restlessness in the elderly – 25–50 mg up to four times daily
Piperazine phenothiazines	Fluphenazine	Initially 2.5–10 mg daily in two to three divided doses adjusted according to response to 20 mg daily
	Perphenazine	Initially 4 mg three times daily to a maximum of 24 mg daily
	Trifluoperazine	Initially 5 mg twice daily increased by 5 mg according to response
Piperidine phenothiazines	Pericyazine	Initially 75 mg daily in divided doses to a maximum of 300 mg daily
Substituted benzamide	Sulpiride	200–400 mg twice daily, maximum of 800 mg daily in patients with predominantly negative symptoms and 2.4 g daily in patients with mainly positive symptoms
Thioxanthenes	Flupentixol	3–9 mg twice daily, maximum 18 mg daily
	Zuclopenthixol	Initially 20–30 mg daily in divided doses to a maximum of 150 mg daily

Thioxanthenes

These have activity similar to that of the piperazine phenothiazines. Flupentixol (flupenthixol) is indicated for schizophrenia and other psychoses, except where there is mania or motor hyperactivity or in confusional states; it is also useful in low doses in depression. It is used mainly as depot injections. Zuclopenthixol is indicated for schizophrenia, especially with agitated, aggressive or hostile behaviour. It, too, is used mainly as depot injections. Zuclopenthixol acetate injection is useful for the short-term management of acute psychosis and mania.

Substituted benzamides

This is a structurally distinct group of drugs with a lower incidence of side-effects, particularly tardive dyskinesia. Sulpiride, at high doses, can control positive symptoms; at lower doses (less than 800 mg per day) it has an alerting effect useful for the treatment of negative symptoms (antipsychotics – type and dosage – are illustrated in Table 18.7).

Atypical antipsychotics

All conventional antipsychotics are targeted primarily at the D_2 receptor and are effective against positive symptoms (delusions and hallucinations) but have little impact on negative symptoms (e.g. lack of motivation and social withdrawal) and have potentially debilitating side-effects. These are very distressing for patients and contribute to poor compliance with treatment. It has been estimated that 40–65% of schizophrenic patients will discontinue oral antipsychotic therapy within 6 weeks of starting treatment, mainly because of extrapyramidal side-effects.

In recent years, several new antipsychotic drugs, termed atypical antipsychotics because of their low propensity for causing extrapyramidal symptoms, have been introduced. The first was clozapine, which differs from conventional antipsychotics in having a relatively weak affinity for D_2 receptors while affecting a number of other neuroreceptors (serotonergic, histaminergic, muscarinic, adrenergic). It improves both positive and negative symptoms and reduces hostile and aggressive behaviour and suicidality. Clozapine causes few extrapyramidal symptoms. However, the risk of neutropenia in the first year of treatment is 2–3% and haematological monitoring is a mandatory condition of treatment. This is coordinated by the Clozaril Patient Monitoring Service. Initiation must be as a hospital inpatient. Leucocyte and differential blood counts must be normal before treatment commences and must be monitored weekly for the first 18 weeks, then fortnightly. Patients who have received clozapine for a year or more and have stable blood counts may have their blood monitoring reduced to every 4 weeks. Drugs which depress leucopoiesis (such as co-trimoxazole and carbamazepine) should be avoided. Conventional antipsychotics should be tapered off before starting clozapine. The dose of clozapine should be titrated gradually upwards with the patient being observed for side-effects including:

- postural hypotension (due to α-adrenergic block)
- sedation (due to histaminergic block)
- tachycardia (due to cholinergic block)
- fever (may be due to neutropenia but usually unexplained and settles despite continued treatment).

Excess sedation sometimes responds to alterations in the timing of the daily dose. For example, early morning hangover may be reduced by giving the last dose of the day at 8 p.m. Care should be taken to distinguish true drug-induced sedation from lack of motivation, often seen in schizophrenia, or simple inactivity due to boredom. Hypersalivation can be alleviated by simple measures such as propping up the pillows at night, although anticholinergic medication is usually required. Where postural hypotension occurs, the patient should be advised not to stand up quickly. Dietary advice and exercise may be helpful to avoid constipation and weight gain. Seizures are dose-related and the incidence may be increased by the rapid upward titration of the dose – hence it is important to increase the dose slowly. Tachycardia, where persistent, can be alleviated by beta-blockers.

The dose regimen for clozapine is 12.5 mg once or twice on the first day then 25–50 mg on the second day, and then, if well tolerated, gradually increased in steps of 25–50 mg over 14–21 days to 300 mg daily in divided doses (larger dose at night, up to 200 mg daily may be taken as a single dose at bedtime). If necessary there may be further increased steps of 50–100 mg once (preferably) or twice weekly. The usual antipsychotic dose is 200–450 mg daily (maximum 900 mg daily), with subsequent adjustment to usual maintenance of 150–300 mg. Lower doses should be used in the elderly and special-risk groups. Other atypical antipsychotics include risperidone, olanzapine, quetiapine, amisulpride and zotepine.

Risperidone

Risperidone was the first of a newer class of antipsychotic agents, the benzisoxazoles.

Mode of action. Risperidone binds strongly to the 5-HT_2 receptor and less strongly to the D_2, histamine H_1, and α_1- and α_2-adrenergic receptors. The main clinical features of risperidone are thought to be due to its balance of 5-HT_2 and D_2 receptor antagonism. As a D_2 antagonist, risperidone relieves positive symptoms by countering the dopaminergic overactivity that causes them. 5-HT_2 antagonism may reduce negative and affective symptoms. Antagonism at 5-HT_2 receptors modifies dopaminergic transmission, reducing the effect of D_2 antagonism and lowering the risk of extrapyramidal side-effects. α_1-adrenergic receptor antagonism may cause hypotension. α_2-adrenergic receptor antagonism may reduce the sedative effect.

Pharmacokinetics. Risperidone is rapidly absorbed after oral administration and reaches peak plasma concentration within 2 hours. The half-life of the antipsychotic metabolite is approximately 24 hours. Excretion is mainly in the urine.

Side-effects. Side-effects with risperidone are less severe than with typical antipsychotics, particularly with regard to extrapyramidal side-effects. It is unlikely to cause extrapyramidal side-effects at doses less than 6 mg/day. It is prone to cause nausea, abdominal pain, hypotension and sedation. Akithisia is common.

Dose. 2 mg in one or two divided doses increasing by 2 mg on the second and third days; usual range 4–8 mg daily (maximum 16 mg daily). Reduced dosing is required in the elderly.

Olanzapine

Mode of action. Olanzapine exhibits affinities for serotonin 5-HT_2, dopamine D_1, D_2, D_3, D_4, D_5, histamine H, α_1- and α_2-adrenoceptors.

Pharmacokinetics. Olanzapine is well absorbed after oral administration, reaching peak plasma concentrations in 6–8 hours. It is metabolised in the liver. Mean elimination half-life ranges from 32–52 hours.

Side-effects. Frequent side-effects are somnolence and weight gain. Occasional side-effects include dizziness, increased appetite, peripheral oedema, orthostatic hypotension and transient anticholinergic effects. Blood pressure should be monitored in the elderly.

Dose. 10 mg daily adjusted to the usual range of 5–20 mg daily; doses of 15 mg daily or greater only after reassessment.

Quetiapine

Mode of action. Quetiapine exhibits a higher affinity for serotonin (5-HT_2) receptors in the brain than it does for dopamine D_1 and D_2 receptors. It also has a high affinity for histaminergic and adrenergic α_1 receptors.

Pharmacokinetics. Quetiapine is well absorbed after oral administration and has an elimination half-life of approximately 7 hours.

Side-effects. The most frequent and significant side-effects are drowsiness, dizziness, constipation, postural hypotension, dry mouth and liver enzyme abnormalities.

Dose. 25 mg twice daily on day 1, 50 mg twice daily on day 2, 100 mg twice daily on day 3, 150 mg twice daily on day 4, then adjusted according to response; usual range 300–450 mg daily in two divided doses: maximum 750 mg daily. Reduced dosing is required in the elderly.

Amisulpride

Mode of action. Amisulpride binds selectively with a high affinity to D_2- and D_3-dopaminergic receptors producing dopamine release responsible for its disinhibitory effects. It has no affinity for serotonin, α-adrenergic histamine H_1 and cholinergic receptors.

Pharmacokinetics. Amisulpride is readily absorbed. The elimination half-life is approximately 12 hours.

Side-effects. Common side-effects include insomnia, anxiety, agitation, drowsiness, constipation, nausea, dry mouth and weight gain.

Dose. Acute psychotic episode, 400–800 mg daily in divided doses adjusted according to response: maximum 1.2 g daily.

Zotepine

Mode of action. Zotepine binds to serotonin (5-HT_2), α_1-adrenoceptors and histamine H_1 receptors. It inhibits noradrenaline (norepinephrine) reuptake and is antagonistic to D_1 and D_2 receptors.

Pharmacokinetics. Zotepine is well absorbed and undergoes extensive first-pass metabolism. Peak plasma levels are achieved after 2–3 hours and elimination half-life is around 14 hours.

Side-effects. The most common side-effects include constipation, dry mouth, dyspepsia, elevated liver function tests, agitation, anxiety, depression, weight increase, asthma, hypotension and tachycardia.

Dose. Initially 25 mg three times daily increased according to response at intervals of 4 days to a maximum of 100 mg three times daily. In the elderly, initially 25 mg twice daily increased according to response to a maximum of 75 mg twice daily.

Cautions. In the prescribing of atypical antipsychotics caution is required in renal and hepatic impairment.

Antipsychotic depot injections

Long-acting depot injections are used for maintenance therapy especially when compliance with oral treatment is unreliable. Depot injections are esters of an antipsychotic molecule with a long-chain fatty acid, dissolved in vegetable oil. The oil retards the release of the depot drug and prolongs the duration of action. Once administered by deep intramuscular injection, the depot is slowly released into the bloodstream and is hydrolysed into the active drug and the inactive fatty acid. The rate at which the active drug is released depends on the concentration and volume of the injection. Intramuscular depot preparations are used for maintenance therapy for schizophrenia and other psychoses. The most significant clinical advantage of depot antipsychotics is that they aid patient compliance. Depot injections are given every 1–4 weeks. A test dose should be administered to assess the patient's sensitivity to drug and vehicle, and susceptibility to side-effects, which may be prolonged.

Side-effects of depot preparations

Depot antipsychotics have side-effects similar to those of oral antipsychotics. There tends to be a greater incidence of extrapyramidal side-effects because a much higher dose is given as a single injection. All depot antipsychotics can cause weight gain. Erythema, swelling, nodules and pain at the injection site may develop.

There are currently five depot antipsychotics available (see Table 18.8). As with oral antipsychotics, the drugs differ with respect to their side-effect profiles. Pipotiazine has indications similar to those of fluphenazine. Haloperidol decanoate probably has a more potent antipsychotic action than fluphenazine. Flupentixol is probably a slightly less potent antipsychotic than fluphenazine. As flupentixol has mood-elevating effects it should be avoided in aggressive, agitated patients. Zuclopenthixol may have a specific indication for aggressive and agitated patients as it does not have stimulant effects.

Table 18.8 Equivalent doses of depot antipsychotics

Antipsychotic	Dose (mg)	Interval (weeks)
Flupentixol decanoate	40	2
Fluphenazine decanoate	25	2
Haloperidol decanoate	100	4
Pipotiazine palmitate	50	4
Zuclopenthixol decanoate	200	2

Compliance with medication

Poor compliance is a major problem and is due to factors which include:

- denial of illness
- time taken for therapeutic effect
- side-effects of medication
- complexity of regimen
- poor social support
- poor relationship between patients and service providers
- meeting of patient's expectations
- level of professional supervision
- influence of family and friends.

Every effort requires to be made to improve compliance such as:

- simple drug regimens
  - tablets organised in blister packs
  - the use of depot medications
- improved social support
- improved professional supervision of care
- patient/carer education/information.

MANIC–DEPRESSIVE DISORDERS

The commonest disorder of mood is depression. Mania is much less common, but many patients with mania will also experience severe depression, although there is enormous variation in frequency, sequence and duration between patients. Where the symptoms are serious or psychotic, the term manic–depressive disorder or bipolar affective disorder is used. Lifetime risk for bipolar disorder is less than 1 in 100 and it is equally common in males and females. Cycle length refers to the length of time between the onset of one episode and the onset of the next. This can range from months to years. There is a high risk of recurrence in bipolar illness and the severity tends to increase with successive episodes. Bipolar illness causes immense personal pain and disruption of families and carries a 10–15% lifetime risk of death by suicide.

Diagnosis and clinical features of mania

The diagnosis of mania requires the detection of mood change together with other characteristic symptoms. Simple cyclical changes in mood, without additional morbid symptoms and major changes in behaviour, are recognised as a personality trait and described as cyclothymia. A person with moderately exaggerated mood swings may be described as having a cyclothymic personality which is not an illness. Cyclothymia is an apparent antecedent of bipolar illness. The symptoms required for diagnosis of mania are as follows:

- Mood – there is an abnormally elevated mood characterised by euphoria, unwarranted optimism, overconfidence, and the mood eventually changes from euphoria to irritability and aggressiveness.
- Talk – accelerated mental processes cause a flight of ideas with rapid speech; the patient jumps rapidly from subject to subject and may appear quite incoherent.
- Thought – inflated self-esteem, hyperactivity of thought with delusions of wealth, power and influence (counterpart of the depressive's delusions of worthlessness).
- Cognition – impaired concentration, short attention span.
- Behaviour – reduced sleep without tiredness, restless, demanding, loud, behavioural disinhibition with inappropriate laughter/dancing/singing, excessive libido, wearing of flamboyant clothes/make-up.

Attacks are extremely disruptive, financially, socially and domestically. Overconfidence causes patients to undertake wildly ambitious commitments. The resulting impairment of judgement may cause business failure, excessive spending or generosity, and sexual promiscuity.

Management

Patients may require compulsory admission to a psychiatric unit and detention under an appropriate section of the Mental Health Act (1983) because of loss of judgement resulting in a risk to both themselves and others. Severe manic states used to be associated with significant mortality from exhaustion, dehydration and hyperthermia, but modern practice has reduced this risk considerably.

Drug treatment

The aims of treatment are to control behaviour, terminate the episode and minimise recurrence with prophylactic therapy. In an acute attack of mania, treatment with an antipsychotic drug is usually required. Mood stabilisers may be given concurrently with the antipsychotic drug and treatment with the antipsychotic gradually tailed off as symptoms recede. Patients who demonstrate a recurrent pattern must be assessed for maintenance lithium therapy.

Lithium

Lithium salts are used in the prophylaxis and treatment of mania, in the prophylaxis of manic–depressive illness (bipolar affective disorder) and in the prophylaxis of recurrent depression (unipolar illness or unipolar depression). The body handles lithium in a manner very similar to that of sodium and it is thought to enter neurones in the brain, decreasing their excitability.

Pharmacokinetics. Lithium is well absorbed from the gastrointestinal tract. It is not protein bound and is distributed throughout the body water. Peak plasma concentrations are achieved within 1–2 hours of oral ingestion, 3–6 hours with a controlled-release preparation. Elimination is by the kidneys.

Investigations prior to lithium treatment. Lithium has a narrow therapeutic index, and since it is almost completely renally excreted it is essential to have a baseline measure of renal function. Plasma urea and electrolyte levels should then be measured routinely, and creatinine clearance estimation is desirable in the elderly, since lithium will be retained if the kidneys are not functioning properly. Hypothyroidism can present as depression and lithium can induce clinical hypothyroidism, making it important to monitor thyroid function. A full blood count should be done because anaemia can present as depression and lithium can induce a leucocytosis. An ECG should be carried out as lithium should be avoided in cardiac disease.

Dose. The initial dose of lithium carbonate is 400 mg (200 mg in the elderly). Since the elimination half-life may be in excess of 24 hours in some individuals, a serum lithium level (blood taken 12 hours post-dose) should be checked after 5–7 days. The dose is increased as necessary to achieve a serum level in the therapeutic range (0.4–0.6 mmol/L for prophylaxis and 0.6–1.0 mmol/L for treatment of acute episodes). Lithium levels should be determined weekly until they are stable. Thereafter they should be checked every 3 months along with plasma creatinine and electrolytes. Thyroid function tests should be checked every 6 months. Lithium is widely prescribed in elderly patients, and levels in this group of patients should be monitored more frequently since an increased half-life can lead to increased levels of lithium.

Side-effects. The commonest clinical problems are tremor, polyuria, polydipsia and weight gain. It may be worth lowering the dose to try to reduce these symptoms as they may all affect compliance. Lithium inhibits the response of the distal tubule to vasopressin (antidiuretic hormone) resulting in polydipsia and polyuria. Nephrogenic diabetes insipidus occurs infrequently and can be relieved by the use of loop diuretics. Increased body weight may result from lithium-induced thirst and increased fluid intake. It is exacerbated by consumption of high-calorie drinks. Nausea and diarrhoea usually pass after 2–3 weeks of treatment but may be signs of impending intoxication. Nausea may be worse with conventional-release tablets as higher concentrations of lithium are released in the stomach. Diarrhoea may be worse with sustained-release preparations since more lithium is released in the lower gastrointestinal tract. Dry mouth and a metallic taste may also be experienced.

Toxicity. Overdosage, usually with plasma concentrations over 1.5 mmol/L, may be fatal, and toxic effects include:

- early symptoms: nausea, vomiting, tremor, blurred vision, polyuria, polydipsia
- symptoms of severe toxicity/intoxication: convulsions, cardiac arrhythmias, impaired consciousness, coma, oliguria, anuria.

If these potentially hazardous signs occur, treatment should be stopped and plasma-lithium concentrations determined. Any predisposing condition which may have precipitated intoxication should be identified and treated. Appropriate supportive and corrective measures for complications of toxicity, e.g. continuous ECG, rehydration, should be instituted.

If there is acute poisoning, induced emesis with ipecacuanha is of benefit if carried out within 3 hours of ingestion.

In mild to moderate intoxication, intravenous sodium chloride solution 0.9%, 1–2 litres every 6 hours, is given. This is of most benefit if the problem is volume depletion or hyponatraemia. If severe, e.g. 4 mmol/L, haemodialysis should be initiated.

Drug interactions. Lithium toxicity is made worse by sodium depletion; thus, concurrent use of diuretics is hazardous and should be avoided. Lithium is reabsorbed in the proximal tubules in the same proportions as sodium and water. If anything occurs to produce sodium depletion in the body, e.g. use of diuretics, diarrhoea, vomiting, there is a compensatory attempt by the body to reabsorb sodium at the level of the proximal tubule. In someone taking lithium this means a corresponding reabsorption of lithium and hence a raised serum lithium level. Caution is required when prescribing a diuretic to a patient stabilised on lithium. The severity of increase of lithium levels is greater with thiazides than with loop diuretics. Bendroflumethiazide (bendrofluazide), 2.5 mg daily, has been shown to increase lithium levels by 20–25%.

Dietary salt restriction can cause an increase in serum lithium as sodium and lithium ions are reabsorbed. Conversely, an excess of sodium can cause expansion of intracellular fluid and an excretion of sodium and hence lithium.

THINKING ABOUT STARTING A FAMILY?

Because lithium can affect the unborn baby do NOT become pregnant without first talking to your doctor. If you are pregnant tell your doctor now.

KEEP YOUR TABLETS IN A SAFE PLACE WELL OUT OF THE REACH OF CHILDREN

PLEASE RECORD YOUR BLOOD LEVEL OF LITHIUM

DATE TAKEN	BLOOD LEVEL	DAILY DOSE

LITHIUM TREATMENT CARD

CARRY THIS CARD WITH YOU AT ALL TIMES. SHOW IT TO ANY DOCTOR OR NURSE WHO TREATS YOU AND ANY PHARMACIST YOU BUY MEDICINES FROM

NAME ....

PREPARATION OF LITHIUM ....

Should a different proprietary product be prescribed, the card must be suitably endorsed.

(A)

HOW SHOULD I TAKE THE TABLETS?

Swallow each tablet whole or broken in half, with water. Do NOT chew or crush it. Try to take the dose at the same time each day.

WHAT SHOULD I DO IF I MISS A DOSE?

Do NOT double your next dose. If you find you have missed a few doses, start taking your usual dose on the day you remember and tell your doctor.

WHY MUST I HAVE A BLOOD TEST?

This is to check the amount of lithium in your blood. It is very important to have the correct amount because too much can be dangerous. Take the blood test ABOUT 12 HOURS AFTER the last dose of lithium.

CAN I DRINK ALCOHOL?

It is safe to drink SMALL quantities.

CAN I TAKE OTHER MEDICINES WITH LITHIUM?

Some medicines can change the amount of lithium in the blood. These include diuretic (water) tablets and capsules, some pain killers and some indigestion mixtures and laxatives. So check with your doctor or pharmacist before taking other medicines.

Please note: it is safe to take paracetamol but not ibuprofen.

WHAT ELSE ALTERS THE LITHIUM LEVEL?

The level can be altered by the amount of fluids you drink, changes in the amount of salt in your food, sweating more than usual (in hot weather, fever or infection), severe vomiting, severe diarrhoea and a low salt diet. Check with your doctor if any of these things happen.

SIGNS OF A HIGH LITHIUM LEVEL

Vomiting, severe diarrhoea, unusual drowsiness, muscle weakness and feeling very giddy may mean that your level of lithium is too high. Stop taking the tablets and talk to your doctor IMMEDIATELY.

DOES LITHIUM HAVE SIDE EFFECTS?

Some slight effects (such as sickness, shaking) may occur at first but they usually wear off if blood tests are normal. Discuss this with your doctor. Some patients may gain weight but this can be prevented with a sensible diet.

HOW LONG WILL I HAVE TO TAKE LITHIUM?

Lithium is a way of preventing illness so you may have to take it for many years. Never stop taking the tablets without asking your doctor.

(B)

Figure 18.3 Lithium treatment card. (A) Front. (B) Reverse.

Some NSAIDs are known to affect the control of lithium treatment by reducing the extent of elimination from the body and thus causing an increase in serum lithium level. Aspirin may be used safely, having no effect on plasma lithium levels.

Counselling of patients

Advice and information should be given to the patient on commencement of lithium therapy. This is essential to provide the patient with an understanding of the drug action and side-effects, and also to improve compliance. Advice and information given to the patient would be as follows:

- swallow tablets whole; do not chew (this would affect the modified-release mechanism)
- always take the same brand of lithium tablets (this will ensure consistent plasma levels); if in doubt, ask your pharmacist
- lithium will not have an immediate effect; it may be up to 14 days before benefits are apparent
- therapy may be lifelong, and it is important to keep taking lithium even though you may be feeling better
- information regarding common side-effects
- reason for monitoring levels/taking bloods and the importance of attendance at the lithium clinic when requested to do so
- importance of maintaining fluid intake, particularly in hot weather or following exercise – if weight gain is a problem, use low-calorie drinks
- dietary intake of sodium should not be subject to fluctuations
- over-the-counter drugs containing sodium or NSAIDs should be avoided
- sickness/diarrhoea due to risk of sodium depletion
- advice on contraception where appropriate.

Every patient taking lithium should have a lithium card (Fig. 18.3), provided by the pharmacist, which reinforces the advice and information given.

Carbamazepine

Carbamazepine may be used for the prophylaxis of manic–depressive illness in patients unresponsive to lithium. It seems to be particularly effective in patients with rapid cycling manic–depressive illness (four or more affective episodes per year).

Mode of action. Carbamazepine exerts its effect through depression of neuronal synaptic transmission.

Pharmacokinetics. It is well absorbed. Carbamazepine is metabolised by the liver. The half-life is 7–24 hours on regular administration.

Dose. Starting dose 100–200 mg twice daily, increasing gradually until symptoms are controlled or a total daily dosage of 800 mg is reached. The usual dosage range is 400–600 mg in divided doses.

Side-effects. Dizziness, drowsiness, nausea and vomiting, headache, confusion, visual disturbances, rash, inappropriate antidiuretic hormone-secretion causing water intoxication, hyponatraemia and blood dyscrasias. Full blood counts are required, probably 3-monthly but at least annually. In overdose, seizures, chorea-like movements, nystagmus and liver damage may occur.

Interactions. Carbamazepine is an enzyme inducer, and concomitant administration with some drugs, e.g. theophylline and haloperidol, leads to decreased plasma level. The therapeutic benefits of carbamazepine have not yet been related to the serum levels achieved. Serum levels are measured to ensure safety and compliance rather than to assure efficacy.

DEPRESSION

About 60–70% of adults will, at some time, experience depression or worry of sufficient severity to influence their daily activities. Approximately 1.5% of the population in Britain is treated for depressive illness each year. Episodes of major depression are about twice as common among women as men, peak in middle age and are commonly associated with adverse social and economic circumstances such as unemployment, divorce or separation, inadequate housing and lower social class. Having a first-degree relative with depressive illness is associated with a fivefold increase in the risk of developing a similar illness. For the majority of people episodes of depression are short-lived but a minority experience a range of severe psychological and clinical symptoms which may persist.

Major depression

Criteria have been developed to identify people who are categorised as having a major depressive episode. Termed the DSMIII-R criteria, these are summarised in Box 18.2.

The ICD 10 criteria are similar.

Major depression is diagnosed when at least five of the symptoms (which must include symptoms 1 or 2, or both) have been present over a minimum duration of 2 weeks.

The term bipolar disorder is used to indicate at least one episode of mania (i.e. manic–depressive disorder). Depression may be further classified as mild, moderate or severe according to the intensity of the symptoms.

Box 18.2 Summary of DSMIII-R criteria for major depression

1. Depressed mood for most of the day, nearly every day
2. Marked diminished interest or pleasure in all or almost all activities most of the day nearly every day
3. Marked weight loss or gain, or decrease or increase in appetite
4. Insomnia or hypersomnia nearly every day
5. Psychomotor agitation or retardation nearly every day
6. Fatigue or loss of energy nearly every day
7. Feelings of worthlessness or excessive inappropriate guilt
8. Diminished ability to think or concentrate, or indecisiveness
9. Recurrent thoughts of death, or suicidal ideation or attempt
10. Feelings of hopelessness

Differential diagnosis

For depression to be diagnosed, certain other conditions may have to be ruled out:

- normal sadness
- anxiety neuroses with or without phobic or obsessional symptoms
- schizophrenia
- dementia (chronic organic brain syndrome)
- organic brain lesion
- other drug treatment, e.g. β-blockers.

Treatment

There is no evidence that very mild depressive symptoms respond to pharmacological treatment. Such symptoms are best managed with psychological support, encouragement and explanation to ensure that a clinical depression does not develop. Other psychological approaches include dynamic psychotherapy and cognitive therapy. Dynamic psychotherapy aims to change interpersonal dynamics which may contribute to an individual's vulnerability to developing depression, whereas cognitive therapy aims to alter cognitions, that is, the way in which an individual interprets adverse circumstances.

For more severe symptoms, treatment with an antidepressant drug is the preferred option.

The choice of antidepressant is influenced by many factors including the clinical presentation, response to treatment during previous episodes, side-effect profile and cost. Antidepressants with sedative properties may be desirable in some patients but not in others, for example if retardation is marked. Previous good response to an antidepressant would make the same antidepressant a logical choice in subsequent episodes. Conversely, previous poor response would militate against the reuse of the same drug or one from the same class.

The side-effect profile should be borne in mind where there is pre-existing physical illness. For example, tricyclic antidepressants have a membrane-stabilising effect and should therefore be avoided in patients with cardiac conduction abnormalities. Anticholinergic side-effects are also undesirable in those with angle-closure glaucoma or prostatic hypertrophy. In recent years with the introduction of newer antidepressants, such as the selective serotonin reuptake inhibitors (SSRIs), a major cost factor has been introduced. These are considerably more expensive than tricyclics. A balancing factor may be less expenditure in treating tricyclic overdoses and lower drop-out rates from treatment leading to improved therapeutic outcomes. There is a need, however, for more detailed pharmacoeconomics to be undertaken.

Care plan

The choice of antidepressant drug and the starting dose should be tailored to the individual patient's needs. The dose should be titrated against both clinical symptoms and side-effects. Care should be taken to ensure that a therapeutic dose is reached. The patient should be counselled about both the anticipated effects and side-effects of the drugs prescribed. Particular attention should be paid to the expected time of clinical effect and the overall duration of treatment.

Tricyclic and related antidepressants

Mode of action

Tricyclic antidepressants are thought to exert their clinical effect by blocking the reuptake of amines, e.g. noradrenaline (norepinephrine), 5-hydroxytryptamine (5-HT), dopamine, into the presynaptic neurone and thus increasing the amounts available in the synaptic cleft.

Pharmacokinetics

Tricyclic antidepressants are rapidly absorbed and extensively metabolised in the liver. They have a long action and may need to be given only once a day. Patients differ widely in the extent to which they

Table 18.9 Adverse effects of tricyclic antidepressants

Antidepressant	Average dose (mg/day)	Relative side-effects				
		Anticholinergic	Cardiac	Nausea	Drowsiness	Danger in overdose
Amitriptyline	75	XXX	XXX	XX	XXX	XXX
Clomipramine	75	XXX	XX	XX	XX	X
Dosulepin (dothiepin)	75	XX	XX	–	XXX	XXX
Doxepin	75	X	XX	X	XX	XX
Imipramine	75	XX	XX	XX	X	XX
Lofepramine	140	XX	X	XX	X	–
Maprotiline	75	XX	XX	XX	X	XXX
Mianserin*	90	X	–	–	XXX	X
Trazadone	150	X	X	XXX	XX	X

Higher doses may be required for severe depression.
* Full blood count recommended every 4 weeks for the first 3 months.
XXX = high incidence/severity; XX = moderate; X = low; – = very low/none.

absorb or metabolise antidepressants, and dosage should always be adjusted to the individual's clinical response. There appears to be some evidence of a 'therapeutic window'.

Response

A patient is unlikely to experience any improvement in mood for at least 2 weeks. Treatment should be monitored at the optimum dose or maximum tolerated dose for at least 4–6 weeks to allow for a full therapeutic trial. The typical pattern of response to an antidepressant is:

- sleep pattern may start to improve after a few days and concentration after about a week
- lifting of mood may be delayed 2 weeks or more
- when response commences, good days will be followed by bad but after several weeks there will be more good days than bad ones.

Adverse effects (Table 18.9)

The patient should be reassured that mild anticholinergic side-effects are common initially but if these are found to be intolerable they should be discussed rather than treatment discontinued. Patients who experience blurred vision need to know that this effect is reversible. It is not the time to buy new glasses. Patients should also be advised to stand up slowly if they feel dizzy and let their doctor know if they develop a rash. Patients with depression have very poor concentration so it is important that they receive written information to support verbal advice.

Other anticholinergic side-effects may be dry mouth and constipation. More serious and occurring less frequently are failure to pass urine, closed-angle glaucoma, jaundice, depression of the white blood cell count, convulsions, arrhythmias and tachycardia.

Many tricyclic antidepressants have sedative properties so that they can be prescribed at night to help treat insomnia in the short term. This also helps to alleviate the anticholinergic side-effects. The return of a more normal sleep pattern results as depression is alleviated. Taking more than one tricyclic antidepressant at the same time is not recommended. There is no evidence that side-effects are minimised. Examples of tricyclic and related antidepressants are listed in Table 18.9.

If a therapeutic response is obtained, an average course of antidepressants would be for 6 months to 1 year and should be given for at least 3 months after recovery. Care must be taken in withdrawing antidepressants following treatment. Reduction in dosage should be carried out gradually over a period of about 4 weeks, otherwise withdrawal symptoms will be experienced. These include gastrointestinal symptoms of nausea, vomiting and anorexia accompanied by headache, dizziness and insomnia. Panic, anxiety and motor restlessness may also occur.

A tricyclic or related antidepressant should not be started until 2 weeks after stopping a monoamine-oxidase inhibitor (MAOI). Conversely, an MAOI should not be started until at least a week after a tricyclic or related antidepressant has been stopped.

Choice of drugs

All tricyclic antidepressants have approximately equal clinical efficacy and the choice of which tricyclic to use in a particular patient is determined by the side-effect profile. Agitated and anxious patients tend to respond best to more sedative products whereas withdrawn and apathetic patients will obtain more benefit from less sedating compounds.

Clomipramine is useful in the treatment of depression linked with anxiety and is used in obsessional compulsive disorders, phobic anxiety states and panic disorder. Lofepramine is useful in the elderly. Mianserin has been reported for serious bone marrow suppression leading to leucopenia, agranulocytosis and aplastic anaemia. This would normally occur in the first 6 weeks of treatment and is more common in the elderly, requiring regular blood counts to be carried out. Weight gain is common with all tricyclic antidepressants.

Monoamine-oxidase inhibitors (MAOIs)

Mode of action

Monoamine oxidase has a variety of isoenzymes which have been classified as type A (present in the gut and liver) and type B (present in the brain). The different isoenzymes have different selectivities for amine substrates:

- monoamine oxidase A – metabolises 5-hydroxytryptamine (5-HT) and noradrenaline (norepinephrine)
- monoamine oxidase B – metabolises phenylethylamine and benzylamine
- dopamine and tyramine are metabolised to both the type A and type B enzymes.

Monoamine-oxidase inhibitors inhibit the action of monoamine oxidase, resulting in an accumulation of monoamines such as 5-hydroxytryptamine, noradrenaline (norepinephrine) and dopamine within the synapse. It is this effect that is thought to be the primary action of MAOIs in relieving depression. The MAOIs are used much less frequently than other antidepressants because of dietary and drug interactions. They are used to treat atypical depression with associated anxiety and obsessional, hysterical or hypochondriacal symptoms. They can also be used to treat resistant depressions.

Pharmacokinetics

The MAOI antidepressants are readily absorbed from the gut, extensively metabolised and excreted mainly as metabolites in the urine and faeces.

Response

The dose needs to be gradually built up to a therapeutic level. There will be a time lag of 4–6 weeks to achieve a full antidepressant effect.

Choice

The drugs of choice are phenelzine or isocarboxazid, which are less stimulant and therefore safer than tranylcypromine. Monoamine-oxidase inhibitors are generally administered in divided doses with the last dose given before the late afternoon to prevent insomnia because of their alerting effect. Phenelzine – 15 mg three times daily increased where required up to four times daily after 2 weeks (hospital patients, maximum 30 mg three times daily) then reduced gradually to lowest possible maintenance dose. Isocarboxazid – initially up to 30 mg daily in single or divided doses increased after 4 weeks if necessary to a maximum of 60 mg daily for up to 6 weeks under close supervision and then reduced to a maintenance dose of 10–40 mg daily.

Side-effects

The MAOIs, especially tranylcypromine, can cause anticholinergic side-effects. They are very alerting, causing sleep disturbance. To avoid this, the last dose should be taken in the early afternoon. Other side-effects include weight gain, sexual dysfunction, dizziness, postural hypotension, liver damage, dry mouth, constipation, headache, tremor and ankle oedema.

Interactions

Hypertensive crisis is a rare but severe side-effect. It is due to MAOIs preventing metabolism of tyramine in tyramine-rich food or drink. A hypertensive crisis may also arise with sympathomimetic drugs.

Tyramine. Irreversible MAOIs block the ability of monoamine oxidase to inactivate tyramine in the gastrointestinal tract and liver for a long period of time. The tyramine is present in foods such as cheese, salted fish, broad bean pods, Bovril, Oxo, Marmite, shrimp paste, pâté and drinks including red wine, beer, ale, and non-alcoholic beers and lagers. Excess tyramine enters the bloodstream and releases noradrenaline (norepinephrine) from its storage sites located in the sympathetic nerve endings. This can cause vasoconstriction and an increase in blood pressure which can result in a potentially fatal reaction characterised by severe hypertension associated with severe headache, sweating, flushing, nausea, vomiting and palpitations. Patients on MAOIs are restricted to a low-tyramine diet. They are given a treatment card and counselled (Fig. 18.4).

Sympathomimetics. Sympathomimetics such as pseudoephedrine and phenylpropanolamine, which release noradrenaline (norepinephrine) at nerve endings,

TREATMENT CARD

Carry this card with you at all times. Show it to any doctor who may treat you other than the doctor who prescribed this medicine, and to your dentist if you require dental treatment.

INSTRUCTIONS TO PATIENTS
Please read carefully

While taking this medicine and for 14 days after your treatment finishes you must observe the following simple instructions:-

1. Do not eat CHEESE, PICKLED HERRING OR BROAD BEAN PODS.
2. Do not eat drink BOVRIL, OXO, MARMITE, or ANY SIMILAR MEAT OR YEAST EXTRACT.
3. Eat only FRESH foods and avoid food that you suspect could be stale or 'going off'. This is especially important with meat, fish, poultry or offal. Avoid game.
4. Do not take any other MEDICINES (including tablets, capsules, nose drops, inhalations or suppositories) whether purchased by you or previously prescribed by your doctor, without first consulting your doctor or your pharmacist.
   NB *Treatment for coughs and colds, pain relievers, tonics and laxatives are medicines.*
5. Avoid alcoholic drinks and de-alcoholised (low alcohol) drinks.

Keep a careful note of any food or drink that disagrees with you, avoid it and tell your doctor.

Report any unusual or severe symptoms to your doctor and follow any other advice given by him.

Figure 18.4 MAOI treatment card.

may be potentiated by MAOIs. A severe hypertensive crisis may result. An early warning symptom may be a throbbing headache. Sympathomimetics are present in many cough mixtures and decongestant nasal drops, and patients must be warned not to use these medicines. The danger of the reaction persists for up to 14 days after treatment with MAOIs has been discontinued.

Dopamine receptor agonists. Levodopa may cause similar hypertensive reactions in patients taking non-selective MAOIs and should be avoided.

Tricyclic antidepressants. Since tricyclic antidepressants inhibit noradrenaline (norepinephrine) reuptake by nerve endings, the combination of tricyclics with MAOIs is hazardous. MAOIs should not be started until at least 2 weeks after tricyclics and related antidepressants have been stopped and 2 weeks after cessation of selective serotonin reuptake inhibitors (5 weeks for fluoxetine). Similarly, other antidepressants or another MAOI should not be given to patients for 14 days after treatment with a previous MAOI has been discontinued.

Selective monoamine-oxidase inhibitors

Since the transmitters considered to play a role in depression are serotonin, noradrenaline (norepinephrine) and dopamine, the antidepressant effects are thought to depend largely or exclusively on inhibition of MAO-A.

Drugs which reversibly affect mainly MAO-A are known as reversible inhibitors of MAO-A (RIMAs) as distinguished from the previously discussed irreversible MAOI. A RIMA, which preferentially inhibits MAO-A, interferes less with the metabolism of tyramine. Reversible inhibition of an MAO-A does not provoke an increase in blood pressure for two reasons. First, by preferentially inhibiting MAO-A, it leaves MAO-B free to metabolise ingested tyramine. Second, when an excess of tyramine is ingested, the RIMA inhibitor will dissociate with MAO-A allowing the enzyme to metabolise the excess. Patients should avoid ingesting large quantities of tyramine while prescribed an RIMA but they do not have to adhere to an MAOI diet. An example of this type of drug is moclobemide.

Moclobemide

Moclobemide is comparable in its effect to the tricyclic antidepressants and the MAOIs. The usual dosage range is 300–450 mg daily in two or three divided doses. There is 95% absorption but extensive first-pass metabolism results in an oral bioavailability of 45–60%. The half-life is 1–2 hours.

Moclobemide is well tolerated, largely devoid of anticholinergic effects, postural hypotension or weight gain. The main side-effects include dizziness, headache, dry mouth, tremor, insomnia and nausea.

Withdrawal. Moclobemide can be stopped almost immediately without the requirement to reduce the dose slowly over a number of weeks.

When transferring from other antidepressants to moclobemide, the washout period depends on the half-life of the parent drug or the active metabolite, as shown in Table 18.10.

Table 18.10 Washout periods of antidepressants

Drug	Washout period
MAOIs	14 days
Amitriptyline	4–5 days
Imipramine	3–4 days
SSRIs (except fluoxetine)	14 days
Fluoxetine	5 weeks

Selective serotonin reuptake inhibitors (SSRIs)

Mode of action. SSRI antidepressants inhibit the neuronal reuptake of serotonin (5-hydroxytryptamine) by blocking the action of the uptake pump, allowing the 5-HT to remain longer in the synaptic cleft, thereby enhancing its action. SSRIs differ from tricyclic antidepressants in having a more selective action in the uptake of serotonin, producing less muscarinic receptor blockade and being free from membrane-stabilising effects in the heart. As a result they are less likely to cause anticholinergic and cardiotoxic effects.

Pharmacokinetics. SSRIs are rapidly absorbed and food has little effect on absorption. Peak plasma concentrations are reached within 8 hours and steady-state concentrations within 2 weeks (2–6 weeks in the case of fluoxetine). SSRIs are metabolised in the liver, the metabolites having little or no activity with the exception of *N*-desmethylfluoxetine, the main metabolite of fluoxetine. Metabolites are excreted mainly in the urine. Fluoxetine has a half-life of 1–3 days and that of desmethylfluoxetine is 1–2 weeks. The half-lives of the other SSRIs are less than 24 hours.

Selection of SSRIs

The dose range for each single SSRI is the same for all groups of patients. Fluoxetine and paroxetine are generally administered as a single dose in the morning. Fluvoxamine and sertraline, at therapeutic doses, tend to be given in two divided doses. Citalopram can be given as a single dose either in the morning or the evening. Table 18.11 gives details of doses.

All SSRIs appear to be clinically equivalent but they differ in their half-lives and thus have differing lengths of action. They may be considered as a first-line choice for those patients with heart disease, those at increased risk of overdose, the elderly and for those unable to tolerate tricyclic antidepressants or MAOI antidepressants.

Patients with impaired hepatic and renal function should be monitored when commenced on SSRIs. The drugs should be discontinued when dysfunction is severe. Care should be taken in patients with seizure disorders and these drugs should be avoided in patients with unstable epilepsy.

Table 18.11 5-hydroxytryptamine reuptake inhibitors

Drug	Average daily dose/range (mg)
Citalopram	20–60
Fluoxetine	20
Fluvoxamine	100–200
Paroxetine	20–40
Sertraline	50–100

Side-effects. The most common unwanted effects are nausea, dyspepsia, dry mouth, headache, somnolence, insomnia and dizziness. In general, the SSRI antidepressants have a much reduced incidence and severity of side-effects compared to the tricyclic antidepressants. They do not cause weight gain and there may even be a slight weight loss. Paroxetine may be the most suitable for patients with renal and/or hepatic impairment.

Withdrawal. Withdrawal of SSRIs should be undertaken slowly. An SSRI or related antidepressant should not be started until 2 weeks after stopping an MAOI. Conversely, an MAOI should not be started until at least a week after an SSRI or related antidepressant has been started (2 weeks in the case of paroxetine and sertraline, at least 5 weeks in the case of fluoxetine).

Related antidepressants

Newer antidepressants are venlafaxine, nefazodone, mirtazapine and reboxetine.

Venlafaxine

Mode of action. The antidepressant effect of venlafaxine is due to blocking the reuptake of both noradrenaline (norepinephrine) and serotonin. There is also a weak effect on dopamine reuptake.

Pharmacokinetics. Venlafaxine hydrochloride is well absorbed after oral administration. The half-life for venlafaxine is about 5 hours and, for its metabolite *O*-desmethylvenlafaxine, about 11 hours. Venlafaxine undergoes extensive metabolism in the liver and is excreted primarily in the urine. For patients with moderate hepatic impairment or moderate renal impairment the dose should be reduced by 50%.

Dosage. Initially, 75 mg daily in two divided doses, the second dose no later than early evening, increased if necessary after several weeks to 150 mg daily in two divided doses. In severely depressed patients, a maximum of 375 mg daily then gradually reduced.

Side-effects. The most common side-effect in the short term is nausea. Other side-effects include dizziness, dry mouth, sweating, constipation, anorexia, insomnia, nervousness and impotence. Side-effects are dose-related and occur most often during the first week of therapy, decreasing in incidence shortly thereafter.

Withdrawal. If taken for more than 6 weeks, withdrawal should be over at least a week.

Nefazodone

Mode of action. Nefazodone has a dual action. It both inhibits serotonin reuptake presynaptically and blocks serotonin type 2 ($5\text{-}HT_2$) receptors postsynaptically.

Pharmacokinetics. It is rapidly absorbed, reaching peak plasma concentrations after 1–3 hours, and has an elimination half-life of 2–4 hours. It is metabolised primarily in the liver.

Dosage. Initially 100 mg twice daily, increased after 5–7 days to 200 mg twice daily. Maximum dose is 300 mg twice daily (in the elderly, maximum dose 100–200 mg twice daily).

Side-effects. Nefazodone has positive effects on the quality and quantity of sleep. The most frequent side-effects are asthma, dry mouth, nausea, somnolence and dizziness.

Mirtazapine

Mode of action. Mirtazapine enhances the neurotransmission of serotonin and noradrenaline (norepinephrine).

Pharmacokinetics. Mirtazapine is well absorbed, reaching peak plasma levels after 2 hours. The mean elimination half-life is 20–40 hours.

Dose. Initially 15 mg daily at bedtime increased to 45 mg daily where required.

Side-effects. Main side-effects are restlessness, insomnia and hypomania.

Reboxetine

Mode of action. Reboxetine is a highly selective and effective inhibitor of noradrenaline (norepinephrine) reuptake.

Pharmacokinetics. Reboxetine is well absorbed with a peak plasma level after 2 hours. The elimination half-life is about 13 hours.

Other antidepressant drugs

Flupentixol

In low doses, flupentixol has antidepressant properties and is licensed for this using the oral route. The usual daily dose is 1–3 mg daily in divided doses, with the last dose being given prior to 1600 hours because it may have an alerting effect. The elderly may require lower doses. Side-effects tend to be fewer because of the low doses employed. If no response is obtained after 1 week at the maximum dose, then it should be discontinued.

Tryptophan

Tryptophan is a precursor of serotonin and is generally used in combination with tricyclic antidepressants and other antidepressants to increase central 5-HT levels. Tryptophan is at present available only on a named-patient basis owing to reports associating it with eosinophilia–myalgia syndrome, characterised by eosinophilia, muscle weakness and skin rashes. It is sometimes used in patients for whom no alternative treatment is suitable.

Combination therapy

Combination therapy is generally reserved for resistant depressions or depressions that have not completely resolved using monotherapy. Some of the more commonly used combinations are as follows:

1. Lithium + tryptophan + clomipramine or phenelzine – these triple combinations are used in severe resistant depression. Tryptophan enhances the action of clomipramine or phenelzine on 5-HT sites and improves 5-HT absorption. Lithium also affects 5-HT and is a mild antidepressant in its own right.
2. Tricyclic antidepressants and MAOIs – used in the treatment of severe resistant depression; it is advisable to start both together at low doses and build up the dose according to side-effect and clinical response. Most problems arise if the tricyclic antidepressant is added to the MAOI. Generally, doses less than the full antidepressant doses of either agent are required.
3. Lithium + antidepressants – used in the treatment of depressed patients with a bipolar illness and as an augmented treatment with tricyclic antidepressants.

OBESITY

Obesity is associated with many health problems including diabetes mellitus and cardiovascular disease.

The main treatment of the obese individual is a suitable diet and increased physical activity with appropriate support and encouragement. Drugs should never be used as the sole treatment of obesity. The individual should be monitored on a regular basis and drug treatment should be discontinued if weight loss is less than 5% after the first 12 weeks or if the individual regains weight at any time whilst receiving drug treatment.

Drugs specifically licensed for the treatment of obesity are orlistat and sibutramine. Orlistat may be appropriate for those who have a high intake of fat whereas sibutramine may be selected for those who cannot control their eating. Orlistat is a gastric and pancreatic lipase inhibitor which causes a reduction in fat absorption by increasing fat excretion. Orlistat or sibutramine should only be prescribed as part of an overall treatment plan for the management of obesity in people aged 18–75 (orlistat) or 18–65 (sibutramine) who meet the following criteria.

- body mass index (BMI) of 30 kg/m^2 or more without associated co-morbidities
- BMI of 28 kg/m^2 (orlistat) or 27 kg/m^2 (sibutramine) or more in the presence of significant co-morbidities.

120 mg of orlistat is taken immediately before, during or up to 1 hour after each main meal. The most common side-effects are gastrointestinal, e.g. fatty stools, faecal urgency and flatulence.

The starting dose of sibutramine should normally be 10 mg/day. Continuation of this therapy beyond 4 weeks should be supported by evidence of a 2 kg weight loss and beyond 3 months should be supported by evidence of a loss of at least 5% of initial body weight from the start of drug treatment. Dosage may be increased to 15 mg/day after 4 weeks. Sibutramine therapy should be stopped if there is an inadequate response.

Since the use of sibutramine may increase blood pressure of some individuals, blood pressure must be checked regularly in all those for whom it is prescribed. If blood pressure increases, continuation of sibutramine must be reconsidered taking into account the risks and benefits of the effects of treatment on cardiovascular risk profile for the individual. Sibutramine is not recommended for individuals whose blood pressure before the start of therapy is above 145/90 mm mercury. Treatment is not recommended beyond 12 months.

It is important for patients taking either orlistat or sibutramine that arrangements exist for appropriate health professionals to offer advice, support and counselling on diet, physical activity and behavioural strategies.

NAUSEA AND VERTIGO

Nausea and vomiting

Anti-emetics relieve nausea and vomiting from a variety of causes. The group of nuclei known collectively as the vomiting centre is located in the medulla oblongata in the brain stem and can receive stimuli from various sources. The nausea response can be initiated when the upper GI tract sends nerve impulses to the vomiting centre along the vagus and sympathetic nerves. This can be stimulated, for example, by irritation of mucosal receptors in the GI tract, radiation therapy injury of the GI mucosa or malignant disease of the GI tract.

Another collection of nuclei called the chemoreceptor trigger zone (CTZ) is located in the area postrema. Activation of the CTZ can stimulate the vomiting centre, which, in turn, causes nausea or initiates emesis. Motion sickness results from stimulation of the vestibular apparatus of the ear, which activates the vomiting centre via the CTZ. People who know they may experience motion sickness under certain circumstances can use an anti-emetic prophylactically to avoid this.

Labyrinthitis resulting from inflammation of the vestibular apparatus of the ear causes nausea, vomiting, dizziness and hearing loss. Ménière's disease, which involves dilatation of the endolymphatic channels in the cochlea, also produces nausea as well as dizziness, tinnitus and hearing loss.

Cancer chemotherapy can directly or indirectly (through the CTZ) stimulate the vomiting centre, causing severe nausea and vomiting. Narcotics can cause nausea and vomiting either by stimulating the CTZ or sensitising the vestibular apparatus of the ear.

Nausea and vomiting are frequent and often distressing side-effects connected with anaesthesia and surgery. Various factors may be involved including inhalation agents, premedication, postoperative pain, opioid analgesia and movement.

The main neurotransmitters in the area postrema, thought to have a role in emesis are:

- acetylcholine
- histamine
- dopamine
- 5-hydroxytryptamine.

The actions of certain anti-emetics indicate that acetylcholine and histamine are more important in motion sickness than in other types of emesis. Many anti-emetics are antidopaminergic and this may lead to the occurrence of extrapyramidal reactions.

Drug treatments

Hyoscine
Hyoscine acts on the vomiting centre in the medulla where it has an antimuscarinic action. Its efficacy in motion sickness is due to an effect on the vestibular apparatus. Hyoscine is available as tablets, slow-release tablets and in a transdermal presentation.

Phenothiazines
The phenothiazines are dopamine antagonists and act centrally by blocking the CTZ. They are rapidly absorbed after oral administration. Rectal or parenteral administration is required if vomiting has already started. Prochlorperazine, perphenazine and trifluoperazine are less sedating than chlorpromazine. Long-term use is limited by side-effects including extrapyramidal reactions and antimuscarinic effects. Patients should be advised about drowsiness and warned not to drive or operate machinery. Side-effects include hypotension, cholestatic jaundice, skin rash and leucopenia. The sedative effects are potentiated by alcohol and other sedative drugs.

Metoclopramide
Metoclopramide blocks peripheral and central dopamine receptors when in high doses and it also acts on peripheral and central 5-HT_3 receptors, which is of value in the prevention of nausea and vomiting associated with cytotoxic drug therapy. Metoclopramide also reduces oesophageal reflux and enhances gastric emptying, which is useful in treating gastric hypomotility found in migraine. Side-effects are usually mild, transient and reversible on discontinuation of therapy. CNS side-effects include dizziness, drowsiness, anxiety and depression. Extrapyramidal symptoms may also occur, including akathisia, parkinsonism and acute dystonia.

Domperidone
Domperidone acts on the CTZ and has anti-emetic properties, and its effects on gastrointestinal motility are similar to those of metoclopramide. It causes little extrapyramidal side-effects and is less sedating than metoclopramide; it is therefore useful in treating patients with Parkinson's disease where nausea and vomiting associated with levodopa or bromocriptine are troublesome.

Selective 5-HT_3 antagonists
The 5-HT_3 antagonists, including ondansetron, granisetron and tropisetron, act peripherally on vagus nerve endings and centrally in the CTZ. They have no action on other receptor types. The lack of therapeutic activity on dopamine receptors indicates that, unlike metoclopramide, anti-emetic activity can be achieved without dose-limiting extrapyramidal side-effects. These drugs are used mainly to treat nausea and vomiting in patients on highly emetogenic chemotherapy such as cisplatin, although ondansetron and granisetron are also licensed for use in postoperative vomiting. A single intravenous dose is recommended before chemotherapy. If vomiting is not adequately controlled, the drug should be continued orally or intravenously for up to 5 days. Side-effects of 5-HT_3 antagonists include constipation and headache.

Drug treatment of nausea and vomiting in particular situations

Motion sickness. Hyoscine is the most effective drug for the prevention of motion sickness. It is available both in tablet form and as a transdermal patch providing a slow continuous absorption into the bloodstream. A 300 microgram tablet is taken 30 minutes before the start of the journey, or a 500 microgram patch is applied to a hairless area of skin behind the ear 5–6 hours before a journey and replaced after 72 hours if necessary. Side-effects such as drowsiness, blurred vision, dry mouth and urinary retention do not occur to any great extent at the doses used.

Antihistamines. Antihistamines act on the vestibular apparatus, the vomiting centre and the CTZ. Cinnarizine, cyclizine, dimenhydrinate and promethazine are effective. The first dose should be taken 30 minutes before the journey commences (2 hours for cinnarizine). The latter two are more sedating. They potentiate CNS depressants such as alcohol, phenothiazines and benzodiazepines. The sedative effect and the times of administration of these four drugs are shown in Table 18.12.

Drowsiness may affect performance of skilled tasks such as driving or operating machinery. Effects of alcohol are enhanced.

Drug-induced nausea and vomiting. Lowering the dose or withdrawal of the drug should be considered. If the drug has to be continued, choice of treatment depends on drug-induced emesis. Local gastric irritation may be reduced by increasing dosage frequency and lowering the dose, and also by taking the drug with food.

Table 18.12 Administration and sedative effect of some antihistamines

Antihistamine	Taken before journey	Sedative effect
Cinnarizine	2 hours	Mild
Cyclizine	0.5 hour	Mild
Promethazine	0.5 hour	Moderate

Domperidone is used for nausea and vomiting induced by drugs such as levodopa and bromocriptine in the treatment of Parkinson's disease. Central effects such as opiate-induced vomiting may be treated with a phenothiazine such as prochlorperazine. Cyclizine is often effective, and a combination of cyclizine and morphine is available as Cyclimorph.

Postoperative vomiting. Postoperative nausea and vomiting may cause electrolyte imbalance and dehydration. Patients may have difficulty with food and fluid intake, and oral drug therapy can be disrupted. Metoclopramide or a phenothiazine can be used. More recently, ondansetron has been used to treat nausea and vomiting where not controlled by less expensive drugs.

Pregnancy. Drug therapy of vomiting in pregnancy should be reserved for severe cases and, where possible, treatment should be avoided during the first trimester. Vomiting is usually most troublesome during this period, reaching a peak at about 10 weeks. Promethazine has been widely used and appears to be free from teratogenic effects.

Cytotoxic drug therapy. Nausea and vomiting occur frequently during the treatment of cancer with cytotoxic drugs or irradiation. Not all cytotoxic agents cause vomiting but those that frequently do include cisplatin, doxorubicin, cyclophosphamide and nitrosoureas. Prochlorperazine may be effective in mild to moderate cases. Metoclopramide in higher doses is also effective, but dosage is limited by side-effects. Nabilone, an oral synthetic cannabinoid with anxiolytic properties, has been used but is limited by side-effects (drowsiness, hallucinations, psychosis, blurred vision and depression). Vomiting due to highly emetogenic drugs can often be alleviated by parenteral corticosteroids (dexamethasone and methylprednisolone). Adding a sedative such as lorazepam may help, and combination with high-dose metoclopramide is often effective. When vomiting persists, 5-HT_3 antagonists are effective. Dexamethasone has been shown to enhance the efficacy of ondansetron and high-dose metoclopramide. When given in combination with ondansetron, a single dose of dexamethasone sodium phosphate 20 mg in 50 mL of 0.9% sodium chloride is given as a single 15-minute infusion starting 30 minutes before, for example, cisplatin.

Vestibular disorders

Acute labyrinthine disorders are distressing for the patient. The symptoms of nausea, vomiting and vertigo usually respond to prochlorperazine. Antihistamines and phenothiazines may be helpful in treating chronic vertigo. Age-related loss of postural stability should not be treated with agents (notably phenothiazines) whose side-effects include postural hypotension, mental confusion and parkinsonism. Betahistine and cinnarizine are useful in treating Ménière's disease. In an acute attack, cyclizine or prochlorperazine may be given rectally or by intramuscular injection.

MIGRAINE

Migraine affects at least 10% of the population of the UK. Attacks generally start in the teens or 20s. After puberty, migraine affects more women than men. During the reproductive period about 20% of women suffer, particularly those in their early 40s. Headache is only one symptom of migraine which has been defined as episodic headaches lasting between 2–72 hours with each attack accompanied by visual and/or gastrointestinal disturbance. Migraine's most common accompanying symptoms are photophobia, nausea and vomiting.

Migraine is classified into two main types:

- migraine without aura (common migraine)
- migraine with aura (classical migraine).

Only 10% of attacks are preceded by an aura. Patients who experience an aura can start their migraine treatment during this phase. Visual aura takes the form of blind spots. Other symptoms are sensory disturbances such as 'pins and needles' in one arm moving up to the face.

Triggers

Several factors need to be present to trigger a migraine attack. The triggers are not the same for everyone. The triggers are:

- Hormonal factors (women)
  - pregnancy
  - oral contraception
  - hormone replacement therapy
  - menstruation
- Environmental factors
  - bright or flickering lights
  - overexertion
  - travel
- Emotional factors
- Head and neck pain
- Insufficient food – missed meals
- Specific foods
  - cheese
  - chocolate
  - caffeine
  - citrus fruits.

Treatment

Early treatment during attacks with effective drugs is of the utmost importance as the efficacy of oral medication during migraine is impaired by gastric stasis. Patients should carry medication at all times. A drop in blood sugar precedes a migraine attack and food is an important part of treatment. If patients feel too nauseous, the attack is being treated too late. For many, sleep is the best natural remedy, and applications of hot and cold compresses can help to ease the pain.

Drug treatment

This includes analgesics, anti-emetics, ergotamine and the 5-HT_1 agonists – sumatriptan, zolmitriptan, naratriptan, rizatriptan. Simple analgesics such as paracetamol and aspirin may be insufficient. There are specific over-the-counter migraine preparations such as Migraleve (contains buclizine, paracetamol and codeine). Where these are unsuccessful, an anti-emetic with an effect on gastric motility is used with analgesics. Metoclopramide by mouth, or if vomiting is likely, by intramuscular injection, relieves the nausea.

The value of ergotamine is limited by difficulties in absorption and by its side-effects and is little used now owing to more effective preparations (the triptans) becoming available. It should be used no more than twice a month.

Sumatriptan is available as a subcutaneous auto-injector device for self-administration, a nasal spray and also in tablet form. It is a 5-HT_1 agonist which appears to be of considerable value in the treatment of an acute attack. Side-effects include sensations of tingling, heat, heaviness, pressure or tightness in any part of the body, flushing, dizziness and drowsiness. Naratriptan, zolmitriptan and rizatriptan are 5-HT_1 agonists more recently introduced. They are contraindicated in patients with ischaemic heart disease, previous myocardial infarction or uncontrolled hypertension. Tolfenamic acid is effective as an acute treatment for migraine attacks.

Prophylaxis

Some patients require prophylactic medication taken daily to prevent migraine, usually given if the patient has more than two migraine attacks per month. Drugs used are listed in Table 18.13.

Clonidine and methysergide have been used but the former is probably little better than a placebo and the latter has dangerous side-effects, e.g. fibrosis of the heart valves and pleura.

Table 18.13 Drugs used to prevent migraine

Drug	Class	Dose
Amitriptyline	Tricyclic antidepressant	10–50 mg at night
Cyproheptadine	Antihistamine with serotonin antagonist and calcium-channel-blocking properties	4 mg at night
Pizotifen	Antihistamine and serotonin antagonist	0.5–3 mg daily
Propranolol	Beta-blocker	10–40 mg three times daily

EPILEPSY

The term 'neurone' describes the nerve cell and its processes. The neurones behave like a small electrical source and, when nerve impulses are generated, the impulses pass along the axon to the neuromuscular junction and from there they energise the muscle fibres. During an epileptic seizure the nerve impulses generated are greatly in excess of normal and are uncoordinated. An epileptic seizure can be defined as a sudden, brief abnormal discharge of cerebral neurones which is accompanied by a disturbance of behaviour, emotion, motor function or sensation.

The manifestation of a seizure depends on which neurones are involved and how far and how quickly the discharge spreads or extends. A generalised seizure is a seizure that occurs simultaneously throughout the cortex, whereas a partial seizure begins in a specific group of cortical neurones and may then spread. If a partial seizure spreads to involve the whole cortex, then this is referred to as a secondary generalised seizure. A seizure results from an imbalance of the excitatory and inhibitory mechanisms within the brain, either in one specific area owing, for example, to scar tissue or brain tumours, or in a generalised fashion owing to genetic factors. A diagnosis of epilepsy is usually considered when an individual has had two or more seizures in a short interval.

Anticonvulsants act to prevent the spread of neuronal excitation by exerting a stabilising effect on excitable cell membranes or by enhancing the activity of neurotransmitters such as gamma-aminobutyric acid (GABA) which inhibit the spread of seizure activity by blocking synaptic transmission.

Classification

Many different terms have been used to describe the various types of epilepsy. A classification has been produced by the International League Against Epilepsy.

In this classification, seizures are divided into two types: generalised and partial (or focal). An abbreviated version is as follows.

Generalised seizures

- *Absence seizures.* This type of seizure occurs most commonly in childhood, often resolving during puberty. Absence seizures consist of brief episodes of unconsciousness with little or no motor accompaniment.
- *Myoclonic seizures.* These consist of single or multiple sudden or uncontrollable jerks.
- *Tonic–clonic seizures.* The most commonly encountered seizure type, this disorder is characterised by a sudden loss of consciousness followed by muscle rigidity (the tonic phase) which, in turn, is followed by a period of jerking of the limbs (clonic phase). The patient then enters a deep coma, with consciousness usually being fully regained within 1 hour. There may be a period of confusion prior to full recovery. Urinary and faecal incontinence may occur during the tonic phase.

Partial (focal) seizures

- *Simple partial seizures.* These seizures result from a focal epileptic discharge in a localised area of the brain. A simple partial seizure may be motor (e.g. abnormal movement of limb), sensory (e.g. abnormal sensation) or both. It is not accompanied by unconsciousness and is usually of short duration. The nature of the symptoms depends largely on the anatomical site of seizure discharge. A partial seizure is often preceded by abnormal symptoms (an aura) such as an unpleasant taste or smell.
- *Complex partial seizure.* This type of seizure may have a simple partial onset followed by impaired consciousness as it spreads throughout the brain to become secondarily generalised. This may result in bizarre or inappropriate behaviour (e.g. lip smacking, tearing of clothing).

Treatment

Drug treatment aims at suppressing seizures completely without producing troublesome side-effects. Anticonvulsants have a fairly narrow therapeutic index, and dosages must be carefully tailored in order to maximise efficacy while minimising adverse effects. A major cause of treatment failure is poor compliance. It is essential that the patient understands the importance of regular medication. For improved compliance, once-a-day dosage would be preferable but this may not be possible because of too short a half-life. Most antiepileptic drugs can be given twice daily at the most.

Medication should be initiated with a single drug and very often at reduced dosage, gradually increasing until the clinically effective level is reached. This is in order to minimise toxic effects. If this drug fails to provide adequate control of seizures, another drug will be substituted. A second drug should be added to the regimen only if seizures continue despite high plasma concentrations or toxic effects. In order to attain the correct dose, plasma drug concentrations should be monitored where appropriate, e.g. phenytoin.

Some antiepileptic drugs are more effective than others in certain forms of epilepsy. For example, sodium valproate and ethosuximide are more effective than phenytoin and carbamazepine in the treatment of absence seizures. However, there is little evidence to suggest whether sodium valproate or ethosuximide is the most effective drug for the treatment of absence seizures. It is therefore worth considering the differences in toxicity when choosing a drug.

Drugs of choice in the treatment of particular types of epilepsy are listed in Table 18.14.

Carbamazepine

Carbamazepine is a drug of choice for simple and complex partial seizures and for tonic–clonic seizures.

Table 18.14 Drugs of choice in treatment of epilepsy

Type of epilepsy	First choice	Other major drugs
Absence seizures	Ethosuximide	Sodium valproate
Myoclonic seizures	Sodium valproate	Clonazepam Ethosuximide
Tonic–clonic seizures	Carbamazepine	Phenytoin Sodium valproate Phenobarbital Primidone Lamotrigine Vigabatrin
Simple partial seizures	Carbamazepine	Phenytoin Sodium valproate Vigabatrin Lamotrigine Phenobarbital Gabapentin Topiramate Oxcarbazepine Levetiracetam
Complex partial seizures	Carbamazepine	Phenytoin Phenobarbital

Mode of action. This is not entirely clear but the drug appears to affect the characteristics of the membrane that controls electrical excitability, providing a stabilising effect on the neuronal membrane.

Pharmacokinetics. Carbamazepine is slowly absorbed from the gastrointestinal tract. Following absorption, it is widely distributed in body tissues and is highly plasma-protein-bound. Carbamazepine induces enzymes in the liver which increase its own metabolism and that of some other drugs. The half-life of carbamazepine after a single dose is 24–36 hours and this falls to 10–20 hours on regular dosing. As a result, dose requirements are likely to increase with time as carbamazepine clearance increases. The full effect of the enzyme induction may not be seen until several weeks after commencement of therapy.

Dose. Side-effects are minimised by introducing the drug at a low dose (100 mg twice daily) and increasing in increments of 200 mg every 1 or 2 weeks until optimal clinical effects are obtained. The usual dose is 0.8–1.2 g daily in divided doses although in some cases 1.6–2 g daily may be required.

Side-effects. Common side-effects include diplopia, dizziness, ataxia, headache, rashes, nausea and hyponatraemia. If serum sodium falls below 120 mmol/L, the patient may experience confusion, peripheral oedema and more seizures. Fluid retention may occur, particularly at higher doses, owing to stimulation of vasopressin production.

Drug interactions. The drug is a powerful inducer of liver enzymes, and its own clearance rate increases – with the result that the half-life may reduce significantly over the first few weeks of treatment. Carbamazepine induces metabolism of several other drugs given concurrently, e.g. other antiepileptics, oral contraceptives. Metabolism of carbamazepine is inhibited by certain drugs including ciprofloxacin, verapamil and diltiazem, which may result in increased carbamazepine levels and toxicity. Caution should be exercised in hepatic or renal impairment, cardiac disease, glaucoma, breast-feeding and pregnancy.

Phenytoin

Phenytoin is particularly effective in treating generalised tonic–clonic and partial seizures.

Mode of action. Phenytoin alters ion movement across cell membranes, affecting the electrical excitability and stabilising excitable cells.

Pharmacokinetics. Phenytoin is slowly absorbed following oral administration and poorly absorbed after intramuscular administration. The intravenous route is essential if parenteral therapy is required. Phenytoin is rapidly distributed to all tissues, with highest concentrations occurring in the liver and adipose tissue. It is extensively bound to plasma protein.

The pharmacokinetics of phenytoin are important as the relationship between dose and plasma level is very variable, with the result that seizure control is related to plasma level but not to dosage. The capacity of the liver to metabolise the drug may become saturated at or about the therapeutic range. Small increases in dosage will then produce large increases in plasma level as the additional drug cannot be metabolised. Therapeutic monitoring is therefore of great importance in the use of phenytoin.

Dose. The dosage range of phenytoin is 200–600 mg/day depending on serum concentrations. It should be started at a dose of 200 mg/day and then adjusted according to measured serum concentrations. The target range for phenytoin plasma levels in the treatment of epilepsy is 10–20 mg/L. Dose-related toxicity is more common at levels over 20 mg/L.

Side-effects. Phenytoin, although a highly effective antiepileptic, is generally less suitable for many patients compared with carbamazepine because of a high incidence of side-effects and a difficulty in dosage optimisation because of its complex pharmacokinetics. Side-effects, which may limit its use in children and women, are gingival hyperplasia, hirsutism, acne and coarsening of facial features. Phenytoin is also associated with deficiencies of calcium, vitamin D and folic acid; hence, replacement therapy may be required. Dose-related adverse effects include nausea, vomiting, drowsiness, nystagmus, diplopia and ataxia. These problems may be minimised if phenytoin plasma levels are maintained within the drug's therapeutic range (10–20 mg/litre).

Acute idiosyncratic reactions include rashes, Stevens–Johnson syndrome, blood dyscrasias (such as agranulocytosis or aplastic anaemia) and immunological reactions (such as systemic lupus erythematosus and hypersensitivity reactions).

Sodium valproate

Sodium valproate is effective against all types of seizures but particularly tonic–clonic seizures, absence seizures and myoclonic seizures, being the drug of choice in myoclonic seizures.

Mode of action. Sodium valproate produces a significant increase in gamma-aminobutyric acid, which probably accounts for its anticonvulsant action.

Pharmacokinetics. It is well absorbed, strongly protein bound and metabolised in the liver. Plasma concentrations are not a useful indicator of efficacy and therefore routine monitoring is not required.

Dose. Initially 600 mg daily given in two divided doses, increasing by 200 mg/day at 3-day intervals to a maximum of 2.5 g daily in divided doses. The full pharmacological action may not occur for some weeks after steady-state concentrations have been reached. Liver dysfunction has occurred in association with valproate and it is contraindicated in acute liver disease or where there is a history of severe hepatic dysfunction.

Side-effects. The main side-effects include gastric irritation, nausea, weight gain, alopecia and tremor.

Ethosuximide

Ethosuximide is the drug of choice in simple absence seizures.

Mode of action. Ethosuximide appears to reduce the frequency of absence seizures by depressing nerve transmission in the motor cortex and increasing the seizure threshold for stimulus.

Pharmacokinetics. Ethosuximide is well absorbed from the gastrointestinal tract and widely distributed throughout body tissues, plasma protein binding being negligible. It is metabolised in the liver with approximately 25% excreted unchanged in the urine.

Dose. Initially 500 mg daily increased by 250 mg at intervals of 4–7 days to a usual dose of 1–1.5 g daily.

Side-effects. Side-effects include nausea, vomiting and weight loss. The neurological complaints are ataxia, dizziness, drowsiness, headache, euphoria, lethargy and confusion. Haematological, genitourinary and hypersensitivity reactions can occur.

Lamotrigine

Lamotrigine is an antiepileptic for partial seizures and secondarily generalised tonic–clonic seizures that are not satisfactorily controlled by other anticonvulsants.

Mode of action. Lamotrigine acts by inhibiting the release of glutamate, the excitatory neurotransmitter, which results in reduced levels of glutamate in the CNS and so blocks voltage-sensitive sodium channels to stabilise neuronal membranes. Lamotrigine also has weak antifolate activity which may be responsible for part of its anticonvulsant activity.

Pharmacokinetics. Lamotrigine is well absorbed following oral administration. Plasma protein binding is 55%, and the drug is primarily metabolised by the liver. The half-life is 24 hours. Concomitant administration with liver-enzyme-inducing drugs (phenytoin, carbamazepine or phenytoin) increases the metabolism and elimination rate of lamotrigine and reduces the half-life to 14 hours. Conversely, sodium valproate inhibits drug-metabolising enzymes in the liver, reducing the metabolism of lamotrigine whose half-life rises to 60–70 hours when the drugs are co-administered. Because of the increased half-life, lower doses of lamotrigine are given when used with sodium valproate.

Dose. It is important not to confuse the different combinations.

Monotherapy: initially 25 mg daily for 14 days then 50 mg daily for a further 14 days; usual maintenance as monotherapy: 100–200 mg daily in one or two divided doses (up to 500 mg daily has been required).

Adjunctive therapy with valproate: initially 25 mg every other day for 14 days then 25 mg daily for a further 14 days; usual maintenance with valproate: 100–200 mg daily in one or two divided doses.

Adjunctive therapy without valproate: initially 50 mg daily for 14 days then 50 mg twice daily for a further 14 days; usual maintenance without valproate: 200–400 mg daily in two divided doses.

Cautions. Closely monitor (including hepatic, renal and clotting parameters) and consider withdrawal if rash, fever, influenza-like symptoms, drowsiness or worsening of seizure control develop, especially in first month of treatment. Use with caution in the elderly.

Side-effects. Common side-effects are rashes in 2–3% of patients (dose-related), minor CNS effects (including diplopia), blurred vision, dizziness, drowsiness, unsteadiness, headache and gastrointestinal upsets. It may also act as a psychostimulant, particularly in patients with learning disabilities, which may be beneficial.

Phenobarbital and other barbiturates

Mode of action. Phenobarbital enhances the action of gamma-aminobutyric acid by binding to a site on the gamma-aminobutyric acid receptor–channel complex that is distinct from the binding sites of either gamma-aminobutyric acid or benzodiazepine.

Phenobarbital is effective in treating partial and generalised tonic–clonic seizures but ineffective in absence seizures. Its efficacy is similar to that of carbamazepine or phenytoin, but the drug is used less often because of adverse effects.

Dose. The dosage range is usually 60–180 mg/day, given at night because of sedation.

A response should be seen within 2–3 weeks of therapy at the maximum tolerated dose. If this is ineffective, then another anticonvulsant should be tried. Its use is generally restricted to patients who cannot tolerate or do not respond to the other first-line drugs.

Side-effects. The main side-effect of phenobarbital is sedation which may not resolve with continued treatment. Other common side-effects are fatigue, listlessness, tiredness in adults and insomnia; hyperkinesia and aggression in children, along with impairment of mood, memory and learning in both groups. Tolerance to these effects can develop but also to the anticonvulsant effect, requiring ever-increasing doses of phenobarbital to be prescribed. Withdrawal can lead to a temporary increase in seizure frequency.

About 25% is excreted unchanged in the urine with the remaining 75% metabolised. There is no useful relationship between plasma concentration and efficacy, and so routine plasma level monitoring is unnecessary. Phenobarbital is an enzyme inducer.

Primidone is metabolised to phenobarbital and phenylethylmalonamide, both of which have anticonvulsant activity. It has efficacy similar to that of phenobarbital but has more side-effects, and withdrawal of the drug usually leads to temporary exacerbation of seizures.

Vigabatrin

Vigabatrin is effective for use in chronic epilepsy not satisfactorily controlled by other antiepileptics. It is useful in tonic–clonic and partial seizures but has prominent behavioural side-effects in some patients.

Mode of action. Vigabatrin is an irreversible gamma-aminobutyric acid inhibitor which acts to increase levels of gamma-aminobutyric acid, the inhibitory neurotransmitter in the central nervous system.

Pharmacokinetics. Vigabatrin is well absorbed. It is not metabolised or protein bound. Since it is primarily excreted unchanged by the kidneys, dosage must be reduced in the elderly and those with reduced renal function.

Dose. With current antiepileptic therapy, initially 1 g daily in single or two divided doses, then increased according to response in steps of 500 mg; usual range 2–4 g daily – above 4 g daily (maximum 6 g daily) only in exceptional circumstances with close monitoring for adverse effects.

Side-effects. Mild CNS side-effects, such as drowsiness, fatigue, dizziness, nervousness, irritability, depression and headache, are most frequently reported and wear off with continued therapy. Weight gain and minor gastrointestinal side-effects have also been reported. However, neurotoxicity, psychosis and behaviour disturbances, especially in the young and in patients with learning disability, have been reported and may limit its use.

Benzodiazepines

Clonazepam is occasionally used in tonic–clonic or partial seizures but its sedative side-effects may be prominent. Clobazam may be used as adjunctive therapy in the treatment of epilepsy, but the effectiveness of these and the benzodiazepines may wane considerably after weeks or months of continuous therapy.

Mode of action. Benzodiazepines exert their anticonvulsant effect by increasing the actions of gamma-aminobutyric acid and thus prevent the abnormal activity from spreading.

Dose.

Clonazepam. 1 mg (elderly, 500 micrograms) initially at night for 4 nights, increased over 2–4 weeks to a usual maintenance dose of 4–8 mg daily in divided doses.

Clobazam. 20–30 mg daily; maximum 60 mg daily.

Side-effects. Sedation is the main side-effect. Other common side-effects include fatigue, irritability and muscle hypotonia.

Oxcarbazepine

Oxcarbazepine is indicated for the treatment of partial seizures with or without secondary generalised tonic–clonic seizures; also as monotherapy or adjunctive therapy in adults and in children of 6 years and older.

Mode of action. Oxcarbazepine exerts its effect by stabilising hyperexcited neural membranes.

Dose. Initially 300 mg twice daily increased according to response to a maximum of 2.4 g daily.

Side-effects. Fatigue, dizziness, headache, somnolence, nausea and vomiting are very common. Asthenia, constipation, diarrhoea, abdominal pain, hyponatraemia and rash are common.

Levetiracetam

Levetiracetam is licensed for the adjunctive treatment of partial seizures.

Mode of action. The mode of action of levetiracetam is unknown.

Dose. Initially 500 mg twice daily to a maximum of 1.5 g twice daily.

Side-effects. Common side-effects are drowsiness, asthenia and dizziness.

Gabapentin

Gabapentin is used as adjunctive treatment of partial seizures with or without secondary generalisations not satisfactorily controlled with other antiepileptics.

Mode of action. Gabapentin is structurally related to gamma-aminobutyric acid but has an unknown mechanism of action.

Pharmacokinetics. The bioavailability of gabapentin at normal dose range is 50–80%. There is reduced bioavailability with increasing doses. A clinical consequence of decreasing absorption with increasing doses is that it may protect the patient from overdosage. Gabapentin is rapidly absorbed from the gastrointestinal tract and peak plasma concentrations are obtained in 1–3 hours. It is not bound to plasma proteins, resulting in a large volume of distribution. Gabapentin is not metabolised and is excreted mainly unchanged via the kidneys. It has a half-life of 5–7 hours. Antacids reduce the bioavailability of gabapentin and co-administration is not recommended.

Dose. The dosage range is 900–1200 mg daily, up to a maximum of 2400 mg daily, in a minimum of two divided doses. The dose must be reduced in patients with impaired renal function.

Side-effects. Gabapentin is safe and well tolerated, and most side-effects subside spontaneously or on dosage reduction. The most common side-effects are somnolence, dizziness, ataxia, fatigue, nystagmus, headache, tremor, nausea and/or vomiting, and rhinitis.

Topiramate

Topiramate is used as adjunctive treatment of partial seizures with or without secondary generalisation not satisfactorily controlled with other antiepileptics.

Mode of action. Topiramate markedly enhances the activity of gamma-aminobutyric acid at some types of gamma-aminobutyric acid receptors and also inhibits glutamate receptors. Mechanisms of action of antiepileptics are summarised in Figure 18.5.

Pharmacokinetics. Topiramate is rapidly and well absorbed following oral administration, with peak plasma concentrations occurring within 2–3 hours. The half-life is 21 hours and twice-a-day administration is adequate. Topiramate is poorly bound to plasma proteins, not extensively metabolised and is excreted largely unchanged in the urine.

Dose. The dose is gradually increased from 100 mg daily to a usual dose of 200–600 mg daily in two divided doses; the maximum is 800 mg/day.

Side-effects. Side-effects include ataxia, impaired concentration, confusion, dizziness, fatigue, paraesthesia, somnolence, abnormal thinking, agitation, emotional lability (with abnormal behaviour), depression, nephrolithiasis.

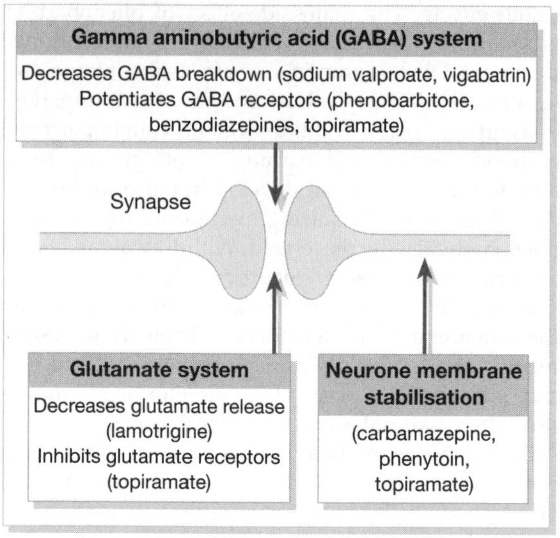

Figure 18.5 Mechanism of action of antiepileptic drugs.

Acetazolamide

Acetazolamide is a carbonic anhydrase inhibitor which is used as an adjunct therapy to other anticonvulsants, particularly carbamazepine. The exact mechanism of action is unknown but acetazolamide may act by causing carbon dioxide accumulation or reducing the oedema resulting from hyponatraemia due to carbamazepine. It has been used to treat tonic–clonic, absence and complex partial seizures. It is of limited efficacy as rapid tolerance to the anticonvulsant effect develops.

Dose. 0.25–1 g daily in divided doses.

Side-effects. Flushing, headache, drowsiness, dizziness and paraesthesia of the extremities may be experienced.

Withdrawal of anticonvulsants

Withdrawal of anticonvulsant medication must be done slowly and in a staged dose reduction manner. If the dose is reduced too quickly or the time between each reduction is too short, then the likelihood of withdrawal seizures is increased. Even with a very slow and gradual reduction and withdrawal of phenobarbital/primidone, withdrawal seizures may occur months after either of these drugs is actually stopped. The changeover from one antiepileptic drug regimen to another should be done with care, building up the second drug to a therapeutic range while gradually decreasing the first.

Driving

Epilepsy sufferers may drive a motor vehicle (not heavy goods or public service) provided they have had a seizure-free period of 2 years or, if subject to attacks only while asleep, have established a 3-year period of asleep attacks without awake attacks. Patients affected by drowsiness should not drive or operate machinery.

Status epilepticus

Status epilepticus occurs when a seizure lasts for more than 30 minutes or there are recurrent episodes without recovery of consciousness between attacks. Status epilepticus may be precipitated by a variety of conditions, such as a brain tumour, infection (for example, meningitis), alcohol, reduction in or non-compliance with anticonvulsant medication, trauma, or may be due to some metabolic abnormality such as hypoxia or ischaemia.

It is a medical emergency and requires urgent treatment aimed at stopping seizures as quickly as possible. A nurse must stay with the patient. An airway should be established and patients should be in a physical environment where they cannot hurt themselves. Diazepam emulsion 10–20 mg should be administered intravenously over 3–6 minutes. This is repeated in 30 minutes if necessary, which may be followed by intravenous infusion to a maximum of 3 mg/kg over 24 hours. Caution should be exercised because of the risk of respiratory depression. Small doses of diazepam can be administered by rectal solution.

To prevent recurrence of seizures after the initial diazepam injection, phenytoin may be given by slow intravenous injection in a dose of 15 mg/kg with ECG monitoring in case of cardiac arrhythmias. If status epilepticus continues or returns, clomethiazole may be given by slow intravenous injection, monitoring respiration carefully, particularly if following on diazepam. Paraldehyde may be given when other agents have failed to control seizures. Some 5–10 mL should be given by deep intramuscular injection. The dose may be repeated after 1 hour. Paraldehyde may cause muscle necrosis. Doses of 10 mL should be split into 2 mL, 3 mL and 5 mL doses in separate muscles. When preparing paraldehyde for administration, contact with rubber and plastics should be avoided.

Phenobarbital can be given in a dose of 50–200 mg by slow intravenous injection, i.e. over about 5 minutes. This may be repeated after 6 hours if necessary. Prolonged sedation or respiratory depression may be a problem.

Once seizures have been abolished, an appropriate oral regimen should be instituted immediately and loading doses of the particular anticonvulsant may have to be given, particularly if non-compliance has been a precipitating factor.

PARKINSON'S DISEASE

Parkinson's disease is a degenerative condition which affects a large number of people, particularly older people. The deterioration of health and quality of life caused by Parkinson's disease has a major impact not only on the sufferers but also on their family and carers. There is insufficient knowledge about the causes of Parkinson's disease to develop widespread strategies to prevent the disease and there is no known cure.

The key symptoms of idiopathic Parkinson's disease are:

- tremor, present when the patient is at rest and when severe 'pill rolling' may be seen
- rigidity; on standing the patient may exhibit stooped posture, arms slightly bent, weight on ball of foot, knees flexed
- bradykinesia
  - general slowness in daily activities
  - difficulty initiating movement, particularly walking
  - difficulty in rising from a chair
- walking problems
  - the patient's weight is on the ball of the foot and there appears to be a loss of heel strike
  - reduction in length of stride
  - the patient leans forward before commencing to walk and flexes the knees to prevent falling forward
- balance problems
  - frequent falls can occur
  - difficulty in turning.

Other features of Parkinson's disease include excessive salivation, dysphagia – frequently in older people, anxiety, depression and a fixed staring appearance.

Onset of Parkinson's disease is usually insidious and progression is slow. Many patients notice a resting tremor, usually affecting the hands initially. The tremor disappears on movement and during sleep, and may be worse under stress. Bradykinesia is reflected in immobile features and a fixed, staring appearance. Along with rigidity, it is responsible for the typical abnormalities of gait; difficulty in starting and finishing steps with resultant shuffling; a stooped head, fixed neck, upper extremities and knees and a lack of

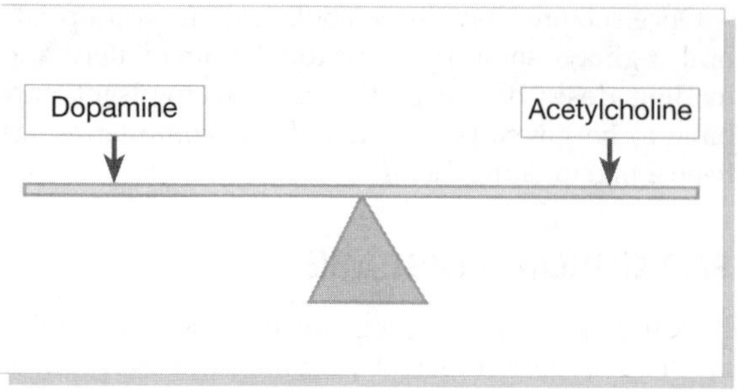

Figure 18.6 Dopamine and acetylcholine in balance.

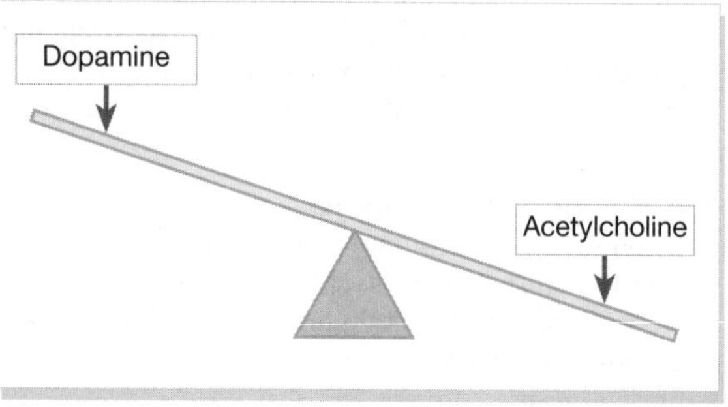

Figure 18.7 Dopamine deficiency with resultant cholinergic overactivity leading to symptoms of the disease.

normal arm swing. Frequent falls may result from loss of postural reflex leading to postural imbalance.

Dopamine, working in balance with another chemical messenger, acetylcholine, is responsible for the mechanisms which control programmes of movements (Fig. 18.6). Imbalances in the neurotransmitters lead to movement disorders. In Parkinson's disease, degeneration of certain cells in the substantia nigra leads to a deficiency in the production of dopamine so that the normal balance between the neurotransmitters, dopamine and acetylcholine, is altered (Fig. 18.7).

The symptoms of Parkinson's disease do not appear until some 80% of the capacity to produce dopamine has been lost. The level of dopamine will continue to fall over subsequent years. However, each person with Parkinson's disease is very different, and the rate and character of the progression may vary greatly from one person to another. The disease usually presents in middle or old age.

Drug treatment

The main aim of drug therapy is to restore the balance between dopamine and acetylcholine. This can be achieved by:

- replacing dopamine
- use of dopamine agonists to stimulate surviving dopamine receptors
- prolonging action of dopamine by inhibiting metabolism
- use of antimuscarinic drugs.

Replacing dopamine

Administration of dopamine is ineffective since it cannot cross the blood–brain barrier into the brain cells where it is required to produce an effect. It is necessary to give its precursor, levodopa, which crosses the blood–brain barrier and is subsequently broken down to dopamine by the enzyme dopa decarboxylase. However, levodopa requires to be given in high concentrations since over 90% is decarboxylated in the liver and gut before it reaches the brain. This results in peripheral side-effects such as nausea, vomiting, anorexia and postural hypotension.

Levodopa is rarely given alone. It is usually given in combination with an inhibitor of extracerebral dopa decarboxylase, such as carbidopa (Sinemet) or benserazide (Madopar). This prevents the peripheral degradation of levodopa to dopamine and so increases effective brain levels. This allows the dose of levodopa to be reduced markedly, resulting in a reduction in side-effects.

Levodopa is the drug of choice in the treatment of Parkinson's disease and is tolerated by most patients, who experience considerable improvement for several years, especially where stiffness and slowness of movement are concerned. It is initiated at low doses (50–100 mg twice daily with benserazide) since some feelings of nausea are common because of stimulation of the dopaminergic receptors in the chemoreceptor trigger zone. These are usually mild and pass as the body adjusts to the drug. Taking levodopa with or after meals helps to minimise these effects.

Domperidone, a dopamine antagonist which does not cross the blood–brain barrier, may be useful in controlling nausea where this is severe (doses of 10–20 mg domperidone 1 hour before levodopa preparations are effective). The dosage regimen of levodopa is gradually increased, the final dose being a compromise between increased mobility and incidence of side-effects.

The relatively short half-life of levodopa (2–3 hours) has led to the development of controlled-release preparations which can be given less frequently and the use of which evens out the peaks and troughs associated with conventional levodopa therapy.

There is a small percentage of people who cannot tolerate levodopa because of severe sickness or other side-effects such as confusion, hallucinations and mood swings.

Levodopa usually provides very effective control of Parkinson's disease for a number of years, after which a deterioration in response often occurs. This is probably related to increasing degeneration of nigrostriatal neurones.

Interactions can occur with drugs which affect central monoamines, and MAOIs should be withdrawn at least 14 days before instituting levodopa treatment. Antipsychotic drugs, such as the phenothiazines, should not be administered concurrently as they would exacerbate the disease. Caution should be exercised in patients with open-angle glaucoma.

Dopamine agonists

Dopamine agonists (bromocriptine, cabergoline, lisuride, pergolide) are ergot derivatives which act by direct stimulation of surviving dopamine receptors. They are usually used in conjunction with levodopa to smooth out control of symptoms in patients whose response to treatment is beginning to fluctuate. Treatment is begun at low dosage, taken with food and gradually increased to a maintenance dose. The use of dopa agonists allows a reduction in the levodopa dosage and the effects of the combination should be carefully balanced. Drop-out rates can be high owing to adverse effects. Gastrointestinal upset, postural hypotension, dizziness and headache are common. With bromocriptine, patients are best advised to refrain from excessive alcohol consumption as alcohol may reduce tolerance of the drug and lead to increased side-effects.

Ropinirole is a dopamine agonist which is a non-ergot derivative, in contrast to the other available oral agonists discussed above. Ropinirole is indicated for the treatment of Parkinson's disease, either alone or in combination with levodopa, to control 'on–off' fluctuations and permit a reduction in the daily dose of levodopa. It is the only dopamine agonist licensed for monotherapy, the others being licensed only as adjunctive therapy.

Ropinirole is rapidly absorbed, with bioavailability of approximately 50%. It has a half-life of about 6 hours. The initial dose is 250 micrograms three times daily increased weekly to 3 mg daily; the usual dose range is 3–9 mg. The most common side-effects are nausea, somnolence, leg oedema, abdominal pain, vomiting and syncope. When used as an adjunct to therapy the most common side-effects are dyskinesia, nausea, hallucinations and confusion.

Prolongation of dopamine action

Selegiline is a drug which prolongs the action of dopamine at the receptor by inhibiting its enzymatic degradation. It is a monoamine oxidase B inhibitor and its use therefore does not involve dietary restriction. Use of selegiline may help to reduce the dose of levodopa in early stages of the disease. The dose is 10 mg in the morning or 5 mg at breakfast and midday. It is given in the morning as it is partly metabolised to amfetamine, which may cause insomnia. Selegiline can cause hypotension, nausea, vomiting, confusion and agitation, and the side-effects of levodopa may be increased. To avoid initial confusion and agitation in the elderly it may be appropriate to start treatment with a dose of 2.5 mg daily.

Catechol-O-methyl transferase (COMT) inhibition

Entacapone acts by preventing the breakdown of levodopa because of inhibition of the enzyme catechol-*O*-methyl transferase. This results in an increase in the availability of levodopa to the brain and a reduction in the levels of the metabolite 3-*O*-methyldopa which competes with levodopa for transport across the blood–brain barrier. Entacapone thus prolongs the clinical response to levodopa. A 200 mg dose is given with each dose of levodopa (with dopa-decarboxylase inhibitor) up to a maximum of 10 doses per day. Because of increased dyskinesia, concurrent levodopa may need to be reduced by about 10–30%.

Side-effects experienced may include dyskinesia, nausea, diarrhoea, abdominal pain, fatigue and insomnia. The urine may be coloured brown.

Pramipexole is indicated as an adjunct to levodopa in advanced Parkinson's disease.

End of dose and 'on–off' effects

In excess of 50% of parkinsonian patients experience fluctuations in motor response after 5 years of levodopa treatment. Two of the most common side-effects of levodopa therapy are the 'end of dose' deterioration and 'on–off' phenomena.

The duration of the beneficial response to each dose of levodopa becomes progressively shorter and may be reduced from an initial 4–6 hours to as little as 30 minutes with a return of symptoms towards the end of each dose, such as early morning immobility, dystonia and start hesitation. End-of-dose effects appear to be the result of failing levodopa plasma levels as they can be abolished by levodopa infusions. This condition may respond to the administration of smaller doses of levodopa at more frequent intervals with the first dose on waking and last dose at bedtime.

Adjunctive treatment may also be considered at this stage. Bromocriptine or selegiline are both useful in conjunction with levodopa for smoothing out the effects of end-of-dose deterioration. Controlled-release preparations of Sinemet or Madopar can also be used.

'On–off' effects are sudden fluctuations in disability which can occur, involving rapid and abrupt alterations between periods of good mobility and periods of hypokinesia, tremor and dyskinesia. This may last for only a few seconds or up to several minutes, or even hours, before normal function returns. Apomorphine has been used to overcome this effect. There is also some evidence that dietary manipulation may improve 'on–off' effects since there is competition for transport across the blood–brain barrier between levodopa and certain dietary amino acids.

Apomorphine

Apomorphine can reduce and sometimes reverse these disabling 'off' period phenomena. The rapid and reliable onset of action of apomorphine can be used to advantage when oral doses of levodopa become progressively less effective and less predictable. The aim of treatment is to optimise the delicate balance between an effective response and minimal side-effects. The complex nature of apomorphine therapy necessitates that it should be initiated in specialist centres.

Apomorphine is a directly acting dopamine agonist with no opiate or addictive properties. It is not used orally because it undergoes extensive first-pass metabolism to an inactive metabolite. Treatment with apomorphine is usually administered either by intermittent subcutaneous injections or by continuous waking day subcutaneous infusion.

Following a single subcutaneous dose, apomorphine has an onset of action of between 5 and 15 minutes. The effect usually lasts for about 1 hour.

Since apomorphine is a potent emetic, pretreatment with domperidone is necessary for at least 3 days before initiating therapy. A dose of 30 mg every 8 hours is given. Domperidone is a peripherally acting dopamine antagonist, unlike metoclopramide or prochlorperazine which have both peripheral and central effects. It does not cross the blood–brain barrier to act as an antagonist at central dopamine receptors with consequent detrimental effects on motor performance. Domperidone can usually be withdrawn gradually over several weeks to 6 months, although some patients may need to continue taking a low dose. In addition, it appears to counteract some of the other peripheral effects of apomorphine, such as postural hypotension.

After initiation of domperidone, all existing antiparkinsonian medication is stopped overnight to provoke an 'off' period. The lowest or 'threshold' dose of apomorphine that produces a definite motor response may be determined as follows:

- 1.5 mg apomorphine is injected subcutaneously and the patient is observed for 30 minutes for motor response.
- If there is no response, or a poor response, 3 mg is injected subcutaneously 40 minutes after the first dose with increase in dose incrementally every 40 minutes until a response is seen. Patients not responding to a 7 mg dose are classified as non-responders. The maximum dose for a subcutaneous bolus injection is 10 mg.
- Finally, antiparkinson's therapy is started and continued using apomorphine at the dose determined above when required for 'off' periods.

The drug may be given by repeated single subcutaneous injections in doses of 3–30 mg daily, titrated against response. The maximum total daily dose quoted in the data sheet is 100 mg.

If patients require many daily injections, apomorphine may be administered by continuous daytime subcutaneous infusion via syringe driver. The manufacturers recommend that infusions should start at a rate of 1 mg/hour. Infusions may be increased in steps of not greater than 0.5 mg/hour at intervals of not less than 4 hours, to a maximum of 4 mg/hour.

Side-effects. Stimulation of the chemoreceptor trigger zone by apomorphine commonly results in nausea and vomiting. Other side-effects include hypotension, bradycardia, sweating and respiratory depression. Drowsiness is common but usually resolves over the first few weeks of treatment.

Since apomorphine can cause hypotension, care should be taken in patients with pre-existing cardiac disease or in patients taking antihypertensive medication.

Antimuscarinic drugs

Antimuscarinic drugs (e.g. benzatropine, orphenadrine, procyclidine, trihexyphenidyl) may be used in Parkinson's disease to reduce the relative excess of acetylcholine, and, as a result, reduce to some extent the tremor, rigidity and sialorrhoea. All are given in gradually increasing doses until an optimal balance of efficacy and side-effects is obtained (see Table 18.15).

The most common adverse reactions are dry mouth, constipation, blurred vision, tachycardia and dizziness. The antimuscarinics are contraindicated in urinary retention and glaucoma, and interactions may occur with antihistamines and tricyclic antidepressants.

Table 18.15 Dosages of antimuscarinic drugs

Drug	Initial dose	Maintenance dose
Benzatropine	0.5–1 mg	1–4 mg
Orphenadrine	150 mg in divided doses	150–300 mg
Procyclidine	2.5 mg three times daily	10–20 mg
Trihexyphenidyl (benzhexol)	1 mg	5–15 mg

They can be useful for younger patients in the early stages when symptoms are mild. When treatment of mild symptoms is initiated with antimuscarinic drugs, levodopa is added or substituted as symptoms progress.

Drug-induced parkinsonism

The features of drug-induced parkinsonism are the same as those of the idiopathic disease. There may be tremor, rigidity, bradykinesia, expressionless face, dysphagia and drooling. This occurs to some degree in all patients treated with antipsychotic drugs, although there is a wide variation between patients. The following have a high propensity for causing extrapyramidal effects:

- piperazine phenothiazines, e.g. fluphenazine, trifluoperazine
- butyrophenones, e.g. haloperidol, droperidol
- diphenylbutylpiperidines, e.g. pimozide.

Chlorpromazine has a lower propensity. Metoclopramide blocks dopamine receptors and also enhances the action of acetylcholine.

Drug-induced parkinsonism does not always require treatment and it is reversible on dose reduction or drug withdrawal. Severe cases may require treatment with antimuscarinics but the routine use of these drugs should be avoided as they add to the antimuscarinic side-effects of antipsychotic drugs. Because of the tendency of antipsychotics to accumulate, side-effects may be very prolonged lasting days or weeks after the drug has been withdrawn.

Care of the patient with Parkinson's disease

The symptoms of Parkinson's disease are fairly familiar to the general public. It follows therefore that when a diagnosis is made the patient will be concerned and those involved must give every encouragement to patients and those who are close to them.

Education of the patient and participation in treatment are important from the outset, since treatment is likely to be prolonged and eventually problematic. Plans and objectives should be formulated in conjunction with the patient. Physiotherapy can assist in posture and walking, and regular exercise is important to maintain mobility. Occupational therapists can offer a wide range of helpful appliances. Constipation may be a concern for sufferers but a high-fibre diet usually controls symptoms. In the UK, The Parkinson's Disease Society is recommended as a source of support.

SUBSTANCE DEPENDENCE

Alcohol dependence

There are few drug treatments that reliably maintain abstinence in patients with alcohol dependence. Disulfiram can help to reduce a patient's drinking but, in general, its use needs to be supervised (for example, by the patient's partner) to help ensure adherence to therapy. Disulfiram gives rise to extremely unpleasant systemic reactions after the ingestion of even small amounts of alcohol because it leads to accumulation of acetaldehyde in the body. This occurs because disulfiram inhibits the enzyme responsible for the oxidation of acetaldehyde, a metabolite of alcohol. Reactions can occur within 10 minutes and last several hours.

The dose is 800 mg as a single dose on the first day, reducing over 5 days to 100–200 mg daily. It should not be continued for longer than 6 months without review. Reactions include flushing of the face, throbbing headache, palpitations, tachycardia, nausea, vomiting and, with larger doses of alcohol, arrhythmias, hypotension and collapse.

Patients taking disulfiram should be instructed to avoid all substances containing alcohol such as tonics, elixirs and gargles. They should also not apply alcohol-containing substances such as after-shave lotion, rubbing alcohol, and liniments because the skin may absorb the alcohol. Alcohol should be avoided for at least a week after stopping disulfiram.

Benzodiazepines are also used in the management of withdrawal. Chlordiazepoxide or diazepam is given orally 4-hourly. The final dose should be determined by regular clinical monitoring of the patient's level of distress, the aim being a calm patient. Close monitoring is essential to avoid overdosage. Caution should be exercised in liver dysfunction, which is associated with reduced clearance of benzodiazepines, and airways dysfunction may be associated with respiratory depression.

Acamprosate is a newer preparation which, in combination with counselling, may be helpful in maintaining abstinence in alcohol-dependent patients. Therapy should be initiated as soon as possible after abstinence has been achieved. The recommended treatment period is 1 year.

The mechanism of action of acamprosate is uncertain. It has gamma-aminobutyric acid (GABA) agonist properties and glutamate antagonist properties. It is thought that, in chronic alcohol dependency, glutamate receptors increase and disrupt the excitatory/inhibitory balance between glutamate and GABA neurotransmission. Acamprosate may act by stimulating GABA inhibitory transmission and antagonise excitatory amino acids, particularly glutamic acid.

Cigarette smoking

Around 1 in 4 adults in the UK smoke cigarettes. It is notoriously difficult to stop smoking but success rates are increased where nicotine products or amfebutamone/ bupropion are used as an aid to smoking cessation in combination with motivational support.

Amfebutamone/bupropion

Mode of action. Developed originally as an antidepressant, its mode of action in smoking cessation is not entirely clear. Amfebutamone/bupropion may increase levels of dopamine and adrenaline (epinephrine) in the brain thereby counteracting the reductions in these neurochemicals that result from nicotine withdrawal.

Pharmacokinetics. Amfebutamone/bupropion is readily absorbed following oral administration with peak plasma concentrations in 3 hours. The elimination half-life is about 20 hours.

Dose. It is recommended that treatment is started while the patient is still smoking and that a target stop date is set within the first 2 weeks of treatment, preferably in the second week. The initial dose is 150 mg to be taken daily for 3 days, increasing to 150 mg twice daily. If at 7 weeks no effect is seen, treatment should be discontinued.

Side-effects. The most common side-effects are dry mouth and insomnia. Amfebutamone/bupropion is contraindicated in patients with epilepsy.

Nicotine replacement

Five types of nicotine replacement are available in the UK: chewing gum, transdermal patches, inhalator, a sublingual tablet and a nasal spray. To use nicotine replacement, smokers are advised to set a date and a time for quitting smoking and from that point onwards to use the replacement product instead of cigarettes, generally for up to 3 months.

Counselling

The effectiveness of smoking cessation initiatives is increased where counselling and support are provided in addition to the medication. In this way the patient can be advised of the difficulties that will be experienced and the ways in which these can be anticipated and action taken to minimise their effect on the smoking cessation initiative. This can take the form of regular counselling both at the outset and during the course of the medication. A helpline may be available to deal with issues as they arise. A few examples of guidance are as follows:

- Clean your home and car to get rid of the smell of cigarettes.
- Get a piggy bank to save the money you currently spend on cigarettes.
- Get rid of smoking 'bits and pieces', e.g. ashtrays, lighters.
- Keep busy and plan your activities.
- Keep your hands active, e.g. doodle.
- Change your routine around the times and places you normally smoke.
- Chew sugar-free gum or suck sugar-free sweets.
- Have a counsellor or friend you can ring for support.
- Take up a new hobby or activity.
- Reward yourself for no longer smoking.
- If you have a lapse, try again. Remember you can still become a non-smoker.

Opioid dependence

Drug misuse, even with some degree of dependence, may not be in itself an indication to prescribe controlled drugs. Simple reassurance and the prescription of non-controlled drugs may be helpful and effective in alleviating the patient's anxiety about withdrawal.

Prescribing a substitute drug where appropriate can be a useful tool to change the behaviour of some misusers, either towards abstinence or towards intermediate goals such as a reduction in injecting or sharing of injecting equipment. A flexible plan should be agreed for stabilisation/maintenance which may range from a week to many months. Important factors are length of use, stability of lifestyle and the patient's wishes and motivation. Goals for ultimate reduction/withdrawal and rate of reduction need to be discussed and regularly reviewed. An agreement or 'contract' should be established based on the agreed goals and when these will be reviewed.

Methadone

Methadone mixture (1 mg/mL) can be substituted for opioids. It may be prescribed for daily dispensing of up to 14 days, allowing the client to collect medication from a community pharmacy on a daily basis. A 'drop in the mouth' arrangement entails the client consuming the dose in the pharmacy, supervised by the pharmacist. This avoids 'bingeing' or the medication being sold. The client should be seen every 2 weeks by a nominated GP and not left repeat prescriptions.

Methadone is a synthetic compound with properties similar to those of morphine. It is well absorbed from the gastrointestinal tract and has a bioavailability of 80–90%. The half-life is 1–2 days and once-daily dosing is sufficient. The initial dose is based on previous consumption. The dose is then titrated against signs of withdrawal, for example, tachycardia, mydriasis, perspiration and sensations of discomfort. The ability to drive or operate machinery may be severely affected. Methadone is less sedating than the other opiates. Nausea may occur.

Interactions. Rifampicin, carbamazepine, phenobarbital and phenytoin accelerate the metabolism of methadone by induction of enzymes, leading to a reduced effect. Methadone may increase plasma concentration of zidovudine.

Contraindications. Methadone is contraindicated in respiratory depression, obstructive airways disease or during an acute asthma attack.

Urine testing. A urine sample should be taken before starting on methadone to establish whether the patient is using opiates – and also while on prescription for evidence of both taking methadone and not taking other drugs.

Lofexidine

Noradrenergic neuronal hyperactivity is the pathway responsible for the signs and symptoms of opiate withdrawal. Lofexidine is an alpha-noradrenergic agonist which significantly reduces opiate withdrawal symptoms without the adverse sedative and hypotensive effects of clonidine.

Dose. Initial dosage should be one 200-microgram tablet twice daily. The dose may be increased by increments of 200–400 micrograms per day up to a maximum of 2.4 mg (12 tablets) per day, according to the patient's response. Where no opiate use occurs during detoxification, a duration of treatment of 7–10 days is recommended. At the end of treatment, dosage should be reduced gradually over a period of at least 2–4 days to minimise any risk of blood pressure elevation.

Interactions. Lofexidine may enhance the CNS depressive effects of alcohol, barbiturates and other sedatives.

Side-effects. These comprise drowsiness and, if affected, patients should be advised not to drive or operate machinery. It may cause dryness of mucous membranes, especially of the mouth, throat and nose.

Precautions. It should be used with caution in cardiac disease, cerebrovascular disease, chronic renal failure and marked bradycardia.

Naltrexone

Naltrexone is an opioid antagonist. It blocks the action of opioids such as diamorphine and precipitates withdrawal symptoms in opioid-dependent subjects. Since the euphoric action of opioid agonists is blocked by naltrexone, it is given to former addicts as an aid to prevent relapse. The patient should be narcotic-free 7–10 days prior to treatment as verified by urinalysis. Liver tests are required before and during treatment.

Buprenorphine

Buprenorphine can be used as substitution therapy for patients with moderate opioid dependence.

ALZHEIMER'S DISEASE

Symptoms

Alzheimer's disease is characterised by an insidious onset with a gradual but relentless decline in memory and other aspects of cognitive function that is sufficient to impair activities of daily living. An early feature is memory impairment for recent events and poor retention of new information. Memory for more distant events is usually preserved in the early stages. Language problems (aphasia) occur and are sometimes quite prominent even in the early stages of the disease. As Alzheimer's disease progresses, there are increasing changes in behaviour.

Acetylcholinesterase-inhibiting drugs

Degeneration of cholinergic neurones and associated loss of cholinergic neurotransmission appear to contribute significantly to the cognitive decline seen in Alzheimer's disease. Acetylcholinesterase is the chemical which breaks down acetylcholine, and inhibition of this process results in a boost to the cholinergic system in Alzheimer's disease.

Table 18.16 Drugs used in the treatment of Alzheimer's disease

Drug	Starting dose	Dose titration	Maximum dose	Side-effects
Donepezil	5 mg once a day at bedtime	Reviewed after 1 month, increased to 10 mg daily if well tolerated	10 mg daily (some local protocols keep dose at 5 mg)	Diarrhoea, muscle cramps, fatigue, nausea, vomiting, insomnia
Galantamine	4 mg twice daily for 4 weeks	After 4 weeks, initial maintenance dose is 8 mg twice daily, for at least 4 weeks, then consider increase to maintenance dose of 12 mg twice daily	12 mg twice daily	Asthenia, anorexia, dizziness, nausea, somnolence, vomiting
Rivastigmine	1.5 mg twice daily	Increased in steps of 1.5 mg twice daily at minimum fortnightly intervals	6 mg twice daily	Nausea, vomiting, diarrhoea, abdominal pain, dyspepsia, anorexia, fatigue, somnolence

Donepezil, rivastigmine and galantamine are acetylcholinesterase inhibitors prescribed for patients with Alzheimer's disease (Table 18.16). Treatment should be initiated and supervised by a specialist experienced in the management of dementia. Benefit is assessed by repeating the cognitive assessment at around 3 months. Up to half the patients given these drugs will show a slower rate of cognitive decline.

FURTHER READING

[Anonymous] 1999 Drug treatment for schizophrenia. Effective Health Care 5:1–12

[Anonymous] 1999 Nicotine replacement to aid smoking cessation. Drug and Therapeutics Bulletin 37:52–54

[Anonymous] 2000 Bupropion to aid smoking cessation. Drug and Therapeutics Bulletin 38:73–75

Burn D 2000 Parkinson's disease: treatment. Pharmaceutical Journal 264:476–479

Burn D 2000 Parkinson's disease: an overview. Pharmaceutical Journal 264:333–337

Dawson A 2000 Migraine. Pharmaceutical Journal 265:519–523

Fabetti A E 2000 Risperidone for control of agitation in dementia patients. American Journal of Health-System Pharmacists 57:862–870

Hart Y 2000 Rational drug choice in epilepsy management. Prescriber 11:45–61

Jones R 2000 Alzheimer's disease. Pharmaceutical Journal 264:846–850

Michael T 1999 Epilepsy treatment – the established drugs. Pharmaceutical Journal 262:432–435

Michael T 1999 Epilepsy – new treatments. Pharmaceutical Journal 262:470–473

Nash E M, Sangha K S 2001 Levetiracetam. American Journal of Health-System Pharmacists 58:195–199

Thomas H, Rai G 2001 The aetiology and pathology of dementia. Hospital Pharmacist 8:33–40

Thomson F C, Fraser K, Kelly S J et al 2001 Drug treatment in dementia. Hospital Pharmacist 8:41–49

Thornett A 2000 Current approaches to depression management. Prescriber 11:49–58

Worrel J A, Marken P A, Beckman S E et al 2000 Atypical antipsychotic agents: a critical review. American Journal of Health-System Pharmacists 57:238–257

CHAPTER CONTENTS

19

Drug treatment of infections

INTRODUCTION

The discovery of sulphonamides in the 1930s, followed by penicillin in the 1940s, heralded a new era in the treatment of infections. Since then a large number of drugs have been produced which either kill or inhibit the growth of bacteria, fungi or viruses. These drugs, in tandem with the patient's natural immunity, have cured many infectious diseases which previously often proved fatal. It should be noted that where immunity is impaired due to prolonged illness, old age or the use of cytotoxic drugs, infections are more difficult to eradicate. As organisms become resistant to chemotherapy, a continuing search is necessary for new drugs and modifications of those already in use.

CLASSIFICATION OF BACTERIA

Bacteria can be broadly classified according to cell shape (Fig. 19.1), that is:

cocci – spherical
bacilli – straight rods
vibrios – curved rods
spirochaetes – spiral, flexible filaments
spirilla – spiral, non-flexible filaments.

Subdivision of these categories is based on the Gram stain. This staining technique was developed by Christian Gram in 1884. A heat-fixed smear of bacteria is stained successively with a solution of crystal violet (or related dye) and iodine. This is then treated with an organic solvent such as acetone. The cells of some bacteria, termed Gram-negative bacteria, are rapidly decolorised. The treatment with organic solvent is normally followed by counterstaining with, for example, fuchsin or safranin. Gram-positive cells retain the deep purple conferred on them by the initial staining with crystal violet and iodine, whereas Gram-negative cells, which had been decolorised, exhibit the red colour of the counterstain. As a result, Gram-positive and Gram-negative cells can be readily distinguished under the microscope.

Microorganisms are also classified as aerobes – those that can live and grow in the presence of oxygen – or as anaerobes – those that can live and grow without oxygen. These three factors:

- cell structure
- reaction to Gram stain
- aerobe/anaerobe

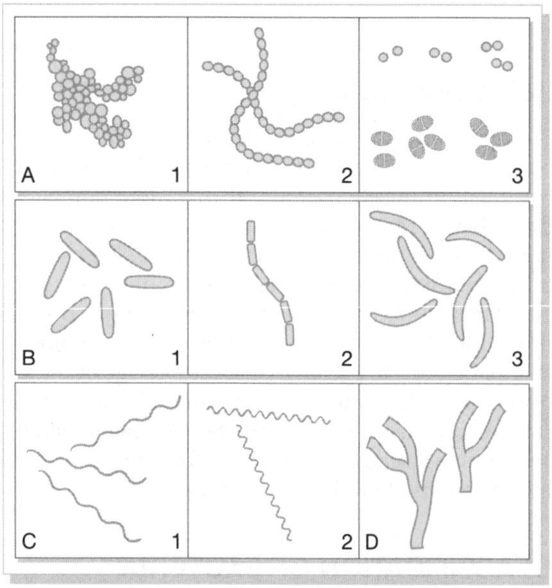

Figure 19.1 Bacteria – examples of cell shapes. **A.** Cocci (spherical bacteria): 1. staphylococci; 2. streptococci; 3. diplococci. **B.** (1–3) Bacilli. **C.** (1, 2) Spirochaetes. **D.** Actinomyces.

can be used in the classification of infectious bacteria (Table 19.1).

MICROBIOLOGY

Serious infections can be life-threatening, and decisions require to be made on the most appropriate therapy. For example:

- Viral infections should not be treated with antibacterials.
- Samples should be taken for culture and sensitivity testing.
- Knowledge of prevalent organisms (see Table 19.2) and their current sensitivity will help the selection of an antibacterial before bacteriological confirmation is available.
- The dose should take account of age, weight, renal function and severity of infection.
- Life-threatening infections require intravenous therapy.
- Duration of therapy must be appropriate; a single dose of an antibacterial may cure uncomplicated urinary tract infections; in many cases a 5-day course is sufficient. However, in certain infections such as tuberculosis or chronic osteomyelitis it is necessary to treat for prolonged periods.

Other factors affecting the choice of antibiotic include:

- known allergies or hypersensitivities of the patient
- site of infection
- toxicity of chosen antibiotic
- cost.

Table 19.1 Classification of infectious bacteria

Gram-positive aerobes		Gram-negative aerobes	
Cocci, e.g. *Staphylococcus aureus* *Staphylococcus epidermidis* *Streptococcus pneumoniae* Viridans streptococci	Bacilli, e.g. *Corynebacterium diphtheriae* *Listeria monocytogenes*	Cocci, e.g. *Neisseria meningitidis* *Neisseria gonorrhoeae*	Bacilli, e.g. *Haemophilus influenzae* *Klebsiella pneumoniae* *Escherichia coli* *Enterobacter* species *Proteus* species *Pseudomonas aeruginosa* *Legionella* species *Campylobacter* species
Gram-positive anaerobes		**Gram-negative anaerobes**	
Cocci, e.g. *Peptococcus*	Bacilli, e.g. *Clostridium tetani* *Clostridium perfringens*	Cocci, e.g. *Veillonella* species	Bacilli, e.g. *Bacteroides* species *Fusobacterium* species

It is essential to obtain specimens for microbiological investigation before antimicrobial therapy is initiated so that the antibiotic therapy can be reassessed if an organism is identified. Conventional laboratory techniques for identification require at least 18 hours of incubation in appropriate media to allow detectable numbers of bacteria to grow. However, more rapid techniques help in diagnosis before culture results are available. The most valuable is a Gram-stained smear of blood or aspirate from the site of infection.

An identification of organisms from culture is followed by sensitivity tests. Filter paper discs impregnated with known concentrations of antibiotic are placed onto an agar culture plate containing the individual strain of organism isolated in the culture process. The degree of sensitivity of the organism to the antibiotic is assessed by the size of inhibition zones around the discs after further incubation. Results are reported back to the prescriber, indicating antibiotics effective in treatment.

Table 19.2 Causative pathogens in some common bacterial infections

Respiratory infections	
Exacerbation of chronic bronchitis	*Haemophilus influenzae* *Streptococcus pneumoniae*
Pneumonia	*Streptococcus pneumoniae* *Staphylococcus aureus* *Haemophilus influenzae*
Urinary tract infections	*Escherichia coli (E. coli)* *Proteus* spp. *Klebsiella* spp. *Streptococcus faecalis* *Pseudomonas*
Venereal disease	
Gonorrhoea	*Neisseria gonorrhoeae*
Non-specific urethritis	*Chlamydia*
Skin/soft tissue infections	
Intravenous catheter site	*Staphylococcus aureus* *Staphylococcus epidermidis*
Surgical wound	*Staphylococcus aureus* Gram-negative rods
Furuncle	*Staphylococcus aureus*
Endocarditis	
Acute	*Staphylococcus aureus* *Streptococcus pyogenes* Gram-negative bacilli
Subacute	*Streptococcus* spp. *Staphylococcus epidermidis* Gram-negative bacilli
Septicaemia	*Staphylococcus aureus* *Streptococcus pneumoniae* Coliforms *Enterobacter* spp.
Meningitis (adults) (many organisms may cause meningitis in neonates)	*Streptococcus pneumoniae* *Neisseria meningitidis*
Food poisoning	Salmonellae *Clostridium perfringens*

ANTIBACTERIAL DRUGS

Antibacterial drugs act by a number of mechanisms (Fig. 19.2). They can be either bactericidal (kill bacteria) or bacteriostatic (arrest the growth of bacteria) (Box 19.1). Bacteriostatic agents, since they do not kill bacteria, rely upon the host's immune and cell defence mechanisms to clear the bacteria. If these defence mechanisms are compromised, a bactericidal drug may be preferable.

Minimum inhibitory concentration (MIC) of antibiotics

As a guide to the sensitivity of a specific microorganism to an antibiotic, the MIC is utilised. This is the lowest concentration of antibiotic which will inhibit the growth of a given strain of microorganism under controlled conditions. The lower the concentration, the more potent

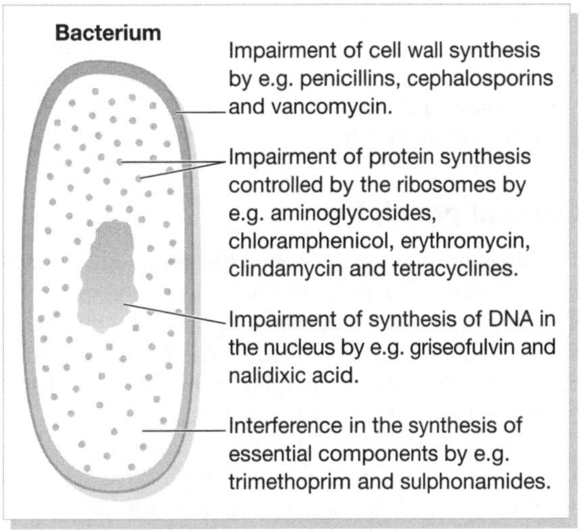
Bacterium
Impairment of cell wall synthesis by e.g. penicillins, cephalosporins and vancomycin.
Impairment of protein synthesis controlled by the ribosomes by e.g. aminoglycosides, chloramphenicol, erythromycin, clindamycin and tetracyclines.
Impairment of synthesis of DNA in the nucleus by e.g. griseofulvin and nalidixic acid.
Interference in the synthesis of essential components by e.g. trimethoprim and sulphonamides.

Figure 19.2 Actions of antibacterial drugs.

Box 19.1 Some bactericidal and bacteriostatic drugs

Bactericidal drugs
Aminoglycosides
Cephalosporins
Penicillins

Bacteriostatic drugs
Tetracyclines
Trimethoprim
Erythromycin
Chloramphenicol

the antibiotic. However, the MIC is determined in a homogeneous culture system in vitro. In vivo, the drug may have to pass from the plasma into infected tissue to destroy bacteria. The penetration of antibiotics into abscess cavities may be poor, and surgical drainage is often necessary. In either case, higher doses would be required in vivo to achieve the MIC compared with in vitro.

Minimum bactericidal concentration (MBC) is the lowest concentration of antibiotic which will kill a given strain of bacterium under controlled conditions.

Control of antibiotic usage

Since the rates of resistance are proportional to antibiotic use, the unnecessary use of antibiotics contributes to the spread of resistance. Many hospitals have adopted antibiotic policies and guidelines which are aimed at reducing the induction of resistance through controlling the range and use of anti-infective agents. Good antibiotic prescribing requires information about the probable cause and the antibiotic susceptibility of the infective agent. This can be obtained by taking appropriate specimens for culture and prescribing according to the results.

General principles

The objective of drug therapy in the treatment of infectious disease is to assist the body in overcoming the infecting organism. This is accomplished by the use of an anti-infective agent which is toxic to the causative organism while the normal biochemical functions of the patient are not seriously impaired.

When selecting the anti-infective agent, consideration must be given to the dose, route and frequency of administration. The dosage regimen for antibiotics excreted primarily by the kidneys will be decided according to the type of infection to be treated and the toxicity of the drug. The dose of antibiotics with a narrow therapeutic spectrum, such as the aminoglycosides, requires to be titrated according to the serum concentration. This is in order to maintain an effective therapeutic level but avoid toxic effects due to too high a level. Where renal dysfunction is present – which results in a longer half-life – dosage schedules should be lowered accordingly to prevent toxicity.

Route of administration

If the infection is severe, the general condition of the patient may be poor. Oral absorption may therefore be ineffective owing to nausea, vomiting or gastric stasis. In these instances, antibiotics are commonly administered by injection. After the infection is under control, appropriate concentrations will be maintained by the oral route as this is more cost-effective and easier to administer.

Many antibiotic injections are presented as a sterile powder requiring reconstitution prior to administration. The nurse should refer to the manufacturer's product insert and to local policies in order to reconstitute the drug with correct diluent and the correct volume. Strict aseptic technique should be followed. It is advisable to discard any remaining solution after the initial dose has been withdrawn to avoid possible contamination or deterioration of the remaining solution.

Routine prophylaxis

Routine antibiotic prophylaxis in surgical patients is needed only for those procedures associated with a high risk of postoperative infection (e.g. vaginal or colorectal surgery) or prosthetic insertions. Normally, prophylactic antibiotic treatment should not be extended beyond 48 hours following surgery and should be given parenterally. Intravenous administration during induction, or intramuscular administration 30 minutes before surgery, usually ensures effective blood levels of antibiotic at the time when anticipated bacteraemia is likely to be highest. When gastrointestinal function is unimpaired during the postoperative period, oral administration of antibiotics provides an optimum non-invasive approach.

Allergic responses

An accurate history of previous allergies is essential before antibiotics are administered. This applies particularly to penicillins with which anaphylactic shock occasionally occurs. Patients with a history of asthma, hay fever and eczema are more likely to experience severe reactions to penicillins. Some patients allergic to penicillins will also be allergic to cephalosporins. If patients are not allergic to penicillins, they are safe drugs.

Monitoring the patient's response

The patient's response to antibiotic therapy is monitored with regard to (i) controlling the infection and (ii) adverse effects.

Specific toxic effects of antibiotics should be noted, for example hearing or renal impairment in patients receiving aminoglycosides. Phlebitis can occur on intravenous administration, and the nurse should monitor the patient's veins carefully for evidence of redness, swelling or pain and report these to the doctor. Where blood samples are taken, the doctor should ensure that times are recorded accurately so that maximum and minimum drug concentrations during the dosing interval can be accurately estimated.

Superinfection

Superinfection may occur as a result of:

- Proliferation of a resistant microorganism in place of the original sensitive microorganism at the site of infection.
- Proliferation of a resistant microorganism in the alimentary tract owing to suppression of the normal flora by antibiotic therapy. The broader the spectrum, the greater is the possibility of superinfection developing. Tetracyclines and ampicillin are examples. Pseudomembranous colitis results as an overgrowth of *Clostridium difficile* in the bowel presenting as watery diarrhoea, abdominal cramping, fever and leucocytosis. The most common treatment is oral vancomycin.
- Drugs interfering with the immune response of the body, for example, corticosteroids and other immunosuppressive agents. Oral candidiasis, caused by *Candida albicans*, is the commonest example. This can be treated effectively with nystatin suspension.

Bacterial resistance to antibiotics

The resistance of bacteria to antibiotics is a problem that has continued to grow in parallel with the development of new antibiotics. Bacterial resistance reflects antibiotic use and is more of a problem where controls on antibiotic use are lax. The sensible use of antibiotics guards against this. There are several mechanisms by which resistance may emerge.

Selection

An antibiotic will eliminate the sensitive organisms within a bacterial population, and the resistant forms will proliferate.

Mutation

Resistance to an antibiotic may develop as a result of the spontaneous appearance of mutants during the process of cell division. These mutants will then proliferate.

Transferred resistance

Resistance may be acquired by the transfer of genetic material which confers antibiotic resistance from one organism to another. This may be achieved by (i) *transduction*, involving the transfer of genes contained within bacteriophages (viruses which infect bacteria); (ii) *conjugation*, involving the transfer of genes contained within plasmids. Transfer of plasmids is not confined to the same species and they can be passed from, for example, *Escherichia coli* to *Salmonella*. Either way, new DNA enters the bacterium and codes for a mechanism which confers resistance. Such mechanisms involve:

- Enzymatic inactivation of the antibiotic. The bacterium produces enzymes that inactivate the antibiotic by altering its chemical structure. For example, the enzymes responsible for destroying penicillins and cephalosporins are called β-lactamases; these enzymes are found in Gram-negative bacteria such as *Escherichia coli, Salmonella* spp. and *Pseudomonas* spp. and in Gram-positive bacteria, e.g. staphylococci. These enzymes open up the β-lactam ring of the penicillin, which is the portion responsible for antimicrobial activity. Aminoglycoside resistance is often due to a similar mechanism where bacteria produce enzymes that alter the chemical structure of the aminoglycoside.
- Altered permeability of the bacterium to the drug. Some bacteria reduce the permeability of their cell membrane to antibiotics such as aminoglycosides or tetracycline so that less antibiotic is able to enter and bind to its target.
- Formation of alternative metabolic pathway. Sulphonamides and trimethoprim act by inhibiting the folate metabolic pathways within bacteria. However, where bacterial enzymes are produced that are much less inhibited by these two agents, resistance occurs.

The general spread of antibiotic resistance is most likely to occur in an environment in which there is a significant use of antibiotics and the opportunity to move from one host to another exists. In an environment where little use is made of antibiotics there will be no selective advantage for the resistant bacteria. Where antibiotics are used in low dose there will be greater opportunity for resistance to develop and spread, since strains will survive at low dose which would have been eliminated at a higher dose. An example of this is the huge increase in the level of resistance in *Salmonella* due to the use of low-dose antibiotics as growth-enhancers in farm animals. The cost of resistance is measured not only in terms of failure of therapy but also in the increased costs of more expensive drugs needed to combat the resistant bacteria.

In parts of the USA, there are now pneumococci that are 100% resistant to penicillin as well as to erythromycin, cefalexin, methicillin and all other antibiotics except vancomycin. Other examples of resistance emerging in the last 15 years include tuberculosis resistant to isoniazid and rifampicin, multidrug-resistant salmonella, vancomycin-resistant enterococcus and methicillin-resistant *Staphylococcus aureus* (MRSA).

Methicillin-resistant *Staphylococcus aureus* (MRSA)

Approximately 30% of the population carry the organism *Staphylococcus aureus* (*S. aureus*). This is a bacterium that is normally found in the nose and on skin. Although most healthy people are unaffected by it, it does have the potential to cause infection in those who have severely reduced resistance, e.g. some ill patients in hospital.

MRSA is a form of *S. aureus*. It is transmitted in the same way and causes the same range of infections as other strains of *S. aureus*. However, it has developed resistance to the more commonly used antibiotics. This makes infections caused by MRSA more difficult and costly to treat and every effort should be made to prevent its spread.

The majority of individuals are *colonised* where the organism lives harmlessly on the body with no ill effects as opposed to *infected* which is when the organism penetrates tissue and causes disease.

In order to control and minimise the spread of MRSA there must be compliance with the following:

- universal infection control precautions, e.g. thorough hand hygiene
- cleaning of an acceptable standard
- adherence to infection control policies, e.g. isolation, clinical waste, laundry
- education on infection control policy
- strict adherence to antibiotic policy
- minimal movement of patients and staff between wards, units and hospitals.

Treatment of MRSA infection

Patients who demonstrate clinical signs of infection will require treatment with the appropriate antibiotics. The agent used will depend on the site of infection (Table 19.3). Some of these organisms are sensitive only to vancomycin or teicoplanin. Strains may be susceptible to rifampicin, sodium fusidate, tetracyclines, aminoglycosides and macrolides. Treatment is guided by the sensitivity of the infecting strain.

Table 19.3 Decolonisation

Site	Treatment
Nasal carriage only	Nasal decolonisation only
Throat carriage	Nasal and throat decolonisation
Axilla or groin carriage	Nasal and body decolonisation

Nasal decolonisation

Nasal carriage treatment is to apply with a cotton bud, mupirocin 2% nasal ointment three times daily to the inner surface of each nostril for 5 days. Where mupirocin resistance is encountered, second-line treatment is with neomycin and chlorhexidine cream (Naseptin) provided the organism is neomycin susceptible.

Throat decolonisation

First-line treatment is chlorhexidine gluconate using the mouthwash (0.2%), spray (0.2%) or gel (1%) as appropriate. Oral hygiene is very important as teeth and dentures may harbour MRSA. Where this treatment is unsuccessful, oral trimethoprim (200 mg twice daily) and sodium fusidate tablets (500 mg three times daily) should be used for 5 days. In the event of resistance or patient intolerance an alternative is a combination of oral rifampicin (600 mg once daily) and co-trimoxazole (two tablets twice daily) for 5 days. Rifampicin or sodium fusidate should not be used alone because resistance may develop rapidly.

Skin decolonisation

Treatment consists of a direct application of 4% chlorhexidine to all skin using a damp disposable cloth daily for 5 days using the chlorhexidine as a soap substitute and then rinsing it off. The hair should be washed with chlorhexidine twice during the 5-day period. Alternatively, 2% triclosan or 7.5% povidone-iodine could be used. Hair conditioners and body lotions can be used after treatment if required.

Linezolid and quinupristin with dalfopristin

Linezolid and the combination of quinupristin and dalfopristin are active against MRSA but these antibacterial drugs should be reserved for organisms resistant to other antibacterials or for patients who cannot tolerate other antibacterial drugs. Linezolid is available both orally (600 mg every 12 hours) and by intravenous infusion. Thrombocytopenia, anaemia, leucopenia and pancytopenia have been reported and weekly monitoring of full blood counts is recommended. Quinupristin with dalfopristin is available as an intravenous infusion.

THE PENICILLINS

The penicillins are bactericidal and interfere with cell wall synthesis in growing and dividing bacteria. Lysis and cell death result from weakening of the cell wall. Penicillins are excreted in the urine in therapeutic concentrations.

The most significant and adverse effect of the penicillins is hypersensitivity which manifests as rashes and, on occasion, anaphylaxis. Allergy to one penicillin indicates allergy to them all, since the hypersensitivity is related to the basic penicillin structure.

Excessively high serum levels due to either very high doses or renal failure in patients given normal doses may give rise to encephalopathy, a rare but serious toxic effect due to cerebral irritation. The penicillins should not be given by intrathecal injection as this can cause encephalopathy which may be fatal. A second problem is accumulation of electrolyte since most injectable penicillins contain either sodium or potassium.

Diarrhoea often occurs during oral penicillin therapy.

Benzylpenicillin and phenoxymethylpenicillin

Benzylpenicillin (penicillin G) is readily inactivated by gastric acid juice and is given by injection. It diffuses into most of the body tissues but does not pass the blood–brain barrier unless the meninges are inflamed; neither does it penetrate well into the pleural cavity nor into the synovial or ocular fluids. It is inactivated by bacterial penicillinases. Penicillinases are enzymes which inactivate penicillin by attacking part of the penicillin molecule known as the β-lactam ring. This structure is an essential part of penicillins and cephalosporins, and the family of enzymes involved is known as the β-lactamases. Notable producers of penicillinase are staphylococci.

Benzylpenicillin is effective in a wide range of infections, including those shown in Table 19.4.

Phenoxymethylpenicillin (penicillin V) has a similar but less active antibacterial spectrum. It is indicated principally for respiratory infections in children, streptococcal tonsillitis and continued treatment following benzylpenicillin injection. It is used as a prophylactic against reinfection after recovery from rheumatic fever. Phenoxymethylpenicillin is not destroyed in the stomach and is quickly but unpredictably absorbed from the small intestine. Absorption is superior when administered on an empty stomach. Phenoxymethylpenicillin is not suitable for the treatment of severe conditions where high blood levels of penicillin are necessary.

The dose range and side-effects of benzylpenicillin and phenoxymethylpenicillin are shown in Table 19.5.

Penicillinase-resistant penicillins

Some organisms are resistant to penicillin because of their ability to produce the enzyme penicillinase, which destroys penicillin. Flucloxacillin is available for treatment of staphylococcal infections where resistant organisms are particularly common (see Table 19.6). Flucloxacillin is available in oral as well as injectable form and is well absorbed.

Table 19.4 Infections for which benzylpenicillin is effective

Organism	Disease
β-haemolytic streptococci	Septicaemia, tonsillitis
Viridans streptococci	Subacute bacterial endocarditis
Streptococcus pneumoniae	Pneumonia
Neisseria meningitidis	Meningococcal meningitis
Clostridium tetani	Tetanus
Clostridium perfringens	Gas gangrene
Treponema pallidum	Syphilis
Neisseria gonorrhoeae	Gonorrhoea
Borrelia burgdorferi	Lyme disease

Table 19.6 Penicillinase-resistant penicillin

Drug	Adult dose range	Notes
Flucloxacillin	Oral: 250 mg 6-hourly at least 30 minutes before food. Intramuscular: 250 mg 6-hourly. Slow intravenous injection or infusion: 0.25–1 g every 6 hours	Side-effects as for benzylpenicillin. Doses can be doubled in severe infections

Table 19.5 Benzylpenicillin and phenoxymethylpenicillin

Drug	Adult dose range	Onset of peak serum levels	Side-effects
Benzylpenicillin	By IM or slow IV injection or by infusion: 2.4–4.8 g daily in four divided doses. Bacterial endocarditis – slow IV injection or by infusion: 7.2 g daily in divided doses. Meningitis – slow IV injection or by infusion: 2.4 g every 4 hours	15–30 minutes	Sensitivity reactions including urticaria, fever, joint pains, anaphylactic shock, diarrhoea after oral administration
Phenoxymethylpenicillin	500 mg–1 g every 6 hours half an hour before food	30–60 minutes	As for benzylpenicillin

Broad-spectrum penicillins

This group includes ampicillin and amoxicillin. The main difference between ampicillin and amoxicillin is in absorption from the gut. Less than half the dose of ampicillin is absorbed from the gut and this is decreased by the presence of food. About 40% passes into the large bowel, and diarrhoea, a common side-effect, is thought to be caused by a disturbance of the large bowel flora. Amoxicillin is better absorbed, producing higher plasma and tissue concentrations, absorption not being affected by the presence of food in the stomach. Both of these drugs are inactivated by penicillinases, including those produced by almost all staphylococci, 50% of *E. coli* strains and 15% of *Haemophilus influenzae* strains. They should not be used for hospital patients without checking sensitivity.

Co-amoxiclav is a combination of amoxicillin and a β-lactamase inhibitor, clavulanic acid. The clavulanate molecules penetrate the bacterial cell and combine with the β-lactamase molecules. This inactivates the β-lactamases, leaving the amoxicillin free to exert a full bactericidal effect. This makes the combination active against penicillinase-producing bacteria that are resistant to amoxicillin – *Staphylococcus aureus*, *E. coli* and *Haemophilus influenzae* as well as many *Bacteroides* and *Klebsiella* species. The broad-spectrum penicillins are summarised in Table 19.7.

Antipseudomonal penicillins

Ticarcillin is active against *Pseudomonas aeruginosa*, *Proteus* spp. and *Bacteroides fragilis* and, because of its combination with clavulanic acid, is active against penicillinase-producing bacteria.

Piperacillin has a broad spectrum and is active against *Pseudomonas aeruginosa*. These drugs are used in pseudomonal septicaemias. In those life-threatening conditions, it is preferable to give them in combination with an aminoglycoside such as gentamicin as this combination is synergistic. This group of penicillins can be given only by injection.

The antipseudomonal penicillins are summarised in Table 19.8.

CEPHALOSPORINS AND CEPHAMYCINS

The cephalosporins were first obtained from a mould cultured from the sea near a Sardinian sewage outfall in 1945. The cephalosporins are related to the penicillins – both have a β-lactam ring which confers on them a similar mode of action. They act, like the penicillins, by inhibiting bacterial cell-wall synthesis.

The cephalosporins are broad-spectrum antibiotics. They are used in the treatment of septicaemia, pneumonia, meningitis, biliary tract infections, peritonitis and urinary tract infections. All have a similar antibacterial spectrum, although individual agents have differing activity against certain organisms. Although cephalosporins are resistant to the penicillinase β-lactamases, cross-resistance between penicillinase-resistant penicillins and cephalosporins occurs.

The principal side-effect of the cephalosporins is hypersensitivity, and about 10% of penicillin-sensitive patients will be allergic to cephalosporins. Allergic

Table 19.8 The antipseudomonal penicillins

Drug	Adult dose range	Side-effects
Piperacillin	IM, IV injection and infusion: 100–150 mg/kg daily in divided doses doubled for serious infections	As for benzylpenicillin
Ticarcillin with clavulanic acid	IV injection or infusion: 15–20 g daily in divided doses	As for benzylpenicillin

Table 19.7 Broad-spectrum penicillins

Drug	Indications	Adult dose	Side-effects
Amoxicillin	As for ampicillin, plus typhoid fever and endocarditis prophylaxis	Oral: 250–500 mg every 8 hours. IM: 500 mg every 8 hours. IV: 500 mg every 8 hours, increased to 1 g every 6 hours	As for ampicillin
Ampicillin	Urinary tract infections, otitis media, sinusitis, chronic bronchitis, gonorrhoea	Oral: 0.25–1 g every 6 hours at least 30 minutes before food. IM, IV: 500 mg every 4–6 hours	Nausea, diarrhoea, rashes
Co-amoxiclav	Infections due to β-lactamase-producing strains (where amoxicillin alone not appropriate) including respiratory tract infections, genitourinary and abdominal infections, cellulitis, animal bites and severe dental infections	Expressed as amoxicillin 250–500 mg every 8 hours. IV injection or infusion: 1 g every 8 hours	As for ampicillin

reactions include rashes, pruritus, urticaria, fever and anaphylaxis. Other side-effects include diarrhoea, nausea, vomiting, erythema multiforme, eosinophilia and transient hepatitis.

Oral cephalosporins

The oral 'first-generation' cephalosporins, cefalexin, cefradine and cefadroxil and the 'second-generation' cephalosporins, cefaclor and cefprozil, have a similar antimicrobial spectrum. They are useful for urinary tract infections which do not respond to other drugs or which occur in pregnancy, respiratory tract infections, otitis media, sinusitis, and skin and soft tissue infections. Cefaclor has good activity against *H. influenzae* but it is associated with protracted skin reactions especially in children. Cefadroxil has a long duration of action and can be given twice daily; it has poor activity against *H. influenzae*. Cefuroxime axetil, an ester of the 'second-generation' cephalosporin cefuroxime, has the same antibacterial spectrum as the parent compound; it is poorly absorbed.

Cefixime has a longer duration of action than the other cephalosporins that are active by mouth. It is presently only licensed for acute infections.

Cefpodoxime is more active than the other oral cephalosporins against respiratory bacterial pathogens and it is licensed for upper and lower respiratory tract infections.

The side-effects of the oral cephalosporins include diarrhoea, nausea and vomiting, abdominal discomfort, headache and allergic reactions such as rashes, pruritus and urticaria.

Eight oral cephalosporins are listed in Table 19.9.

Table 19.9 Oral cephalosporins

Drug	Adult dose
Cefaclor	250–500 mg every 8 hours
Cefadroxil	0.5–1 g twice daily
Cefalexin	250 mg every 6 hours; 1–1.5 g every 6 or 8 hours for severe infections
Cefixime	200–400 mg daily as a single dose or in two divided doses
Cefpodoxime	Upper respiratory tract infections: 100 mg twice daily with food (200 mg twice daily in sinusitis)
	Lower respiratory tract infections (including bronchitis and pneumonia): 100–200 mg twice daily with food
Cefprozil	500 mg daily for upper respiratory tract infections. Acute bronchitis: 500 mg every 12 hours
Cefradine	250–500 mg every 6 hours
Cefuroxime axetil	250 mg twice daily

Parenteral cephalosporins

In general, cefradine and cefazolin have been replaced by newer cephalosporins. Cefuroxime and cefamandole are less susceptible than first-generation cephalosporins to inactivation by penicillinase and have greater activity against *Haemophilus influenzae* and *Neisseria gonorrhoeae*.

Cefoxitin is active against bowel flora including *Bacteroides fragilis*, and because of this is recommended for abdominal sepsis such as peritonitis.

Cefotaxime, ceftazidime and ceftriaxone are third-generation cephalosporins. They have a markedly increased activity against certain Gram-negative bacteria. However, they are less active than cefuroxime and cefamandole against Gram-positive bacteria, most notably *Staphylococcus aureus*, and superinfection may occur with resistant bacteria. Ceftazidime possesses good activity against *Pseudomonas* and is also active against other Gram-negative bacteria. Ceftriaxone requires only once-daily administration owing to its longer half-life. It has potent bactericidal activity against a wide spectrum of Gram-positive and particularly Gram-negative organisms. Indications include serious infections such as septicaemia, pneumonia and meningitis. Cefpirome has been recently introduced for treating urinary tract, lower respiratory tract and skin infections, bacteraemia and infections associated with neutropenia.

Parenteral cephalosporins are summarised in Table 19.10, and some other β-lactam antibiotics are given in Table 19.11.

TETRACYCLINES

The most commonly used members of the tetracycline family are chlortetracycline, demeclocycline, doxycycline, minocycline, oxytetracycline and tetracycline.

Mode of action. The tetracyclines are generally bacteriostatic rather than bactericidal in action. They inhibit protein synthesis in bacterial ribosomes in susceptible organisms, thus preventing production of polypeptides.

Uses. Tetracyclines have a broad antimicrobial spectrum and demonstrate activity against most Gram-positive organisms that are sensitive to the penicillins and also against some Gram-negative organisms that are not susceptible to the penicillins. Table 19.12 lists some of the infectious diseases for which tetracyclines may be indicated. They are also used for the treatment of exacerbations of chronic bronchitis because of their activity against *Haemophilus influenzae*. Microbiologically, there is little to choose between the various tetracyclines. Minocycline is an exception since it has a

Table 19.10 Parenteral cephalosporins

Drug	Indications	Dose
Cefamandole	See cefotaxime	0.5–2 g every 4–8 hours
	Surgical prophylaxis	1–2 g 30–60 minutes before surgery and then 1–2 g 6-hourly for up to 3 days
Cefazolin	See cefotaxime. Surgical prophylaxis	0.5–1 g every 6–12 hours
Cefotaxime	Infections due to sensitive Gram-positive and Gram-negative organisms	1 g every 12 hours. Increased for life-threatening infections up to 12 g in divided doses
Cefoxitin	See cefotaxime. Surgical prophylaxis, more active against Gram-negative organisms	1–2 g every 6–8 hours, increased to maximum 12 g daily in divided doses
Cefpirome	See cefotaxime	1–2 g every 12 hours
Cefradine	See cefotaxime. Surgical prophylaxis	0.5–1 g every 6 hours. Increased in severe infections
Ceftazidime	See cefotaxime. Active against *Pseudomonas aeruginosa*	1 g every 8 hours. Increased in severe infections
Ceftriaxone	See cefuroxime	1 g daily. Severe infections 2–4 g. Gonorrhoea: 250 mg as a single dose. Once-daily dosing facilitates a single dose in surgical prophylaxis – 1 g
Cefuroxime	See cefotaxime	750 mg every 6–8 hours. Increased in severe infections
	Surgical prophylaxis	1.5 g IV at induction followed by 750 mg 8 and 16 hours later (orthopaedic)
	More active against *H. influenzae* and *N. gonorrhoeae*	Gonorrhoea: 1.5 g IM as single dose

Table 19.11 Other β-lactam parenteral antibiotics

Drug	Indications	Side-effects	Dose
Aztreonam	Gram-negative infections, including *Pseudomonas aeruginosa, Haemophilus influenzae, Neisseria meningitidis, Neisseria gonorrhoeae*	Nausea, vomiting, diarrhoea, abdominal cramps, mouth ulcers, urticaria and rashes	1 g every 8 hours or 2 g every 12 hours
Imipenem with cilastatin (cilastatin inhibits inactivation of imipenem by kidney enzymes)	Aerobic and anaerobic Gram-positive and Gram-negative infections, surgical prophylaxis	Nausea, vomiting, diarrhoea, fever, anaphylactic reactions, allergic reactions, blood disorders	IM: 500–750 mg every 12 hours. IV infusion: 1–2 g daily in divided doses
Meropenem	Aerobic and anaerobic Gram-positive and Gram-negative infections	Nausea, vomiting, diarrhoea, abdominal pain	500 mg–1 g every 8 hours; meningitis: 2 g every 8 hours

Table 19.12 Main indications for the use of tetracyclines

Disease	Organism
Infections caused by chlamydia	
psittacosis	*Chlamydia psittaci*
lymphogranuloma venereum	LGV chlamydiae
trachoma	*Chlamydia trachomatis*
non-specific urethritis	*Chlamydia* and *Ureaplasma* spp.
Q fever	*Coxiella burnetii*
Typhus diseases	*Rickettsia* spp.
Mycoplasma pneumonia	*Mycoplasma pneumoniae*
Brucellosis (doxycycline with rifampicin)	*Brucella abortus*
Lyme disease	*Borrelia burgdorferi*

broader spectrum of activity, is active against *Neisseria meningitidis* and has been used in the prevention of meningococcal meningitis as an alternative to rifampicin. Tetracyclines may also be used in the treatment of acne vulgaris (p. 443).

Pharmacokinetics. The tetracyclines in general are reasonably well absorbed (about 70%), minocycline and doxycycline being absorbed to a greater extent (about 90%). The concomitant administration of milk, agents such as antacids containing aluminium, magnesium or calcium, and iron salts reduces absorption from the gastrointestinal tract because of the formation of insoluble chelates and should be avoided. The tetracyclines are widely distributed to body tissues and are taken up in teeth and bone, especially growing bone and teeth

Table 19.13 Dosages of tetracyclines

Drug	Dose
Demeclocycline	150 mg every 6 hours
Doxycycline	200 mg initially then 100 mg daily
Minocycline	100 mg twice daily
Oxytetracycline	250–500 mg 6-hourly
Tetracycline	Oral: 250–500 mg 6-hourly

during the early stages of calcification. This can cause both discoloration and enamel hypoplasia in teeth and decreased growth of long bones. Tetracyclines should therefore not be given in pregnancy or to children under 12 years of age.

Approximately 50% of most tetracyclines are excreted in the urine unchanged. Renal failure causes decreased clearance and accumulation, resulting in toxicity. Minocycline and doxycycline are exceptions, being metabolised mainly in the liver, and doxycycline is the tetracycline of choice in compromised renal function.

Adverse effects. Tetracyclines commonly produce gastrointestinal adverse effects, e.g. nausea, vomiting and diarrhoea. A rarely occurring condition is superinfection with *Clostridium difficile*, resulting in pseudomembranous colitis. Oral superinfection with *Candida albicans* may result in thrush. Overgrowth in the bowel may cause diarrhoea. Treatment consists of stopping the administration of tetracycline and, in severe cases, treatment with nystatin. Minocycline, in addition, can cause dizziness, vertigo and severe exfoliative rashes.

Dosage. The dosages of the tetracyclines (see Table 19.13) vary, and this is partly accountable to different half-lives, e.g. oxytetracycline, tetracycline 8 hours, demeclocycline 14 hours, minocycline and doxycycline 18 hours.

AMINOGLYCOSIDES

This group of drugs includes amikacin, gentamicin, neomycin, netilmicin, streptomycin and tobramycin.

Mode of action. The aminoglycosides are bactericidal. The mechanism is not fully understood but they inhibit the synthesis of bacterial protein by binding to ribosomes within the organism.

Uses. The aminoglycosides are active against some Gram-positive and many Gram-negative organisms. Examples of bacteria which are sensitive to the aminoglycosides are given in Table 19.14.

Table 19.14 Examples of bacteria which are sensitive to aminoglycosides

Bacteria	Disease	Aminoglycoside
Gram-positive cocci	Streptococcal endocarditis	Gentamicin in combination with penicillin G
Gram-negative bacilli	Infections due to *Escherichia coli*, *Klebsiella pneumoniae*, *Proteus*, *Pseudomonas*	Amikacin, gentamicin, tobramycin
Mycobacteria	Tuberculosis	Streptomycin

Gentamicin is the most important aminoglycoside and is used for the treatment of serious infections including septicaemia, meningitis, pyelonephritis and endocarditis. The main indication for amikacin is the treatment of serious infections caused by Gram-negative bacilli resistant to gentamicin. Neomycin is not significantly absorbed following oral administration and is used for bowel sterilisation prior to bowel surgery. The aminoglycosides are effective agents for the local treatment of infections of the external ear and conjunctiva. Neomycin, which is too toxic for parenteral administration, framycetin and gentamicin are commonly used. Neomycin is also used, in combination with chlorhexidine, for attempted eradication of staphylococci in the nasal passage.

Pharmacokinetics. The aminoglycosides are poorly absorbed from the gastrointestinal tract and must be given by injection for systemic infections. They have a narrow therapeutic spectrum and plasma concentration monitoring ensures that optimal therapeutic levels are maintained, thus preventing toxicity and ensuring efficacy. Plasma concentrations should be measured approximately 1 hour after injection (peak level) and just before the next dose (trough level).

Parenterally administered aminoglycosides are excreted almost entirely by the kidneys. Care should be taken with dosage and, where possible, treatment should not exceed 7 days in order to minimise side-effects. Doses should be reduced in renal failure.

Adverse effects. The important side-effects are ototoxicity and, to a lesser degree, nephrotoxicity. These occur most commonly in the elderly and in patients with renal failure because of elevated serum levels, i.e. trough levels greater than 2 micrograms/mL and peak levels greater than 12 micrograms/mL (gentamicin). Long duration of treatment is also a causative factor. Gentamicin tends to cause vertigo and ataxia while neomycin causes deafness. Neomycin is too toxic for systemic use. Aminoglycosides should be avoided in pregnancy as they cross the placenta and cause damage to the eighth nerve of the fetus. Aminoglycosides may impair neuromuscular transmission

Table 19.15 Dosages of aminoglycosides

Drug	Dose
Amikacin	IM, slow IV injection or IV infusion: 15 mg/kg daily in two divided doses
Gentamicin	IM, slow IV injection or intravenous infusion: 2.5 mg/kg daily in divided doses 8-hourly (monitor serum level, and creatinine clearance in renal impairment)
Neomycin	1 g every 4 hours for bowel sterilisation
Netilmicin	IM, slow IV injection or IV infusion: 4–6 mg/kg daily; for urinary tract infection 150 mg as single daily dose for 5 days; gonorrhoea 300 mg as a single dose
Tobramycin	IM, slow IV injection or IV infusion: 3 mg/kg daily in divided doses every 8 hours; urinary tract infection, by IM injection 2–3 mg/kg daily as a single dose

and should not be given to patients with myasthenia gravis.

Interactions. Aminoglycosides should not be given with furosemide (frusemide) as this may potentiate the ototoxic and nephrotoxic effects.

Dosages. The dosages of aminoglycosides are summarised in Table 19.15.

MACROLIDES

This group of drugs includes erythromycin, clarithromycin and azithromycin.

Erythromycin

Mode of action. Erythromycin is classified as a bacteriostatic drug but it may be bactericidal in high concentrations or against highly susceptible organisms. Erythromycin inhibits protein synthesis in susceptible organisms by binding to ribosomes and inhibiting polypeptide synthesis. Resistance is rarely observed during successful short-term treatment.

Uses. Erythromycin has an antibacterial spectrum similar to that of benzylpenicillin and is used for infections in which benzylpenicillin would be the treatment of choice but where the patient is sensitive to penicillin. Erythromycin is indicated for respiratory infections, whooping cough, Legionnaire's disease (*Legionella pneumophila*), chlamydia and mycoplasmas.

Pharmacokinetics. Erythromycin may be administered orally or by injection. Oral formulations containing the erythromycin base are enteric-coated as the base is decomposed by gastric acid. The enteric coating breaks down in the higher pH of the duodenum and the erythromycin is absorbed. The stearate, and ethylsuccinate forms of erythromycin are not acid-labile. They dissociate in the duodenum, liberating active erythromycin which is absorbed. Following absorption, erythromycin is widely distributed in the tissues. It penetrates the meninges only when they are inflamed. The drug is excreted primarily in the bile. Erythromycin may be given intravenously as the lactobionate.

Adverse effects. Erythromycin is one of the safest and least toxic of the antibiotics. The most common side-effects of the oral erythromycins are gastrointestinal and are dose-related. These include nausea, vomiting, diarrhoea and abdominal discomfort after large doses. Azithromycin and clarithromycin cause fewer gastrointestinal side-effects than erythromycin. The intravenous injection of erythromycin causes venous irritation and thrombophlebitis, particularly in high doses. It is recommended that the drug be well diluted and infused slowly over 20–60 minutes to minimise these effects, or, alternatively, to use clarithromycin.

Dosage. Orally, 250–1000 mg four times daily; intravenously 25–50 mg/kg daily.

Clarithromycin

Clarithromycin is a derivative of erythromycin with similar actions and uses. It is acid stable and so has a greater degree of bioavailability.

Adverse effects. Headache, rash and gastrointestinal disturbances are side-effects. Care is necessary in renal and hepatic impairment.

Dosage. Clarithromycin is given in doses of 250 mg twice a day for 7 days, doubled in severe infections, with treatment continued if necessary for 14 days. It may also be given by intravenous infusion in divided doses of 1 g daily for 5–7 days.

Azithromycin

Azithromycin is chemically related to erythromycin but it is more acid-stable. It is well absorbed after oral administration, giving high tissue levels which decline slowly and so permit single daily doses. It is effective in many soft tissue infections, bronchitis and atypical pneumonia. Such pneumonia, caused by *Mycoplasma* and similar organisms, is becoming more common and resistant to many antibiotics. The invading organisms migrate to the phagocytes, and azithromycin appears to be concentrated in the phagocytes to a greater degree than erythromycin.

Adverse effects. Gastrointestinal disturbances are the main side-effect. It is contraindicated in hepatic disease.

Dosage. It is given in single daily doses of 500 mg for 3 days, 1 hour before or after food.

CLINDAMYCIN

Clindamycin acts by inhibiting bacterial protein synthesis. It has restricted use owing to the significant side-effects, in particular pseudomembranous colitis, which may be fatal. The drug should be immediately discontinued if diarrhoea or colitis develops.

Clindamycin is active against Gram-positive cocci (streptococci, penicillin-resistant staphylococci), Gram-negative bacilli (*Bacteroides*) and Gram-positive bacilli (*Clostridium* spp.). Because of the adverse effects, clindamycin is generally reserved for staphylococcal bone and joint infections, peritonitis and endocarditis prophylaxis, and topically for severe acne.

Adverse effects. Adverse effects due to clindamycin include abdominal discomfort, nausea, vomiting, diarrhoea and pseudomembranous colitis, jaundice and blood dyscrasias. It may cause thrombophlebitis following an intravenous injection.

Dosage. Oral therapy, 150–450 mg every 6 hours. Deep intramuscular injection, 0.6–2.7 g daily in two to four divided doses. Single dose above 600 mg by intravenous infusion only.

OTHER ANTIBIOTICS

A number of other antibiotics are described in Table 19.16.

SULPHONAMIDES AND TRIMETHOPRIM

The first of the sulphonamides was used in the treatment of infections in the 1930s. However, the importance of sulphonamides in this role has decreased in recent years as a result of increasing bacterial resistance and replacement by more effective and less toxic antibiotics.

A combination of trimethoprim one part and sulfamethoxazole five parts (co-trimoxazole) has been used because of the synergistic activity of these drugs. However, co-trimoxazole is associated with rare but serious side-effects including blood dyscrasias notably bone-marrow depression and agranulocytosis, especially in the elderly. Its use is therefore restricted. It is the drug of choice in *Pneumocystis carinii* infection and it is also indicated for toxoplasmosis and nocardiasis. Trimethoprim can be used alone for urinary and respiratory tract infections and for prostatitis, shigellosis and invasive salmonella infections. Although similar to co-trimoxazole, the side-effects of trimethoprim are less severe and occur less frequently.

Mode of action. The sulphonamides are bacteriostatic and act by preventing the conversion of para-aminobenzoic acid to folic acid. Trimethoprim blocks bacterial folic acid synthesis at the stage immediately following that blocked by the sulphonamides, as shown in Box 19.2.

Pharmacokinetics. Individual sulphonamides differ markedly in their absorption, distribution and excretion. Sulfamethoxazole and sulfadiazine are generally well absorbed. Metabolism is very variable, the major route being acetylation in the liver. Variability is due to the fact that the population can be divided into two groups – those which acetylate the drug rapidly and those which acetylate slowly. This characteristic is genetically determined. The acetylated drug, which is excreted in the urine, has a low solubility and there is a danger that it will precipitate in the urine (crystalluria). Renal damage may occur due to precipitation in the renal tubules. Crystalluria may cause pain and haematuria. Anuria can occur if the renal pelvis or the ureters become completely occluded. A high intake of fluid helps to minimise this side-effect.

Trimethoprim is rapidly absorbed. It is excreted mainly in the urine, and dosages should be reduced in renal failure. Crystalluria does not occur.

Adverse effects. Allergic reactions are common, their incidence increasing with increased dosage. These include maculopapular skin rashes, drug fever and photodermatitis. Occasionally blood dyscrasias may occur, including thrombocytopenia, agranulocytosis and leucopenia. Crystalluria, which was a problem with the older, less-soluble sulphonamides, does not occur with sulfamethoxazole. Nausea, vomiting and diarrhoea may occur. Special care should be taken where folate may be deficient, e.g. the elderly, chronic sick and those on prolonged treatment or high doses. Because of the possibility of jaundice and kernicterus (deposition of bilirubin in the brains of neonates), sulphonamides should not be given to pregnant women particularly in the third trimester or to newborn or premature infants. Side-effects which may occur with trimethoprim include nausea, vomiting, pruritus and rashes.

The dosages of co-trimoxazole and trimethoprim are summarised in Table 19.17.

TUBERCULOSIS

Tuberculosis is an infection caused by the bacterium *Mycobacterium tuberculosis*. In humans, the lung is the most common site of infection, although numerous other areas (meninges, bones, joints, peritoneum, genitourinary tract, skin) may also become infected.

Tuberculosis is spread by airborne droplets, from coughing and sneezing, which contain viable bacilli. These are inhaled and lodge in the alveoli where the bacilli rapidly multiply. On primary infection, the bacilli

Table 19.16 Other antibiotics

Indications	Pharmacokinetics	Adverse reactions	Dose
Chloramphenicol Only for life-threatening infections because of toxicity, e.g. meningitis due to *Haemophilus influenzae*, typhoid fever. Eye drops useful for bacterial conjunctivitis	Well absorbed from GI tract	Blood disorders, including aplastic anaemia caused by severe depression of bone marrow activity, nausea, vomiting, diarrhoea. 'Grey syndrome' in neonates, i.e. vomiting, respiratory depression, cyanosis and collapse associated with a reduced ability of the infant to metabolise and excrete choramphenicol	50 mg/kg daily in four divided doses
Colistin Bacterial in action, it is active against Gram-negative organisms, including *Escherichia coli*, *Klebsiella* spp. and *Pseudomonas aeruginosa*	Not absorbed from the GI tract so must be given IM or IV for treatment of systemic infections. However, it is toxic and seldom used systemically	Nephrotoxicity is the most serious adverse effect. Allergic manifestations, paraesthesia, vertigo, apnoea and muscle weakness occur less frequently	Oral for bowel sterilisation: 1.5–3 million units every 8 hours. IM, IV injection or infusion: 2 million units every 8 hours
Sodium fusidate Infections due to penicillin-resistant staphylococci, particularly osteomyelitis, often in conjunction with a second antistaphylococcal antibiotic to prevent resistance, e.g. flucloxacillin	Well absorbed, widely distributed in body tissues, including bone. Metabolised in liver and excreted in bile	Nausea, vomiting, skin rashes	Oral: 0.5–1 g every 8 hours. IV infusion: 0.5 g over 6 hours three times daily
Teicoplanin Bactericidal against most Gram-positive organisms. Serious Gram-positive infections, including endocarditis, treatment of staphylococcal infections of bone and joint	Longer half-life than vancomycin and requires only once-daily dosing. Available as IM and IV injection, low nephrotoxic, ototoxic and allergenic potential – routine serum monitoring not required	No significant enhanced renal toxicity when used with aminoglycosides. Nausea, vomiting, diarrhoea, rash, fever, anaphylaxis, blood disorders, tinnitus, local thrombophlebitis	By IM injection, IV injection or infusion: 400 mg initially, 200–400 mg daily
Vancomycin Bactericidal activity against aerobic and anaerobic Gram-positive bacteria. Drug of choice in antibiotic-related pseudo-membranous colitis (*Clostridium difficile*). Alternative to penicillins in infective endocarditis. Also used IV for other serious infections caused by Gram-positive cocci including multiresistant staphylococci (e.g. MRSA)	Very poorly absorbed from the GI tract. Widely distributed in body tissues following IV infusion. Almost completely eliminated unchanged in the urine. It has a long duration of action and can be given every 12 hours. Accumulates in renal failure, necessitating a modified dosage schedule and serum concentration monitoring (below 30 micrograms/mL). Dose should be reduced in the elderly	Ototoxic and nephrotoxic, which are dose related. Extravasation causes necrosis and thrombophlebitis. After parenteral administration may get nausea, chills, fever, urticaria, rashes, tinnitus (discontinue use). It is important to administer as an infusion. Severe flushing of the upper body ('red man' syndrome) can occur if given as a bolus	Oral: 125 mg 6-hourly. IV infusion: 500 mg every 6 hours

Box 19.2 The action of trimethoprim

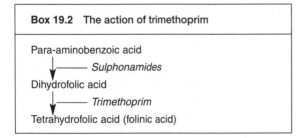

Para-aminobenzoic acid

↓—— *Sulphonamides*

Dihydrofolic acid

↓—— *Trimethoprim*

Tetrahydrofolic acid (folinic acid)

Table 19.17 Dosages of co-trimoxazole and trimethoprim

Drug	Dose
Co-trimoxazole	1–2 tablets twice daily; IM or IV infusion: 960 mg every 12 hours
Trimethoprim	Oral: 200 mg twice daily; slow IV injection or infusion: 150–250 mg every 12 hours

multiply rapidly in the lungs and spread to the lymph nodes and to the bloodstream. The organism is thus distributed throughout the body where it can remain viable but dormant for many years, particularly in the lungs, bones, lymphatic system and kidneys.

Primary infection is usually controlled by the host's immune system. The bacteria become engulfed by macrophages which coalesce to form a mass of cells – a tubercle or granuloma. The bacilli contained in the granuloma may survive and remain dormant for many years. The granuloma may break down in later years, leading to pulmonary or extrapulmonary clinical disease.

Widespread disease following primary infection is rare, although susceptible groups such as young infants, the immunocompromised, or malnourished and debilitated patients may be at risk.

Signs and symptoms

Primary tuberculosis is usually a mild asymptomatic illness which resolves spontaneously without problems. The onset of post-primary disease is slow. When symptoms occur they include chronic cough, sometimes with blood-streaked sputum (haemoptysis), malaise, weight loss, fever, night sweats, anorexia, anxiety and depression.

Diagnostic tests

The discovery of *Mycobacterium tuberculosis* by either microscopy of sputum smears or by culture is diagnostic of active tuberculosis. Tuberculin testing is an adjunct to diagnosis. The two tests used are as follows.

Mantoux test

This consists of the intradermal injection of 1, 10 or 100 units of tuberculin purified protein derivative (PPD) in 0.1 mL. (10 units is the normal dose.) The reaction is read 48–72 hours after injection; a positive reaction, indicating the presence of antibodies, is demonstrated by an induration of 10 mm or more in diameter.

Heaf (multiple puncture) test

A syringe gun with six needles arranged in a circle is used to puncture the skin to which a drop of tuberculin PPD, 100 000 units/mL, has been applied. The reaction is read 3–10 days later; a positive result is indicated by a solid induration of at least 5 mm.

Tuberculin testing should not be carried out within 4 weeks of receiving a live viral vaccine since response to tuberculin may be inhibited.

Drug treatment of tuberculosis (Table 19.18)

The treatment of tuberculosis has two phases – an initial phase using at least three drugs, and a continuation phase with two drugs. Recommended regimens of the Joint Tuberculosis Committee of the British Thoracic Society for the treatment of tuberculosis in the UK are given below.

Initial phase

In order to reduce the population of viable bacteria rapidly and to prevent emergence of resistant bacteria, at least three drugs are given concurrently in the initial phase. This involves the daily use of isoniazid, rifampicin and pyrazinamide. Ethambutol is added where drug resistance to isoniazid is a possibility. This regimen should be continued for at least 8 weeks.

Continuation phase

This follows the initial phase, and treatment with isoniazid and rifampicin is continued for a further 4 months.

METRONIDAZOLE AND TINIDAZOLE

Most bacteria can be divided into two groups, those that survive and grow in the presence of oxygen (aerobes) and those that survive and grow in the absence of oxygen (anaerobes). Metronidazole is an antimicrobial drug with high activity against anaerobic bacteria and protozoa (see Table 19.19). Indications include trichomonal vaginitis, bacterial vaginosis, *Entamoeba histolytica* and *Giardia lamblia* infections. It is also used for surgical and gynaecological sepsis in which its activity against colonic anaerobes, especially *Bacteroides fragilis*, is important. Metronidazole is also effective in the treatment of antibiotic-associated colitis (pseudomembranous colitis). Metronidazole by the rectal route is an effective alternative to the intravenous route when oral administration is not possible. Intravenous metronidazole is used for the treatment of established cases of tetanus.

Metronidazole has no action against aerobic organisms and so, in mixed infections, combined treatment with an additional antibiotic is required. Metronidazole also has applications in the oral treatment of infected leg ulcers and pressure sores. It is also used locally as a 0.8% gel (Metrotop) in the control of malodorous fungating tumours associated with anaerobic bacteria, by application to the cleaned area once or twice daily.

Tinidazole has similar actions, uses and side-effects to those of metronidazole with the advantage of a longer plasma half-life. The dose is 2 mg initially, followed by 500 mg twice a day.

Table 19.18 Drugs used in the treatment of tuberculosis

Drug	Adult dosage	Adverse effects/interactions	Comments
Ethambutol	15 mg/kg daily	Optic neuritis, colour blindness and restriction of visual fields. These are related to plasma levels and are more common where excessive dosage is used. Therapy should be discontinued where these adverse effects are experienced	Reduce dosage in renal failure. Patients should be advised to seek medical advice if they experience visual disturbance
Isoniazid	300 mg daily	Well tolerated and side-effects not usually serious. Skin reactions may occur. Persistent nausea and vomiting may indicate liver damage. Peripheral neuropathy may occur, particular where diabetes, alcoholism, renal failure or malnutrition are present, in which case 10 mg of pyridoxine should be given daily. Some epileptic patients treated with phenytoin experience symptoms of phenytoin toxicity when given isoniazid and rifampicin. Appears to be related to inhibition of metabolism in slow acetylators of isoniazid	Elimination by acetylation in the liver. Check hepatic function before commencing treatment
Rifampicin	Under 50 kg – 450 mg daily; over 50 kg – 600 mg daily	Anorexia and nausea may occur. Hepatotoxicity is a serious side-effect and alcoholics, the elderly and patients with pre-existing liver disease are at risk. Concurrent administration of rifampicin with oral contraceptives increases the metabolism of oestrogen and progestogen, which may result in contraceptive failure. Alternative contraceptive methods should be used. Anticoagulant effects of warfarin are reduced by concurrent administration of rifampicin owing to increased metabolism of the anticoagulant	Monitor liver function tests. Caution in pregnancy. Patients should be advised that rifampicin colours the urine, stools and tears. Soft contact lenses may become permanently discoloured
Pyrazinamide	Under 50 kg – 1.5 g daily; over 50 kg – 2 g daily	Liver damage, hyperuricaemia	Monitor liver function tests. Readily absorbed and penetrates well into CSF, making it particularly useful in tuberculous meningitis. Should not be given to patients with gout

Products are available containing various combinations of the above drugs, which may aid compliance.

Table 19.19 Metronidazole

Mode of action	Uses/dosage	Pharmacokinetics	Important adverse effects and interactions
Has high activity against anaerobic bacteria and protozoa. It is reduced to active metabolites which interfere with nucleic acid function of the organism	*Anaerobic infections* Oral: treated for 7 days, 800 mg initially then 400 mg every 8 hours. By rectum: 1 g every 8 hours for 3 days then 1 g every 12 hours. IV infusion: 500 mg every 8 hours *Bacterial vaginosis* Oral: 400 mg twice daily for 7 days or 2 g as single dose *Giardiasis* 2 g daily for 3 days *Amoebiasis* Oral: 400–800 mg three times daily for 5–10 days *Acute ulcerative gingivitis* Oral: 200 mg every 8 hours for 3 days *Pseudomembranous colitis* Oral: 400 mg three times daily *Surgical prophylaxis* Oral: 400 mg every 8 hours, started 24 hours before surgery then continued postoperatively by IV infusion or by rectum	Well absorbed after oral and rectal administration. Effective serum concentrations are reached in 1–3 hours and maintained for 8–10 hours. Excreted mainly in the urine. Crosses placental barrier and appears in the milk of nursing mothers	The most common reactions to metronidazole therapy are rash, pruritus, urticaria, nausea, furry tongue, dry mouth, metallic taste in the mouth, headache and dizziness. Patients are advised to avoid taking alcohol when receiving metronidazole as disulfiram-like reaction may occur resulting in abdominal cramps, nausea, vomiting, headaches and flushing. Caution in pregnancy and breast-feeding

QUINOLONES

The original quinolone antibiotic is nalidixic acid which has been available for 30 years. More recently, molecular changes have produced fluorinated quinolones with a broader antibacterial spectrum and better pharmacokinetics.

Mode of action. The quinolone antibiotics are bactericidal. They act by inhibiting the enzyme DNA gyrase which is required by the bacterial DNA.

Uses. The spectrum of microbiological activity of the quinolone antibiotics is one of high activity against Gram-negative bacteria, slightly less activity against Gram-positive bacteria and little or no activity against anaerobes. Examples of the quinolones are summarised in Table 19.20.

Pharmacokinetics. The quinolones are well absorbed following oral administration. Antacids decrease their absorption. They are eliminated in three ways:

- secreted into the gut lumen and excreted in the faeces
- metabolised by the liver
- excreted as unchanged drug via the kidneys.

No differences have been found in serum half-lives in the elderly. Patients taking ciprofloxacin should ensure adequate fluid intake to minimise the risk of crystalluria.

Adverse drug reactions. Side-effects of the quinolones commonly involve the central nervous system – headache, dizziness, sleep disorders and less frequently restlessness, hallucinations, confusion. Patients should be advised of this since performance of skilled tasks, e.g. driving, may be impaired. Because of these adverse reactions, the drugs should be used with caution in patients with a history of epilepsy. They may induce convulsions in patients with or without a history of convulsions, and taking NSAIDs concurrently may potentiate this. Gastrointestinal side-effects including nausea, vomiting, abdominal pain and diarrhoea may occur. Allergic reactions to the quinolones include rash and anaphylaxis. Photosensitivity reactions consisting of erythema on exposed skin surfaces may occur. Blood disorders including eosinophilia, leucopenia and thrombocytopenia have been noted. Other side-effects include an increase in blood urea and creatinine, arthralgia and myalgia.

Since weight-bearing joints of juvenile animals have suffered cartilage damage when quinolones were administered, caution should be exercised in children and adolescents. Care should be taken where hepatic or renal impairment exists and also in pregnancy and breast-feeding.

URINARY TRACT INFECTIONS

Bladder urine is normally sterile, although transient small numbers of bacteria may be present after micturition or sexual intercourse. This occurs because of retrograde flow up the urethra. It is far more likely to happen with women because of the length of the urethra and the increased number of organisms resident on the surfaces surrounding the orifice. The first step in the development of UTI is colonisation of the periurethral mucosa, commonly by *Escherichia coli* from faeces.

To initiate infection, bacteria present in the urine must adhere to the urothelial cells on the bladder surface. One of the more important host defence mechanisms is the continual renewal of the surface by shedding cells

Table 19.20 The quinolones

Drug	Indications	Dose
Ciprofloxacin	Particularly active against Gram-negative bacteria including *Campylobacter*, *Neisseria*, *Pseudomonas*, *Salmonella*, *Shigella*. Less activity against Gram-positive bacteria such as *Strep. pneumoniae* and *Strep. faecalis*. Used for infections of the respiratory tract (but not first choice for pneumococcal pneumonia), urinary tract, gastrointestinal system, gonorrhoea and septicaemia	Oral: 250–750 mg twice daily. Gonorrhoea: 250 mg as a single dose. Available as intravenous infusion
Levofloxacin	Greater activity against pneumococci than ciprofloxacin	Oral: 250–500 mg daily for 7–14 days. IV infusion: 500 mg (over at least 60 minutes) once or twice daily for community-acquired pneumonia
Nalidixic acid	Uncomplicated urinary tract infections	500 mg–1 g every 6 hours
Norfloxacin	Uncomplicated urinary tract infections	400 mg twice daily
Ofloxacin	Infections of urinary tract, lower respiratory tract, gonorrhoea	200–400 mg daily. Gonorrhoea: 400 mg as a single dose. Available as an IV infusion

together with attached bacteria and mucus. Urine does not normally support the growth of bacteria because of the large variation in pH, osmolality and the antibacterial substances present.

In managing patients with urinary tract infection, the infection is often classified as simple (uncomplicated) or complicated. One way to define a complicated UTI is as one that fails to respond to a short course of antibiotics. Symptoms commonly associated with lower UTIs (e.g. cystitis) include:

- urgency
- frequency
- pain or burning on micturition (dysuria)
- cloudy or malodorous urine
- suprapubic pain.

Patients with acute pyelonephritis may also present with loin pain, tenderness, fever, chills, nausea and haematuria (see Box 19.3).

UTI is predominantly a disease of females from the age of 1 until about the age of 50, most neonatal cases of UTI occurring in males. UTIs again become a problem for males after the age of 50 when prostatic obstruction, urethral instrumentation and surgery influence the infection rate. In general, 10–20% of the elderly living at home have bacteriuria, and up to 40% in long-stay hospitals. The reasons for higher UTI rates in older people include the high prevalence of prostatitis in males, poor bladder emptying and faecal incontinence.

Box 19.3 Terms associated with urinary tract infections

Bacteriuria. Presence of bacteria in the urine. Asymptomatic bacteriuria exists if colony counts exceed 10^5/mL in a patient without urinary tract infection (UTI) symptoms.
Pyelonephritis. Inflammation of the kidney with pain, tenderness, bacteriuria, pyuria and fever.
Pyuria. White blood cells in the urine.
Urethritis. Inflammation of the urethra with dysuria.
Prostatitis. Inflammation of the prostate.

Causes

Most organisms involved are bowel commensals, the commonest being *Escherichia coli*. Less common causes include *Proteus* and *Klebsiella* spp. *Staphylococcus epidermidis*, *Pseudomonas aeruginosa* and *Enterococcus faecalis* infection may occur following catheterisation or instrumentation. Whenever possible, a specimen of urine should be collected for culture and sensitivity testing before starting antibacterial therapy. The antibacterial selected should reflect local antibacterial sensitivity, which needs to be reviewed regularly.

Treatment

Table 19.21 outlines the drugs used according to the degree of infection being treated.

Nitrofurantoin

Nitrofurantoin is bacteriostatic. It acts by inhibiting a number of bacterial enzymes essential for bacterial function.

Table 19.21 Treatment of urinary tract infections

Condition	Uncomplicated infection	Serious infection (pending culture results or in primary treatment failure)	Notes
Acute pyelonephritis		Cefotaxime, ciprofloxacin, augmentin, gentamicin, cefuroxime	Best treated initially by injection, especially if the patient is vomiting or severely ill
Cystitis	Trimethoprim, cefradine, nalidixic acid, nitrofurantoin for 5–7 days	Ciprofloxacin, augmentin	Long term therapy may be required in selected patients to prevent recurrence of infection. Trimethroprim, nitrofurantoin and cefalexin has been recommended for long-term therapy
(in pregnancy)	Cefradine, amoxicillin	Nitrofurantoin	
Prostatitis	Trimethoprim	Ciprofloxacin, cefotaxime	Can be difficult to cure and requires treatment for several weeks with an antibiotic which penetrates prostatic tissue

Apart from nitrofurantoin, details of the drugs in this table have appeared in earlier pages.

Pharmacokinetics. Nitrofurantoin is rapidly and well absorbed following oral administration at a dosage of 50 mg four times daily with food. About 40% of the dose appears unchanged in the urine.

Adverse reactions. Nausea and vomiting are common but this can be reduced by administering with food and lowering the dose. Mild allergic reactions may occur. Long-term therapy occasionally results in peripheral neuropathy which is dose-related. It occurs as a result of renal failure, and patients with this condition should not be given nitrofurantoin. Other adverse effects include arthralgia, agranulocytosis, thrombocytopenia and aplastic anaemia.

FUNGAL INFECTIONS

Two general types of fungal infection exist:

- topical infections affecting the skin and mucous membranes
- systemic infections.

The patient's underlying condition may predispose to fungal infection, for example (i) a severely immunocompromised patient, (ii) a patient receiving antibiotic therapy that eliminates normal flora, (iii) a patient who wears dentures.

Topical infections are more common and include candidiasis and infections by dermatophytes. The causative organism in candidiasis is usually *Candida albicans*, a yeast which may be found in up to 50% of healthy mouths and about one-third of adult vaginas. Infection caused by this organism is usually superficial, for example invasion of the superficial layers of the epidermis of the mouth or vagina, or very occasionally skin which has become damp and macerated, as in the nappy area. This condition is commonly referred to as thrush. Vaginal thrush is an opportunistic infection which affects women predominantly of childbearing age because *Candida* thrives in the low pH and abundant glycogen present in the urine at this time. The initially harmless *Candida* is transformed into a pathogen either by local changes in the vagina or by lowered immune resistance. Pregnancy and diabetes are two predisposing factors.

Vulval pruritus and vaginal discharge are the usual presenting symptoms. Dysuria may be severe, especially when there is local excoriation and maceration due to scratching. Painful intercourse (dyspareunia) may occur and may be severe. When present, the discharge is usually thick and white or creamy.

Oral candidiasis presents in different forms, denture stomatitis being the most common. Acute pseudomembranous candidiasis is the form commonly referred to as oral thrush. The infected epithelium proliferates rapidly, producing the characteristic soft, creamy yellow plaques, which can occur on any mucosal surface of the mouth. Steroid inhalers are a common cause of thrush by thinning the oral mucosa and suppressing inflammatory reaction. Patients should be advised to rinse out the mouth following administration to help prevent this.

Dermatophytes cause many common infections which are named according to the affected part of the body:

- tinea pedis – athlete's foot
- tinea capitis – scalp ringworm
- tinea corporis – body ringworm
- tinea unguium – nail infection (onychomycosis).

Tinea versicolor is a fungal infection of the horny layer of the skin which shows as oval, light-brown patches in fair-skinned people.

Antifungal drugs

The treatment of fungal infections is outlined in Table 19.22. Clotrimazole, econazole, ketoconazole and miconazole are applied topically to treat fungal skin infections. Treatment should continue for 10–14 days after the lesions have healed.

VIRUSES

Viruses are much smaller than bacteria, consisting essentially of a core of nucleic acid in a protective protein envelope. They possess only one of the two classes of nucleic acids as carriers of their genetic information, either ribonucleic acid (RNA) or deoxyribonucleic acid (DNA). These organisms have no enzymes of their own such as are necessary for internal metabolism. It is for this reason that they are resistant to antibiotics which act by blocking some stage of microbial metabolism.

Viruses can be regarded as intracellular parasites. Since new proteins, not present in the normal cell, are synthesised in virus-infected cells, this offers the possibility of selective inhibition of viral replication by chemical agents. The majority of virus infections resolve spontaneously in immunocompetent persons.

Antiviral agents

The only therapeutic approach to viral illness until recently was prevention by immunisation. Examples of vaccines include those against rubella, poliomyelitis and yellow fever. There are now a small number of

Table 19.22 Drugs used to treat fungal infections

Mode of action	Pharmacokinetics	Indications	Dose	Adverse effects
POLYENE ANTIFUNGAL DRUGS				
Amphotericin				
Alter permeability of cell membranes resulting in loss of essential cell constituents	Poorly absorbed from GI tract. May be administered orally as suspension, tablets or lozenges for treatment of superficial candida infections. Administered by IV infusion to treat systemic infections	Active against most fungi and yeasts (*Aspergillus*, *Candida* spp., *Cryptococcus*, *Coccidioides*, *Histoplasma*)	Intestinal candidiasis: 100–200 mg every 6 hours. Lozenges given four times daily are used to treat oral candidiasis. IV infusion in glucose: 250 micrograms–1 mg/kg daily. (It is precipitated from solutions containing cations such as sodium or potassium)	When given parenterally toxicity is common and close supervision is necessary. Renal impairment occurs owing to renal vasoconstriction and a direct effect on the tubules resulting in diminished renal plasma flow giving rise to acidosis and hypokalaemia. Other adverse reactions include nausea, vomiting, febrile reactions, headache, anaemia, blood disorders, rash, anaphylactoid reactions. Fever is common and may be reduced by intravenous hydrocortisone at start of treatment. Lipid formulations of amphotericin (Abelcet, AmBisome and Amphocil) are significantly less toxic and are recommended when the conventional formulation of amphotericin is contraindicated because of toxicity, especially nephrotoxicity
Nystatin				
As for amphotericin	Not absorbed after oral or topical administration. Too toxic for parenteral use	Principally used for *Candida albicans* infections of GI tract, skin, vagina and respiratory tract	Oral: intestinal candidiasis, 500 000 units every 6 hours; oral or peri-oral candidiasis: 100 000 units four times daily	Usually unimportant – may experience nausea, vomiting and diarrhoea at higher doses
TRIAZOLE ANTIFUNGAL DRUGS				
Fluconazole				
Alters cell membrane permeability	Absorbed by mouth. Effective parenterally	Mucosal and systemic candidiasis; cryptococcal infections including meningitis	Oral: single dose of 150 mg for vaginal candidiasis. 50–100 mg daily in oropharyngeal candidiasis. 200–400 mg daily orally or by IV infusion for systemic candidiasis or cryptococcal meningitis	GI side-effects. Caution in pregnancy, breast-feeding and renal impairment

Itraconazole				
As for fluconazole	As for fluconazole	Mucosal candidiasis and dermatophyte infections	Oral preparations only. Oral candidiasis: 100 mg daily for 15 days. Vaginal candidiasis: 200 mg twice daily for 1 day. Tinea pedis and corporis: 100 mg daily	GI side-effects. Caution in pregnancy and breast-feeding
IMIDAZOLE ANTIFUNGAL DRUGS				
Ketoconazole				
Increases membrane permeability. Also inhibits cellular enzymes	Poorly absorbed after local application. Widely distributed parenterally	Systemic mycoses, serious candidiasis, resistant dermatophyte infections of skin and finger nails	200 mg orally once daily with food until at least 1 week after symptoms have cleared	GI side-effects, rashes, pruritus. Contraindicated in hepatic impairment. Avoid in pregnancy and porphyria. Monitor liver function
Miconazole				
As for ketoconazole	As for ketoconazole	Oral, intestinal and systemic fungal infections	5–10 mL in the mouth after food four times daily. Continue for 2 days after symptoms clear	Nausea, vomiting
OTHER ANTIFUNGAL DRUGS				
Flucytosine				
Penetrates certain fungal cells where it is converted to fluorouracil and alters protein synthesis	Well absorbed and widely distributed. Undergoes little metabolism	Systemic yeast and fungal infections	By IV infusion: 200 mg/kg daily in four divided doses. Reduce dose in renal impairment	GI reactions, rashes, thrombocytopenia, leucopenia. Caution in pregnancy and breast-feeding
Griseofulvin				
Binds to keratin and makes it resistant to fungal infection. Must be continued until all infected tissue has been shed and replaced	Absorption variable. It is improved if given after food	Dermatophyte infection of the skin, nails and hair where topical therapy is ineffective	0.5–1 g daily for up to a year depending on site of infection	Well tolerated. Headache, GI side-effects or hypersensitivity may occur. Caution in breast-feeding
Terbinafine				
Interferes with fungal sterol biosynthesis, at an early stage. This leads to deficiency in ergosterol and to intracellular accumulation of squalene resulting in fungal cell death	Well absorbed orally. Rapidly diffuses through dermis and concentrates in the stratum corneum. Distributed into nail plate within first few weeks of commencing therapy. Metabolites excreted predominantly in urine	Dermatophyte infection of the nails. Ringworm infection	250 mg daily up to 3 months or longer, depending on site of infection	GI effects, headache, rash, arthralgia, myalgia

Table 19.23 Drugs used to treat viral infections

Mode of action	Use	Pharmacokinetics	Adverse effects	Dose
Aciclovir				
Aciclovir enters all cells. It is changed by a virus-specific enzyme, thymidine kinase, to the active derivative aciclovir triphosphate. This then inhibits DNA polymerase, an enzyme necessary for viral growth, and disrupts viral replication	Active against herpes virus if started early. It is used IV for the treatment of systemic infections of herpes simplex and varicella-zoster; topically for treating herpes infections of the skin and mucous membranes (including genital herpes); as an ointment in herpes simplex eye infections. Used in the immunocompromised for prophylaxis and for prevention of recurrence	15–30% absorbed orally, but this results in therapeutic serum concentration levels. Widely distributed throughout the body. There are a number of metabolites formed either in the liver or in cells infected by the herpes virus; the active aciclovir triphosphate is formed in the latter. The half-life increases as renal function deteriorates and dosage needs to be adjusted in patients with renal impairment	Headache can occur with oral administration as can GI reactions such as nausea, vomiting and diarrhoea. Local reactions at the injection site particularly with inadvertent extravasation can occur. These include irritation, phlebitis, inflammation and pain	Must be started at the onset of infection to be effective. Viral herpes simplex treatment: 200–400 mg five times daily. Herpes zoster (shingles): 800 mg five times daily for 7 days. By IV infusion over 1 hour: 5–10 mg/kg every 8 hours. Cream or eye ointment to be applied every 4 hours
Famciclovir				
Converted in vivo to penciclovir triphosphate which inhibits replication of viral DNA	Treatment of herpes zoster and genital herpes	Rapidly and extensively absorbed following oral administration	Well tolerated. Headache and nausea have been reported	Herpes zoster: 250 mg three times daily for 7 days
Valaciclovir				
Converted in vivo to aciclovir	Treatment of herpes zoster and herpes simplex	Well absorbed orally and almost completely converted to aciclovir	Headache, skin rashes, GI disorders	Herpes zoster: 1 g three times daily for 7 days. Herpes simplex: 500 mg twice daily for 5–10 days

therapeutic agents available to treat certain viral infections (Table 19.23).

Inosine pranobex has been used orally for herpes simplex infections but its effectiveness has not been established. The dose is 1 g four times daily for 7–14 days. It does not act directly on the viruses but is of value mainly as an immunostimulant by increasing the proliferation of T and B cells, which is depressed during viral infections. Inosine pranobex is well tolerated but care is necessary in gout and renal impairment as it increases uric acid levels.

IMMUNE SYSTEM CELLS

The human immune system protects the body against foreign objects, such as microorganisms. It comprises many different cells that are spread throughout the body, each playing different roles and moving around the body as needed.

Blood cells

There are two major types of cell in the blood. The most common are red blood cells or erythrocytes which carry oxygen to the body tissues and carry away carbon dioxide. The other group is the white blood cells or leucocytes. These are the immune cells.

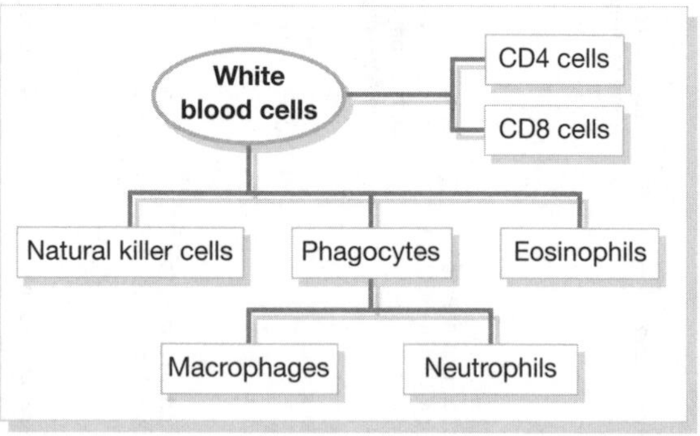

Figure 19.3 White blood cells.

Some white blood cells recognise specific foreign organisms to which the body has been exposed in the past. These specific immune cells are called lymphocytes. Other white blood cells are non-specific and can attack a range of different foreign organisms: these include neutrophils, eosinophils and natural killer cells (see Fig. 19.3).

Lymphocytes

There are two different types of lymphocyte. B lymphocytes (sometimes just called B cells) produce antibodies. An antibody is a protein that can lock onto a distinctive part of a specific foreign organism. When this happens, the antibody signals to other immune cells to attack the organism.

T lymphocytes (sometimes just called T cells) are called different names depending on the molecules on their surface. They are white blood cells that play important roles in the immune system. There are two main types of T cell. One type has molecules called CD4 on its surface; these 'helper' cells orchestrate the body's response to certain microorganisms such as viruses. The other T cells, which have a molecule called CD8, destroy cells that are infected and shut down the immune response once the infection has been dealt with.

HIV is able to attach itself to the CD4 molecule allowing the virus to enter and infect these cells. Even while a person with HIV feels well and has no symptoms, billions of CD4 T cells are infected by human immunodeficiency virus (HIV) and are destroyed each day, and billions more CD4 T cells are produced to replace them.

Other immune cells

Natural killer cells attack tumour cells and virus-infected cells in a way similar to that of lymphocytes. However, while each lymphocyte can recognise and attack cells infected by only one specific virus, natural killer cells can attack a wider range.

Phagocytes are cells that attack and destroy foreign cells by engulfing them. There are two main different types of phagocyte:

- Macrophages roam the blood and the body tissues, killing organisms that can cause AIDS-related diseases and cells infected by viruses.
- Neutrophils leave the blood to go to tissues where infection or inflammation is developing. They mainly attack bacteria and fungi.

Eosinophils engulf organisms too large for phagocytes.

Uses of CD4 counts

The number of CD4 cells in a cubic millimetre of blood is used as a marker in HIV. A normal count in a healthy, HIV-negative adult can vary but is usually between 600 and 1200 CD4 cells/mm^3.

Most people with HIV find that their CD4 count falls over time. This often happens at a variable rate and so the count can still be quite stable for long periods. It is useful to have the CD4 count made regularly for two reasons:

- to monitor the immune system and help decide whether and when to take anti-HIV drugs and treatments to prevent infections
- to help monitor the effectiveness of any anti-HIV drugs being taken.

If the CD4 count is persistently below 500, the immune system is slightly weakened and the patient is at a gradually increasing risk of infections the further it falls. If it drops below 200, there is increased risk from serious infections and the patient is diagnosed as having the acquired immune deficiency syndrome (AIDS). At this point, to try to prevent infections, drugs such as co-trimoxazole for pneumocystis pneumonia are given. Likewise, if the CD4 count starts to drop rapidly or falls below a certain point, or if symptoms develop, anti-HIV drugs are considered.

One effect of anti-HIV drugs is to improve the state of the immune system. This is crudely reflected in an increase in the CD4 count.

HUMAN IMMUNODEFICIENCY VIRUS (HIV)

The virus multiplies extremely rapidly and this continues throughout the course of the disease. At one time it was thought that after the initial infection, there was a long incubation period before the virus started multiplying. It is now known that in the apparently latent period, the virus is breeding at a rate of billions per day but is kept in check by the immune system. However, over time, the virus slowly destroys the immune system's ability to produce the CD4 lymphocytes, and resistance to it falls. This takes an average of about 10–11 years but varies – some people (about 20%) develop AIDS within 5 years of HIV infection; others (about 5%) seem to resist the virus much longer than 10 years. It is now possible to measure the number of viruses in the blood and this gives a good guide to the speed of progression. The higher the virus count per mL of blood, the faster the progression. During this very rapid multiplication, genetic 'errors' or mutations occur, and unfortunately this often leads to new strains which are resistant to drugs.

Anti-HIV therapy

Anti-HIV drugs interfere with the way the virus tries to reproduce itself inside a human cell. Although anti-HIV drugs cannot kill the virus completely, they reduce the chance of infected cells producing new HIV particles which could go on to infect even more cells. There is currently no cure, only a slowing of the progression of HIV infection.

The anti-HIV drugs that are currently available fall into two main categories:

- reverse transcriptase inhibitors
- protease inhibitors.

Treatment is aimed at reducing the plasma viral load as much as possible and for as long as possible; it should be started before the immune system is irreversibly damaged. The need for early drug treatment should, however, be balanced against the development of toxicity. Commitment to treatment and strict adherence over many years are required; the regimen chosen should take into account convenience and patient tolerance. The development of drug resistance is reduced by using a combination of drugs; such combinations should have synergistic or additive activity while ensuring that their toxicity is not additive. Testing for resistance to antiviral drugs particularly in therapeutic failure should be considered.

The optimum time for initiation of antiviral treatment will depend primarily on the CD4 cell count; the plasma viral load and clinical symptoms may also help. Initiating treatment with a combination of drugs which includes two nucleoside reverse transcriptase inhibitors with *either* a non-nucleoside reverse transcriptase inhibitor *or* one or two protease inhibitors is recommended.

Deterioration of the condition (including clinical and virological changes) may require either switching therapy or adding another antiviral drug. The choice of an alternative regimen depends on factors such as the response to previous treatment, tolerance and the possibility of cross-resistance.

Reverse transcriptase inhibitors

Once HIV has locked onto and invaded a human cell, it uses an enzyme called reverse transcriptase (RT) to convert its genetic code into the same form as the genetic code of human cells (DNA). This viral DNA then merges with the human DNA, converting the cell into a factory for making the building blocks of new virus.

There are two different classes of anti-HIV drug that target reverse transcriptase. The nucleoside reverse transcriptase inhibitors are zidovudine, didanosine, abacavir, zalcitabine, lamivudine and stavudine. The benefit of combination therapy is that when resistance develops to one, another of the group may still work, and a combination of two of these drugs will act for longer than one alone since the virus has to develop two forms of resistance.

The reason for the development of resistance has been the high mutation rate of the virus, which leads to resistant strains. Combination therapy using several drugs is more effective in dealing with this. However, treatment will inevitably result in eventual resistance, and the best management involves monitoring viral levels and changing drug combination when required. This will improve symptoms and survival in the short term but does not yet mean that the disease can be cured.

The best combination depends on previous treatment and individual patient factors, but will usually be at least two and often three drugs (e.g. two reverse transcriptase inhibitors and a protease inhibitor). Choice will take into account long-term considerations, such as preserving efficacy for advanced disease by avoiding early use and hence earlier resistance.

The other class is non-nucleoside reverse transcriptase inhibitors (NNRTIs). Like the nucleoside analogues, they also attack RT, but in a different way. The NNRTIs include efavirenz and nevirapine (Table 19.24).

Nucleoside reverse transcriptase inhibitors

Didanosine

Mode of action. After didanosine enters the cell it is converted to its active metabolite, dideoxyadenosine

Table 19.24 Non-nucleoside reverse transcriptase inhibitors

Drug	Dose	Cautions	Contraindications	Side-effects
Efavirenz	600 mg once daily	Hepatic and severe renal impairment, pregnancy, elderly, mental illness	Breast-feeding	Rash, dizziness, headache, fatigue, sleep disorders, nausea, ataxia, vertigo
Nevirapine	200 mg once daily for first 14 days then if no rash, 200 mg twice daily	Hepatic and renal impairment, pregnancy, rash	Breast-feeding	Rash, hepatitis, nausea, vomiting, headache, fatigue

triphosphate (ddATP). ddATP inhibits the viral enzyme reverse transcriptase, so inhibiting viral nucleic acid replication.

Pharmacokinetics. Didanosine (DDI) is active orally. However, it is acid-labile so that all oral formulations must contain buffering agents designed to increase gastric pH. It is rapidly absorbed after oral administration, maximum concentrations occurring within an hour of administration. Taking food with DDI reduces the absorption by as much as 50% and so it should be given at least 30 minutes before a meal. Although the half-life is 1.4 hours, active metabolites of DDI remain within the cell for much longer so that twice-daily dosing is sufficient.

Dose. Adult under 60 kg: 125 mg every 12 hours; 60 kg and over: 200 mg every 12 hours; on an empty stomach.

Cautions. Extreme caution is needed where there is a history of pancreatitis; it is also associated with the development of toxic peripheral neuropathy where therapy should be suspended until resolution of symptoms; hyperuricaemia has occurred and treatment should be suspended if there is significant elevation in uric acid level; liver enzymes should be monitored, and didanosine is contraindicated where hepatic abnormalities have occurred due to previous didanosine treatment; also contraindicated in breast-feeding.

Side-effects. The most serious adverse effects are pancreatitis, peripheral neuropathy and asymptomatic hyperuricaemia. Other side-effects include nausea, vomiting, diarrhoea and dry mouth.

Lamivudine

Mode of action. Lamivudine is a nucleoside analogue, metabolised intracellularly to lamivudine 5-triphosphate. Its main mode of action is as a chain terminator of HIV reverse transcription. It is not recommended for use in monotherapy. Lamivudine in combination with zidovudine is highly synergistic, reducing HIV viral load and increasing the CD4 count, which, in turn, slows the progression of the disease.

Pharmacokinetics. Lamivudine is well absorbed from the gut, with oral bioavailability between 80 and 85%. Maximum serum concentrations are reached in about an hour. It is excreted largely unchanged in the urine. Reduced dosage may be required in renal dysfunction.

Dose. 150 mg every 12 hours (not taken with food).

Side-effects. Side-effects commonly reported are headache, malaise, fatigue, nausea, diarrhoea, vomiting, abdominal pain, insomnia, cough, nasal symptoms and musculoskeletal pain.

Stavudine

Mode of action. Stavudine is a thymidine analogue. It is phosphorylated by cellular kinases to stavudine triphosphate, which inhibits HIV reverse transcriptase by competing with the natural substrate, thymidine triphosphate. It also inhibits viral DNA synthesis by causing DNA chain termination. Stavudine is indicated when zidovudine is not appropriate.

Pharmacokinetics. Stavudine is well absorbed after oral administration. It should be taken an hour before food or on an empty stomach. The clearance of stavudine decreases as creatinine clearance decreases; therefore it is recommended that the dosage be adjusted in patients with reduced renal function. Zidovudine may inhibit the intracellular phosphorylation of stavudine and is therefore not recommended to be used in combination with stavudine.

Dose. Adult under 60 kg: 30 mg every 12 hours; 60 kg and over: 40 mg every 12 hours.

Cautions. Caution should be exercised in patients with a history of peripheral neuropathy or pancreatitis. Stavudine should be suspended if peripheral neuropathy develops – characterised by persistent numbness, tingling or pain in the feet or hands. If symptoms resolve satisfactorily, resumption of treatment with stavudine at 50% of the previous dosage may be considered.

Side-effects. The major clinical toxicity is dose-related peripheral neuropathy requiring dose modification. Pancreatitis, occasionally fatal, has been reported. Other undesirable effects include headache, chills/fever, malaise, diarrhoea, constipation, nausea, vomiting, chest pain, dyspnoea, insomnia, depression and rash.

Zalcitabine

Mode of action. Zalcitabine is converted to the active metabolite dideoxycytidine-5-triphosphate (ddCTP) by cellular enzymes. It inhibits the replication of HIV by competitive inhibition of viral DNA synthesis. Zalcitabine is indicated in advanced HIV infection in adults intolerant of zidovudine or in whom zidovudine has failed.

Pharmacokinetics. Well absorbed but absorption rate is reduced when administered with food. Largely excreted unchanged in the urine.

Dose. 750 micrograms every 8 hours.

Cautions and side-effects. Similar to those for stavudine.

Zidovudine

Mode of action. The phosphorylation of zidovudine to zidovudine triphosphate is catalysed by thymidine, thymidylate and related kinases. Zidovudine triphosphate acts as an inhibitor of and substrate for the viral reverse transcriptase. The formation of further proviral DNA is blocked by incorporation of zidovudine triphosphate into the chain and subsequent chain termination.

Pharmacokinetics. Zidovudine is well absorbed from the gut with a bioavailability of 60–70%. It is excreted in the urine as the glucuronide.

Dose. 500–600 mg daily by mouth in two to three divided doses. For patients temporarily unable to take zidovudine by mouth, an intravenous infusion is available.

Side-effects. The most serious adverse reactions include anaemia (which may require transfusions), neutropenia and leucopenia. These occur more frequently at higher dosages (1200–1500 mg/day) and in patients with advanced HIV disease (especially when there is poor bone marrow reserve prior to treatment) and particularly with CD4 counts less than 100 cells/mm^3. Dosage reduction or cessation of therapy may become necessary. Blood tests are advised at least every 2 weeks for the first 3 months then at least once a month. Other adverse events recorded include somnolence, diarrhoea, dizziness, sweating, dyspnoea, flatulence, taste perversion, chest pain, loss of mental acuity, anxiety, urinary frequency, depression, generalised pain, chills, cough, urticaria, pruritus and an influenza-like syndrome.

Protease inhibitors

Protease is an HIV enzyme. After HIV has successfully merged its DNA with the human cell's DNA, the cell produces a string of protein. Protease cuts this protein string into smaller proteins that can be used to construct new HIV particles. By blocking protease, protease inhibitors help to prevent an infected cell from producing new infectious viral particles.

The protease inhibitors include amprenavir, indinavir, nelfinavir, ritonavir and saquinavir (Table 19.25). Combining a protease inhibitor with two nucleoside analogues has significant anti-HIV effects and their use is indicated in progressive or advanced HIV infection, in combination with nucleoside analogues.

Protease inhibitors are generally associated with fewer and milder toxic side-effects. Side-effects appear to be more severe in the later stages.

Opportunistic infections

There is a group of infections which the body normally easily controls but which can cause serious disease in people whose immune system is impaired by HIV (or other forms of immunosuppression such as anti-rejection drugs after transplants). These are called cytomegalovirus infections, and they particularly attack the eye (this is known as CMV retinitis) and can

Table 19.25 Protease inhibitors

Drug	Dose	Cautions	Contraindications	Side-effects
Amprenavir	Body weight over 50 kg: 1.2 g every 12 hours; under 50 kg: 20 mg/kg every 12 hours	Hepatic impairment, pregnancy, diabetes, haemophilia	Breast-feeding	Rash, nausea, vomiting, diarrhoea, flatulence, headache, fatigue
Indinavir	800 mg every 8 hours (600 mg every 8 hours if receiving concurrent ketoconazole or in hepatic impairment)	Hepatic impairment; ensure adequate hydration to reduce risk of nephrolithiasis; haemophilia, pregnancy, metabolism of many drugs inhibited	Breast-feeding	Nausea, vomiting, diarrhoea, abdominal discomfort, dry mouth, taste disturbances, headache, dizziness, insomnia, myalgia, rash, nephrolithiasis, dysuria, haematuria, crystalluria, proteinuria, elevated liver enzymes, blood disorders
Nelfinavir	1.25 g twice daily	Hepatic and renal impairment, diabetes, haemophilia, pregnancy	Breast-feeding	Diarrhoea, nausea, vomiting, flatulence, rash, hepatitis, neutropenia
Ritonavir	600 mg every 12 hours	Hepatic impairment, haemophilia, pregnancy; metabolism of many drugs inhibited	Severe hepatic impairment; breast-feeding	Nausea, vomiting, diarrhoea, abdominal pain, taste disturbances, dyspepsia, anorexia, vasodilatation, headache, dizziness, asthenia, rash, raised liver enzymes
Saquinavir	600 mg every 8 hours	Severe hepatic or renal impairment, haemophilia, pregnancy	Breast-feeding	Diarrhoea, mucosal ulceration, abdominal discomfort, nausea, headache, peripheral neuropathy, asthenia, rash

lead to blindness. Another infection seen commonly in AIDS (and used as one of the defining infections) is a form of pneumonia caused by *Pneumocystis carinii*. Different methods can be used to treat these infections some of which are very expensive.

The drugs used in opportunistic infections (HIV-positive patients) are described below.

Pneumocystis pneumonia

Pneumonia caused by *Pneumocystis carinii* occurs in immunosuppressed or severely debilitated patients. It is the commonest cause of pneumonia in AIDS. Co-trimoxazole (see p. 275) in high dosage is the drug of choice for the treatment of pneumocystis pneumonia.

Atovaquone is available for AIDS patients who are intolerant of, or who do not respond to, co-trimoxazole. The dose is 750 mg twice daily with food. Trimetrexate has a similar use. It is a potent dihydrofolate reductase inhibitor and must be given with calcium folinate.

Pentamidine isethionate is an alternative to co-trimoxazole and is particularly indicated for patients with a history of adverse reactions or who have not responded to co-trimoxazole. Pentamidine isethionate is a potentially toxic drug that can cause severe hypotension during or immediately after administration. Other severe reactions include hypoglycaemia, pancreatitis and arrhythmias. It can be given by intravenous infusion but can also be administered by inhalation, which reduces side-effects.

Dose. By intravenous infusion: 4 mg/kg daily for at least 14 days (reduced in renal impairment).

By inhalation of nebulised solution, 600 mg daily for 3 weeks; secondary prevention, 300 mg every 4 weeks, or 150 mg every 2 weeks.

Cytomegalovirus (CMV)

Three drugs are in use at present – ganciclovir, cidofovir and foscarnet. Large doses are required to control the infection. Two have to be given intravenously at least twice a day (cidofovir weekly or biweekly). After the spread of infection has been halted, lower maintenance doses are given. Maintenance ganciclovir can be given as capsules but foscarnet has to be given by intravenous infusion. No drug cures the CMV infection; they only suppress it. Resistance is inevitable over time. However, CMV retinitis is a late feature of AIDS.

These drugs have a limited effect on the HIV as well. However, they have severe toxicity and side-effects. Those of ganciclovir are less than those of foscarnet but ganciclovir does affect the bone marrow, as does AZT, and the combination is often too toxic. Monitoring of blood counts and serum creatinine is required. Hydration and pre-treatment with probenecid is required for cidofovir.

MALARIA

There are four malaria parasites that infect humans, by far the most hazardous being *Plasmodium falciparum*, which causes malignant malaria; this can rapidly progress from an acute fever to severe multiorgan disease, leading eventually to cerebral malaria with coma and death. Falciparum malaria usually presents within 3 months of acquiring the infection and, once successfully treated, it does not relapse.

Infection with *Plasmodium vivax*, benign malaria, can present many months after exposure and may relapse for years after the initial infection. It is a less severe illness than that caused by *P. falciparum*. Benign malaria is caused less commonly by *P. ovale* and *P. malariae*.

Most of Africa south of the Sahara is highly malarious, the risk decreasing in southern Africa. Many popular tourist destinations in South-East Asia are low-risk. However, Vietnam, Cambodia and the Thai–Cambodian border are high-risk areas where multidrug-resistant falciparum malaria is transmitted. Melanesia and parts of South America are also malarious.

Protection

It is important to reduce the chance of an infective bite as much as possible, e.g. travellers should sleep in screened accommodation and use aerosols or vaporisers to eliminate mosquitoes.

Chemoprophylaxis

Drug regimens should be started at least 1 week before departure and continued without interruption for 4 weeks after return. This ensures therapeutic blood concentrations before travelling and enables unwanted effects to be dealt with before departure. The continued use of drugs after returning home will deal with infection contracted at the end of the trip. The drugs used in prophylaxis are chloroquine, proguanil and pyrimethamine, either alone or in combinations, depending on the risk factor and the emergence of resistant strains. Mefloquine or doxycycline used alone for short-term travellers is also an option for certain areas of the world.

For those intending travelling to areas where malaria is endemic, the most up-to-date information should be sought on the current chemoprophylaxis.

THREADWORMS (PINWORMS)

The only commonly occurring helminth infection in the UK is enterobiasis. This is caused by the threadworm *Enterobius vermicularis*, also known as pinworm, which is estimated to have affected up to 40% of children by the time they are 10 years old. It is also contracted by adults, but the incidence is lower. Threadworms are initially acquired through swallowing eggs which hatch and mature in the small intestine. After copulating, the males die, and the females migrate to the caecum and anus at night to lay their eggs in the perianal area, attaching them to the skin with a sticky, highly irritant fluid. Some eggs hatch there and return to the rectum to mature. The intense itching caused by the sticky secretion provokes scratching by the host, and eggs are transferred onto the fingers.

Infestation is passed on or perpetuated through picking up eggs on the fingers and being transmitted on fingers to the mouth often via food eaten with unwashed hands. Washing the hands and fingers with the aid of a nail brush before each meal and after each visit to the toilet is essential. Infection is transmitted either by direct contact between individuals or from contaminated surfaces or objects as, under suitable conditions, eggs can remain viable for several weeks outside the human host. Infection is recognised by sighting the whitish worms, about 10 mm in length, on the stools after defecation and sometimes around the anus, and also from the intense perianal itching that they cause.

Anthelmintics are effective in threadworm infections, and their use should be combined with hygienic measures to break the cycle of autoinfection. All members of the family require treatment.

Adult threadworms do not live longer than 6 weeks, and for development of fresh worms, ova must be swallowed and exposed to the action of digestive juices in the upper intestinal tract. A bath taken immediately after rising will remove ova laid during the night. Enterobiasis is treated with mebendazole or piperazine.

Mebendazole

Mode of action. Mebendazole is a benzimidasole derivative which disrupts parasite energy metabolism by causing selective destruction of cytoplasmic microtubules in tegumental and intestinal cells; it irreversibly inhibits glucose uptake and causes immobilisation and death of the parasite within 3 days of administration. It also binds to tubulin, a protein required by the parasite for the uptake of nutrients. It is poorly absorbed from the human gastrointestinal tract, and the small proportion of a dose that is absorbed is almost entirely eliminated from the body following first-pass metabolism in the liver.

Dose. Adults and children over 2 years: a single dose of one 100 mg tablet. Treatment failures are rare but reinfection is possible, in which case a second dose should be given after 2–3 weeks. Mebendazole is not recommended for children under 2 years.

Piperazine

Mode of action. Piperazine acts by blocking the response of worm muscle to acetylcholine, and by interfering with the permeability of cell membranes to ions which regulate cell resting potential. Flaccid paralysis results and the paralysed worms are then expelled from the gut by peristalsis. Piperazine is readily absorbed from the gastrointestinal tract but is almost completely metabolised and excreted through the kidney within 24 hours.

Dose. Piperazine phosphate is presented as a powder in sachets containing 4 g, together with standardised senna which acts as a laxative to facilitate the expulsion of the paralysed worms. *Dose for threadworms*: adults and children over 6 years, one sachet; children 1–6 years, two-thirds of a sachet; infants 3 months to 1 year, one-third of a sachet. The dose should be stirred into a small glass of water or milk and drunk immediately. Because the life cycle of the threadworm is about 30 days, and some worms may be in the larval stage when the first dose is taken, a second dose should be taken after 14 days to eliminate the possibility of reinfection.

Piperazine citrate is available as a syrup, containing the equivalent of 750 mg piperazine hydrate per 5 mL. *Dosage for threadworms:* adults and children over 12 years: 15 mL daily for 7 days; children 7–12 years, 10 mL; children 4–6 years, 7.5 mL; children 2–3 years, 5 mL. For infants and children under 2 years, piperazine citrate should only be given on medical advice.

HANDWASHING

The single most important measure in the prevention of cross-infection is handwashing. Depending on the procedure to be carried out, three levels of handwashing are employed in patient care:

- social
- hygienic hand disinfecting
- surgical.

In all cases, while working with patients, nurses should have short clean nails free of nail varnish and should not wear jewellery or a wrist watch.

The hands should be made *socially clean* by using soap and water, and drying with a paper towel *before* and *after* handling/serving food or working with patients.

Any procedure which requires to be carried out using an aseptic technique, such as the dressing of a wound or the insertion of a urinary catheter, involves *hygienic hand disinfection*.

Surgical handwashing, used prior to surgery, is not discussed.

Most handwash preparations are a formulation of chlorhexidine gluconate available in different strengths. They are considered suitable as they combine detergency with antiseptic properties. They remove and kill transient organisms on the skin and also have some effect on bacteria in deeper layers of the skin. Organisms on the skin include Gram-positive ones such as *Staphylococcus aureus* and Gram-negative ones such as *Escherichia coli*, both of which are common causes of hospital infection. Regular use of an antiseptic handwash has a cumulative effect and an extremely low level of resident organisms can be achieved. For each handwash, the hands should be wetted first before the handwashing agent is applied using an elbow dispenser. All surfaces are lathered, including the wrists. Particular attention should be paid to both the palms and the backs of the hands, the thumbs and fingers as well as between the fingers. Both hands should be cleaned thoroughly; right-handed people tend to clean the left hand more thoroughly and vice versa. Scrubbing the hands is not advocated as this action creates disturbance to the resident flora and can cause trauma. The hands and wrists are rinsed under running water to remove lather and the taps turned off with the elbows or, if necessary, holding a paper towel. Careful drying of the hands with a paper towel is essential to protect the skin from possible breakdown, to make it harder for microorganisms to thrive, and to facilitate putting on gloves. The exact timing of handwashing prior to undertaking an aseptic procedure must be left to the discretion of the nurse. The wearing of gloves does not obviate the need for thorough handwashing.

FURTHER READING

Alcorn A 1997 Is 'undetectable' viral load the optimal aim of treatment – and is it realistic? AIDS Treatment Update Issue 59:1–5

Bloom S 1995 Toohey's medicine: a textbook for students in the health care professions, 15th edn. Churchill Livingstone, Edinburgh

Dawson C, Whitfield H 1996 Urinary incontinence and urinary infection. British Medical Journal 312:961–964

De Cock K M 1997 Guidelines for managing HIV infection. British Medical Journal 315:1–2

Gillespie S 1997 Guide to prophylaxis and diagnosis of malaria. Prescriber 8:19–24

Goodyer L 2000 Malaria. Pharmaceutical Journal 264:405–410

King E 1997 To stay or to switch. AIDS Treatment Update 58:1–3

Klepser M E, Marangos M N, Patel K B et al 1995 Clinical pharmacokinetics of newer cephalosporins. Clinical Pharmacokinetics 28:361–384

Lewis D A 1995 Antibacterial agents: trimethoprim and cotrimoxazole. Prescribers Journal 35:25–36

McMichael A 1996 How HIV fools the immune system. MRC News 69:12–15

Nathwani D 1994 Antibacterial agents – semisynthetic penicillins. Prescribers Journal 34:59–73

Patel R 1996 Valaciclovir: a new drug for genital herpes. Prescriber 7:116–119

Percival A 1997 Increasing resistance to antibiotics – a public health crisis? Hospital Pharmacist 4:193–196

Pietronic M, Davidson R 1996 Treatment for worm infections seen in the UK. Prescriber 7:33–51

Shetty N 1997 A guide to today's use of penicillins in practice. Prescriber 8:49–70

Wise R 1994 Antibacterial agents: oral cephalosporins. Prescribers Journal 34:110–115

Wood M J 1994 Antibacterial agents: macrolides. Prescribers Journal 34:151–156

CHAPTER CONTENTS

20

Drug treatment of endocrine disorders

The endocrine system regulates the inner environment of the body, adjusting and correlating the activities of the various body systems. This regulation is possible through chemical agents which act as messenger substances: hormones. Hormones are secreted by endocrine or ductless glands which are situated in various parts of the body (see Fig. 20.1). They are released directly into the blood which carries them, some attached to a transport protein, to their target organ or tissue where they

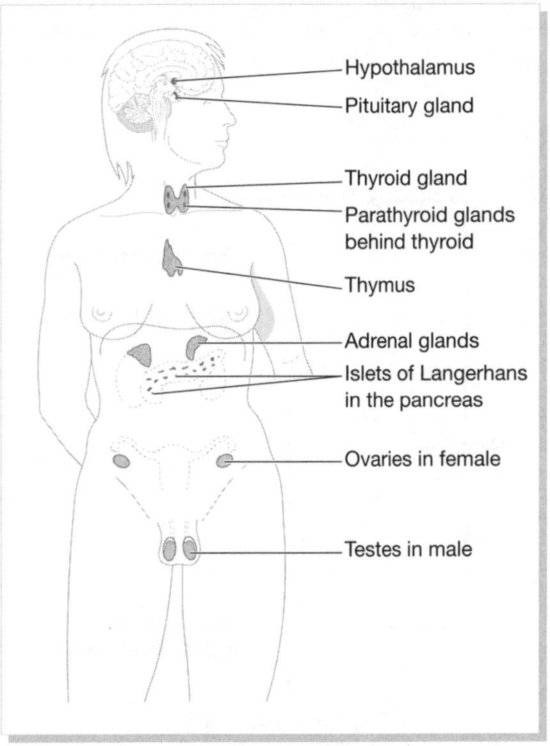

Figure 20.1 The endocrine glands. (After Waugh A, Grant A 2001 Ross and Wilson Anatomy and physiology in health and illness, 9th edn. Churchill Livingstone, Edinburgh.)

act upon specific receptor mechanisms on the surface of the cell or in the cell cytoplasm, producing their characteristic effects, such as the stimulation or inhibition of enzymatic processes.

Some hormones are released in response to internal or external stimulation. Others follow a 24-hour (circadian) rhythm or an even longer rhythm such as the menstrual cycle. In health, a constant blood level of levothyroxine sodium (thyroxine sodium) is maintained.

HORMONAL REGULATION

Although each ductless gland produces a hormone with specific functions, there is an integrated relationship between the activities of the several ductless glands. If these relationships are disturbed by a disease process the consequences can be far-reaching.

The hypothalamus and the pituitary gland together form the central control unit for the production and secretion of many hormones. The hypothalamus produces 'releasing' and 'inhibiting' hormones which influence the anterior lobe of the pituitary gland to release corresponding hormones, the trophic hormones, some of which affect target cells in the body directly while others do so through the intermediary of a second endocrine organ such as the thyroid, the adrenal cortex and the gonads. The second endocrine organ, in turn, produces a third specific hormone such as levothyroxine sodium (thyroxine sodium), corticosteroids or sex hormones, which influences various other body functions.

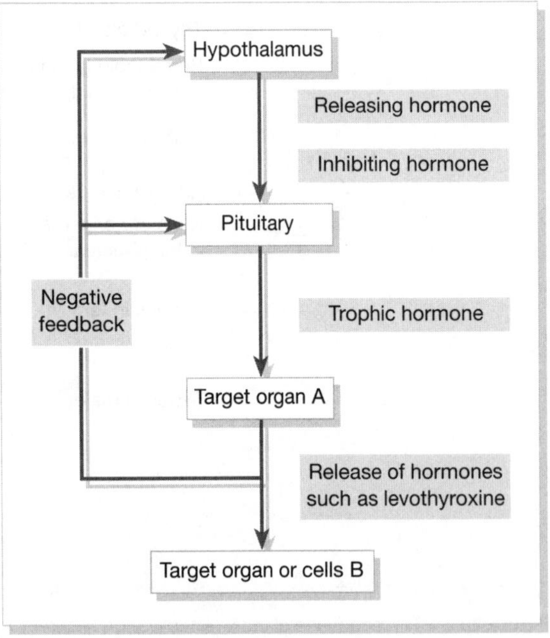

Figure 20.2 Negative feedback mechanism.

Chemoreceptors in the hypothalamus register the blood hormone level and react accordingly by either increasing or decreasing hormone production. If the blood hormone level is low, more hormone is secreted; if the blood hormone level is high, hormone production is reduced (negative feedback) (see Fig. 20.2). Not all hormonal activities, however, follow this mechanism.

HYPOTHALAMUS AND PITUITARY GLAND

The hypothalamus forms the base of the diencephalon (the base of the brain). It is responsible for the coordination of nervous and endocrine systems and therefore many basic life functions such as cardiovascular, respiratory and alimentary functions, sexual behaviour and reproduction. It is connected to the pituitary gland, a small endocrine gland of great importance, by the hypophyseal stalk or infundibulum. The pituitary gland lies almost completely surrounded by bone in the base of the skull. It consists of three parts, the adenohypophysis (anterior lobe), the median eminence and the neurohypophysis (posterior lobe).

The adenohypophysis (see Fig. 20.3) synthesises and releases seven known trophic hormones. These are somatotrophin (STH) which is involved in prepubertal body growth; prolactin which stimulates the growth and secretory activity of the female breasts during pregnancy; melanocyte-stimulating hormone which causes an increase in cutaneous pigmentation; adrenocorticotrophic hormone (ACTH) which governs the secretions of some of the hormones by the adrenal cortex; thyrotrophin (TSH) which stimulates thyroid activity; follicle-stimulating hormone (FSH) or human menopausal gonadotrophin, which stimulates growth of ovarian follicles and secretion of oestrogen in the female and spermatogenesis in the male; and luteinising hormone (LH) which stimulates the production of progesterone in the corpus luteum of the follicle (female) and activates androgen secretion by the Leydig cells of the testis (male).

The neurohypophysis (see Fig. 20.4) hormones vasopressin (antidiuretic hormone (ADH)) and oxytocin are produced in the hypothalamus and secreted (neurosecretion) directly into the bloodstream of the infundibulum and posterior lobe of the pituitary gland from where they can be released into the body.

Vasopressin controls the reabsorption of water by the kidney tubules. In large doses it causes vasoconstriction of the smooth muscles with a concomitant rise

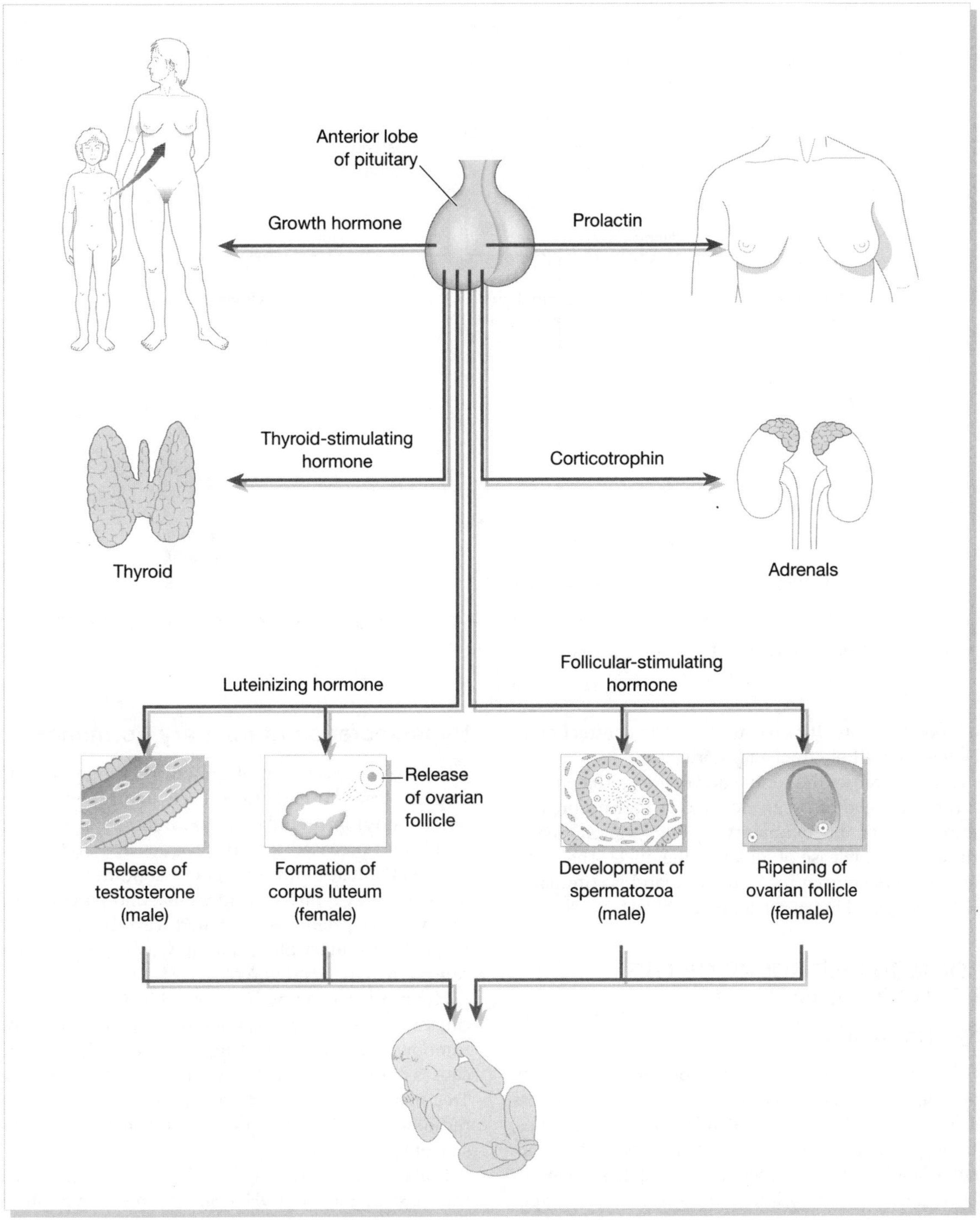

Figure 20.3 Hormones released by anterior pituitary.

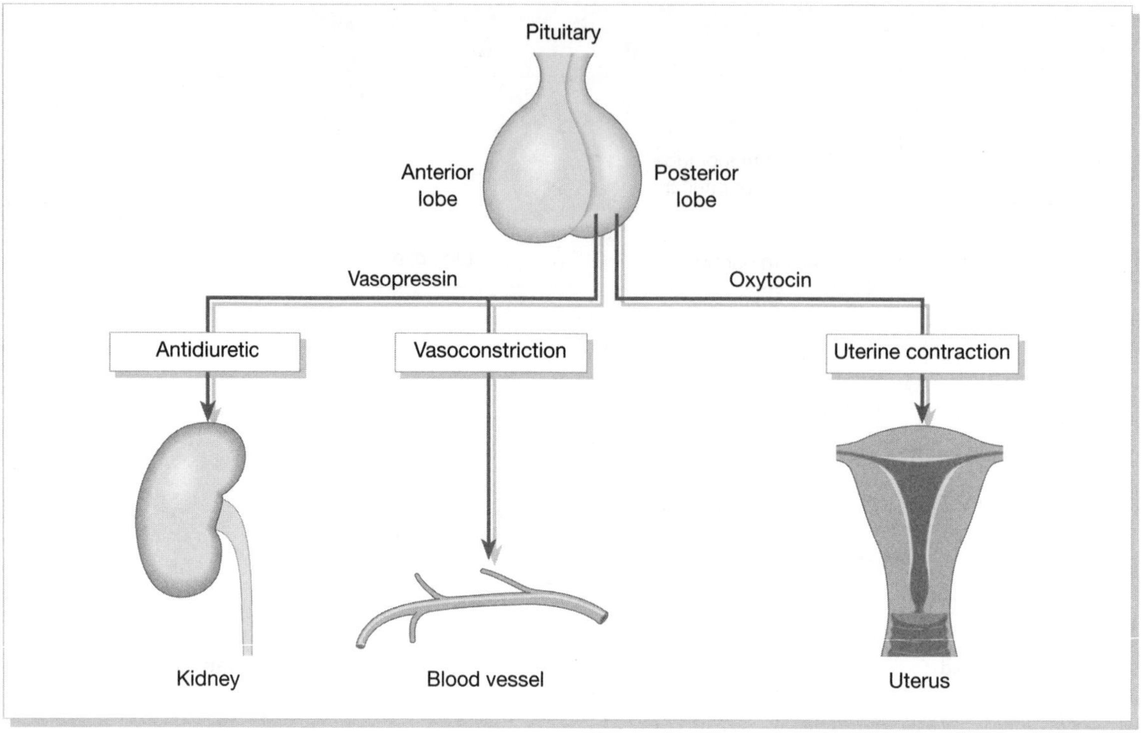

Figure 20.4 Hormones released by posterior pituitary.

in blood pressure. It also causes muscle contraction in the gastrointestinal tract and uterus.

Oxytocin causes the contraction of the uterine muscle towards the end of pregnancy and at parturition, and contraction of the mammary smooth muscle which stimulates the release of milk into the ducts. The secretion of oxytocin from the pituitary gland is stimulated by the baby sucking at the mother's breast.

COMMON DISORDERS OF THE PITUITARY GLAND

Hypopituitarism

Reduced secretion of pituitary hormones caused by tumour, trauma, etc. often results in a progressive loss of function of organs stimulated by trophic hormones, starting with growth hormone deficiency in children, then gonadotrophin deficiency, which causes amenorrhoea and anovulatory infertility in women and impotence and reduced spermatogenesis in men. At a later stage, levels of ACTH and eventually TSH decrease, resulting in hypothyroidism (see p. 300) and Addison's disease (see p. 305).

Hypersecretion of pituitary hormones

The excessive secretion of growth hormone (somatotrophin) leads to gigantism (excessive growth of the whole body) in prepubertal children and acromegaly in adults (increased size of tongue, lips and organs such as the heart and liver); both conditions are usually caused by a pituitary adenoma, and patients tend to have other problems associated with abnormal function of the pituitary gland such as Cushing's syndrome caused by hypersecretion of ACTH.

Hyperprolactinaemia may be due to a variety of causes such as prolactinoma (prolactin-secreting tumour), trauma and drugs. Hyperprolactinaemia causes infertility in women and impotence in men. Treatment usually consists of a combination of surgery, radiotherapy and drug treatment depending on the size of the tumour.

Diabetes insipidus occurs either when there is failure of secretion of ADH from the neurohypophysis (cranial diabetes insipidus) or when ADH secretion is adequate but the kidney fails to respond (nephrogenic diabetes insipidus). This causes a reduced reabsorption of water in the kidney tubules and an increased output of very dilute urine (up to 40 L/day). The loss of water has to be replaced by increased drinking (polydipsia).

MAIN DRUG GROUPS

Hypothalamic hormones, anterior pituitary hormones, and anti-oestrogens

Hypothalamic hormones

Gonadorelin

Gonadorelin is the gonadotrophin-releasing hormone secreted by the hypothalamus.

Use. The uses of gonadorelin are outlined below:

- amenorrhoea and infertility due to abnormal release of endogenous gonadorelin (after a negative response to anti-oestrogens and exclusion of any other causes)
- diagnostic purposes for the assessment of pituitary function.

Administration and dose. For the assessment of pituitary function in adults 100 micrograms is given by intravenous or subcutaneous injection. Gonadorelin analogues are used in the treatment of endometriosis, infertility and anaemia due to uterine fibroids. Breast cancer and prostate cancer may be treated with gonadorelin analogues (see p. 346).

Anterior pituitary hormones

Corticotropins

Tetracosactide is a synthetic anterior pituitary hormone and has the same physiological properties as ACTH but a shorter duration of action. It stimulates the biosynthesis of glucocorticosteroids, mineralocorticosteroids and androgens in the adrenal cortex.

Use. Tetracosactide and its slow-release form are used for diagnostic purposes to investigate adrenocortical insufficiency. Tetracosactide (250 micrograms) is given as an intramuscular or intravenous injection for a 30-minute test. The depot preparation is used for a 5-hour test (1 mg by intramuscular injection) in cases where the 30-minute test has been inconclusive or the functional reserve of the adrenal cortex is being tested. Owing to the variable and unpredictable therapeutic response, tetracosactide is no longer used as a therapeutic agent. Corticosteroids (p. 305) are preferred in the treatment of such conditions as Crohn's disease.

Contraindications and adverse effects. As a polypeptide, tetracosactide may cause allergic reactions, and in severe cases anaphylactic shock (see p. 136). It should not be used in patients with known hypersensitivity to tetracosactide.

Gonadotrophins

There are three known human gonadotrophins, two of which, FSH and LH, are secreted by the pituitary gland, whereas chorionic gonadotrophin (CG) is secreted by the placenta and has LH-like properties. CG for therapeutic use is obtained from the urine of pregnant women, and FSH and LH are extracted from the urine of menopausal women (HMG human menopausal gonadotrophin). HMG comprising 75 units of FSH and 75 units of LH is known as menotrophin. Urofollitropin contains 75 units of FSH but no LH.

Use. Gonadotrophins are used in the following conditions:

- secondary female infertility due to the absence of follicle-ripening or ovulation (FSH and LH followed by CG)
- women undergoing superovulation for in vitro fertilisation (FSH and LH or in conjunction with CG)
- male infertility due to deficient spermatogenesis associated with hypopituitarism (FSH, LH and CG)
- delayed puberty in men due to hypogonadotrophic hypogonadism (FSH, LH and CG)
- cryptorchidism (CG).

Administration and dose. As glycoproteins, which would be destroyed in the digestive system, gonadotrophins must be given parenterally and are generally given intramuscularly. They are available as powder for reconstitution with Water for Injections. The dose depends on the indication and the individual circumstances, e.g. responsiveness of the ovaries to exogenous gonadotrophins; therefore, it is impossible to set a uniform dosage scheme.

Examples for dose regimens are as follows. Female infertility: daily administration of 75–150 units HMG, increasing gradually until oestrogen levels start to rise then reach pre-ovulatory oestrogen levels, followed by a single dose of CG (5000 units intramuscularly) 2 days later. Cryptorchidism: CG 500–4000 units intramuscularly three times a week.

Contraindications and adverse effects. Gonadotrophins are contraindicated in ovarian, pituitary and testicular tumours.

- CG can cause precocious puberty when used in cryptorchidism.
- CG can cause fluid retention so that careful monitoring is advised in patients with cardiac failure, migraine, renal dysfunction, hypertension and epilepsy.

• CG can also cause gynaecomastia, ovarian hyperstimulation with multiple ovulations, ovarian enlargement and even rupture.

• HMG (FSH and LH) can cause ovarian hyperstimulation with an increased risk of multiple pregnancies, fluid retention and oliguria.

Somatropin (synthetic human growth hormone)

Somatropin, a biosynthetic human growth hormone, has replaced growth hormone of human origin which has been implicated as a cause of CJD.

Use. Growth hormone is used in the treatment of short stature in children with hypopituitarism whose epiphyses have not yet fused, and in short stature associated with Turner syndrome.

Administration and dose. Like other peptides, somatropin must be given parenterally by subcutaneous or intramuscular injection. It is available as powder for reconstitution for SC or IM injection.

The dose is determined on an individual basis depending on the condition being treated.

Contraindications and adverse effects. These are as follows:

• Use of somatropin is contraindicated in patients with fused epiphyses.

• Lipoatrophy at the injection site may occur; it can be prevented by varying the injection site.

• Somatropin may influence glucose tolerance, and patients with diabetes mellitus might have to change the dosage of their hypoglycaemic drugs.

Anti-oestrogens

Anti-oestrogens act as antagonists to oestrogens at the relevant chemoreceptors in the hypothalamus, preventing the inhibitory effects of oestrogens on the gonadotrophin-releasing hormone gonadorelin. This causes an increased release of gonadotrophins from the pituitary gland and, by stimulating the ovaries, ovulation in women with anovulatory cycles.

Use. Anti-oestrogens are used in the treatment of anovulatory infertility attributed to dysfunction of the hypothalamo-pituitary–ovarian axis or when the cause is unknown. Before considering treatment with an anti-oestrogen other causes of infertility should be excluded. Appropriate treatment should first be given to other treatable endocrine disorders, such as hyperprolactinaemia and pituitary tumours. To make a successful outcome of the treatment more likely, the patient should also have an adequate level of endogenous oestrogens. Some anti-oestrogens such as tamoxifen are used in breast cancer (see p. 346).

Drugs used in this group are:

- clomifene citrate
- tamoxifen.

Administration and dose. Both drugs are available as tablets. Clomifene is given generally as a dose of 50 mg/day for 5 days (tamoxifen 20 mg daily for 4 days) starting on the fifth day (second day for tamoxifen) of the cycle and at any time in women who are not menstruating. If there is no ovulation after the first course, the dose may be increased to 100 mg/day (40 mg then 80 mg for tamoxifen) for 5 days starting 30 days after the first course. If no ovulation has occurred after the third course, treatment should be stopped and a new evaluation of the cause of infertility should take place.

Contraindications and adverse effects. Liver disease, abnormal uterine bleeding and pregnancy are contraindications for treatment with anti-oestrogens. To exclude pregnancy, careful monitoring of basal temperature throughout the cycle is necessary. Adverse effects are usually dose-related and include hot flushing, rashes, breast discomfort and weight gain. If visual side-effects and ovarian hyperstimulation occur, treatment should be withdrawn immediately.

Multiple pregnancy, mostly twins, occurs in about 8% of successful pregnancies induced with anti-oestrogen treatment. Patients have to be made aware of this possibility and the risks associated with multiple pregnancies. It is recommended that clomifene should not normally be used for more than six cycles because of the possible increased risk of ovarian cancer.

Posterior pituitary hormones

Vasopressin (antidiuretic hormone ADH)

The use of vasopressin, a peptide with antidiuretic and vasoconstrictor properties, has declined since the development of more selective semisynthetic analogues desmopressin and terlipressin. Desmopressin has no vasoconstrictor effect but it has an increased antidiuretic activity and a longer duration of action than vasopressin (synthetic porcine vasopressin); terlipressin is used for its vasoconstrictor effects.

Use. The uses are as follows:

- treatment of pituitary diabetes insipidus (desmopressin and vasopressin); for long-term treatment, desmopressin is preferred
- diagnosis of diabetes insipidus (desmopressin)
- primary nocturnal enuresis in adults and children (desmopressin)
- treatment of bleeding oesophageal varices (vasopressin, terlipressin).

Administration and dose. *Pituitary diabetes insipidus.* In acute cases, such as after a head injury, vasopressin or desmopressin are used as intramuscular or subcutaneous injection; because of its much longer duration of action desmopressin has to be given only once a day (1–4 micrograms). For long-term maintenance treatment, desmopressin is available as nasal spray (10 micrograms/metered spray) or nasal solution (100 micrograms/mL). Oral treatment of diabetes insipidus (in adults and children) with desmopressin tablets (200 micrograms) requires careful monitoring and dosage adjustment.

Oesophageal varices. For the initial treatment of bleeding oesophageal varices, vasopressin is given as an intravenous infusion (20 units diluted in 100 mL glucose 5% w/v). Terlipressin is given as a single intravenous dose of 2 mg which can be repeated every 4–6 hours.

Contraindications and adverse effects. These are outlined as follows:

- Despite its reduced vasopressor effects, desmopressin, like all vasopressins, has to be used with extreme caution in patients with cardiovascular problems.
- Water retention and water intoxication may occur following large doses.
- In low doses, nausea, abdominal cramps and a rise in blood pressure may occur.
- Nasal preparations may cause nasal congestion and local ulceration.

Patients on nasal preparations have to be counselled on the proper use of the device. Improper use will result in unsatisfactory response.

Oxytocin

Oxytocin is used in obstetrics (see p. 317).

Dopamine receptor stimulants

Bromocriptine is chemically related to ergotamine and is a stimulant for dopamine receptors in the brain. It also inhibits the release of prolactin and growth hormone from the pituitary.

Use. The uses are outlined as follows:

- treatment of prolactin-secreting tumours of the pituitary gland (prolactinoma) and acromegaly alone or in conjunction with surgery and radiotherapy
- galactorrhoea, hyperprolactinaemic infertility
- suppression of lactation after childbirth (only if simple analgesia will not suffice)
- in the treatment of idiopathic Parkinson's disease
- cyclical breast pain and cyclical menstrual disorders.

Administration and dose. Bromocriptine is available as 1 mg and 2.5 mg tablets and 5 mg and 10 mg capsules. There is a great difference in the dosage range depending on the condition to be treated and the individual response to treatment. In most indications, apart from suppression and prevention of lactation, the optimum dosage is achieved by gradual introduction of bromocriptine. In this way optimum response and minimum side-effects can be properly balanced.

Contraindications and adverse effects. Bromocriptine is contraindicated in hypertension after childbirth, toxaemia of pregnancy and known hypersensitivity reactions to bromocriptine or other ergot alkaloids. Adverse effects are numerous and dose-related, and can usually be reduced by dose adjustment:

- gastrointestinal disturbance
- hypotensive reactions at the beginning of the treatment
- ovulation in hyperprolactinaemic women; this effect may be desired – as in the treatment of hyperprolactinaemic women; if the effect is undesired, patients should be advised on the use of contraception
- dry mouth, leg cramps, cardiac arrhythmias
- peptic ulceration in acromegaly patients.

Cabergoline has similar actions and uses to bromocriptine but may be better tolerated in some patients than bromocriptine. Quinagolide is a similar drug given in smaller doses than both bromocriptine and cabergoline.

THYROID GLAND

The thyroid gland is situated anteriorly in the lower part of the neck. It consists of two side lobes connected by a narrow region, the isthmus. The gland is made up of two types of secretory cell: the thyroid follicles secreting the hormones levothyroxine sodium (thyroxine sodium) and liothyronine sodium, and the parafollicular cells, which secrete thyrocalcitonin (calcium-lowering hormone). Levothyroxine and liothyronine are derivatives of the amino acid tyrosine. They are formed in the thyroid follicles by incorporating circulating iodine, stored and transported in the plasma almost entirely bound to levothyroxine sodium-binding globulin. After secretion, the minute unbound (free) hormone fraction diffuses into tissues and exerts its hormonal

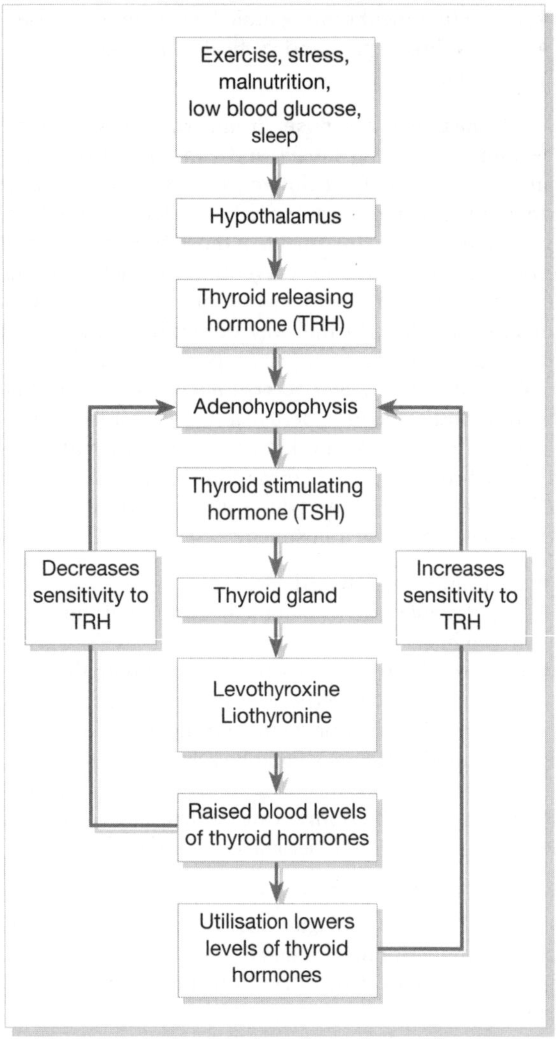

Figure 20.5 Production and regulation of thyroid hormones.

activity after conversion of levothyroxine into the more potent and more rapidly metabolised liothyronine.

Production of hormones is stimulated by TSH, which is released from the pituitary gland in response to hypothalamic thyrotrophin-releasing hormone (TRH). The production is regulated by negative feedback through circulating concentrations of free liothyronine (Fig. 20.5).

Levothyroxine and liothyronine increase the oxygen consumption of almost all metabolically active tissues; this means an increase in the metabolic rate. They also affect growth and maturation, especially brain and skeletal development.

COMMON DISORDERS OF THE THYROID GLAND

Hypothyroidism (thyroid deficiency)

Hypothyroidism results from a reduced secretion by the thyroid gland, irrespective of the cause. The most common causes of primary hypothyroidism are thyroid failure following radioactive iodine-131 (^{131}I) therapy and surgical treatment; thyroid failure associated with Hashimoto's thyroiditis or an autoimmune disease; and congenital thyroid failure (congenital hypothyroidism or cretinism). Hypothyroidism due to pituitary failure (secondary hypothyroidism) is much less common.

Hypothyroidism causes a reduction in the basal metabolic rate and affects most systems in the body. Symptoms vary in range and severity. They may include goitre, bradycardia, depression, iron-deficiency anaemia, infertility, constipation and dermatological symptoms.

In children with hypothyroidism the dominant features are reduction in growth and arrest of pubertal development.

Severe hypothyroidism in the adult is called myxoedema and is marked by a thickening and swelling of the skin. Hypothyroid coma is the severest form of thyroid deficiency and a medical emergency. The patient has a reduced level of consciousness and a body temperature which may be as low as 25°C.

Hyperthyroidism

Hyperthyroidism (thyrotoxicosis) results from exposure of the body tissues to excess circulating levels of free levothyroxine and/or free liothyronine. It is a common disorder which affects women more than men.

It is very important to establish the cause of hyperthyroidism to be able to provide adequate treatment. The most common conditions are:

- Graves' disease
- toxic multinodular goitre
- toxic solitary nodule (autonomous thyroid hormone-secreting adenoma).

Hyperthyroidism causes an increase in the basal metabolic rate and affects almost every system in the body. It presents with a wide variety of symptoms and severity. Symptoms include:

- an increase in body temperature
- tachycardia
- restlessness
- vomiting and diarrhoea
- loss of libido and infertility
- pruritus

- ocular symptoms such as exophthalmos in Graves' disease
- goitre.

Thyrotoxic crisis ('thyroid storm') is a life-threatening increase in the severity of the clinical features of thyrotoxicosis and requires immediate treatment. It is very unusual but may occur after subtotal thyroidectomy, within a few days after ^{131}I therapy, or may be precipitated by infection in a patient with hyperthyroidism which is inadequately controlled by antithyroid drugs.

Treatment includes intravenous propranolol (to control cardiac symptoms) intravenous hydrocortisone, oral iodine solution and an antithyroid drug.

Non-toxic goitre

Non-toxic diffuse goitre may be caused by iodine deficiency, drugs such as lithium carbonate, Hashimoto's thyroiditis or Graves' disease. It is usually easy to make the right diagnosis and provide adequate treatment. The simple goitre is of unknown aetiology and usually requires no treatment.

Drugs and thyroid function

Drugs can influence thyroid function in different ways. Some drugs, e.g. androgens, oestrogens, salicylates, alter thyroid function tests. Some drugs may induce thyroid disease. Those which induce hypothyroidism include antithyroid drugs, lithium, sulphonylureas, amiodarone; those which cause hyperthyroidism include iodides and levothyroxine.

Thyroid disease can alter the distribution, metabolism and elimination of some drugs such as digoxin. Thyroid disease may also alter the pharmacodynamic effects of some drugs such as cardiac glycosides and warfarin.

MAIN DRUG GROUPS

Thyroid hormones

Levothyroxine and liothyronine are the naturally occurring thyroid hormones. Liothyronine with a half-life of 1–2 days has a much faster onset of action than levothyroxine with a half-life of 7 days. Levothyroxine reaches its maximum effect after about 10 days. The difference in the onset of action is important for the therapeutic use of thyroid hormones.

Use. Because of its rapid and more potent effect, liothyronine is used in the treatment of acute hypothyroid states. In the treatment of hypothyroid coma, liothyronine as injection is the treatment of choice, usually in conjunction with other measures such as intravenous corticosteroids, intravenous fluids, slow rewarming using blankets and foil, with broad-spectrum antibiotic cover and oxygen.

Levothyroxine is normally the drug of choice for routine replacement therapy in hypothyroidism of any cause. In congenital hypothyroidism, treatment has to begin as soon as possible after birth to prevent irreversible brain damage.

Thyroid hormones are also used to suppress the release of thyroid-stimulating hormone from the pituitary gland in the treatment of non-toxic diffuse goitre, Hashimoto's thyroiditis and thyroid carcinoma, and in combination with antithyroid drugs to prevent the development of a goitre in hyperthyroid patients.

Administration and dose. A dose of 20 micrograms of levothyroxine is equivalent to 100 micrograms of liothyronine. Dosage for replacement therapy is individual and is usually started slowly with a dose of 50 micrograms of levothyroxine and then increased to a dose of 100–200 micrograms daily. In the elderly, and patients with ischaemic heart disease, the initial dose should be 25 micrograms/day.

When first treating severe hypothyroidism, liothyronine is used as an initial dose of 5 micrograms, increased to 60 micrograms at weekly intervals. When a dose of 60 micrograms is reached, treatment should switch to low-dose levothyroxine increased by 50 micrograms at 4-week intervals up to 200 micrograms if required.

The dose can be monitored by the clinical response of the patient but serum liothyronine and TSH levels should be measured at intervals. The correct dose of liothyronine is that which restores serum TSH concentration to normal.

For the treatment of myxoedema coma, 5–20 micrograms of levothyroxine are given by slow intravenous injection, repeated at 12-hour intervals or more frequently if necessary.

Contraindications and adverse effects. These are as follows:

- Thyroid hormones should be used with caution in patients with cardiovascular problems, prolonged myxoedema or adrenal failure (in the elderly).
- Adverse effects are dose-related and usually disappear on reduction of dosage or withdrawal of treatment. Especially in the early stages of treatment, patients may suffer from anginal pain, cardiac arrhythmias or myocardial infarction. Patients with a pre-existing heart condition are especially at risk.
- Other side-effects include gastrointestinal disturbance, tremors, restlessness, excessive loss of weight and muscular weakness.

Interactions. Levothyroxine sodium (thyroxine sodium) increases the effects of anticoagulants, phenytoin, digoxin and adrenoceptor agonists such as salbutamol, accelerates the response to tricyclic antidepressants and also raises blood sugar levels. The dosage of antidiabetic agents may have to be adjusted.

Patients on replacement therapy should be advised that treatment has to continue for life and follow-up is important, and that tablets should be taken regularly to ensure an adequate level of serum liothyronine and TSH.

Antithyroid drugs

Carbimazole and propylthiouracil

Carbimazole and propylthiouracil prevent the conversion of iodide to iodine, the incorporation of iodine into the prehormonal stages and therefore the production of thyroid hormones.

Use. Carbimazole and propylthiouracil are used:

- in the long-term management of hyperthyroidism
- in the preparation for thyroidectomy in hyperthyroidism
- in the preparation for, and as concomitant therapy with, radio-iodine treatment
- in combination with levothyroxine as a blocking–replacement therapy to prevent the development of goitre and hypothyroidism.

Administration and dose. Carbimazole and propylthiouracil are both available as tablets only. The initial dose of carbimazole is 20–60 mg (propylthiouracil 300–600 mg) daily in two or three divided doses. Carbimazole is not effective until 10–14 days after the beginning of treatment because the thyroid is still releasing its existing hormone reserves for a period of time. After about 3–4 weeks the patient is usually clinically and biochemically euthyroid. The dose may then be reduced progressively to a maintenance dose of between 5 and 15 mg (propylthiouracil 50–150 mg) daily as a single dose. The dose should be determined by clinical status and ideally by the measurement of plasma thyroid hormone levels. Treatment should continue for 12–18 months. If a relapse occurs after discontinuation of treatment, further measures may have to be considered (see Management of hyperthyroidism).

Adverse reactions, side-effects and cautions. The most serious adverse effect of carbimazole and propylthiouracil is bone marrow depression which can lead to agranulocytosis. This is almost always reversible following withdrawal of the drug. Since there is usually no cross-sensitivity between the antithyroid drugs, carbimazole may be successfully substituted by propylthiouracil and vice versa.

Common side-effects are skin rashes and pruritus which are usually self-limiting and do not require withdrawal of the drug.

Both drugs may be used in pregnancy as long as the dose is in the standard range and the woman is monitored regularly. The blocking–replacement regimen must not be used during pregnancy or lactation.

Both drugs are secreted in breast milk but this should not preclude breast-feeding as long as neonatal monitoring is carried out and the lowest dose is used.

Patients should be advised to report sore throats, mouth ulcers, fever or rashes immediately, since these might be early signs of bone marrow depression, and to keep follow-up appointments especially in the initial stages.

Propranolol or nadolol is used for the rapid relief of thyrotoxic symptoms.

Iodine and iodide (in the form of potassium iodide)

Iodine and iodide act by inhibiting the release of levothyroxine and liothyronine from the thyroid into the plasma; they therefore reduce thyroid function very rapidly.

Use. Iodine and iodide are used:

- in the treatment of thyrotoxic crisis (thyroid storm) in conjunction with a beta-blocker (propranolol or nadolol), high doses of antithyroid drugs and corticosteroids to inhibit the peripheral conversion of liothyronine to levothyroxine, and
- to prepare a patient for thyroidectomy by reducing vascularity and friability of the thyroid, and therefore reducing the risk of haemorrhage.

Administration and dose. Iodine and iodide are available as Lugol's solution (aqueous iodine oral solution) which contains 5% iodine and 10% potassium iodide (total iodine 130 mg/mL).

In the treatment of thyrotoxic crisis the dose is 2–3 mL daily, well diluted with milk or water.

Preoperative Lugol's solution has to be given for 10–14 days in a dose of 0.1–0.3 mL three times daily.

Long-term treatment with iodine and iodide is not recommended because its antithyroid action diminishes in time.

Contraindications, adverse reactions and side-effects. Iodine is contraindicated in breast-feeding mothers because it may cause goitre in the infant. Iodine can cause hypersensitivity reactions, conjunctivitis, pain in the salivary glands, bronchitis, gastroenteritis, insomnia and depression.

Management of hyperthyroidism

Short-term treatment. Beta-adrenoceptor blocking agents, propranolol or nadolol, are used to relieve acute symptoms such as tachycardia, tremor and anxiety in the latent period before antithyroid drugs become effective and in conjunction with Lugol's solution for the preparation of patients with mild to moderate hyperthyroidism for surgery.

Long-term treatment. This involves three options:

1. antithyroid drugs for 12–18 months
2. radioactive iodine (^{131}I) for those cases in which drug therapy fails; or
3. surgery in recurrent hyperthyroidism, a large goitre or a single adenoma.

PARATHYROID GLANDS

The parathyroids consist of four small endocrine glands which are situated at the back of the thyroid gland. They produce parathormone (PTH) which is essential for life. Parathormone regulates the metabolism of calcium and phosphorus in the body by action on the kidney, gut and bone (in a dual control mechanism with thyrocalcitonin). It also stimulates the formation of colecalciferol (vitamin D_3), which plays an important part in the mineralisation of bone. The release of PTH from the parathyroid glands depends directly on the blood calcium level.

COMMON DISORDERS OF THE PARATHYROID GLANDS

Hypoparathyroidism

Hypoparathyroidism is a deficiency in parathormone which may be caused by surgical damage to the parathyroids after total or partial thyroidectomy. It results in a decrease of the blood calcium level (hypocalcaemia) and an increase in blood phosphorus (hyperphosphataemia). Hypocalcaemia causes tetany which is characterised by increased tone of skeletal muscles with spasms of the hands, feet and larynx, and generalised convulsions.

Hyperparathyroidism

Hyperparathyroidism (primary) is an increased release of parathormone, usually due to a parathyroid adenoma. The presenting features are due mainly to the raised blood calcium level (hypercalcaemia).

Hypercalcaemia. The most common causes of hypercalcaemia are malignant disease and primary hyperparathyroidism, vitamin D intoxication, and immobilisation (paraplegia in the young and Paget's disease in the elderly). The main features include fatigue, weakness, polydipsia and polyuria, renal stones, nephrocalcinosis, bone changes (osteitis fibrosa), duodenal ulceration and chronic pancreatitis. Some drugs, such as the thiazides and lithium, can also cause hypercalcaemia. Severe hypercalcaemia is an emergency and requires urgent treatment.

MAIN DRUG GROUPS

Calcitonin

Calcitonin lowers the blood calcium level by reducing the renal tubular reabsorption of calcium and increasing its deposition in the bone. By reducing the blood calcium level it also relieves bone pain. Calcitonin is available as synthetic or recombinant salmon calcitonin (salcatonin).

Use. Calcitonin (salmon) (salcatonin) is used for the treatment of:

- hypercalcaemia due to a raised bone turnover such as in Paget's disease of bone and malignancies with bone metastases
- primary hyperparathyroidism
- vitamin D intoxication
- postmenopausal osteoporosis.

Administration and dose. Calcitonin (salmon) (salcatonin) is currently available only as an injection (subcutaneous or intramuscular). The dose depends on the condition treated and its severity. Dose adjustments should be made according to the patient's clinical and biochemical response. Dose regimens may range from 50 units of calcitonin (salmon) (salcatonin) three times a week to 100 units daily in Paget's disease of bone and may be as high as 400 units every 6–8 hours in severe hypercalcaemia.

Adverse effects and cautions. Adverse effects of calcitonin (salmon) (salcatonin) include nausea, vomiting, diarrhoea, flushing, paraesthesia and an unpleasant taste in the mouth. There does not seem to be other serious toxicity. However, calcitonin (salmon) (salcatonin) should be used with caution in pregnancy and breastfeeding. Patients with a history of allergies should undergo a skin test before treatment is undertaken.

Bisphosphonates

Bisphosphonates reduce bone turnover by inhibiting the growth and dissolution of hydroxyapatite crystals and retarding bone resorption and formation. The main indications and dosage regimes are outlined in Table 20.1.

Contraindications, adverse effects and cautions. Bisphosphonates are contraindicated in patients with

Table 20.1 Bisphosphonates

Drug	Preparation	Main indications/dose	Notes
Alendronic acid	5 mg and 10 mg tablets	Postmenopausal osteoporosis: 10 mg daily for treatment; 5 mg daily for prevention. Corticosteroid-induced osteoporosis: 5–10 mg daily	Biochemical monitoring is essential with all these drugs. Higher dose for women not receiving HRT
Disodium etidronate	200 mg and 400 mg tablets	Paget's disease of bone: 5 mg/kg as a single daily dose for up to 6 months (higher doses may be given for shorter periods, up to a maximum of 20 mg/kg daily). Also given with calcium carbonate in the treatment of osteoporosis	Patients should be advised to avoid iron and mineral supplements and antacids
Disodium pamidronate	15 mg, 30 mg and 90 mg injection	Hypercalcaemia of malignancy in dosage determined by serum calcium concentration, by slow IV injection into a large vein. Osteolytic lesions/bone pain: 90 mg every 4 weeks. Paget's disease of bone in various dosage regimens	May be given to coincide with courses of chemotherapy in breast cancer
Risedronate sodium	5 mg and 30 mg tablets	Paget's disease of bone: 30 mg daily for 2 months. In osteoporosis: 5 mg daily	
Sodium clodronate	400 mg capsules, 520 mg and 800 mg tablets, IV solution (for dilution) 30 mg/mL	For osteolytic lesions and bone pain in malignant disease: 1.6 g daily in single or two divided doses up to a maximum of 3.2 g daily (orally). Slow IV administration in hypercalcaemia of malignancy: 300 mg daily for up to 10 days or a single dose infusion of 1.5 g	It is essential to maintain adequate fluid intake during treatment
Tiludronic acid	200 mg tablets	Paget's disease of bone: 400 mg daily as a single dose for 12 weeks	

known hypersensitivities to etidronate, pamidronate or clodronate. Since bisphosphonates are excreted by the kidney they should be used with caution in patients with renal impairment. In higher doses, disodium etidronate causes demineralisation of bone, which can lead to spontaneous fractures. Patients may also experience increased bone pain during the first month of treatment. The adverse effects of bisphosphonates are nausea, diarrhoea and a metallic taste. The bisphosphonates may cause oesophageal reactions, and it is vitally important to ensure the patient takes the tablet in the correct manner. Patients should avoid food for 2 hours before and after oral treatment. Tablets should not be taken with milk, and antacids must be avoided. Patients should sit or stand upright for at least 30 minutes after taking a dose.

TREATMENT OF SEVERE HYPERCALCAEMIA

The initial treatment consists of intravenous fluid replacement with sodium chloride 0.9% solution, 4–6 litres in 24 hours as necessary. Intravenous potassium and magnesium may be needed to correct imbalances. Once the patient has been rehydrated adequately, intravenous furosemide (frusemide), which has a calciuretic effect, may be added. If these measures are insufficient, a bisphosphonate, or salmon calcitonin, may be used to lower the blood calcium level further.

ADRENAL GLAND

Corticosteroids are secreted from the outer layer of the adrenal gland known as the cortex. It is regarded as a separate endocrine gland from the inner section, which is called the medulla. The cortex is divided into three different zones, each of which secretes different hormones as shown in Box 20.1.

Box 20.1 Hormones secreted by the cortex of the adrenal gland

- Outer zone (zona glomerulosa) – mineralocorticoids
- Middle zone (zona fasciculata) – glucocorticoids
- Inner zone (zona reticularis) – glucocorticoids, sex hormones

Mineralocorticoids

These hormones play an important part in regulating mineral salt (electrolyte) metabolism. The hormone with the most physiological importance is aldosterone. The release of aldosterone from the adrenal cortex is controlled by angiotensin, which is formed by renin. Renin is an enzyme released by the kidneys whenever the blood pressure in the afferent arterioles decreases to a certain level. Aldosterone facilitates the reabsorption of sodium by the kidney tubules. When there is an increase

Table 20.2 Properties of corticosteroids

Corticosteroids	Main properties/actions
Mineralocorticoids Fludrocortisone acetate	Fludrocortisone has only minimal anti-inflammatory action and is used solely for its mineralocorticoid activity in Addison's disease. The daily dosage range is 50–300 micrograms per day. If glucocorticoid activity is required, cortisone or hydrocortisone is given concurrently, especially at times of stress and severe illness. Adverse effects are broadly similar to those occurring with glucocorticoids but, as would be expected from the physiology, major problems are oedema, weight gain, hypertension and electrolyte disturbances. Biochemical monitoring is advised
Glucocorticoids Betamethasone Cortisone Dexamethasone Hydrocortisone Methylprednisolone Prednisolone The above glucocorticoids have varying potencies in terms of the anti-inflammatory effects, e.g. 5 mg of prednisolone is equivalent to 20 mg hydrocortisone. Although all the above drugs have broadly similar properties, differences between them influence the choice of drug in particular conditions	*Beneficial properties* Anti-inflammatory action Euphoria* Stimulation of appetite* Protect the body from effects of acute hypersensitivity reactions (see p. 136) Immunosuppression *Adverse effects* Cushing's syndrome (at higher doses over a prolonged period) Diabetes mellitus Infection risk in patients exposed to viral diseases (especially chickenpox) Insomnia/mental disturbances/euphoria Muscle wasting Osteoporosis (of particular concern in older patients) Peptic ulceration/dyspepsia Taste disturbances In children, corticosteroids may suppress growth The use of corticosteroids in pregnancy and in breast-feeding has been reviewed by the CSM and advice issued in the BNF It is vitally important to recognise that prolonged corticosteroid therapy may cause adrenal atrophy. Sudden termination of therapy may be catastrophic. Adrenal insufficiency, hypotension and even death can result (patients on corticosteroid therapy must be carefully assessed prior to surgery). Any changes in dosage levels must be carefully adjusted and a tapering regime adopted if dosage reduction is indicated

* In certain situations these properties may cause problems in the management of patients.

in the amount of aldosterone secreted, there is retention of sodium chloride and hence water, leading to oedema.

Glucocorticoids

The main glucocorticoids are cortisol, also known as hydrocortisone, and corticosterone, which are essential to life. Glucocorticoids have a number of vital functions. They:

- accelerate the breakdown of cellular proteins to amino acids; the amino acids in turn circulate to the liver where they are converted to glucose, a process referred to as gluconeogenesis
- accelerate the mobilisation and breakdown of fats; fat metabolism therefore tends to take over from the usual carbohydrate metabolism
- are essential for maintenance of the blood pressure
- increase their secretion in times of physical or emotional stress
- in high concentration, reduce the number of eosinophils and cause the lymphatic tissues to atrophy, reducing the number of lymphocytes and plasma cells
- have anti-inflammatory properties.

Corticosteroids, like other hormones, are used in both replacement therapy and in the treatment of a wide range of conditions, such as inflammatory bowel disease, asthma, allergies, malignant diseases and skin diseases, both orally and topically. The main properties of corticosteroids are summarised in Table 20.2.

Clinical indications for the use of glucocorticoids (other than replacement therapy)

The use of corticosteroids (glucocorticoids) in certain conditions is dealt with as follows:

- emergency treatment (see p. 137)
- eye diseases (see p. 413)
- diseases of the gastrointestinal tract (treatment of inflammatory bowel disease: see p. 157)
- malignant disease (see p. 346)

Table 20.3 The glucocorticoids

Drug	Dose range*/route	Properties
Betamethasone	Oral: 0.5–5 mg daily. IM or IV: 4–20 mg 6-hourly	Very high glucocorticoid activity. Insignificant mineralocorticoid activity (widely used topically as the valerate)
Cortisone	Oral: 25–37.5 mg daily in divided doses	Has significant mineralocorticoid activity. Not suitable for long-term therapy. Useful for replacement therapy
Dexamethasone	Oral: 0.5–10 mg daily. IV in cerebral oedema: 10 mg initially then 4 mg IM every 6 hours	As betamethasone
Hydrocortisone	Oral: 20–30 mg per day in divided doses. IM or IV: 100–500 mg three to four times daily. Rectal foam: 125 mg	Hydrocortisone is produced by conversion of cortisone in the liver. Hydrocortisone is the active agent and is therefore often preferred to cortisone. Other properties similar to cortisone
Prednisolone	Oral: 10–20 mg daily. IM: 25–100 mg weekly. Rectal foam: 20 mg	Prednisolone is a derivative of hydrocortisone and has predominant hydrocorticoid activity. It is the most commonly used oral glucocorticoid

*Wide variation of dosage will be seen, depending on the condition treated.

- Always carry this card with you and show it to anyone who treats you (e.g. a doctor, nurse, pharmacist or dentist). For one year after you stop the treatment, you must mention that you have taken steroids.
- If you become ill, or if you come into contact with anyone who has an infectious disease, consult your doctor promptly. If you have never had chickenpox, you should avoid close close contact with people who have chickenpox or shingles. If you do come into contact with chickenpox, see your doctor urgently.
- Make sure that the information on the card is kept up to date.

Name	
Address	
Tel	
GP	
Hospital	
Consultant	
Hospital no.	

STEROID TREATMENT CARD

I am a patient on STEROID treatment which must not be stopped suddenly

- If you have been taking this medicine for more than three weeks, the dose should be reduced gradually when you stop taking steroids unless your doctor says otherwise.
- Read the patient information leaflet given with the medicine.

Date	Drug	Dose

Figure 20.6 Steroid treatment card, Department of Health, as cited in BNF.

- palliative care (see p. 475)
- diseases of the respiratory tract (see p. 209)
- skin diseases (see p. 447)
- renal disease (see p. 322)
- rheumatic disease (see p. 403).

Glucocorticoids are powerful drugs which have brought great benefits to patients. The main properties of the commonly used glucocorticoid drugs are summarised in Table 20.3. Adverse effects (see Table 20.2) are significant, but with careful dosage adjustment and other measures these can be minimised. Patient counselling is vitally important. All patients should be encouraged to read the patient information leaflet supplied and given a 'steroid' card (Fig. 20.6). Local therapy has greatly reduced the incidence of systemic side-effects, e.g. the use of corticosteroids that are not absorbed (see p. 210 and p. 447). However, it should be noted that absorption of active ingredient from a topically approved product can occur.

Sex hormones

In both sexes, the adrenal cortex secretes significant amounts of both oestrogens (female hormones) and androgens (male hormones). In the female, the ovaries produce oestrogens and progesterone: oestrogen from the graafian follicles and progesterone from a temporary structure known as the corpus luteum. In the male, testosterone is secreted by the testes. The functions of the sex hormones are described on page 294.

Treatment using sex hormones

Sex hormones are used in replacement therapy when natural secretions are deficient and for the treatment of certain tumours (see p. 347). Long-term therapy with oestrogens requires the addition of a progestogen to reduce the risk of endometrial cancer. The main uses of sex hormones are summarised in Table 20.4.

Table 20.4 Main uses of sex hormones

Drug group	Dosage/clinical indications/side-effects/precautions
OESTROGENS *Estradiol*	Available both in tablet and transdermal form. An implant is also available. Estradiol is used in hormone replacement therapy (HRT) and in the prophylaxis of osteoporosis. Dosage regimens vary according to form of drug used and condition being treated, e.g. implantation: 25–100 mg every 6 months; orally: 1–2 mg daily; transdermally in menopausal symptoms: 50 micrograms/24 hours, change the patch twice weekly with a course of progestogen 12 days a month for patients with an intact uterus. The dose can be adjusted as necessary to control the symptoms
Ethinylestradiol *Mestranol* is available as a composite pack with norethisterone. The tablets are graded in dose and are taken in a specific sequence	In the treatment of menopausal symptoms 10–20 micrograms per day for 21 days orally (ethinylestradiol). Oestrogens must not be given to patients with oestrogen-dependent cancer. The risk of thromboembolic disorders precludes the use of oestrogens in patients with a history of active thrombophlebitis. Nausea, vomiting, weight gain, withdrawal bleeding, oedema and sodium retention may be troublesome
TIBOLONE	This compound has both oestrogenic and progestogenic properties and some weak androgenic activity. Used to treat menopausal symptoms
PROGESTERONE (the naturally occurring hormone). A wide range of compounds with progestogen activity is available including: dydrogesterone, hydroxyprogesterone, medroxyprogesterone, norethisterone	Since progesterones act on tissues sensitised by oestrogens, the drugs are often administered on a cyclical basis with an oestrogen. Dosage regimens vary according to the condition being treated, e.g. dydrogesterone orally in dysmenorrhoea 10 mg twice daily for 5th–25th day of cycle, norethisterone orally in endometriosis 10 mg on 5th day of cycle, increasing if spotting occurs. Injectable preparations are available. Progestogens can cause acne, urticaria, oedema, GI problems and effects on the menstrual cycle. If the woman has an intact uterus, a progestogen must be given. Oestrogen-only preparations are suitable for patients without a uterus
MALE SEX HORMONES *Anabolic steroids* Nandrolone Stanozolol	Related to androgens but have less virilising effects. These drugs have limited use in medicine in osteoporosis and aplastic anaemia. Illegal use by athletes has been well documented. Side-effects are similar to those seen with testosterone
Testosterone is available in a number of forms for use orally or by slow-release IM injection. A transdermal patch is also available	In deficiency states 120–160 mg daily by mouth as the undecanoate compound. Testosterone enantate is given intramuscularly 250 mg every 2–3 weeks. In breast cancer 250 mg intramuscularly every 2–3 weeks. Side-effects are as would be expected from the physiology, e.g. virilism in women and precocious sexual development in men. Caution must be exercised in patients suffering from candida, renal or hepatic impairment. Fertility is not enhanced by testosterone administration
ANTI-ANDROGENS Cyproterone acetate Finasteride	Cyproterone is used in male hypersexuality (50 mg orally twice daily) Finasteride acts to reduce the potency of naturally occurring testosterone. It is of value in benign prostatic enlargement/hyperplasia (5 mg daily, reviewed after 6 months)

HORMONAL CONTRACEPTION

Oral contraceptives

Oral contraception has proved to be a very acceptable and convenient method of contraception for many women. Despite some problems and contraindications, well-managed hormonal contraception is relatively safe and highly effective. Two basic types of routine oral contraceptive products are available. A combined pill containing both an oestrogen and a progestogen (COC) and a progestogen-only pill (POP) are available (Tables 20.5–20.8). Hormonal emergency oral contraception may be required for women who have had unprotected intercourse or experienced failure of a contraceptive barrier device (Table 20.9). The key points relating to the prescribing and contraindications of oral contraceptives are summarised in the above tables.

Infertility treatment

Infertility treatments have been developed during the past 15 years to enable a very high level of success to be achieved. Assisted reproduction treatment (ART) tends to be provided mainly in the private sector but NHS trusts are providing this treatment within budgetary constraints. All treatment programmes must be

Table 20.5 COC: combination oestrogen/progestogen (high strength)

Combination	Dose/contraindications/side-effects/interactions
Oestrogen 50 micrograms (ethinylestradiol or mestranol) with Progestogen 250 micrograms (levonorgestrel)	One tablet daily for 21 days. Subsequent courses repeated after 7 days. Withdrawal bleeding occurs. Absolute contraindications to COC (all strengths) include cardiovascular disease, with particular reference to venous thrombosis or a predisposition to thrombosis; and oestrogen-dependent cancers, e.g. breast cancer. Consult specialist literature for further information
or	
Norethisterone 1 mg (Various combinations are available under different proprietary names)	The COC has an effect on most body systems. As such, side-effects are common (headache, nausea and vomiting, mastalgia and skin complaints). Many of the side-effects are minor and may resolve with time. Enzyme-inducing drugs, e.g. some antibiotics and anticonvulsants, affect the metabolism of oestrogens and progestogens. During periods of intensive therapy with broad-spectrum antibiotics, additional contraceptive precautions may be required (barrier method)

Table 20.6 COC: combination oestrogen/progestogen (standard strength)

Combination	Dose/contraindications/side-effects/interactions
Oestrogen Ethinylestradiol 30 micrograms Ethinylestradiol 40 micrograms	One tablet daily for 21 days, repeating after 7 days. Some packs include tablets of different combinations to be taken in accordance with a schedule clearly defined on the package. Packaging is designed to aid patient compliance. The contraindications etc. are the same as for the high-strength products
Progestogen Levonorgestrel 250 micrograms Levonorgestrel 150 micrograms (Various combination products are available, under different proprietary names. Some courses include dummy tablets to aid compliance)	Some women may choose to have a pill-free time during which cardiovascular risks decline, but these risks return when the pill is started again. Other women may choose to avoid the withdrawal bleed by running three packs together before a 7-day break. It should be noted that if a break is longer than 7 days, ovulation may occur despite re-starting the pill. Careful instructions are given to all patients on the action to take if a pill is forgotten

Table 20.7 Combined oestrogen/progestogen (low strength)

Combination	Dose/contraindications/side-effects/interactions
Oestrogen Ethinylestradiol 20 micrograms *Progestogen* Norethisterone 1 mg *or*	Dose as other COCs. The low-strength product is preferred for older women, or obese women where there are no fundamental contraindications to the use of a COC. In all cases of prescribing oral contraceptives the aim is good cycle control and minimal side-effects. COCs should not be prescribed for women over 50 years of age. Careful clinical examination is essential before commencing COC and health checks during the woman's reproductive life
Desogestrel 150 micrograms	In all cases the COCs act by interfering with secretion of gonadotrophins, which prevents ovulation. There is also progestogenic interference with mucus penetrability by spermatozoa

preceded by a full investigation of both partners. Problems identified in the male partner must be referred to a urologist or endocrinologist. For the female partner, a number of baseline hormonal levels are determined (progesterone, prolactin, estradiol, follicle-stimulating hormone and luteinising hormone). Having determined these levels, it is then necessary to decide on the ovarian stimulation regimen. Screening for viruses such as rubella, hepatitis B and HIV is normally carried out. Common infections such as chlamydia are also screened for. Ultrasound scans are used to identify problems such as fibroids, polyps, or ovarian cysts.

Laparoscopic assessment of disease of the ovaries is also carried out as required. Counselling of both partners is an integral part of the treatment but a key factor in success or otherwise is the woman's age and her ovarian age as determined by the hormone level measurements.

Endometriosis

Endometriosis is regarded as a puzzling condition which creates problems for both GPs and specialists. Essentially, the condition can be defined as the presence of endometrial tissue at ectopic sites which may be at a number of sites in the abdomen. The causes of the condition are not fully understood but a genetic disposition has been confirmed. A factor of significance is the role of endogenous oestrogens. The condition affects mainly women in their 30s and 40s but it can affect women at any time during their reproductive years. No major racial or class factors have been identified. Endometriosis is associated with premenstrual soiling, and infertility. The condition often presents as dysmenorrhoea and pelvic pain. Where extrapelvic sites are involved, there may be soreness, swelling and bleeding.

Treatment options include the improvement of fertility and pain relief. Surgery may be indicated if medical therapy fails. Hormonal treatments are also used and have additional contraceptive effects. If a woman is trying to achieve a pregnancy, dydrogesterone may relieve symptoms without reducing fertility. In the treatment of endometriosis, there is clearly a major risk/benefit aspect to be considered especially when treating subfertile women suffering from a debilitating condition. Medical management should not be used in the asymptomatic or infertile patient. Where drug therapy is indicated, the following drugs may be useful:

- progestogens
- gonadotrophin release inhibitors
- gonadotrophin-releasing hormones
- goserelin – by implantation
- danazol – acts by inhibiting pituitary gonadotrophins
- gestrinone – is similar to danazol, having an antiprogestogen action.

Table 20.9 Emergency hormonal contraception

Drugs	Dose/indications
Tablets containing norgestrel 500 micrograms with ethinylestradiol 50 micrograms	Two tablets are taken as soon as possible after coitus (up to 72 hours) then a further 2 tablets 12 hours later. An alternative product containing 750 micrograms of levonorgestrel is available

Table 20.8 POP (progestogen only)

Drug(s) used	Dose/contraindications/side-effects/interactions
Etynodiol 500 micrograms Norethisterone 350 micrograms Levonorgestrel 30 micrograms *and* Norgestrel 75 micrograms in combination with levonorgestrel 37.5 micrograms	Dose as per prescription, usually one tablet daily (at the same time each day) on a continuous basis, starting on the first day of cycle (contraceptive protection may be lost if delayed by longer than 3 hours) POPs are indicated where there are side-effects to COCs, in older (35+ years) women, especially smokers and patients with hypertension, diabetes mellitus and migraine Contraindications include pregnancy, severe arterial disease, hepatic problems and porphyria. Caution in patients with CVS problems, diabetes mellitus and migraine As with all hormonal contraceptives careful clinical assessment of the patient is required and it is vitally important to take the special wishes/needs of the woman into account Parenteral POPs are available. Administration is by deep IM injection or implantation (consult specialist literature). An intrauterine device which releases levonorgestrel directly into the uterus is also available. 20 micrograms of the drug is released over 24 hours

For the relief of pain associated with endometriosis, NSAID compounds are useful.

THE PANCREAS

In addition to its predominantly exocrine function, the pancreas has two types of cell – alpha and beta – which make up the remaining endocrine part of the gland, known as the islets of Langerhans. Alpha cells secrete the hormone glucagon; beta cells secrete the hormone insulin. In health, insulin and glucagon work in harmony with each other, insulin decreasing the blood glucose level and glucagon increasing it.

When an excess of carbohydrate has been taken in, insulin promotes storage of glucose by accelerating the transport of glucose through the cell membrane. Insulin also converts glucose to glycogen, which is stored in the liver and muscles. It also has the capacity to synthesise protein and to convert glucose to fat. The secretion of insulin is stimulated by a rise in blood glucose reaching the islet cells.

When the blood glucose level is low because of an insufficient intake of carbohydrate or an excessive amount of exercise having been taken, glucagon acts by mobilising the glycogen stores in the liver, converting them into glucose and thus raising the blood glucose level. Glucagon also has the capacity to convert amino acids to glucose in the liver and to increase the conversion of fat to glucose.

Diabetes mellitus

In diabetes mellitus there is an elevation of the blood glucose with consequent glycosuria resulting from an absolute or relative deficiency of insulin. The factors which predispose to the condition are:

- genetic
- Coxsackie virus
- autoimmunity (leading to destruction of islet cells)
- pregnancy
- endocrine disorders (e.g. Cushing's syndrome)
- pancreatic disease
- stress
- obesity
- drugs, e.g. corticosteroids, thiazide diuretics, thyroid hormones and phenytoin.

There is often interaction between the various factors, and social and environmental factors.

There are two types of diabetes. Type 1 diabetes is due to a deficiency of insulin whereas type 2 diabetes is due to a reduced secretion of insulin or the peripheral resistance to the action of insulin. The main characteristics of each type are indicated in Table 20.10.

Diabetes mellitus is a major challenge to all those involved in the care of patients in the hospital or community. It is a multisystem disease which, if not properly controlled, can cause serious renal, neurological, ophthalmological, cardiovascular, metabolic and biochemical disorders. The human toll of the disease is massive as is the economic burden. The incidence of diabetes has reached epidemic proportions in many countries. Diabetes mellitus in children and in pregnancy presents difficult management problems. Diabetic patients facing surgery also need special care.

Diabetes mellitus is characterised by hyperglycaemia and glycosuria. Glycosuria occurs when the glucose concentration in the blood exceeds the capacity of the renal tubules to reabsorb it. The presence of glucose in the glomerular filtrate increases the osmolality which prevents the reabsorption of water. This considerably

Table 20.10 Types of diabetes mellitus

Type 1 diabetes (insulin-dependent diabetes IDDM)	Type 2 diabetes (non-insulin-dependent diabetes NIDDM)
• Genetic predisposition	• Genetic predisposition
• Caused by destruction of islet cells of the pancreas (autoimmunity)	• Caused by resistance to insulin and inadequate secretion of insulin
• Dependent on insulin for life and prevention of major complications	• Not dependent on insulin for survival
	• Behavioural/social factors have significant impact on the development and management of the condition
• Affects younger age group (usually lean people)	• Affects older age group (usually obese people)
• Prone to ketosis	• Resistant to ketosis
	• Associated with hypertension, hyperlipidaemia and atherosclerotic heart disease
• Acute lack of insulin – condition does not deteriorate over time as with type 2 diabetes	• Progressive disorder – becomes more difficult to treat. Should not be considered as 'mild' diabetes

Other types include diabetes due to glucocorticoid therapy, pancreatic destruction, recognised genetic syndromes and gestational diabetes.

increases the volume of urine produced, leading to polyuria. Loss of water and minerals leads to thirst and polydipsia. If the fluid and mineral (electrolyte) loss is not corrected significant complications can ensue. Poor utilisation of glucose triggers the compensatory mechanisms of glycogenolysis (breakdown of glycogen) and gluconeogenesis (breakdown of protein). Lipolysis (breakdown of fats) also occurs leading to a raised fasting plasma concentration of non-esterified fatty acid (NEFA). In severe insulin deficiency, high levels of NEFA lead to the accumulation of ketone bodies and the dangerous condition of ketoacidosis. The chain of events leading to ketoacidosis is summarised below:

- Lipolysis → plasma concentration of NEFA rises.
- Fatty acids are normally broken down in the liver to give acetylcoenzyme A.
- Levels of acetylcoenzyme A exceed the body's ability to clear it.
- Acetylcoenzyme A forms acetoacetic acid.
- Acetoacetic acid is converted into acetone (ketone bodies).
- Normally the ketone bodies are metabolised but in diabetes mellitus levels accumulate causing a fall in the pH of body fluids.
- The fall in pH is countered to some extent by naturally occurring bicarbonate.
- Bicarbonate levels fall and ketoacidosis results.
- Hydrogen ion concentration increases as does $PaCO_2$.
- Clinically, this may be seen as hyperpnoea.

Diagnosis of diabetes mellitus

Although diabetes mellitus is characterised by an elevated blood glucose and glycosuria, it is essential to differentiate it from other conditions such as renal glycosuria caused by a low renal threshold for glucose. Estimation of the fasting blood glucose concentration and random blood glucose concentrations will normally be sufficient to confirm the diagnosis of diabetes mellitus.

The oral glucose tolerance test (OGTT) may also be used in the diagnosis of diabetes mellitus; it is still required to establish the presence of gestational diabetes (see BNF).

Aims of treatment

The overall aims of treatment can be summarised as follows:

- to lower blood glucose levels
- to achieve and maintain a normal metabolic state
- to avoid hypoglycaemia
- to avoid the complications of the disease
- to avoid acute episodes, e.g. ketoacidosis
- to involve the patient fully in the management programme
- to enable the patient to lead a normal life.

With generally increasing life expectancy, complications are of particular concern in the older patient since ischaemic changes may lead to serious morbidity, e.g. diabetic gangrene. Apart from drug treatment, particular attention must be paid to diet, personal hygiene (especially the feet), exercise and other aspects of lifestyle.

Measuring glycaemic control

This is best achieved by measuring Hb A_{1c} which gives an index of the average blood glucose concentration over the preceding 2 months. Reference ranges vary depending on laboratory methods used. For example the range for people who do not have diabetes is up to 6%. To achieve optimal Hb A_{1c} levels, blood glucose targets of ≤5.9 mmol/L (fasting), 4–7 mmol/L (preprandial) and 7–9 mmol/L (bedtime) are likely to be required.

Major complications

- Ketoacidosis (see above)
- Renal damage – diabetic glomerulosclerosis
- Diabetic retinopathy – a common condition which can cause blindness due to damage to the retinal veins, haemorrhages and exudates in the retina
- Diabetic neuropathy – which may affect the CNS to varying degrees
- Lowered resistance to infection
- Damage to peripheral vasculature (combination of microvascular and macrovascular damage).

All these complications can be ameliorated by effective treatment with insulin or oral agents.

Treatment of type 2 diabetes

Diet is the first line of treatment in type 2 diabetes. Emphasis is placed on weight reduction where indicated and otherwise a 'healthy' high-fibre, low-sugar, low-fat, low-salt diet evenly distributed throughout the day. For many, adherence to the diet is sufficient.

Oral antidiabetic drugs are widely used in the treatment of this condition especially in older, obese patients and where dietary restriction alone has failed. Younger

Table 20.11 Drugs used in the treatment of type 2 diabetes

Drug groups	Mode of action	Dose/notes
Sulphonylureas Chlorpropamide Glibenclamide	These compounds stimulate the synthesis and release of insulin and have other beneficial effects such as increasing the sensitivity of receptors to insulin. It is clear that to achieve benefit these drugs depend on endogenous insulin and a functioning pancreas	These drugs have a prolonged action and may cause problems in older patients who are prone to hypoglycaemia. Other drugs are now preferred. All dosages of these agents must be adjusted in response to the patient's condition. The doses given below may vary from patient to patient
Tolbutamide Gliclazide Glipizide (other similar drugs are glimepiride and gliquidone)		500 mg–1.5 g daily in divided doses 40–80 mg daily up to 160 mg as a single dose. Normally 2.5–5 mg daily. Up to 15 mg may be given as a single dose before breakfast. Maximum daily dose 40 mg. The use of all oral hypoglycaemic agents should be carefully managed. Patients with hepatic or renal insufficiency are at risk of hypoglycaemia. The short-acting tolbutamide may be used if there is renal impairment. Blood disorders have been reported and weight gain may occur with this drug
Biguanides Metformin	Acts by decreasing gluconeogenesis and by increasing peripheral utilisation of glucose. As with the sulphonylureas, it is effective only where there is endogenous insulin	500 mg every 8 hours or 850 mg every 12 hours with food. Avoid in patients with renal problems and a tendency to lactic acidosis; cardiac problems; trauma; infection; and pregnancy. GI problems are common at higher doses
Alpha-glucosidase inhibitors (especially active against the enzyme sucrase acarbose)	Reduce postprandial blood glucose peaks by inhibiting intestinal alpha-glucosidases. This has the effect of delaying the digestion of starch and sucrose into absorbable monosaccharides. The blood glucose profile is smoothed, and fluctuations in blood glucose levels are reduced. These compounds have no stimulatory action on the pancreas. Fasting blood glucose levels are also reduced	50 mg three times daily adjusted if necessary to 100 mg three times daily taken with food. Because of the action of acarbose, dietary carbohydrate is digested in the large bowel. This can lead to GI problems such as flatulence, abdominal distension and diarrhoea. Attention to diet may help to alleviate these symptoms
Thiazolidinediones Pioglitazone Rosiglitazone	Reduce peripheral insulin resistance	To be used under specialist advice only. In combination with another suitable oral agent. Rosiglitazone 4 mg daily increasing to 8 mg daily, depending on response. The side-effects of rosiglitazone include GI problems, headache, anaemia, fatigue, weight gain, oedema and hypoglycaemia. NICE guidance on the use of this agent in combination indicates that this therapy should be offered where other oral therapies have not achieved the desired reduction in blood glucose levels
Repaglinide	Promotes secretion of insulin by an action on the β-cell membrane	Because of the rapid onset of action and short duration of effect, the dose and timing should be related to the patient's meal patterns. Initially 500 micrograms 30 minutes before main meals. Dose adjusted depending on any previous therapy up to a maximum of 16 mg daily. The drug is contraindicated in the presence of ketoacidosis and renal or hepatic impairment. Side-effects include GI disturbances and hypersensitivity reactions

patients or patients with brittle diabetes cannot be treated with oral agents. The range of drugs available is described in Table 20.11.

Many patients with type 2 diabetes may not exhibit any overt symptoms but their hyperglycaemia may be causing vascular damage without the awareness of either doctor or patient. Particular attention needs to be paid to patients with a family history of ischaemic heart disease and blood lipid abnormalities. Hypertension is another major risk factor as is smoking. Regular screening and well-managed therapy can help patients (especially older patients) achieve a better quality of life with reduced incidence of morbidity. Patients with type 2 diabetes who have reached the maximum level of oral therapy and are still hyperglycaemic should be considered for insulin therapy.

A new range of oral antidiabetic compounds has recently been introduced. The thiazolidinediones, pioglitazone and rosiglitazone, reduce blood-glucose levels by reducing the peripheral resistance to insulin. These drugs are used in combination with metformin or if metformin is contraindicated a sulphonylurea is used.

Treatment of type 1 diabetes

Patients suffering from type 1 diabetes are treated by injections of insulin along with a diabetic diet. Parenteral routes must be used as insulin (a protein) is destroyed by the gastric acid and enzymes. For many years, efforts have been made to produce an insulin product utilising more convenient routes of administration, e.g. intranasal insulin. It appears that the parenteral route will remain the mainstay of therapy for the immediate future.

It seems likely that improvements will continue to be made in both insulin formulations and delivery systems. Since some forms of type 1 diabetes may have autoimmunity as a causal factor, immunosuppressants such as ciclosporin may be useful.

Treatment has to be supplemented by careful attention to diet (see under Treatment of type 2 diabetes). Amounts will depend on age and individual nutritional requirements which should be established under the direction and guidance of a dietitian.

The aims of treatment of both forms of diabetes are essentially the same (see p. 311). However, owing to the more brittle and serious nature of this condition more sophisticated insulin dosage regimens and monitoring are often required. Specialist clinics and shared care protocols help to ensure the continuity of care that is vital if the serious complications of diabetes mellitus are to be avoided. The role of the diabetes specialist nurse both in hospital and community practice is of key importance.

Insulins

Great progress has been made with the development of sophisticated insulins designed to achieve good control of blood glucose levels. Insulin can be obtained from the pancreatic tissue of slaughtered animals (bovine or porcine insulins) but insulin with a chemical structure corresponding exactly with that of human insulin is often preferred. Human insulin is prepared by recombinant DNA technology or other biological techniques, e.g. enzymatic modification of porcine insulin. Many patients do well on insulin obtained from animal tissue and the need to change established patterns to human insulin should be carefully evaluated.

A wide range of insulins is available each product being formulated to achieve a specific profile in terms of speed of onset and length of action. In practice a combination of insulins is used, designed to achieve optimal control for the particular patient. The ideal is to achieve a control of blood glucose level corresponding to the non-diabetic physiological profile. Insulin is secreted in the non-diabetic in two ways. About half of the insulin secreted is in response to an intake of food; the remainder is secreted to cover basal requirements (Fig. 20.7).

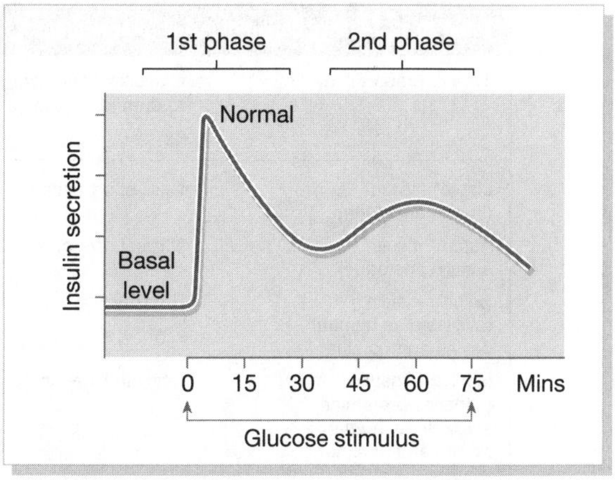

Figure 20.7 Insulin secretion in a non-diabetic.

Insulin formulations (*see Table 20.12*)

Insulin is available as a simple solution which has an immediate or rapid onset with a short duration of action. The onset, duration and peak effects depend on the route of administration. Combined with protamine or a zinc salt, its effect is prolonged. A number of longer-acting preparations of insulin are available. A range of biphasic insulins is also available containing differing proportions of isophane (which contains protamine) and soluble insulins ranging from 10% soluble insulin and 90% isophane insulin to 40% soluble insulin and 60% isophane insulin. The combined use of short-acting and long-acting insulins is the preferred approach to treatment of diabetes mellitus. In acute conditions such as ketoacidosis a soluble, rapid-acting form of insulin must be used. In view of the wide range of preparations available, it follows that great care must be taken in selecting the correct product for the particular patient.

All insulin formulations must be stored between 2 and 8°C. Freezing or exposure to excessive heat will destroy the product. If refrigeration is not available, storage at room temperature for 1 month is acceptable.

All insulins are 100 units per 1 mL and if the packaging is a multidose vial suitable preservatives are included. The mixture of soluble and long-acting insulin is designed for twice-daily administration but dosage levels are always determined in response to the patient's needs. If a ready-mixed preparation of insulin is unsuitable for the patient's needs, certain insulins may be

Table 20.12 Classification of insulin preparations

Type of preparation	Classification according to duration of action	Duration of action following subcutaneous injection		
		Onset	Duration	Peak
Lispro* insulin (insulin analogue)	Ultra-short-acting	Immediate	4 hours	60 minutes
Aspart* insulin (insulin analogue)	Ultra-short-acting	Immediate	4 hours	60 minutes
Soluble insulin (available as human, bovine and porcine)	Short-acting	30 minutes	5 hours	3 hours
Isophane insulin (contains protamine, available as human, bovine and porcine)	Intermediate-acting	90 minutes	16–20 hours	4–12 hours
Lente insulin (contains zinc)	Intermediate-acting Long-acting	120 minutes 4 hours	24 hours Duration greater than 24 hours	6–18 hours
Mixed preparations These are mixtures of soluble and isophane insulin The combinations are fixed, and the choice of product will depend on the needs of the patient	Biphasic	Biphasic onset and duration of action		

*These terms derive from the manipulation of the insulin molecule.
Note 1. Bovine and porcine insulin are satisfactory in use. Studies have failed to support the contention that human insulin may result in loss of awareness of hypoglycaemia.
Note 2. Most insulins should be injected 30 minutes before a meal. Ultra-rapid-acting insulins should be injected immediately before or after food.

mixed in the syringe. The soluble insulin (short-acting) must be drawn up first to avoid the possibility of long-acting insulin (insulin suspension) contaminating the vial of soluble insulin. There is a risk that if insulin suspension were allowed to contaminate the soluble insulin a potentially hazardous interaction would take place that would alter the physiological properties of the soluble insulin. Adjusted dosage levels may be needed during illness or in other stressful situations.

Administration of insulin

In many cases subcutaneous administration using a disposable insulin syringe will meet the patient's needs. The use of a pen injector system and a cartridge of insulin is helpful for many patients.

Pen injector systems have the advantage of portability, greater social acceptability and flexibility of lifestyle. Disadvantages of this means of administration must be appreciated. Patients may be lulled into a false sense of security because of the ease of use. This may lead to poor control of diet. Patients need to understand the adjustment of dosage taking into account blood glucose levels. Cartridges of mixed insulins may not always be appropriate, especially for younger, brittle diabetics whose requirements are more likely to fluctuate. Pens are available in disposable as well as reusable forms.

The constant quest to achieve control of blood glucose levels corresponding to those of a well non-diabetic continues to challenge all those involved in providing care for diabetic patients. Four to six injections daily of a small dose of soluble insulin is an option that would achieve good control but this is not often practicable. Controlled continuous subcutaneous infusion of insulin may be administered using a pump system. Additional doses can be administered to cover meals by the activation of a mechanism incorporated into the pump. An implantable device which releases insulin in response to blood glucose level fluctuations remains an objective for researchers.

Insulin regimens

These will vary widely, taking into account many factors, such as the patient's preferences, lifestyle and delivery device preferred. The regimens include once-daily injections which do not give good control and are rarely used. Twice-daily injections are the most suitable for new patients. A combination of short- and intermediate-acting insulins is injected before breakfast and the evening meal. Pre-mixed preparations are widely used. Multiple injections (up to four daily) can give good control in well-motivated patients who are able and willing to do frequent and regular blood glucose tests. An insulin analogue or soluble insulin is injected before each meal and an intermediate or long-acting insulin is injected to provide background cover. In each case the dose of insulin in units is highly specific to the individual patient's needs.

Some problems of insulin therapy

Hypoglycaemia is always a potential problem. Although many insulin preparations have similar basic characteristics, inadvertent changes may result in severe problems for the patient. Conditions where insulin requirements are reduced include diseases of the adrenal, pituitary or thyroid gland. Reduced doses are also required where there is renal or hepatic impairment, or by the concurrent administration of drugs which have a hypoglycaemic action.

Insulin lispro and insulin aspart are genetically engineered insulins with an immediate onset of action which means they must be administered closer to mealtimes than is required for soluble insulin. They are therefore more convenient in use. In addition, their duration of action is short and, as a result, hypoglycaemia may occur less often than with conventional insulins.

Local side-effects of insulin therapy include local hypersensitivity reactions, lipodystrophy and insulin resistance. Reactions to human insulin are claimed to be less than with insulins of animal origin but in trials no demonstrable advantage has been found.

Treatment of hypoglycaemia

A hypoglycaemic patient is pale and may appear different from usual – acting oddly, possibly aggressive or seeming to be intoxicated. Such patients feel dizzy, begin to tremble and their vision becomes blurred. Beads of sweat appear on the brow and upper lip. Hypoglycaemic attacks are more likely to occur before the midday meal and at night. If hypoglycaemia does occur, whatever the cause, prompt action is required. Diabetics are taught to recognise the onset of hypoglycaemia and to take glucose appropriately. People who are conscious may be given a cup of tea or coffee with one spoonful of sugar and a couple of biscuits. Alternatively, they may chew the Dextrosol tablets (3 tablets = 10 g glucose) they have been taught to carry or eat a richly filled chocolate bar. In hospital, a liquid carbohydrate supplement such as Polycal may be used; 113 mL is removed from the 200 mL bottle and diluted with water to make a 300 mL drink. This is the equivalent of 75 g glucose. A record should be kept of the amount of Polycal given and the time taken by the patient to return to normal.

Hypostop is a gel containing 40% glucose monohydrate (equivalent to 32 g anhydrous glucose). It is used orally for the treatment of hypoglycaemia. The gel is applied to the buccal mucosa followed by external massage of the cheek. This method has been shown to enhance absorption, providing a more rapid rise in blood glucose (5 minutes) than if taken orally (10–15 minutes). The gel is available in a graduated plastic bottle with a dispenser tip. One-third of the contents (10 g glucose) is slowly squeezed from the bottle directly into the mouth. If Hypostop is not available, honey or jam may be used.

Alternatively, glucagon may be given by intramuscular or subcutaneous injection. This is a valuable method for those patients troubled by recurrent hypoglycaemia and for whom a trained family member can give the injection. A kit complete with vial containing the glucagon powder and syringe (with needle attached) containing 1 mL of Water for Injections is available.

If the patient does not respond to oral glucose or to glucagon (within 10 minutes), or if the patient is discovered unconscious, intravenous glucose 50% 20–50 mL should be given. Strong glucose solution is highly irritant to the tissues and must be injected carefully into the vein. The dose may have to be repeated. The nurse should remain with the patient and be ready to provide reassurance and support as the patient regains consciousness.

Blood glucose testing

Whenever possible, self-monitoring of the blood glucose in diabetics is to be encouraged to allow the patient to be independent and to reduce the risk of blood-borne infection. Admission to hospital provides an opportunity for the nurse to check the patient's technique, especially where there is some concern over diabetic control. Some hospital patients are, of course, not well enough to perform this procedure and so the responsibility temporarily falls on the nurse.

A sample of capillary blood may be obtained from the pinna of the ear or from the side of the thumb nail, the former being the more vascular.

Apart from reasons of cleanliness, the patient's ear/hand should be washed with soap and warm water and dried before carrying out the blood test so as to improve the circulation and allow blood to be more easily obtained. An alcohol swab is not used to clean the skin as the alcohol from the swab may create a false reading. Since the maintenance of an optimum blood glucose level is highly dependent on the use of biochemical tests, it is essential to follow the manufacturer's instructions implicitly.

Reagent strips used for measuring plasma glucose levels may be read against a colour chart or by using a meter specially designed to record the result accurately. Since colour vision may be impaired in diabetics, the glucometer is a considerable advantage for self-monitoring. There are several different kinds of glucometer. Each type has its own reagent strip.

Role of the nurse in the management of diabetes mellitus

Nurses play a vital role at all stages in the management of diabetes. The routine screening of patients attending any clinic is performed with a view to identifying previously undiagnosed diabetes. Assisting in the assessment and diagnosis of suspected diabetes, including carrying out the oral glucose tolerance test, for example, is another important part of the nurse's role. Once diabetes is diagnosed and treatment agreed, the day-to-day management of the condition and the education of patients (and their families) are left largely in the hands of nurses. On no other occasion are the nurse's teaching skills more greatly drawn upon than during the period between confirmation of the diagnosis and discharge from hospital. The challenge for nurses is to have patients who are both competent and confident in managing their condition. Such an opportunity lends itself to a planned programme of teaching using different teaching methods, including explaining, demonstrating with the help of visual aids, supervising practice and providing suitable written information. Subject areas to be covered are detailed in Table 20.13.

In any clinical setting at any time, the nurse may be involved with the diabetic patient and so it is essential that all nurses have a grasp of the condition and an understanding of the aims of treatment. Nurses in accident and emergency departments and acute medical wards will, from time to time, have to care for the acutely ill diabetic patient. Especially with the insulin-dependent diabetic, the need to be observant, adhere to correct procedures, maintain high standards of hygiene and keep meticulous records cannot be overemphasised. Diabetic prescribing and recording sheets should reflect an accurate diabetic 'picture'. This can be achieved by combining into a single document, blood glucose and glycosuria test results. Other biochemical recordings may also be relevant, e.g. ketonuria. The document must give details of the hypoglycaemic agent(s) (oral or parenteral) prescribed and a record of administration.

Table 20.13 Areas to cover in a teaching programme for new diabetics

Subject area	Detail
Anatomy and physiology	A clear understanding of: the pancreas, the blood and the tissues carbohydrate metabolism
The disorder itself	What has gone wrong with the pancreas and why treatment is essential
Controlling the blood glucose level	Administration of insulin or oral antidiabetic agent as appropriate: prescriptions supplies storage (especially insulin) equipment aids to administration dosages timing frequency sites of administration technique
Controlling the diet	An understanding of the different classes of food and the need to avoid pure sugars
	Knowledge of dietary exchanges
	The need to eat regularly, including snacks between meals and before bedtime
	Importance of trying to eat, even if feeling unwell
Monitoring the disorder	The importance of keeping careful records of: blood glucose readings urinalysis insulin administered hypoglycaemic episodes and action taken
The patient's self-care	How to recognise hypoglycaemic reactions
	The importance of meticulous care of the feet
	The importance of attending clinics as arranged: diabetic clinic dietetic clinic eye clinic chiropody
	Encouragement of healthy lifestyle with adequate sleep, minimisation of stress and reduced exposure to infections where possible
	Advice and encouragement to allow the continuation of normal activities such as schooling, work, sport, travel
	The benefits of carrying some indication that the patient is diabetic, e.g. card, medical pendant/bracelet
	What to do when feeling unwell
	Sources of help: medical nursing dietetic pharmaceutical financial

The aim for nurses in primary care is to maximise quality of life for the diabetic, prevent long-term diabetic complications and increase longevity. Increasingly, health authorities are utilising the skills of nurses specialising in care for diabetics. The importance of close liaison between diabetic clinic and general practitioner cannot be overstressed. Similarly, good communication between nurses and doctors is paramount.

In summary, nurses play an especially full part in the diagnosis, treatment and care of the diabetic patient. It is, however, in their teaching role that there is the greatest potential to contribute to maximum independence and otherwise good health for diabetics.

DRUGS USED IN OBSTETRICS

Prostaglandins of the E series have an action on smooth muscle and are used for a number of purposes in obstetric practice. They are used to induce abortion, induce or augment labour and to minimise blood loss. A summary of the main products is given in Table 20.14. Ergometrine maleate, either alone or in combination with oxytocin, is used in obstetric practice. The main indication for ergometrine is postpartum haemorrhage. The dosage and route of administration will depend on the nature of the risk involved. For example, intravenous administration (125–250 micrograms) is required in high-risk situations. Intravenous infusion oxytocin is also used as an alternative. In domiciliary practice, 500 micrograms orally three times daily is advised. Ergometrine has a high incidence of side-effects but is a valuable drug in obstetric practice.

Premature labour

Beta$_2$-adrenoceptor stimulants (see p. 144) are used in uncomplicated premature labour to inhibit premature delivery. The use of these drugs is intended to provide

Table 20.14 Prostaglandins

Product	Presentation/administration	Actions/uses	Precautions/side-effects
Alprostadil injection Prostin VR sterile solution	Injection. 1 mL contains 500 micrograms alprostadil	Used to temporarily maintain the patency of the ductus arteriosus until corrective surgery can be performed in infants	See specialist literature. A specially formulated injection of alprostadil is available for the treatment of erectile dysfunction
Carboprost as trometamol salt (tromethamine salt) Hemabate sterile solution	Solution for IM injection containing 250 micrograms per 1 mL	Treatment of postpartum haemorrhage due to uterine atony which is refractory to conventional drugs (ergometrine/oxytocin)	Side-effects and precautions are similar to those of other prostaglandins
Dinoprostone Prostin E2 sterile solution	Sterile solution – each mL contains 10 mg dinoprostone. Diluted to produce 100 micrograms per mL before use	Oxytocic. Sometimes used in the therapeutic termination of pregnancy by the extra-amniotic route. Specialist use only. Consult product literature	Potentiates effect of oxytocin. Caution should be exercised in patients with asthma, epilepsy, glaucoma, disordered hepatic, renal or cardiovascular function, and hypertension. Side-effects include GI disturbances, hypersensitivity. Consult literature
Dinoprostone gel Prostin E2 vaginal gel	Sterile gel containing 1 mg or 2 mg dinoprostone per 2.5 mL in a syringe	Induction of labour where there are no fetal or maternal contraindications	Side-effects and precautions are similar to those of other prostaglandins Notes: 1. Refrigerated storage is generally required for prostaglandin preparations 2. As with all prostaglandins, avoid contact with skin. Wash off any skin contamination with soap and water
Dinoprostone vaginal tablets Prostin E2 vaginal tablets	Vaginal tablets containing 3 mg dinoprostone. An oral tablet of 500 micrograms is also available	Oxytocic, used for the induction of labour where there are no fetal or maternal contraindications. One tablet is inserted high in the posterior fornix. A second tablet may be inserted after 6–8 hours if labour is not established	Not to be used if the patient is sensitive to prostaglandins or where oxytocic drugs are contraindicated. Contraindicated if prolonged contraction of the uterus would be dangerous, e.g. history of caesarean section or uterine surgery. Undesirable effects similar to those of other prostaglandins

Table 20.15 Drugs used in the treatment of premature labour

Drug	Dosage	Precautions/side-effects
Ritodrine	Tablets 10 mg; injection 10 mg/mL IV infusion 50 micrograms per minute, increasing to 150–350 micrograms/minute and continued according to effect on contractions IM injection 10 mg every 3–8 hours for up to 40 hours after contractions have ceased Continue orally 10 mg 30 minutes before the termination of the infusion, repeated every 2 hours for 24 hours then 10–30 mg every 4–6 hours. Maximum dose 120 mg daily	Particular caution is needed in patients with cardiac problems, hypertension and electrolyte disorders. The drug is contraindicated in eclampsia and severe pre-eclampsia, and where there are uterine problems, e.g. infection, placenta praevia. Side-effects include nausea, vomiting, sweating, tremor and electrolyte disturbances. Great care must be taken to avoid fluid overload (volume of infusion fluid is kept to a minimum)
Salbutamol	Injection 50 micrograms/mL and 500 micrograms/mL Solution for IV infusion 1 mg/mL to be diluted before use. Dose 10 micrograms/minute, increasing to a maximum of 45 micrograms/minute until contractions have ceased **or** 100–250 micrograms by IV or IM injection. Then orally 4 mg every 6–8 hours	See page 207
Terbutaline	Tablets 5 mg Injection 500 micrograms/mL. Dose by IV infusion 5 micrograms/minute for 20 minutes, increasing according to the dosage schedule. 20 micrograms/minute should not be exceeded. Once contractions have ceased, the oral or SC route is used	See page 207

a delay in delivery of about 48 hours, during which time other measures can be taken to improve perinatal health. Following successful preventive therapy, oral therapy is used for maintenance of the situation. The drugs available have significant side-effects and there are potential drug interactions. The available drugs are briefly described in Table 20.15.

FURTHER READING

Harrison P T C 2001 Endocrine disrupters and human health. British Medical Journal 323:1317–1318

Hindmarsh P 2002 Commentary: exogenous glucocorticoids influence adrenal function, but assessment can be difficult. British Medical Journal 324:1083

Mason P 2002 Diet and diabetes. Pharmaceutical Journal 268:499

Murray J S, Jayarajasingh R 2001 Deterioration of symptoms after start of thyroid hormone replacement. British Medical Journal 323:332–333

Olivarius N A F, Henning B-N 2001 Randomised controlled trial of structured personal care of type 2 diabetes mellitus. British Medical Journal 323:970–975

Pickup J, Keen H 2001 Continuous subcutaneous insulin infusion in type 1 diabetes. British Medical Journal 322:1262–1263

Pollock A M, Sturrock A 2001 Thyroxine treatment in patients with symptoms of hypothyroidism but thyroid function tests within the reference range: randomised double blind placebo controlled crossover trial. British Medical Journal 323:891–895

Prentice A 2001 Endometriosis. British Medical Journal 323:93–95

Shaw K 2001 Oral antidiabetic drugs in type 2 diabetes. Prescriber 12:65–79

Sackey G H 2000. Recurrent generalised urticaria at insulin injection sites. British Medical Journal 321:1449

CHAPTER CONTENTS

21

Drug treatment of genitourinary disorders

ANATOMY AND PHYSIOLOGY

The major excretory function of the production of urine is performed by a structure consisting of secretory organs (two kidneys) and a system which conveys the urine (two ureters) to a collection and temporary storage organ (the bladder). Urine is discharged from the bladder via the urethra (see Fig. 21.1).

A longitudinal section of the kidney (see Fig. 21.2) indicates the structures visible to the naked eye. At the microscopic level the kidney is made up of nephrons which, in health, are responsible for maintaining the fluid and electrolyte balance.

In health, the intake and output of fluids and electrolytes are maintained in a state of balance by the kidneys. The kidneys also excrete the products of metabolism, urea, creatinine and uric acid. Many drugs are also excreted by the kidneys in the urine. Renal function is subject to a number of control mechanisms, such as the production of antidiuretic hormone produced by the pituitary gland. The adrenal cortex produces aldosterone which also influences renal activity.

Production of urine

Urine is produced in the kidney within the nephron, of which there are about 1 million in each kidney. Each nephron is a functional unit which consists of a cup-shaped capsule and a tortuous tubule and ends as a reservoir for the urine (see Fig. 16.2). The tubule walls are one epithelial cell thick and at certain points are flattened to allow them greater permeability. Lying within each capsule in close proximity to the capsule wall is a cluster of intertwining arterial capillaries known as the glomerulus. Arterial blood enters the glomerulus via the afferent arteriole and leaves via the efferent arteriole. The autonomic nervous system provides the nerve supply. Essentially there are three phases in urine production.

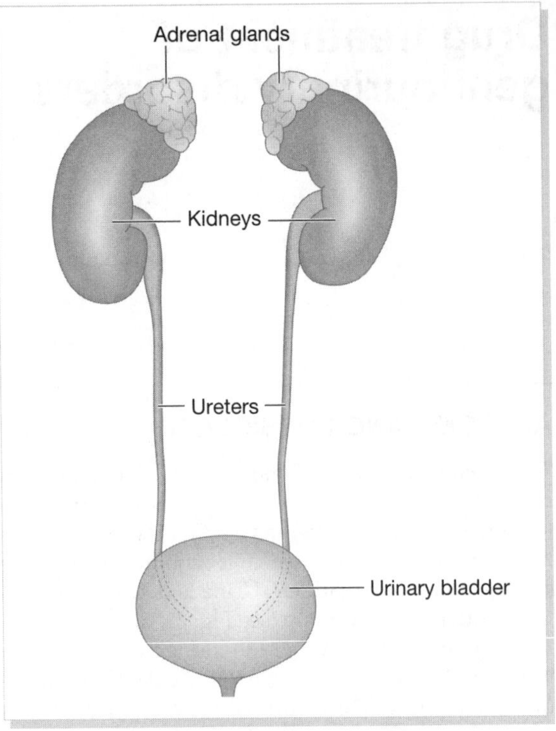

Figure 21.1 The urinary system. (From Waugh & Grant 2001 Ross and Wilson Anatomy and physiology in health and illness, 9th edn. Churchill Livingstone, Edinburgh.)

Glomerular filtration

Water and most small molecules filter through the semi-permeable walls of the glomerulus and the glomerular capsule because the blood pressure in the glomerulus is greater than the pressure of the filtrate within the glomerular capsule. Large molecules and large cells (e.g. erythrocytes) and plasma proteins remain in the capillaries.

Tubular reabsorption

Constituents (such as glucose, sodium and potassium) which have filtered through the glomerulus into the tubules but which the body still requires are reabsorbed. This process ensures that fluid and electrolyte balance and blood pH are maintained. Selective reabsorption is regularised by both the autonomic nervous system and by hormones. Water reabsorption is regulated by the action of antidiuretic hormone on the distal part of the tubule; the parathyroid hormone and calcitonin regulate the reabsorption of calcium and phosphate. Aldosterone influences the reabsorption of sodium and the excretion of potassium.

Tubular secretion

Substances which were not given sufficient time to filter through the glomerular wall are cleared from the

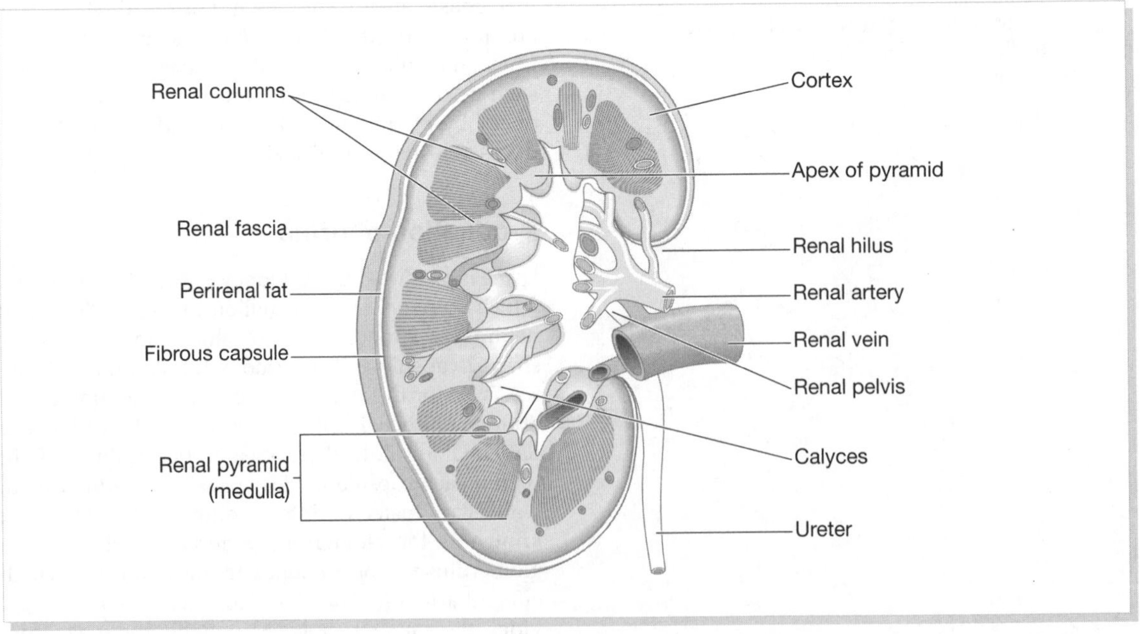

Figure 21.2 Longitudinal section of kidney.

body by secretion into the convoluted tubules. Some drugs are excreted in this way (see p. 119).

Excretion of urine

From the collecting tubule the urine is received into the renal pelvis before passing into the ureter and thence to the bladder. The smooth muscle of the bladder wall comes under the influence of the autonomic nervous system. The external urethral sphincter is under voluntary control and only when it is released will micturition occur. Depending on fluid intake and other factors, a healthy adult will pass 1–2.5 litres of urine daily.

Water balance

The amount of water excreted in the urine is influenced by the antidiuretic hormone and the level of waste material to be removed from the blood. Antidiuretic hormone is released as part of a feedback mechanism involving the hypothalamus and the posterior pituitary (see p. 298).

Electrolyte balance

Sodium, potassium, calcium and magnesium ions are present in body fluids. For the body to maintain a constant internal environment the concentration of each electrolyte in the body fluids must be maintained (see p. 323). Changes in concentration of electrolytes may result from changes in the amount of water or electrolytes. The amount of sodium and potassium in the urine is regulated by a feedback mechanism dependent on the blood flow through the kidneys (see Fig. 21.3).

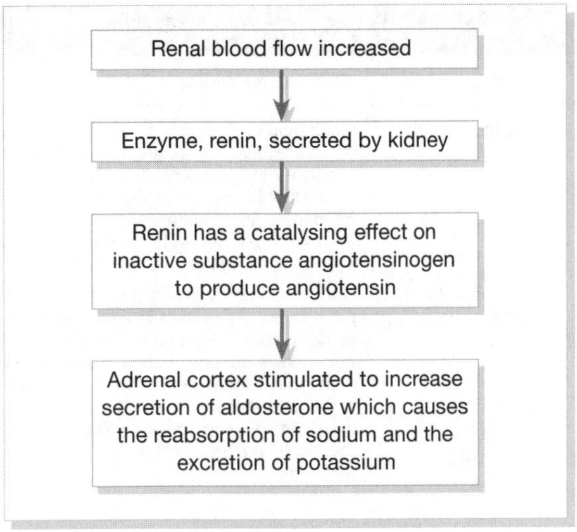

Figure 21.3 Regulation of sodium and potassium.

Other functions of the kidney

In addition to the important functions of fluid and electrolyte control, the kidneys are responsible for the production of erythropoietin (see p. 394) and dihydroxycholecalciferol (a form of vitamin D). Prostaglandins are also produced in the kidneys.

DISEASES OF THE KIDNEYS

In view of the vital functions performed by the kidneys it is evident that any disturbance of renal function will be of major significance for the patient. Any suspected failure of renal function must be investigated by a range of tests including cystoscopy, radiological examination, the use of radioisotopes and scanning techniques. A full chemical examination of the urine is required for the presence of glucose, protein, blood and microorganisms. Chemical analysis of the blood plasma is undertaken to determine the concentration of metabolites such as urea and creatinine. Metabolic acidosis can arise in certain kidney conditions when the excretion of hydrogen ions is diminished. Determination of arterial pH will give an indication of the extent of the acidosis. Table 21.1 gives an outline of kidney dysfunction and kidney failure.

RENAL FAILURE

Renal failure, both acute and chronic, requires a combination of treatment strategies including removal of nephrotoxic substances, specific drug treatment, correction of electrolyte disturbance and dietary measures. Over time, renal function deteriorates leading to complete failure of the kidneys. Renal replacement therapies will then be required.

Acute renal failure (ARF)

If the kidneys are deprived of blood flow by haemorrhage, infection, heart failure or drugs (especially those which cause diarrhoea or vomiting) urinary output will be reduced (less than 50 mL/day), leading to a rise in serum urea and creatinine. Other prerenal causes of failure include atheromatous plaques in the renal blood vessels which reduce the blood supply to the kidneys. Renal causes of ARF may include blocked blood vessels, glomerular nephritis, failure of tubular cells or disturbance of the interstitial cells owing to

Table 21.1 Kidney dysfunction/renal failure		
Condition	Main features/causes	Treatment
Glomerulonephritis (acute)	Inflammation of glomeruli (bilateral). Caused by an immune response to bacterial toxins, especially streptococci. Viral infection may also cause the disease. Histological examination is needed to differentiate various forms of the disease. The main signs are haematuria, hypertension, proteinuria and oedema	Bed rest, low-sodium diet, fluid restriction. Penicillin for streptococcal infection. Most younger patients recover well from the disease. The prognosis is less favourable in the older (40+ years) patients
Glomerulonephritis (chronic)	Chronic glomerulonephritis leads to chronic renal failure. As renal failure develops the levels of body fluids and electrolytes become abnormal. Acid–base balance is disturbed and nitrogenous waste products normally excreted in the urine accumulate. Platelet dysfunction results in bleeding episodes. The hypertension that accompanies the condition may cause retinopathy	Unless this disease is treated either by dialysis or transplantation the prognosis is grave. Treatment is based on dietary control, low protein, high carbohydrate and fat. Fluid intake is not restricted since it is important to achieve a large urinary volume to aid the excretion of the end-products of metabolism. Cardiac failure is a contraindication to a large fluid intake as is salt intake. Acidosis is treated by an appropriate regimen depending on blood chemistry results. An infusion of sodium bicarbonate may be required. Any infection must be treated but care is needed with dosage levels since excretion of the antibiotic may be impaired. GI symptoms must be treated, and bone pain may respond to vitamin D. Hypertension must be carefully managed so as not to cause a fall in renal blood flow. Dialysis and renal transplantation will not be considered in detail in this text. However, these are life-saving methods of dealing with renal failure
Infections (see also Ch. 19)	It may be difficult to determine the extent of an infection of the urinary tract. Any infection of the urinary tract has the potential to involve the kidneys. However, most urinary tract infections are capable of being treated in such a way that the spread of the infection is contained	The antimicrobial treatment of urinary tract infections (UTI) is described in Chapter 19. Approach to treatment depends on a number of factors. Owing to differing anatomical and other features, the approach to the treatment of UTI depends on the sex and age of the patient. Particular care must be taken to prevent kidney damage in children due to vesicoureteric reflux. Careful assessment of the patient is essential, a full history is required, e.g. in men it is important to exclude prostatic malignancy. In pregnant women pyelonephritis must be considered. Advice on prevention, e.g. passing urine after intercourse and vulval hygiene are important
Pyelonephritis (acute)	Acute inflammation of the parenchyma and pelvis of the kidney. The condition may affect one or both kidneys. Many of the infections are due to *E. coli*, but there are other causative organisms, e.g. *Proteus* species. There is a greater degree of prevalence in women than in men, owing to the anatomical differences. Fever, pain, frequency and dysuria are seen	Antimicrobial therapy (see p. 265). Antimicrobial agent should not be delayed until the organism causing the infection has been identified. Treatment should be continued until bacteriological tests are negative. Surgical treatment may be required if the root cause of the infection is a physical obstruction
Pyelonephritis (chronic)	The condition may present with a combination of symptoms, e.g. tiredness, general ill-health and urinary symptoms such as frequency, dysuria and lumbar pain. Careful checks should be made for any mechanical obstruction	Removal of any obstruction and long-term antimicrobial treatment. Suitable changes in antimicrobial therapy should be considered to avoid the possibility of resistance developing
Acute renal failure (ARF)	Renal failure arises from a variety of causes. Disease or drugs, circulatory failure, obstruction and acute renal ischaemia	Water and electrolyte balance must be restored and dietary control exercised (low protein). Acidosis must be treated and hyperkalaemia corrected. Great care must be taken with drug therapy (see p. 120). Haemodialysis or peritoneal dialysis must be considered since acute renal failure is life-threatening. Discussion of these techniques is beyond the scope of this book
Chronic renal failure (CRF)	Primary renal disease, complications of diabetes mellitus, hypertension, UTI, hereditary factors	This is discussed in the text
Nephrotic syndrome	Several kidney diseases are characterised by hypoproteinaemic oedema and proteinurea. The term 'nephrotic syndrome' is used to describe this chemical state	Treatment includes diuretics, corticosteroids, restriction of salt in diet; spironolactone is indicated in hypokalaemia

bacterial infection (pyelonephritis). Failure of tubular cells may be caused by drugs (see p. 141). Interstitial cells may also be damaged by drugs. Postrenal problems, such as blockage of urinary outflow because of prostatic hypertrophy (benign or malignant), may contribute to renal failure. Other postrenal problems include various cancers, urethral stricture and inflammation.

Chronic renal failure may be caused by diseases of the kidney or the multisystem disease diabetes mellitus. Hypertension and long-standing urinary tract infection may also be implicated.

Treatment of renal failure

Renal replacement therapies will be required in cases of severe renal failure. Haemodialysis, peritoneal dialysis (see p. 328), haemofiltration and haemodiafiltration are the main options. Renal transplantation is the replacement therapy of choice since it allows patients to enjoy a good quality of life. However, patients have to take immunosuppressive medication in order to prevent allograft rejection (see Ch. 23).

Drug therapy of renal disease

The kidney has many important physiological functions. If these become disordered, major problems can arise for the patient. Table 21.2 summarises the main treatment of the complications of renal disease.

It is vitally important to ensure that any drug treatment is safe for the patient with chronic renal disease. Analgesics need to be chosen with great care.

Drug dosages must be adjusted with care depending on the severity of renal impairment. Serum creatinine concentrations are a measure of renal function but must be corrected for age, weight and sex, using a nomogram. In mild renal impairment, serum creatinine ranges from 150–300 μmol/litre and in severe renal impairment levels above 700 μmol/litre are seen. Some drugs are best avoided in patients with renal impairment, e.g. acamprosate, acarbose (see BNF).

FLUID AND ELECTROLYTES

Fluid and electrolyte deficiency

Disorders of fluid balance are almost always accompanied by changes in the concentration of plasma sodium, potassium, other electrolytes and urea. Changes in fluid balance also have an effect on electrolyte levels. Such changes may have profound implications for the patient and must therefore be corrected by the administration of water and electrolytes. The volume and chemical content of the fluid, and route of administration depend on the condition being treated and biochemical status of the patient as determined by laboratory tests and clinical findings. The physiological significance of the main electrolytes is summarised in Table 21.3.

In order to enhance understanding of the terms used in the text a series of definitions is given in Table 21.4.

ABNORMALITIES OF ELECTROLYTE LEVELS AND FLUID BALANCE

The main abnormalities of electrolyte levels are closely linked with changes in fluid balance. For example, hypernatraemia is associated with fluid retention; loss of sodium is associated with a reduction in water content of the body. In many cases abnormalities in

Table 21.2 Complications of renal disease and their treatment

Condition	Drug treatment
Acidosis	Sodium bicarbonate corrects decreased bicarbonate levels
Anaemia (see p. 391)	
Calcium/phosphate metabolism (see p. 324). Higher phosphate levels, lower plasma calcium levels arise from the decline in renal function. Renal bone disease may result	Diet (dairy products, eggs, meat, fish), phosphate binders, vitamin D. Phosphate binders include aluminium hydroxide (dangers with long-term use) and calcium carbonate
Hypertension	ACE inhibitors (see p. 186) are valuable but must be used with care if the patient has renal artery stenosis. Other antihypertensive agents are also used (see Ch. 16)
Oedema and electrolyte disturbance	Fluid intake is restricted, as is potassium intake. Hyperkalaemia is a potentially dangerous condition (see p. 327)
Other conditions, restless legs, pruritus and nausea	Clonazepam is used for restless legs. Antihistamines help to relieve pruritus. Standard anti-emetics are used to control nausea

Table 21.3 Physiological significance of the main electrolytes

Electrolyte/normal range	Physiological significance/metabolism
Sodium (Na^+): 137–144 mmol per litre in plasma	Sodium is the most important extracellular cation, making up more than 90% of the total extracellular cations. Sodium accounts for a substantial proportion of the extracellular osmotic pressure. The cell membrane is not readily permeable to sodium ions. However, sodium diffuses slowly into the intracellular compartment according to the concentration gradient. The 'sodium pump' in the cell membrane transports sodium out of the cell. This movement of sodium is important in the establishment and maintenance of the electrical potential of the cell membrane and in the transmission of nerve impulses. A complex process is responsible for the maintenance of the sodium concentration in the body. Intake is normally dietary. Excretion in the urine is controlled by aldosterone and the antidiuretic hormone (ADH)
Potassium (K^+): 3.5–4.9 mmol per litre in plasma (intracellular concentration is of the order of 150 mmol/litre)	Potassium is the most important and abundant intracellular cation. It is present in low concentrations in the extracellular fluid. Potassium is responsible for a major portion of the intracellular fluid's osmotic pressure. Potassium plays a vital role in neuromuscular contraction and cardiac rhythm. Potassium is also important in aspects of carbohydrate metabolism and the synthesis of protein. As with sodium, intake is normally dietary and excretion is in the urine and to a lesser extent in the faeces
Calcium (Ca^{2+}): 2.2–2.6 mmol per litre (total body calcium greatly exceeds the amount present in the extracellular fluid)	Calcium is found in the bones and teeth in combination with phosphate to give strength and rigidity. Most of the calcium in the body is in deposits, with only a small proportion present in plasma (extracellular fluid). Calcium is important in blood coagulation processes, neuromuscular functions and cardiac activity. Intake is mainly dietary (especially dairy products) and excretion is mainly in the faeces. Small amounts are excreted in the urine. Vitamin D and gastric pH influence the absorption of calcium. Regulation of calcium metabolism is by parathyroid hormone, vitamin D and calcitonin
Magnesium (Mg^{2+}): 0.7–1.2 mmol per litre (total body magnesium greatly exceeds the content of the plasma)	Magnesium is present mainly in the bony skeleton; the remainder is found in the intracellular fluid especially in the heart, liver and skeletal muscles. Magnesium is important in enzyme activity – especially in the metabolism of glucose to provide energy. Magnesium also plays a part in the synthesis of protein. The functioning of nervous tissue depends on the presence of magnesium ions. The control mechanisms for magnesium are poorly understood but aldosterone is known to influence renal excretion. Other control mechanisms may be parathyroid hormone and vitamin D. Magnesium is in plentiful supply in a normal diet and the kidney reabsorbs most of the magnesium from the glomerular filtrate
Chloride (Cl^-): 100–106 mmol per litre	Chloride is the most abundant extracellular anion. Low concentrations are present in the intracellular fluid. Chloride plays a key role in the maintenance of the osmotic pressure of the extracellular fluid. Changes in the acid–base balance may influence chloride concentration. Chloride regulation is fundamentally linked with the regulation of the major cations (e.g. sodium) since electrical neutrality must always be maintained. It follows that chloride regulation is influenced by aldosterone, which enhances the tubular reabsorption of chloride and sodium. Intake is mainly dietary (as table salt NaCl). Apart from excretion in the urine some chloride is lost in the sweat and gastrointestinal secretions
Phosphate (PO_4^{2-}): 0.7–1.2 mmol per litre	Phosphate occurs mainly in the intracellular fluid and in combination with calcium is a vital constituent of bones and teeth. Phosphate also helps to maintain acid–base balance by providing a buffer system. Phosphates are vitally important in a number of metabolic processes especially carbohydrate metabolism. Phospholipids are important structural components of cell membranes. Phosphate regulation is linked closely with calcium metabolism. Parathyroid hormone liberates phosphate, and vitamin D probably enhances renal excretion of phosphate. An increase in serum phosphate is associated with a decrease in plasma calcium, and vice versa. Phosphate is widely present in foodstuffs, especially milk and other dairy products. Excretion is via the urine and faeces

electrolyte and fluid balance must be urgently treated by the parenteral (usually intravenous) route. In milder, chronic cases the oral route may be practicable and is always preferred where it can be used. The importance of accurate diagnosis, choice of fluid and concentration of electrolytes cannot be overstated. Accurate monitoring of the changes in plasma and other electrolyte levels achieved by the therapy is a prerequisite. In order to obtain a complete picture of losses of electrolytes from the body it may be necessary to examine faeces, vomitus and aspirate in addition to the blood and urine.

Hyponatraemia (lowered plasma sodium levels)

The main causes of hyponatraemia are:

- excessive sweating in hostile environments, e.g. tropical countries

Table 21.4 Definitions

Term	Definition
Acid–base balance	In health there is a balance between the carbonic acid and bicarbonate (base) content of plasma. Other basic (alkaline) substances in plasma are phosphates and protein
Acidosis (metabolic)	Acidosis has developed when the plasma level of bicarbonate falls to 15 mmol/litre. In severe acidosis the bicarbonate level may fall below 10 mmol/litre
Alkalosis (metabolic)	Alkalosis has developed when the plasma bicarbonate is elevated to 35 mmol/litre. The pH of blood also rises
Anion	Negatively charged ion, e.g. Cl^- or HCO_3^-
Buffering effect	Blood has the property to adjust to the pressure of acids produced by metabolic processes. Hydrogen ions are removed by the carbonic acid/bicarbonate buffer system so that the pH of plasma remains within the normal range 7.37–7.45
Cation	Positively charged ion, e.g. Na^+ or K^+
Electrolyte	A chemical substance that dissociates in water to yield ions (charged particles), e.g. sodium chloride (NaCl) dissociates to yield Na^+ and Cl^-
Isotonic	An isotonic solution has the same osmotic pressure as the comparison solution. The osmotic pressure of plasma is the accepted standard in medicine. A 0.9% w/v solution of sodium chloride is isotonic with plasma. Solutions with a lower osmotic pressure than plasma are hypotonic. Solutions with a higher osmotic pressure are hypertonic
Milliequivalent	1/1000 of the equivalent weight of a substance. This term has been replaced by the millimole
Millimole (mmol)	A mole is the molecular weight of a substance expressed in grams. A millimole is 1/1000 of the molecular weight
Osmolality	A measure of osmotic activity in terms of the concentration of solute particles in a unit of *weight* of solvent
Osmolarity	Also a measure of osmotic activity of a solution but expressed in terms of the concentration of solute particles in a given *volume* of solvent
Osmosis	When two solutions of differing concentration of dissolved solids (solute) are separated by a semipermeable membrane (e.g. cell membrane) water flows to the side of the membrane with the higher concentration of solute. Water flow ceases when the concentrations become equal
Osmotic pressure	The pressure created by the flow of water due to osmosis
pH (hydrogen ion concentration)	A measure of the degree of acidity or alkalinity of a solution. A pH below 7 indicates an acidic pH, whereas a pH above 7 indicates an alkaline solution. pH 7.0 is neutral

- loss of sodium in the urine because of renal disease or poor hormonal control (Addison's disease)
- uncontrolled diabetes mellitus
- chronic uraemia
- over-use of diuretics
- gastrointestinal problems, e.g. diarrhoea, vomiting and intestinal fistula
- loss of fluid owing to trauma, e.g. extensive burns
- side-effects of drugs, e.g. diuretics.

Patients with hyponatraemia may experience nausea, weakness, headache and drowsiness. The degree and nature of the symptoms depend on the level of sodium in the plasma. Concentrations in the region of 120 mmol/litre give rise to weakness; at 90–105 mmol/litre neurological signs and symptoms develop.

Treatment of hyponatraemia

In milder, chronic forms treatment is by the oral administration of sodium usually as chloride in the form of a slow-release tablet. The choice of sodium compound administered depends on the acid–base status of the patient. In acidotic patients, sodium bicarbonate is required whereas in the alkalotic patient sodium chloride is required. In more severe hyponatraemia treatment by parenteral administration of a fluid containing a sodium compound is required. This will also help to correct the fluid loss that almost always accompanies sodium depletion. The administration of sodium parenterally is not without risk. Hypertension and fluid overload must be avoided. Plasma sodium levels must be monitored, and physical signs such as pulse rate and blood pressure give a good indication of the patient's response to the therapy. Fluids commonly used to correct hyponatraemia (and other electrolyte deficiencies) are summarised in Table 21.5.

Hypernatraemia (increased plasma sodium levels)

Just as hyponatraemia is associated with fluid loss, hypernatraemia is accompanied by water retention.

Table 21.5 Fluids used to correct hyponatraemia and other electrolyte deficiencies

Solution/strength	Content (mmol/litre)	Main indications/contraindications
Sodium bicarbonate intravenous infusion 4.2% w/v and 8.4%. Other strengths are available. The 1.26% w/v solution is used as a continuous infusion	150 mmol each of Na^+ and HCO_3^- per litre	Corrections of severe metabolic acidosis. May cause thrombophlebitis at site of infusion. This is a common problem with all long-term intravenous infusion sites
Sodium chloride intravenous infusion 0.45% w/v (hypotonic), 0.9% w/v (isotonic). The term 'normal saline' should not be used as it could be confused with a chemically normal solution, which is much stronger	75 mmol/litre Na^+, 75 mmol/litre Cl^-, 150 mmol/litre Na^+, 150 mmol/litre Cl^-	To correct fluid balance and as a source of sodium and chloride. Must be used with care in patients with reduced ability to handle sodium (e.g. organic heart disease)
Sodium chloride and glucose intravenous infusions. Sterile solutions containing a range of combinations of sodium chloride and glucose are available; e.g. 0.18% w/v sodium chloride and 4% w/v glucose; 0.18% w/v sodium chloride and 10% w/v glucose; 0.9% w/v sodium chloride and 5% w/v glucose		These solutions are a source of sodium, chloride, water and energy. As with all these intravenous infusions the choice of solution, rate of administration, and period of treatment depends on the condition being treated. Combinations of sodium chloride and glucose help to achieve rehydration of both the body cells and the extracellular space
Compound sodium chloride intravenous infusion. Contains in each litre: sodium chloride 8.6 g, calcium chloride dihydrate 330 mg, potassium chloride 300 mg	Sodium 147.5 mmol/litre, potassium 4 mmol/litre, calcium 2 mmol/litre, chloride 150 mmol/litre	Source of water and electrolytes in cases of fluid and electrolyte depletion due to vomiting, diarrhoea, fistula drainage and diabetic acidosis. Prolonged administration may cause metabolic acidosis due to an excess of chloride ions
Sodium lactate intravenous infusions. A number of different formulations containing sodium lactate are available	Sodium lactate M/6 intravenous infusion contains: 167 mmol/litre sodium, 167 mmol/litre lactate. Compound sodium lactate intravenous infusion contains in mmol/litre: sodium 131, potassium 5, calcium 2, chloride 111, lactate 29	Sodium lactate intravenous infusion M/6 has been used to correct metabolic acidosis and as a source of water and electrolytes. All lactate-containing solutions are contraindicated in patients with impairment of lactate utilisation. Also known as Hartmann's solution compound. Sodium lactate intravenous infusion is a source of water and electrolytes. It restores diminished alkali reserves by the slow conversion of lactate into bicarbonate. Sodium lactate infusions are not now advocated in metabolic acidosis owing to the risks of the patient developing lactic acidosis
Potassium chloride and sodium chloride intravenous infusion: 0.15% potassium chloride, 0.9% sodium chloride. A wide range of strengths is available		Fluid replacement, prevention and treatment of potassium deficiency. Care must be taken to avoid cardiotoxicity
Potassium chloride is also available in combination with glucose		The indications are similar to those for potassium chloride and sodium chloride intravenous infusion. The glucose content provides a source of energy
Darrow's intravenous infusion	Sodium 121 mmol/litre, potassium 35 mmol/litre, chloride 103 mmol/litre, lactate 53 mmol/litre	This solution is used to correct mild and moderate potassium deficiency. As with all potassium-containing solutions this infusion is contraindicated in renal disease and where lactate utilisation is impaired

Hypernatraemia results from inadequate renal excretion. The main causes of hypernatraemia are:

- hypoproteinaemia (as in the nephrotic syndrome)
- primary heart failure
- inability to excrete salt and water because of glomerulonephritis
- certain drugs, e.g. corticosteroids, androgens, oral contraceptives
- hepatic cirrhosis.

Treatment of hypernatraemia

The treatment is based on a combination of measures. Underlying disease must be treated, e.g. heart failure by digoxin therapy, and glomerulonephritis by administration of plasma proteins. Restriction of dietary intake of salt and water is always required. Diuretics promote the excretion of salt and water, and are the most important drugs used in the treatment of hypernatraemia.

Hypokalaemia (lowered plasma potassium levels)

Lowered potassium levels occur because of an excessive loss of potassium from the body in the urine or from the gastrointestinal tract. Losses from the gastrointestinal tract result from acute or chronic diarrhoea. Loss from a fistula or gastric aspiration may also be significant.

Use of laxatives and diuretics may cause potassium depletion. It is important to take a full drug history.

Renal loss of potassium is due to a complex range of factors. Primary aldosteronism, Cushing's syndrome and corticosteroid therapy may be implicated. Metabolic or respiratory acidosis is associated with loss of potassium in the urine. Certain renal diseases can cause potassium loss in the urine. A poor diet may also result in mild potassium depletion. Worldwide, hypokalaemia is most often caused by diarrhoea.

The clinical features of potassium depletion (less than 3.5 mmol/litre) include apathy, weakness and mental disturbances. Symptoms increase in severity with decreasing potassium levels. Polyuria and thirst may be seen, and cardiac arrhythmias may occur. Potassium depletion increases the sensitivity of cardiac tissue to digoxin and this may result in toxic reactions. Chloride depletion and metabolic alkalosis are often associated with hypokalaemia.

Treatment of hypokalaemia

As with sodium replacement therapy, the oral route is preferred since it is less likely to cause hyperkalaemia. Potassium chloride is highly irritant to the gastric mucosa. A slow-release tablet formulation or soluble (effervescent) tablet or liquid preparation is often preferred. The dosage will depend on the extent of potassium depletion. A range of potassium-containing solutions is available for intravenous infusion. These are summarised in Table 21.5.

Potassium chloride is available as a concentrated solution for addition to infusion fluids. Great care must be taken with the dosage levels so as to reduce the risk of toxic hyperkalaemia. Wherever possible ready-prepared sterile solutions containing potassium should be used so as to avoid the possible hazards of adding strong potassium solutions (15%) to infusion fluids. All drug additives to infusion fluids must be carefully checked to avoid chemical incompatibility, and care must be taken to ensure adequate mixing. Intravenous infusions of potassium-containing substances are best managed using an infusion pump with adequate controls.

Hyperkalaemia (increased plasma potassium levels)

The commonest cause of this potentially dangerous condition is severe oliguria or anuria. Acute renal failure results in hyperkalaemia. Diabetic ketoacidosis may cause hyperkalaemia. Consequences of hyperkalaemia include muscular weakness, abdominal distension and cardiac disturbances. Pulse irregularities are accompanied by heart block and other irregularities of cardiac function. Hyperkalaemia is a serious condition because of the dangers of cardiac arrest. Levels of 7.5 mmol/litre are very dangerous.

Treatment of hyperkalaemia

Glucose and insulin given together intravenously encourage migration of potassium into cells. The administration of alkali in the form of sodium bicarbonate isotonic solution may be used to correct metabolic acidosis that may develop. The cardiotoxicity of potassium may be reduced by the intravenous administration of calcium gluconate in the form of a 10% solution which improves myocardial stability. Sodium and water deficits must also be corrected. Dietary restriction is necessary and the oral (or rectal) administration of an ion-exchange resin (polystyrene sulphonate) may be required. The choice of the particular ion-exchange resin depends on the patient's condition. A sodium resin should not be used where there is hypernatraemia since the resin liberates sodium as potassium is taken up. Similarly, a calcium resin must not be used where the patient's calcium levels are already too high.

If the above measures fail to control the hyperkalaemia, consideration must be given to peritoneal dialysis or haemodialysis.

Dialysis

Haemodialysis and peritoneal dialysis are based on the same principle. In both, the patient's blood is on one side of a semipermeable membrane and a dialysate solution is on the other. An exchange of metabolites occurs across the membrane. In haemodialysis, blood is diverted out of the body and passed through a dialyser (an artificial kidney) and then returned to the patient. In peritoneal dialysis the fluid is run into the patient's abdominal cavity where the peritoneum acts as the semipermeable membrane. After exchange has taken place, the fluid is drained off.

In haemodialysis, blood is taken from an arterial line, heparinised, pumped through a dialyser then returned to the patient. Metabolites and excess electrolytes pass from the blood, across the semipermeable membrane and into the dialysate. By increasing the pressure of the blood, excess water can be removed from the patient. The duration of a single dialysis is usually about 4 hours, and the haemodialysis process is performed two or three times a week.

In peritoneal dialysis, a semi-rigid catheter is inserted into the abdominal cavity. 1 or 2 litres of warmed dialysate containing an osmotic agent (glucose) are run into the abdomen, left for about 30 minutes and then run into a collecting bag.

In renal failure, haemodialysis is a more rapid treatment than peritoneal dialysis and is essential in hypercatabolic renal failure where urea is produced faster than it can be removed by peritoneal dialysis.

Rehydration therapy

Oral

The oral route is always preferred when it is necessary to replace losses of both water and electrolytes. The BNF describes a wide range of preparations available for oral rehydration therapy (ORT). This approach to rehydration is especially important in countries where diarrhoea is a major health problem. Products available for ORT contain glucose (to enhance absorption of electrolytes) and the three main electrolytes: sodium, potassium and chloride. The choice and dose of formulation depend on the patient's age, severity of the condition and other factors.

Parenteral

If the parenteral route (intravenous) has to be used, a wide range of solutions is available. Since dehydration is almost always accompanied by loss of electrolytes, a fluid containing the necessary electrolytes, often in combination with glucose, will be selected. Where there is no significant loss of electrolytes, a simple solution of glucose in water is used. Between 2 and 10 litres per day may be required to make good the deficit.

DRUG TREATMENT OF DISORDERS OF THE GENITOURINARY TRACT

It is important to note that while drug treatment plays an important role in treating disorders of the genitourinary tract, a combination of treatment strategies may be required. Surgery and/or the use of various appliances may be required in addition to drug therapy. The skills of specialist nurses are increasingly used in the care of patients with urinary problems.

Products used following surgical procedures on the genitourinary tract and other irrigations appear in Table 21.7. Conditions for which patients may derive benefit from drug therapy are discussed below.

Enuresis

Behavioural measures and enuresis alarms are the mainstays of treatment. However, drugs can play an important role.

Imipramine is used to treat nocturnal enuresis in children. A bedtime dose of 25–75 mg is given depending on the age and body weight of the child. Treatment should be for a period of 3 months, including gradual withdrawal as the condition is controlled. Further courses of treatment should not be undertaken without a full physical examination of the child.

Amitriptyline may also be used to treat nocturnal enuresis in children, the dose range being 20–50 mg, depending on the age and weight of the child.

Desmopressin is an analogue of the natural antidiuretic hormone vasopressin (see also p. 298). It is administered as a nasal spray in the treatment of nocturnal enuresis. Tricyclic antidepressants (e.g. amitriptyline) may also be useful but should only be used for a 3-month period. Toxicity and side-effects are of concern.

Enuresis in adults is treated with propantheline (see below).

Urinary incontinence (including benign prostatic hypertrophy)

Urinary incontinence in adults is a common condition which may significantly damage the person's quality of life. Following careful assessment and accurate diagnosis, both drug and non-drug treatment can be very valuable. Non-drug treatment will not be considered here but is often a vital part of patient care.

Urinary incontinence in women arises because of detrusor instability and stress incontinence. In men urinary incontinence is less common. Causes include detrusor instability and bladder disorders.

The presence of infection should always be excluded.

Benign prostatic hypertrophy

A study has shown that benign prostatic hypertrophy (BPH) affects 43% of men aged 60–69 years (Garraway et al 1991). Although this article refers to hypertrophy, the modern term is hyperplasia. This condition presents with frequency and urge incontinence and poor

Table 21.6 Alpha-blockers used in the treatment of urinary retention

Drug	Dose	Notes
Alfuzosin	2.5 mg three times daily, maximum 10 mg daily; elderly initially 2.5 mg twice daily	The first dose may cause collapse due to hypotensive effect; therefore it should be taken on retiring to bed. Patient should be warned to lie down if symptoms such as dizziness, fatigue or sweating develop and to remain lying down until they abate completely
Doxazosin	Initially 1 mg daily; increased if necessary at intervals of 1–2 weeks to a maximum of 8 mg daily; usual maintenance dose 2–4 mg daily	
Indoramin	20 mg twice daily, increased if necessary by 20 mg every 2 weeks to a maximum of 100 mg daily in divided doses	
Prazosin	Initially 500 micrograms twice daily for 3–7 days; usual maintenance (and maximum) dose 2 mg twice daily	As for alfuzosin
Tamsulosin	400 micrograms daily after breakfast	
Terazosin	Initially 1 mg at bedtime; dose may be doubled at weekly intervals according to response; to a maximum of 1 mg once daily; usual maintenance dose 5–10 mg daily	As for alfuzosin

urinary stream and hesitance. The treatment is based on selective alpha-blockers which relax the smooth muscles of the bladder neck and prostate. Bladder outlet resistance is decreased and urinary flow is facilitated (an alternative approach is the use of an anti-androgen). The available drugs are summarised in Table 21.6.

Drug treatment of urinary incontinence

Antimuscarinic drugs may be useful but their side-effects (see p. 258) are often a major source of problems especially for older people. Examples include oxybutynin (including a modified-release formulation), propantheline bromide, propiverine hydrochloride and tolterodine tartrate. Tricyclic antidepressants (see p. 240) may be effective in the management of the unstable bladder. Oxybutynin is widely used in a dose of 5 mg twice daily (older patients) or 5 mg four times daily. It is emphasised that all the above drugs must be used with caution in older patients especially the very frail who have cognitive impairment.

Impotence

Reasons for failure to produce a satisfactory erection include psychogenic, vascular, neurogenic and endocrine abnormalities. Many drugs are also liable to induce impotence.

Alprostadil is a prostaglandin given by intracavernosal injection for the management of erectile dysfunction. The first dose must be given by medically trained personnel. Self-administration may be undertaken only after proper training. The first dose is 2.5 micrograms which is increased depending on response in steps of 5–10 micrograms to obtain a dose suitable for producing an erection not lasting more than an hour. Patients should be instructed to report an erection lasting more than 4 hours which may require treatment by aspiration initially and, if unsuccessful, cautious intracavernosal injection of a sympathomimetic drug (e.g. phenylephrine) with action on alpha-adrenergic receptors. The side-effects of alprostadil include penile pain, prolonged erection and reactions at the injection site. The injection of papaverine into the corpus cavernosum has been found to be an effective treatment for erectile dysfunction but its use has reduced since the introduction of alprostadil and sildenafil. Careful physical examination must be undertaken before any treatment for erectile dysfunction is initiated since the side-effects are a cause of concern, especially in patients with cardiovascular disease.

Sildenafil, the first oral treatment for erectile dysfunction, is available for the treatment of erectile dysfunction in men who have certain specified conditions. The dose is 25–50 mg 1 hour before sexual activity. Subsequent doses should be adjusted according to response. The maximum single dose is 100 mg in a 24-hour period. There are a number of contraindications to the use of this drug, especially cardiovascular disease and deformation of the penis.

Urinary infections

Most infections of the genitourinary tract are treated with systemic antibiotics (see p. 280). In certain

Table 21.7 Sterile solutions used in bladder irrigation

Active ingredient	Strength (all percentages given are w/v)	Pack or presentation	Uses, indications and precautions
Amphotericin	50 micrograms/mL	50 mg vial (powder) made up before use into a solution	Fungal infections
Chlorhexidine	1 in 5000 (0.02%)	100 mL 'Uro-Tainer'. Other pack sizes are available	Used for its mechanical effect. Also has a bacteriostatic action on organisms commonly found in the urinary tract. Inactive against *Pseudomonas* species
Glycine	1.5%	3 L plastic bag	Used in transurethral resection of the prostate gland. Non-haemolytic, weakly ionised. Any glycine absorbed is metabolised; ammonia may be produced, which has toxic effects. Cases of hyponatraemia have been reported but these are rare
Mandelic acid	1%	100 mL 'Uro-Tainer'	Used if resistance to chlorhexidine is encountered. Effective against *Pseudomonas* and *Proteus* species. May cause local irritation
Sodium chloride	0.9%	500 mL or 3 L plastic bag	Used for its mechanical effect. It is also used as a vehicle for certain drugs instilled into the bladder
Sodium citrate	3%	500 mL	Used primarily for the dissolution of blood clots
Solution R	6% citric acid, 0.6% gluconolactone, 2.8% magnesium carbonate, 0.1% disodium edetate	100 mL 'Uro-Tainer'	Used to dissolve existing encrustations. Use between twice and four times a week for 2 weeks, before reverting to Solution G. Should not be used for a period of 10–14 days following prostatic surgery owing to absorption of salts leading to electrolyte imbalance
Solution G (Suby G)	3.23% citric acid	100 mL 'Uro-Tainer'	Use between twice daily and twice weekly to prevent the formation of encrustations. Should not be used for a period of 10–14 days following prostatic surgery owing to absorption of salts leading to electrolyte imbalance
Streptokinase–streptodornase	100 000 units streptokinase with streptodornase 25 000 units	Rubber-capped vial	Used to dissolve blood clots in bladder or urinary catheter. Must not be used where there is active haemorrhage or known sensitivity to the enzymes

conditions, local instillation of antimicrobial agents may be used. Table 21.7 shows the range of products available. Bladder instillations (irrigations or washouts) are of some value but risks of cross-infection, poor antimicrobial action and local irritancy limit their use. Wherever possible systemic therapy, based on the results of microbial sensitivity tests, is preferable.

Malignancy

Instillation of locally acting cytotoxic drugs may be indicated in the treatment of superficial bladder tumours. Doxorubicin, epirubicin, mitomycin and thiotepa are used, made up in sterile water or sodium chloride solution. Any evidence of absorption must be taken into account in selecting the concentration of drug in the irrigating fluid and period of treatment (see p. 349).

Pain

Pain in the urinary tract may be due to a number of conditions. The acute pain of ureteric colic is treated with pethidine or diclofenac (see p. 470). Lidocaine (lignocaine) in the form of a 1% or 2% gel may be useful for urethral pain and prior to male and female catheterisation. Discomfort caused by cystitis may be relieved by alkalinisation of the urine using potassium citrate or sodium bicarbonate. Hyperkalaemia (see p. 327) and hypernatraemia (see p. 325) are possible side-effects of this treatment. Pain due to metabolites of the cytotoxic drug cyclophosphamide can be relieved using mesna (see p. 340).

Urinary frequency

Urinary frequency arises from a number of causes including infection, foreign bodies and malignant

Table 21.8 Parasympathomimetics used in the treatment of urinary retention

Drug	Dose/route	Notes/precautions/side-effects
Bethanechol	10–25 mg three or four times daily, orally, *before* food	If given after food, nausea and vomiting may be caused. Avoid in asthmatic patients and patients with gastrointestinal obstruction. Because of the effect on the eye, blurred vision may occur
Carbachol	2 mg three times daily, orally, *before* food. May also be given by SC injection for postoperative urinary retention, in a dose of 250 micrograms	Similar side-effects and precautions but likely to be more acute than with bethanechol. Carbachol (and bethanechol) must be used with great caution in older patients

disease. Flavoxate is a selective urinary tract antispasmodic. In an oral dose of 200 mg three times daily, it is used in the treatment of dysuria, urgency, nocturia and the incontinence that may result from cystitis and prostatitis. Side-effects include gastrointestinal problems, vertigo, tachycardia and palpitations. Since the drug is an antispasmodic, it must be used with caution in patients with suspected glaucoma (see p. 411).

Flavoxate must not be used in patients with obstructive conditions of the gastrointestinal tract since the antispasmodic action would cause a worsening of the condition. Oxybutynin given orally up to 5 mg four times daily is used to treat urinary frequency. Dosage levels must be carefully adjusted, especially in the older patient. Side-effects are typical of drugs of this type, as are the contraindications.

Urinary retention

Acute urinary retention results from prostatic obstruction or urethral stricture. In women a possible cause is meatal stenosis. Catheterisation is required to reduce the risk of renal damage. Given that the treatment of urinary frequency involves the use of antimuscarinic (atropine-like) drugs, it follows that the treatment of urinary retention may use parasympathomimetics for their muscarinic effects (see p. 146). Parasympathomimetics used include carbachol and bethanechol (see Table 21.8). These drugs have potentially dangerous side-effects such as bradycardia and intestinal colic. Patients with asthma or susceptibility to asthmatic attacks must not be treated with parasympathomimetic drugs owing to the danger of precipitating an acute episode of bronchoconstriction.

Another parasympathomimetic is distigmine which is given orally (5 mg half an hour before breakfast) or by intramuscular injection 500 micrograms 12 hours after surgery to prevent urinary retention. This drug acts by inhibiting the breakdown of acetylcholine (see p. 144) (anticholinesterase). Distigmine is a long-acting drug and should be used with care, especially after surgery, particularly where bowel anastomosis has been carried out.

ADMINISTRATION OF MEDICATIONS INTO THE BLADDER

Bladder irrigation

Indwelling catheters, even when introduced into the bladder under the most rigorous aseptic conditions, are an important source of urinary tract infection. In the course of time, crystallisation around and within the lumen of the catheter further increases the risk of infection by obstructing the flow and causing stasis of urine. Bypassing of urine then follows, leading to discomfort, embarrassment and skin breakdown. Patients who produce haematuric urine can also develop severe drainage problems and discomfort, especially when the catheter is blocked by blood clots. Special responsibility therefore rests with nurses involved in the care of patients with a urinary catheter.

The indications for washing out the bladder are:

- to reduce and treat urinary tract infections
- to prevent and clear obstruction of the eye(s) and lumen of the catheter by debris, crystals or blood clot.

The methods most commonly used for introducing fluid into the bladder are:

- intermittent bladder irrigation, either by instillation from an irrigation device such as the Uro-Tainer, or by mechanical irrigation using a form of suction
- continuous bladder irrigation.

The method used will depend on the reason for carrying out the irrigation.

Intermittent irrigation (Box 21.1)

The Uro-Tainer system

This ready-to-use irrigation device involves a simple technique which is quick and can be mastered by

Box 21.1 Intermittent bladder irrigation

Documentation
- Standard prescribing and recording sheet
- Fluid balance chart

The medicine
- Sterile irrigating solution in either Uro-Tainer or 500 mL bag
- Solution as prescribed, visibly clear and at room temperature

The environment
- As for any aseptic procedure
- Privacy

The nurse and the patient
- Patient identified as corresponding to prescription
- Explanation as to what is involved
- Patient assisted into relaxed position with only catheter exposed; patient kept warm
- Clothes and bedding protected
- Patient made comfortable on completion of procedure

Technique
- Aseptic (gloves not required with Uro-Tainer)
- Observation of returned fluid
- New drainage system attached to catheter after irrigation completed
- All urine measured and recorded
- Administration recorded

Hazards
- Infection

patients or their relatives for use at home. A range of solutions for maintaining patency of a catheter is available. Solution G is weakly acidic and is used for flushing out and for preventing crystal formation, or for dissolving crystals already formed in the catheter. Aqueous chlorhexidine solution (0.02% w/v) has a bacteriostatic action against many of the common urinary tract pathogens. Some clinicians recommend routine use of chlorhexidine solution immediately prior to the removal of all urinary catheters. The solution is left in the bladder until such time as the patient wishes to void.

Clot retention is usually treated by irrigation with sterile sodium chloride solution (0.9% w/v) although, where clots prove to be obstinate, alternative methods of irrigation may have to be employed. Sterile sodium citrate solution 3% may also be used to break up clots. The volume of solution in each Uro-Tainer is 100 mL although the amount instilled into the bladder is not critical, rather the time the solution is left in the bladder, which may be up to half an hour. Gloves are not necessary when this method of irrigation is used. However, thorough handwashing is essential, and care must be taken to connect the catheter and irrigation tubing without contaminating them. A regimen in current use for patients with long-term catheters involves alternate use of a urinary antiseptic, such as chlorhexidine (0.02% w/v), with a decrystallising solution twice a week; for example one solution every Tuesday, the other every Friday.

Mechanical irrigation using suction

In the event of a catheter becoming completely blocked by blood clots, the catheter may be washed out in an effort to break down the clots by a form of suction using a catheter-tipped syringe and sterile irrigating solution. Where blood clots are especially troublesome a large volume of sterile sodium chloride solution (0.9% w/v) will be required. This method is based on first introducing approximately 50 mL of solution, which is left in the bladder. This acts as a physical buffer to allow further volumes of fluid to be instilled under pressure, then withdrawn by suction through the catheter, depending on the severity of the blockage. The nurse wears gloves for this procedure because of the many manipulative processes involved. It may take a considerable time until the catheter drains freely. Patients, who may already be in pain and be losing blood into the bladder, can find this a tedious and uncomfortable experience. They should therefore be kept warm and as comfortable as possible. As with all such procedures the encouragement and support of the nurse are vital throughout.

Continuous irrigation

Continuous irrigation of the bladder may be employed following prostatic surgery to rid the bladder of blood clots and prostatic debris. A three-way catheter, or alternative combination of catheters, is inserted in theatre. This allows one inlet for inflating the catheter balloon and another for the entry of irrigating solution, and an outlet for drainage of the bladder contents. Sodium chloride solution (0.9% w/v) is introduced into the bladder from a 3-litre bag suspended from an infusion stand, via an administration set connected to the catheter. In the immediate postoperative period the control clamp is left open fully to allow for continuous flushing of the bladder and of the eyes of the catheter. After several hours, depending on the degree of haematuria, the rate may be decreased. Volumes of irrigating solution ranging from 15–45 litres may be required to treat the patient during the first 24 hours. The flow of such large volumes of fluid demands frequent attention by the nurse in maintaining input, discarding output and keeping records of both. In urological wards, anticipating needs and finding adequate storage space for large volumes of irrigation solutions can present problems. To some extent, these may be alleviated by active involvement of the ward pharmacist who can, among other things, help to ensure that supply keeps pace with demand.

It should be remembered that hypertension (resulting from absorption of sodium) and perforation of the bladder may each result from this form of irrigation. Nurses in urology wards have particular responsibility therefore to ensure that close monitoring of the blood pressure and pulse (every half-hour at first), fluid balance, and pain is carried out. If the patient complains of pain, no matter how mild, irrigation should not proceed without seeking further advice. While it is important not to alarm junior nursing staff, and hence patients, at this time, the possibility of perforation, especially following transurethral resection of the prostate gland, must never be forgotten.

General principles of bladder irrigation

When using any form of bladder washout the broad principles of medicine administration apply. The details of the solution are checked against the prescription, and the fluid visually examined before use to make sure it is free from any particulate matter. Any container whose contents are not clear should be rejected. In view of the high risk to the patient of microbial contamination, all procedures are carried out using a strictly aseptic technique. Ideally, solutions should be warmed to body temperature before use in a solution-warming cabinet. Improvised methods of warming solutions are not recommended since control of the solution temperature is impossible to achieve. In the absence of a solution-warming cabinet it is probably best to use the solution at room temperature.

Patients with an indwelling catheter which has been on continuous drainage for weeks or months, may have difficulty in tolerating the instillation of volumes of solutions in excess of 50 mL because of reduced bladder capacity or bladder irritability. When the bladder is irritated by infection or is reduced in capacity by tumour, it may be possible to tolerate only very small volumes of fluid. On occasion, a volume as small as 10 mL is as much as the patient can hold. Infected fluid is never re-injected. When the patient indicates that the bladder feels uncomfortable, and as though it cannot take in more fluid, then this must be taken as the maximal amount that can be instilled. As soon as possible following any manipulations of a catheter, the catheter should be attached to a sterile closed drainage system. The drainage tubing should be stiff enough to reduce the likelihood of kinking, and the drainage bag should be adequately supported on a floor stand positioned for ease of observation of the colour, consistency and volume of urine drained. Bag holders can become distorted, for example when lowering the height of the patient's bed. This increases the risk of the tubing becoming kinked. Also, the drainage tap may come into contact with the floor, with obvious risk of contamination.

Details of sterile solutions used in bladder irrigation and some of the drugs used in bladder instillations are given in Table 21.7.

ADMINISTRATION OF VULVAL AND VAGINAL MEDICATIONS

Gynaecological conditions are judged by many women to be a source of extreme embarrassment and fear. Patients express these feelings in different ways. Some are hesitant to ask for further explanation of their condition or treatment, showing a natural reservation about intimate matters. Others fear being thought of as unclean, embarrassed by odour, itching and perhaps staining of underclothes from vaginal discharge. Patients may fear discovery of a malignant condition or that they have developed an infection which has been sexually transmitted. Knowledge of anatomy and physiology of the female genital tract in some instances may be scant and attitudes to bodily functions may have been influenced by folklore.

Nurses working in gynaecological wards and clinics become accustomed to carrying out intimate procedures and discussing very personal issues with their patients. They may need to remind themselves of the importance of maintaining sensitivity to the feelings of each new patient. General ward nurses and district nurses are required to care for patients with gynaecological disorders from time to time, and so they should be ready to turn their attention to the special needs of these patients.

In all cases, embarrassment or attitude on the part of the nurse should never be allowed to interfere with establishing and dealing with the full nature of the problem. Tact, patience and gentleness are essential at all times.

Vulval and vaginal preparations which contain a drug should be prescribed, administered and recorded according to local policy. The genital area should be clean, and traces of previously applied cream should be removed. Whenever possible, the patient should apply the preparation herself. Nurses must guarantee privacy for patients whether they are explaining self-administration or actually carrying out the treatment.

Box 21.2 Insertion of vaginal pessaries

Documentation
- Prescribing and recording sheet

The medicine
- Pessary as ordered, with applicator

The environment
- Privacy, warmth, comfort

The nurse and the patient
- Patient identified
- Patient given explanation of what is involved and advised to empty bladder
- Patient assisted if necessary into supine position, with knees flexed and thighs abducted, or left lateral position with buttocks at edge of bed

Technique
- Nurse attends to own hand hygiene and applies disposable gloves
- Pessary inserted, using applicator, as high as possible along posterior vaginal wall in an upwards and backwards direction for the full length of the vagina
- Patient's vulval area wiped dry and sanitary pad applied to prevent staining of clothes (tampons should not be used in the presence of infection)
- Applicator washed in warm, soapy water, rinsed and dried

Hazards
- Pessary can easily be dislodged and so is best inserted on retiring to bed

It is important to explain to which particular area the treatment is to be directed, the recommended times of administration and the need to complete the course. Disposable gloves should be worn by the nurse when administering vulval and vaginal preparations both to protect the patient and nurse from acquiring infection or the nurse from absorbing any of the medication. Whether nurse or patient carries out the procedure, the hands should be washed before and after. Applicators should be washed in warm soapy water, rinsed and dried. A separate treatment kit should be assigned to the individual patient (Box 21.2).

REFERENCES

Garraway W M, Collins G N, Lee R J 1991 High prevalence of benign prostatic hypertrophy in the community. Lancet 338:469–471

FURTHER READING

Andrews P A 2002 Renal transplantation. British Medical Journal 324:530–533

Barry M J, Roehrborn C G 2001 Benign prostatic hyperplasia. British Medical Journal 323:1042–1045

Berger A 2000 Renal function – and how to assess it. British Medical Journal 321:1444

Gulliford G, Bidmead J 2001 Management of incontinence. Pharmaceutical Journal 267:230–232

Sasi P, English M 2002 Challenges in managing profound hypokalaemia. British Medical Journal 324:269–270

Shakir S A W, Wilton L V 2001 Cardiovascular events in users of sildenafil: results from first phase of prescription event monitoring in England. British Medical Journal 322:651–652

CHAPTER CONTENTS

22 Drug treatment of malignant disease

INTRODUCTION

In spite of the fact that survival rates for many cancers have considerably improved over the past decades, malignant disease remains a major cause of morbidity and mortality. Cancer has existed for thousands of years. It can occur in infants but is more commonly associated with increasing age. Certain cancers show an increased incidence in lower socio-economic groups, and different cancers can affect different populations. Cancer is not one disease; indeed, over 100 different cancers have been identified.

AETIOLOGY

There is no known single cause of cancer, although a number of predisposing factors have been incriminated. These include:

- chemical factors, e.g. tars in tobacco, asbestos, cytotoxic drugs
- physical factors, e.g. sunlight, radiation, chronic trauma/infection
- viruses
- poor diet, low in fruit and vegetables, high in red/processed meat products
- genetic factors, e.g. increased incidence in Down's syndrome
- familial factors, e.g. polyposis coli in families leading to colonic cancer
- geographical factors, e.g. Japanese women who go to live in the USA go from a low risk of developing breast cancer to high risk and have as great a chance of developing it as American women; bowel cancer is almost unknown on the African continent, probably owing to dietary factors.

CLASSIFICATION OF CANCERS

Cancers may be classified in different ways. They may be considered as solid tumours, e.g. lung, liver, or

Table 22.1 Classification of tumours according to tissue of origin

Tissue of origin	Type of tumour
Epithelial tissue	Carcinoma, e.g. of breast, of lung
Connective tissue	Sarcoma, e.g. of bone, of muscle
Lymphatic tissue	Malignant lymphoma, e.g. Hodgkin's disease, non-Hodgkin's lymphoma
Bone marrow	Leukaemia, e.g. myeloblastic leukaemia
Pigment cells	Malignant melanoma

Box 22.1 Spread of some primary tumours

bronchus → brain
breast → bone
testis → lung
colon → liver

'liquid' tumours, i.e. of the blood or lymph. Alternatively, they may be classified according to their tissue of origin (Table 22.1).

SPREAD OF CANCER

Cancer spreads either by direct infiltration of adjacent tissues or by cells from the primary tumour being transported to another often distant site (or sites) in the body where they become established and grow. These secondary deposits are known as metastases. The pathways taken by the metastasising cells include the lymphatic system, the blood, serous cavities and CSF pathways. Different primary tumours tend to show preference for particular secondary sites – see Box 22.1.

Some patients develop a second primary tumour.

PRESENTATION

A malignancy may be an incidental finding when some other condition is being investigated or at a routine check. It otherwise presents in many different ways, ranging from bleeding, swelling and loss of function to anaemia and general malaise depending on the type of tumour and its location. Pain tends to be a feature of more established disease where there is tissue erosion or pressure from metastases.

DIAGNOSIS

The diagnosis of cancer is arrived at through careful history-taking, physical examination, cytological and pathological examination, and various imaging techniques.

TREATMENT

Treatment mainly takes the form of surgery, radiotherapy or chemotherapy, or combinations of these. Much will depend on the stage the cancer has reached, the condition and wishes of the patient, and the sensitivity/resistance of the tumour. Cancer cells, like other living organisms, develop resistance to toxic drugs which may result in treatment failure.

CELL BIOLOGY

In order to appreciate how cancer chemotherapy affects cellular function, it is necessary to have a basic understanding of cell biology. Present in the nucleus of every cell is deoxyribonucleic acid (DNA) which provides the blueprint or template for the chromosomes which carry our genetic characteristics in the form of genes. Also in the nucleus is another acid, ribonucleic acid (RNA), which transmits genetic instructions from the nucleus to the cytoplasm. A cell is stimulated to reproduce in response to the death of another cell. It does this by means of the cell cycle.

Cell cycle

The cell cycle is a continuous process during which some cells are replicating while others are resting. The cycle comprises four discrete phases of activity resulting in the production of two identical daughter cells (Fig. 22.1).

G_1 = RNA synthesis occurs in preparation for DNA synthesis
S = DNA synthesis occurs in preparation for supplying two new cells
G_2 = RNA synthesis occurs in preparation for cell division
M = Cell mitosis occurs, i.e. production of two new cells
G_0 = Resting phase.

The synthesis (S) and mitosis (M) phases are the main points of activity. The G_1 and G_2 phases occupy the gaps between these phases and allow nutrients to be gathered in to supply energy for the immediately following S and M phases respectively.

Once the two new cells have been formed, one will mature and differentiate to become a specialised cell, while the other remains a stem cell which will go into a resting (only from replication) phase known as the

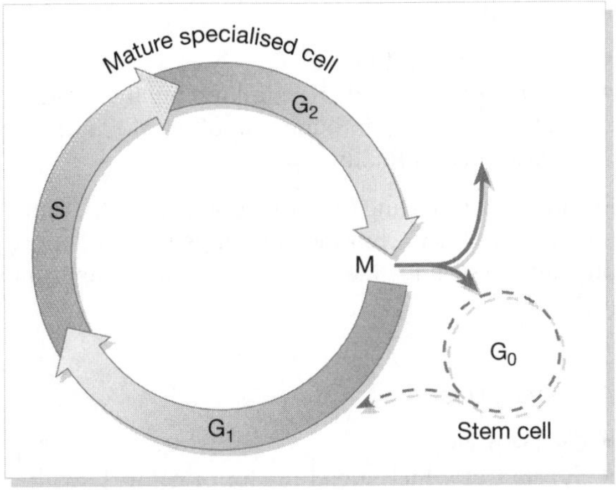

Figure 22.1 Cell life cycle.

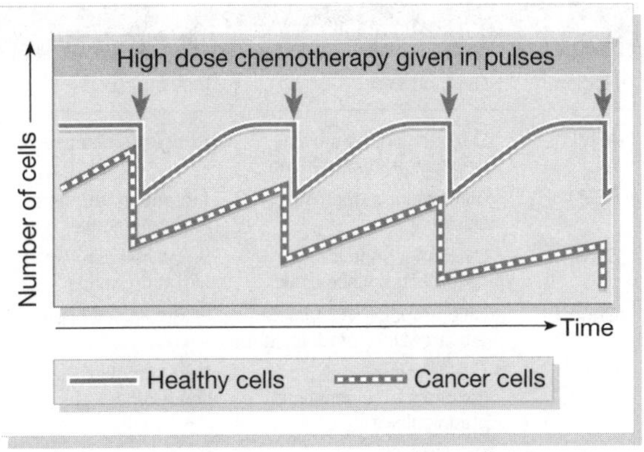

Figure 22.2 Effect of chemotherapy on normal and cancer cells.

G_0 phase. There it will remain until it is stimulated to undergo cell division.

Some cells therefore are 'cycling' and some are resting. Of those 'cycling', at any point in time the cells of any given tissue may be at any stage of the cycle. The time taken for the completion of the cycle varies, depending on the type of tissue. Although malignant cells replicate in exactly the same way as normal cells their cell cycle time is often shorter.

CHARACTERISTICS OF CANCER

Cancer is a problem of abnormal cell growth resulting from an interaction between the causal factor and DNA in a normal cell. The result is that normal control mechanisms are lost and the cancer cells reproduce uncontrollably, invading the surrounding tissues and eventually metastasising to sites distant from the primary tumour.

Malignant cells are therefore not new cells. They are an alteration of existing cells – a change which may have taken place as many as 15 years previously as the result of some insult or combination of effects on the body. The malignant cell behaves in a delinquent way, with no respect for the normal patterns of cell differentiation, growth and control. It is a parasite to the body and as such harms the host, which may ultimately lead to death.

CANCER CHEMOTHERAPY

Cancer chemotherapy is directed towards controlling abnormal cell growth and reducing the number of actively dividing cells. Cytotoxic drugs are used to kill cancer cells but they kill healthy cells as well. All cells, whether they are normal or malignant, are in different stages of the cell cycle at any time or they may be resting (G_0 phase). Chemotherapy drugs are described as being either phase-specific, i.e. they act more powerfully in one specific phase of the cycle, or cycle-specific, i.e. they work equally well killing cells in any or all phases of the cycle. Chemotherapy drugs will not kill cells in the G_0 phase. They are also more effective when the number of cancer cells is small. It is for this reason that chemotherapy is used as adjuvant therapy, i.e. following surgery and/or radiotherapy. High individual doses of chemotherapy will kill a high percentage of cancer cells. Although healthy cells will be destroyed, they will repair themselves quickly and regrow to normal numbers far more quickly than cancer cells following chemotherapy (Fig. 22.2). Intervals between doses are needed to allow normal cells to recover. Repeat doses at intervals are needed to kill those cells which were in the resting phase and therefore protected from chemotherapy. By combining different chemotherapy drugs, e.g. in some cases using four drugs together, remission rates in many situations are hugely increased. Cancer chemotherapy is therefore at its most effective when used:

- where the tumour is small, has been surgically removed or reduced in size with radiotherapy
- in high doses
- intermittently
- in appropriate combinations, often according to internationally agreed protocols (see Table 22.2).

Note: Initial letters of drug names are commonly used to represent the regimen, in some cases forming an acronym, e.g. BEAM. At times, the initial letter of the proprietary name of a drug is used, e.g. MOPP. In spite

Table 22.2 Cancer chemotherapy regimens*

Regimen	Components	Indications
ABVD	Doxorubicin, bleomycin, vinblastine, dacarbazine	Hodgkin's disease
BEP	Bleomycin, etoposide, cisplatin	Advanced teratoma and seminoma
CAV	Cyclophosphamide, doxorubicin, vincristine	Small cell carcinoma of the bronchus
ChlVPP	Chlorambucil, vinblastine, procarbazine, prednisolone	Hodgkin's disease
CHOP	Cyclophosphamide, doxorubicin, vincristine, prednisolone	Non-Hodgkin's lymphoma
CMF	Cyclophosphamide, methotrexate, fluorouracil	Breast cancer
CVP	Cyclophosphamide, vincristine, prednisolone	Non-Hodgkin's lymphoma
MACOP-B	Methotrexate, doxorubicin, cyclophosphamide, vincristine, bleomycin, prednisolone	Non-Hodgkin's lymphoma
MOPP	Chlormethine (mustine), vincristine, procarbazine, prednisolone	Hodgkin's disease

* Consult specialist literature for details of dosage/route of administration, etc. Many other regimens are quoted in the literature.

of changes in names given to drugs, the 'old' acronym still gets used, e.g. CHOP.

The timing of each pulse of treatment is critical to achieving success in eradicating the malignant cells. However, it must always be borne in mind that the patient's normal cells, especially the rapidly dividing ones, are also being damaged. To ensure that the patient can withstand the treatment, regular haematological monitoring is essential. The tissues that are most chemosensitive are the:

- bone marrow
- epithelial lining of the gastrointestinal tract
- skin and hair
- ovaries and testes.

CYTOTOXIC DRUGS

The most commonly used cytotoxic drugs are detailed in Table 22.3.

Cytotoxic drug groups

Cytotoxic drugs fall into four main categories: (1) alkylating drugs; (ii) antimetabolites; (iii) cytotoxic antibiotics; and (iv) vinca alkaloids.

Alkylating drugs

- Phase-specific (M phase)
- Cause breaks in, and cross-linking on, the strands of DNA, resulting in inhibition of or inaccurate replication and finally cell death.

Examples of alkylating drugs include busulfan, carmustine, chlorambucil, chlormethine (mustine), cyclophosphamide, estramustine, ifosfamide, lomustine and melphalan.

Antimetabolites

- Cycle-specific
- Substances which substitute for or compete with intracellular metabolites and become incorporated into the nucleic acids, DNA and RNA, preventing DNA synthesis and leading to cell death.

Examples of antimetabolites include cytarabine, fluorouracil, mercaptopurine, methotrexate and tioguanine.

Cytotoxic antibiotics

- Phase-specific (S phase)
- Act by binding to the DNA helix, inhibiting its synthesis and replication, and disrupting RNA synthesis.

Examples of cytotoxic antibiotics include aclarubicin, bleomycin, dactinomycin, doxorubicin, epirubicin, idarubicin and mitomycin.

Vinca alkaloids

- Phase-specific (M phase)
- Bind to the microtubular proteins which are needed for formation of the mitotic spindle. Because the cell is unable to divide, it dies.

Examples of vinca alkaloids include vinblastine, vincristine, vindesine and vinorelbine.

Calcium leucovorin rescue for patients receiving methotrexate

Calcium leucovorin is chemically related to the essential coenzyme for nucleic acid synthesis. It is used to diminish the toxicity of folic acid antagonists such as methotrexate. The dose of calcium leucovorin will depend on the dose of methotrexate previously administered. As an example, 150 mg would be given in divided doses over 12–24 hours by intramuscular

Table 22.3 Cytotoxic drugs in common use (throughout these tables the abbreviation μg will be used for microgram; this is to save space and is not an endorsement of the use of 'μg' in prescription writing)

Drug name(s)	Classification and mode of action	Main indications	Dose/route/side-effects/precautions
Aclarubicin	Cytotoxic antibiotic. Preferentially inhibits RNA synthesis	Acute non-lymphocytic leukaemia in patients resistant to first-line chemotherapy	175–300 mg/m^2 body surface area over 3–7 days IV via freely flowing peripheral line or central venous line. Side-effects: nausea and vomiting, bone marrow depression. Irritant to tissues. Monitor cardiac function; avoid extravasation
Bleomycin	Cytotoxic antibiotic. Inhibits cell growth and DNA synthesis in tumour cells	Squamous-cell carcinoma of mouth, nasopharynx, larynx, oesophagus, external genitalia or skin	Wide dosage range depending on condition being treated. IV or instillation into cavity. Total dose of 500 units should not be exceeded. Younger men with testicular teratoma may tolerate higher doses. Side-effects: fever, anorexia, nausea, local pain; interstitial pneumonia which may lead to a fatal pulmonary fibrosis (this condition is dose-related and rarely occurs on normal doses); local lesions, skin and mucosa. Chest X-rays carried out weekly. Not to be used in pregnant or breast-feeding women
Busulfan	Alkylating drug. Binds to DNA. Selective action on granulocytopoiesis	Palliative treatment of chronic myeloid leukaemia	60 μg/kg/day, initial maximum dose of 4 mg as a single daily dose, given orally. Treatment continued until leucocyte count has fallen to an acceptable level. Maintenance therapy 0.5–2 mg per day may be instituted following a break in treatment. Side-effects: bone marrow depression, especially thrombocytopenia; interstitial pulmonary fibrosis; skin hyperpigmentation; hepatotoxicity has been seen when used in combination with tioguanine; many other effects/toxicity reactions have been reported; myelosuppression/risk of irreversible bone marrow aplasia. Careful monitoring of blood counts essential. Avoid during pregnancy, especially in the first 3 months owing to possible teratogenic effects
Carboplatin	Platinum-containing compound. Antineoplastic drug with alkylating action	Ovarian cancer (in combination with paclitaxel). Lung cancer (small cell type). This drug is better tolerated than cisplatin	Dose determined according to renal function. Given IV. Toxic side-effects (nephrotoxicity, neurotoxicity, ototoxicity) less of a problem than with cisplatin. Nausea and vomiting less than with cisplatin. Myelosuppression greater than with cisplatin. Aminoglycoside antibiotics increase risk of nephrotoxicity (see BNF)
Carmustine	Alkylating drug	Myeloma, lymphoma, brain tumours	200 mg/m^2 IV every 6 weeks as a single dose or divided into two doses of 100 mg/m^2 on 2 successive days. If given in combination therapy, dosage adjusted. Side-effects: myelosuppression – which may be delayed (this is dose-related), nausea and vomiting; delayed pulmonary fibrosis; renal damage. Gametogenesis is adversely affected. Haematological monitoring essential
Chlorambucil	Alkylating drug	Hodgkin's disease, non-Hodgkin's lymphoma, chronic lymphocytic leukaemia, ovarian cancer	Dosage will depend on condition being treated, e.g. Hodgkin's disease 100–200 μg/kg/day orally for 4–8 weeks. Side-effects: bone marrow suppression; GI disturbances; nausea and vomiting, oral ulceration; hepatotoxicity and jaundice; lung damage has been reported. Haematological monitoring essential. Should not be given to patients who have recently undergone radiotherapy. Dose reduced in presence of hepatic dysfunction
Chlormethine (mustine)	Alkylating drug	Hodgkin's disease	Single dose of 0.4 mg/kg body weight or a course of four daily doses of 0.1 mg/kg IV. Side-effects: very toxic; nausea and vomiting; bone marrow depression – severe; peptic ulcers; thrombophlebitis and venous thrombosis. Often used in combination therapy. Blood counts are essential prior to each treatment. Chlormethine (mustine) is a very irritant drug and must be handled with great care. On no account should it be administered intramuscularly

(*continued*)

Table 22.3 *(continued)*

Drug name(s)	Classification and mode of action	Main indications	Dose/route/side-effects/precautions
Cisplatin	As carboplatin	Metastatic germ cell cancers (seminoma and teratoma), bladder, lung and upper GIT cancers	See specialist literature for dose. Given IV. Cisplatin therapy requires IV hydration. Nausea and vomiting may be severe. Nephrotoxicity is a major problem; renal function must be monitored
Cyclophosphamide	Alkylating drug. Inert until activated in the body by microsomal enzymes in the liver	Chronic lymphocytic leukaemia, lymphomas, soft-tissue and solid tumours	Often used in combination with other drugs. Dose used will depend on condition being treated. Conventional dosage levels are 100–300 mg daily as a single IV or oral dose OR 500 mg–1 g as a singe IV dose weekly. Higher-dose regimens are 30–40 mg/kg as a single IV dose given at intervals of 10–20 days. Side-effects: produces toxic metabolites which can cause haemorrhagic cystitis. Concurrent use of mesna reduces local toxicity. Maintain high fluid intake. As with all cytotoxic drugs, special care must be taken in patients with coexisting disease. Monitoring of haematological and biochemical parameters essential
Cytarabine	Antimetabolite. Inhibits pyrimidine synthesis	Acute myeloblastic leukaemia, acute non-lymphoblastic leukaemia, acute lymphoblastic leukaemia	Dosage according to body surface area. May be used in combination with other drugs. Acute leukaemia: 100–200 mg/m^2 per day or 3–6 mg/kg per day. Duration of therapy depends on clinical findings and bone marrow results. Remission maintenance therapy: 75–100 mg/m^2 per day for 5 consecutive days once a month. Used intrathecally in CNS leukaemias. Side-effects: mild nausea and vomiting; granulocytopenia; infection; haemorrhage due to thrombocytopenia; skin rashes; diarrhoea; gritty eyes; mouth sores. Avoid in pregnancy and lactation. Regular haematological monitoring essential. Renal and liver function monitored. CNS toxicity occurs with high-dosage regimens
Dacarbazine	Exact mechanism of action not known. May have some alkylating action. Inhibits pyrimidine synthesis	Malignant melanoma, soft-tissue sarcomas. Used in combination therapy in Hodgkin's disease (ABVD)	Various dosage schedules recommended, e.g. 2–4.5 mg/kg for 10 days repeated at 4-week intervals IV. Side-effects: anorexia, nausea and vomiting; haemopoietic depression; influenza-like symptoms; alopecia; hepatotoxicity; irritant to tissues. Avoid extravasation. Full haematological monitoring. Nausea and vomiting may be intense but can be reduced by restricting intake of food and drink 4–6 hours prior to therapy
Dactinomycin	Cytotoxic antibiotic. Inhibits cell proliferation by combining with DNA and interfering with RNA synthesis	Paediatric cancer, e.g. Wilms' tumour, rhabdomyosarcoma, carcinoma of testis and uterus on sequential basis with methotrexate	This is a very toxic drug. Dosage should not exceed 15 μg/kg or 400–600 μg/m^2 body surface area. IV for maximum of 5 days. Dosage for children: 15 μg/kg per day IV. Adult dosage: 500 μg/day for 5 days IV. May be used in isolation–perfusion techniques. If seepage of drug into the general circulation can be prevented, higher doses can be given than in systemic therapy. Side-effects: irritant to tissues; nausea and vomiting; possible anaphylaxis; severe haemopoietic depression; oral lesions; anaemia; alopecia. Avoid extravasation. Administer via rubber tube of freely running infusion solution. As with other cytotoxic drugs, may cause established mild infection to become fatal
Docetaxel	Antineoplastic drug which acts by disrupting the microtubular network in cells, which disrupts mitotic and other cellular functions	Advanced metastatic breast cancer where there is resistance to other agents and/or relapse. Given in combination with doxorubicin	1 day prior to treatment commencing, oral dexamethasone (16 mg/day for 5 days) is given if not contraindicated. This reduces the incidence and severity of fluid retention and the risk of hypersensitivity reactions. In monotherapy 100 mg/m^2 is given as a 1-hour infusion every 3 weeks. Close observation of the patient is essential to check for hypersensitivity reactions. Dosage adjustments may be necessary if the neutrophil count falls (see specialist literature)
Doxorubicin	Cytotoxic antibiotic	Acute leukaemias, lymphomas, soft-tissue and osteogenic sarcoma, breast and lung cancer	30–40 mg/m^2 when given in combination therapy. 60–75 mg/m^2 every 3 weeks when used alone. Intravenously via freely running IV infusion. On the basis of body weight, 1.2–2.4 mg/kg as a single dose every 3 weeks. A balance has to be achieved between dosage intervals and resulting toxicity. Dosage must be

			reduced if the patient has had previous therapy with other cytotoxic drugs. Can be given by intra-arterial or intravesical routes. Side-effects: haematological damage; cardiotoxicity – congestive cardiac failure; alopecia; GIT symptoms, nausea and vomiting; causes red colour in urine. Account must be taken of treatment with other cardiotoxic agents. ECG monitoring before and after treatment required. A formulation of doxorubicin inside liposomes provides a delivery system that is claimed to evade detection by the immune system
Epirubicin	Cytotoxic antibiotic	Breast, ovarian, gastric and colorectal cancer, lymphomas, leukaemia and multiple myeloma	75–90 mg/m^2 repeated at 21-day intervals IV. Can also be given by intravesical administration in the treatment of bladder cancer. The side-effect profile and precautions are similar to those of doxorubicin
Estramustine	Alkylating drug. As a combination of estradiol and normustine has oestrogenic action also	Cases of prostatic cancer unresponsive to other therapy	0.14–1.4 g daily in divided doses orally, with meals (avoid milk and milk products). Side-effects: GI problems; gynaecomastia; thromboembolic disorders; bone marrow depression. Use with caution in patients with concurrent disease, e.g. diabetes, hypertension. Haematological monitoring needed
Etoposide	Mitotic inhibitor. Classed along with vinca alkaloids	Small cell lung cancer, resistant non-seminomatous testicular carcinoma and the lymphomas	60–120 mg/m^2 IV daily for 5 consecutive days repeated at not more than 21-day intervals. Twice the IV dose is given orally. Side-effects: myelosuppression; irritant to tissues; alopecia; nausea and vomiting; hypotension due to rapid infusion rate. Avoid extravasation. Haematological monitoring. Liver function monitoring. Affects fertility – contraception advised
Fluorouracil	Antimetabolite. Inhibits cell division by interfering with DNA and RNA synthesis	Colon and breast cancer, malignant skin lesions	IV infusion or injection. By infusion 15 mg/kg at a slow rate over 4 hours (not more than 1 g in 500 mL of fluid) or infuse over 30–60 minutes. Continuous infusion over 24 hours may be preferred. Dose is repeated on successive days to a total of 12–15 g. Toxicity may cause treatment to be discontinued before the full 'course' is given. The dividing line between effective and toxic doses is very fine, so careful monitoring is essential. Side-effects: haematological damage; GI haemorrhage; stomatitis (diarrhoea, nausea and vomiting). Discontinue therapy when signs of toxicity appear (leucopenia and thrombocytopenia). Fluorouracil may be used locally as a 5% cream for superficial premalignant or malignant skin lesions. Applied once or twice daily with occlusive dressing to enhance effect. Avoid contact with mucous membranes or the eyes. Capsules available for oral administration
Hydroxycarbamide (hydroxyurea)	Antineoplastic drug. Acts by interfering with DNA synthesis	Chronic myeloid leukaemia. In combination with radiotherapy in the treatment of cancer of the cervix	20–30 mg/kg daily in single doses orally. Side-effects: anorexia, GI symptoms; myelosuppression; anaemia; alopecia; skin rashes. Monitor renal and liver function. Blood parameters monitored before, during and after treatment. Correct severe anaemia with blood transfusions
Idarubicin	Cytotoxic antibiotic	Acute non-lymphocytic leukaemia (ANLL) and acute lymphocytic leukaemia (ALL). May be used in combination therapy. Also used in advanced breast cancer when first-line therapy has failed	Dosage in ANLL 12 mg/m^2 IV daily for 3 days with cytarabine. Dosage in ALL as a single agent 12 mg/m^2 IV daily for 3 days. Children 10 mg/m^2 IV daily for 3 days. Side-effects: myelosuppression (leucocytes); cardiotoxicity, potentially fatal congestive heart failure; tissue irritancy; causes red coloration of urine. Cardiac function should be monitored. Renal and hepatic function should be monitored. Avoid extravasation. Available as a capsule for oral administration where IV therapy is not practicable
Ifosfamide	Alkylating drug (similar to cyclophosphamide, activated in the liver by microsomal enzymes)	Tumours of lung, ovary, cervix, breast, testis and soft-tissue carcinoma, carcinoma of pancreas, and head and neck tumours	Used in combination therapy and with radiotherapy. Dosage varies according to condition and treatment regimen. Total dose for a course is 8–10 g/m^2 as equal daily doses over 5 days. Courses are repeated at intervals of 2–4 weeks. Side-effects and precautions similar to those of cyclophosphamide. Given with mesna to protect against urethral toxicity. As with many cytotoxic agents, particular attention should be given to mouth care

(*continued*)

Table 22.3 *(continued)*

Drug name(s)	Classification and mode of action	Main indications	Dose/route/side-effects/precautions
Imatinib (Glivec)	Signal transduction inhibitor	NICE advice for treatment of advanced chronic myeloid leukaemia only	Consult specialist literature
Lomustine	Alkylating drug with enzyme-inhibiting properties	Hodgkin's disease, brain tumours, lung tumours, malignant melanoma	Used in combination therapy and with radiotherapy. 120–130 mg/m^2 as a single dose every 6–8 weeks. Side-effects: marrow depression – delayed; nausea and vomiting; loss of scalp hair (infrequent)
Melphalan	Alkylating drug. Prevents cell replication by cross-linking with DNA strands	Myeloma, ovarian adenocarcinoma, in combination therapy to treat breast cancer. Localised treatment of malignant melanoma	Considerable variation in dosage regimens, e.g. in myeloma 150 μg/kg body weight daily orally in divided doses for 4 days repeated at intervals of 6 weeks. Regional perfusion has been used in malignant melanoma. The drug is unstable in infusion fluids. It is preferable to inject slowly via the injection port of a freely running infusion system. Side-effects: bone marrow depression; nausea and vomiting especially with high-dose IV therapy; skin rashes; diarrhoea. Haematological monitoring essential. Avoid in pregnancy and breast-feeding mothers
		Polycythaemia rubra vera	To induce remission 6–10 mg daily for 5–7 days, reducing to 2–4 mg daily to achieve control of the disease
Mercaptopurine	Antimetabolite. Acts by interfering with synthesis of nucleic acid in proliferating cells	Acute lymphoblastic leukaemia and acute myelogenous leukaemia	Adults and children are given 2.5 mg/kg body weight orally. Dosage period of administration will depend on the condition being treated and if given with other drugs. Side-effects: myelosuppression – leucopenia and thrombocytopenia; hepatotoxicity; hyperuricaemia due to cell lysis. Careful blood monitoring essential. Supportive action needed for patient who may develop a relative bone marrow aplasia. Liver function monitoring
Methotrexate	Antimetabolite. Acts during 'S' phase of cell division. Inhibits certain enzyme functions which, in turn, interfere with DNA production. It is a folic acid antagonist	A wide range of conditions: leukaemia, lymphoma, breast cancer, osteogenic sarcoma, lung cancer, head and neck cancer, bladder cancer (has also been used in uncontrolled psoriasis)	Can be administered by all main routes including intrathecal. This is a very important drug in the treatment of many malignant diseases. As a result, a wide range of dosage regimens and routes of administration are employed. (Specialist literature should be consulted for details.) Side-effects: nausea/abdominal distress; stomatitis; leucopenia; anaphylactic reactions (rare); rashes, photosensitivity; bone marrow depression; mucositis; hepatic toxicity; genitourinary toxicity; CNS symptoms – blurred vision; adverse effects of intrathecal administration are complex and may include headache, fever, paraplegia (transient), nerve palsies, convulsions and dementia. Use with great caution in patients with haematological impairment, inflammatory bowel disease and peptic ulcer. Possible dangers from drug interactions, e.g. with NSAIDs (see p. 141), Full laboratory monitoring of patients receiving methotrexate therapy is essential. (*See also Calcium leucovorin rescue for patients receiving methotrexate*, p. 338)
Mitomycin	Cytotoxic antibiotic. In the tissues the drug has an alkylating action, forming a complex with DNA in cancer cells	Breast, stomach, pancreatic, colonic, bladder, rectal and skin cancer	60–150 μg/kg at intervals of 1–6 weeks depending on any drug combination used and bone marrow condition. Also used as an instillation in bladder cancer. Side-effects: myelosuppression; nausea and vomiting; local ulceration due to extravasation; renal toxicity and lung fibrosis. Haematological monitoring. Avoid skin and eye contact. Avoid in pregnancy and breast-feeding
Mitoxantrone	Cytotoxic antibiotic	Advanced breast cancer, non-Hodgkin's lymphoma and adult non-lymphocytic leukaemia. May be useful in liver cancer that cannot be resected	Dosage – consult specialist literature. Reduced dosage in combination therapy. The drug is very irritant and must be handled with care. Careful technique is essential when diluting the drug for IV infusion

Oxaliplatin	As carboplatin	Metastatic colorectal cancer in combination with fluorouracil and folinic acid	See specialist literature for doses (combination therapy). Given IV. Neurotoxic side-effects are dose-limiting. GIT disturbances and ototoxicity may cause problems
Paclitaxel	Similar to docetaxel	Primary ovarian cancer, advanced or where there is residual disease following surgery. Given in combination with cisplatin. Also used in metastatic breast cancer and non-small cell lung cancer where standard therapy has failed	As with docetaxel, premedication is required with a corticosteroid, an antihistamine and an H_2 antagonist. (See specialist literature.) Great care is needed in monitoring this therapy as serious side-effects may arise. Bone marrow suppression, severe cardiac conduction abnormalities have been reported. Peripheral neuropathy frequently occurs; if severe, the dose is reduced by 20%. The usual dose is given IV, 175 mg/m^2 over 3 hours, with a 3-week interval between courses. Dosage adjustments may be required in the light of the neutrophil count. The reconstituted solution is administered through an in-line filter, of pore size not greater than 0.22 μm. PVC bags must not be used because of the leaching of plasticiser. To prevent severe hypersensitivity reactions routine premedication with corticosteroid, an antihistamine and an H_2-receptor antagonist is required. Careful monitoring of this therapy is required because adverse reactions may occur despite premedication. See specialist literature for dosage regimens and precautions in use
Procarbazine	The mechanism of action is unknown	Hodgkin's disease in combination with chlormethine (mustine), prednisolone and vincristine	50 mg daily orally increasing by 50 mg daily to 250–300 mg daily in divided doses. Maintenance dose 50–150 mg daily. Side-effects: nausea, vomiting; myelosuppression; hypersensitivity; rashes; fever, chills; lethargy. As with all cytotoxic therapy, careful monitoring is required
Ralitrexed	Similar to docetaxel	Advanced colorectal cancer where fluorouracil and folinic acid regimens are inappropriate	Dose 3 mg/m^2 IV, repeated every 3 weeks, depending on tolerance. Careful haematological monitoring required as with similar agents. GI toxicity may be severe
Thalidomide	Currently under investigation	Refractory multiple myeloma, renal cell carcinoma, prostate cancer and Kaposi's sarcoma	200 mg orally at bedtime in refractory multiple myeloma, increasing to 400 mg after 14 days. Given in combination with dexamethasone. Side-effects include morning somnolence and tremor. Consult specialist literature
Tioguanine	Antimetabolite, acts by inhibition of purine synthesis	Acute leukaemia, especially acute myelogenous leukaemia and acute lymphoblastic leukaemia. Also chronic granulocytic leukaemia, usually in combination therapy	Dose dependent on combination treatment regimen used. Adults for induction 100–200 mg/m^2 per day as a single or twice-daily regimen over 5–20 days. Similar doses for children with reduction for smaller surface area of child. Side-effects: GI symptoms; stomatitis; hepatotoxicity; bone marrow suppression. Careful monitoring essential
Thiotepa	Alkylating drug	Malignant effusions and bladder cancer. Has been used to treat breast cancer	Dosage levels depend on the white cell count. Parenteral routes used. Mainly used as an instillation into the bladder. Side-effects: myelosuppression; vomiting; headache. Careful blood monitoring is essential; if the white blood cell count falls below 3000 cells/mm^3, the drug is not given
Treosulfan	Alkylating drug	Ovarian cancer. May be used in other neoplasms refractory to conventional therapy	Dosage schedules follow a number of regimens. (See specialist literature for details.) Oral and IV administration is used. Side-effects: bone marrow depression; GI upsets; nausea, vomiting and abdominal pain; alopecia; stomatitis (if capsules chewed). Regular blood counts essential. Avoid extravasation. Since treosulfan is excreted renally dosage should be reduced in older patients
Vinblastine	Vinca alkaloid	Hodgkin's disease, non-Hodgkin's lymphoma. Breast, renal cell and testicular cancer	Adult dose 6 mg/m^2 at weekly intervals. Higher doses may be given in testicular cancer. Only the IV route is used. As with vincristine, inadvertent intrathecal use results in fatality. Side-effects: gastrointestinal; haematological damage; nausea and vomiting; neurological, e.g. paraesthesia; cardiovascular, e.g. myocardial infarction. Avoid eye contamination. Granulocyte counts essential

(*continued*)

Table 22.3 *(continued)*

Drug name(s)	Classification and mode of action	Main indications	Dose/route/side-effects/precautions
Vincristine	Vinca alkaloid	Acute lymphocytic leukaemia, acute myelogenous leukaemia, malignant lymphomas, myeloma, breast cancer and certain paediatric tumours, e.g. Wilms' disease	This is a very potent drug. As with all cytotoxic drugs great care in calculating dosage levels. Accuracy must be ensured in administration. 1.4–1.5 mg/m^2 up to a maximum weekly dose of 2 mg. In children 2 mg/m^2 is the usual dose. Lower doses are used for children weighing less than 10 kg. Under no circumstances must this drug be given intrathecally; deaths have resulted from inadvertent intrathecal use. Side-effects: irritant to tissues; alopecia; neuromuscular reactions; neuritic pain, sensory loss, paraesthesia, difficulty in walking; granulocytopenia; bronchospasm. Avoid eye contamination. The appearance of neuromuscular adverse effects must be carefully watched for and doses reduced if side-effects occur. Careful monitoring of key physiological parameters is required
Vindesine	Vinca alkaloid	Acute lymphoblastic leukaemia in children, advanced carcinoma of the breast	3 mg/m^2 for adults by IV bolus. In children 4 mg/m^2. Subsequently dose based on granulocyte count. If there is no granulocytopenia the dose can be carefully increased. Inadvertent intrathecal injection can be fatal. Side-effects: bronchospasm; nausea, vomiting and other GI effects; paralytic ileus; neurological symptoms; granulocytopenia; alopecia. Daily blood counts. Side-effects can be reduced by appropriate treatment, e.g. reduction of fluid intake, cathartics to avoid ileus, administration of an anticonvulsant, since vindesine lowers blood levels of anticonvulsants. Cardiovascular monitoring is required, especially blood pressure determination
Vinorelbine	Vinca alkaloid	Non-small cell lung cancer and advanced breast cancer	By IV injection only – 25–30 mg/m^2 weekly. Side-effects similar to those of other vinca alkaloids. Can be given by slow bolus injection or short infusion when diluted appropriately

injection, intravenous bolus or intravenous infusion. Following the initial doses, 12–15 mg intramuscularly or 15 mg is given orally every 6 hours for the next 48 hours. Steps should be taken to increase the rate of excretion of the methotrexate, e.g. by alkalinisation of the urine and maintaining the urinary output at a high level. In advanced colorectal cancer combination therapy of calcium leucovorin and fluorouracil is used. Calcium leucovorin at a dose of 200 mg/m^2 is given by *slow* intravenous injection followed at once by fluorouracil 370 mg/m^2 by intravenous injection. The treatment is repeated for 5 consecutive days. Further courses can be given after 21–28 days. Each treatment course must be carefully monitored and any necessary dosage adjustments made.

Other drugs used in the treatment of malignant diseases

Malignant disease is treated by a range of drugs in addition to the cytotoxic drugs previously described. Table 22.4 lists the range together with a brief description of the mode of action, dosage levels and clinical indications, side-effects and precautions in use. Table 22.2 outlines some combination regimens, designed to overcome resistance to therapy with a single agent.

KEY ELEMENTS OF THE TREATMENT OF MALIGNANT DISEASE WITH CYTOTOXIC DRUGS

The treatment of malignant disease with cytotoxic drugs presents many challenges for clinicians, nurses and pharmacists. In order to achieve the best outcome for the patient, and to protect the staff involved, it is vitally important that all those involved in providing anticancer treatment work together within the following framework.

- The importance of discussing the full implications of the treatment with the patient and/or the patient's relatives cannot be overstated.
- Only clinicians having specialised experience and access to full back-up services should initiate and control cytotoxic therapy.
- Where treatment is provided on a shared-care basis with the patient's GP, communications and flow of information must be well managed and clearly understood by all involved.
- All personnel involved in providing the drug therapy must observe the regulations designed to prevent chronic exposure to cytotoxic drugs. These regulations are intended to minimise the risk to handlers of cytotoxic drugs from the known hazards, e.g. teratogenicity. Guidance on the safe handling of cytotoxic drugs is given on page 351.
- Particular attention must be paid to all aspects of drug management such as drug selection, dosage determination, calculation, prescribing, presentation of the drug, route of administration and timing of the administration of individual doses within a course of therapy.
- Every effort must be made to reduce the impact on the patient of foreseeable adverse effects of the therapy. It will often be important to provide advice and support to relatives and carers.
- Without causing unnecessary alarm among staff or patients, a respect for cytotoxic drugs should be engendered in much the same way as is required for radioactive materials. Provided that staff make themselves fully conversant with the guidelines laid down on the safe handling of these drugs and are seen to incorporate the practical measures into their day-to-day work, protection for the user, the patient and all other personnel working near treatment areas should be guaranteed.

DRUG MANAGEMENT IN CYTOTOXIC DRUG THERAPY

The general principles of drug management are discussed in detail in Chapter 7. However, in view of the special importance of drug management in cytotoxic drug therapy the following additional guidance is offered. All the factors listed are not of equal importance but nevertheless must be given full consideration in patients' particular circumstances. Factors in drug selection include:

- condition being treated, stages of disease and prognosis
- regimen to be followed – single or combination therapy (see Table 22.2)
- cost-benefits of the therapy (the escalating costs of newer forms of therapy is of major concern)
- back-up resources available locally
- general condition of the patient – any previous exposure to cytotoxic drugs and/or radiotherapy
- current 'state of the art', consider advice from NICE and/or HTBS
- any coexisting condition that could affect treatment and/or cause complications for the patient
- reproductive status of the patient
- possibility of drug interactions.

Table 22.4 Other drugs used in malignant disease

Drug(s)	Mode of action	Dosage/clinical indications/side-effects/precautions
ANTIBACTERIAL AGENTS	See page 365	Immunosuppression associated with some types of malignant disease and certain cytotoxic drugs may result in the need for antibiotic cover
ASPIRIN	Apoptosis of bowel cancer in vitro	The benefits of the long-term use of aspirin in cardiovascular conditions are well established. Epidemiological evidence indicates that people who take aspirin (or other NSAIDs) have a reduced risk of developing colonic cancer. Further research is required
CORTICOSTEROIDS especially prednisolone	See page 304	Wide variations in dosage. Acute lymphoblastic leukaemia; Hodgkin's disease; non-Hodgkin's lymphoma; breast cancer. Palliation in terminal conditions
HORMONE ANTAGONISTS		
Aminoglutethimide	Acts by inhibiting certain enzymes involved in the conversion in the body of androgens into oestrogens	In advanced breast cancer a course of treatment commencing with 250 mg orally daily, increasing in weekly instalments to 1000 mg daily. The drug has a poorly understood action in advanced prostatic cancer. Usual dose: 750 mg daily. Since the drug interferes with hormone metabolism in the body it is necessary to administer corticosteroids concurrently. Side-effects are very variable but include CNS problems such as dizziness, somnolence and lethargy. Leucopenia, agranulocytosis and other blood dyscrasias may cause problems. Steroidal aromatase inhibitors are now the generally preferred drugs. They are better tolerated and do not need corticosteroid replacement therapy
Cyproterone	An anti-androgen which competes with testosterone at prostatic receptors	Given orally 100 mg three times daily in the treatment of prostatic carcinoma. Adverse effects include impotence and gynaecomastia. Hepatotoxicity is associated with long-term use. Short courses only
Formestane (other drugs with similar indications/actions are anastrozole, extramestane and lentrozole)	Has been shown to be as effective as aminoglutethimide for the treatment of breast cancer in postmenopausal women resistant to tamoxifen treatment. The side-effect profile is better than that of aminoglutethimide and drug–drug interactions are less likely. An aromatase inhibitor which blocks the conversion of androgens to oestrogens. In premenopausal women with functioning ovaries oestrogen levels are largely unaffected	By deep IM injection 250 mg every 2 weeks. Higher doses have been used on a trial basis. Local reaction at injection site; vary injection site. CNS disturbances and GI problems
Gonadorelin-like substances (see p. 297) buserelin, goserelin	Prostatic cancer cells require androgens for continued growth and development. Goserelin deprives the cancer cells of androgens by inhibition of pituitary LH secretion, which causes a fall in serum testosterone	Used in advanced prostatic cancer in the form of a biodegradable implant. A 4-weekly implant of 3.6 mg (depot) maintains the fall of testosterone levels to the castrate range. Patients at risk of developing ureteric obstruction or spinal cord compression. Should be monitored closely during the early stages of therapy. Side-effects include flushes, decrease in libido and a temporary increase in bone pain
Tamoxifen	Some patients suffering from breast cancer have tumours that have receptors which are oestrogen-positive. Such patients are likely to respond to treatment with an oestrogen receptor antagonist	Tamoxifen is a widely used oestrogen antagonist. The main indication for the use of this drug is in breast cancer both in post- and premenopausal women. The dose in breast cancer is 20 mg per day by mouth. Side-effects include hot flushes, vaginal bleeding, GI disturbances and skin rashes. Dosage reduction may relieve the side-effects

DRUGS USED TO TREAT NEUTROPENIA Filgrastim	Human granulocyte-colony stimulating factor (G-CSF). Haematopoietic growth factor for the mobilisation of peripheral blood progenitor cells (PBPC)	Regulates the production and release of functional neutrophils from the bone marrow. Used in conjunction with chemotherapy to reduce the incidence and severity of neutropenia and febrile neutropenia. Also used in myelo-ablative therapy. Dose will depend on the patient's condition. A typical dose is 5 μg/kg/day SC or IV. Course dependent on neutrophil count. Consult specialist literature
Lenograstim	Human granulocyte-colony stimulating factor (G-CSF). Stimulates production of neutrophils. Also used to mobilise stem cells prior to harvesting	May be given by IV infusion following bone marrow transplantation. Dose 19.2 million units/m^2 daily from day 1 to day 28 (max.) in accordance with neutrophil count. For cytotoxic-induced neutropenia, given SC in same dose. For other dosage regimens, consult specialist literature
DRUGS USED TO TREAT HYPERCALCAEMIA (see p. 304)	Hypercalcaemia is a common complication of some cancers. The cause of this condition is thought to relate to the ectopic production of a peptide which has a parathyroid hormone-like action. Another cause of hypercalcaemia may be local breakdown of bone (osteolysis)	
Octreotide	Acts by inhibiting the release of growth hormone and other hormones in the GIT. Because of its diverse effects it has been found useful in patients with severe secretory diarrhoea that can occur in VIPomas	Has been used to treat hypercalcaemia resistant to the bisphosphonates. Dosage levels vary but are of the order of 50 μg once or twice daily SC
INTERFERONS (alfa, beta and gamma). The alfa form of interferon is normally used in antitumour treatment regimens. Three forms of interferon alfa are available. All are complex proteins with slightly different structures, but very similar actions	The mode of action of interferon alfa is based on a direct antiproliferative effect on the life cycle of normal and malignant cells. The decrease in cell growth rate may be great enough to result in a cytotoxic effect. In addition, interferon alfa modulates the activity of the immune system	Dosage levels vary according to the condition being treated, e.g. hairy cell leukaemia: 3 megaunits (MU) IM or SC daily. Depending on response, maintenance doses may be given three times weekly. Interferons can be self-administered by SC injection. IV injection is reserved for high doses that may be required in the treatment of malignant melanoma. Conditions treated with interferon alfa include chronic myeloid leukaemia, hairy cell leukaemia, lymphomas and certain solid tumours (consult specialist literature for doses). Side-effects include influenza-like symptoms, fever, chills, etc., CNS effects including depression, confusion, dizziness, drowsiness, somnolence or even coma. Effects on blood pressure and CVS have been reported. Anorexia, nausea, diarrhoea and vomiting. Reduction in white blood cell count and platelet count may result in the need to suspend treatment to allow the counts to recover to pretreatment levels. Electrolyte disturbances may be associated with anorexia and dehydration. Skin reactions may occur at the site of injection and mild to moderate alopecia has been reported. As with other drugs used in the treatment of malignant disease, careful laboratory monitoring is needed during treatment, e.g. standard haematological tests, biochemical profile, urinalysis. Adequate hydration of the patient should be maintained
INTERLEUKIN-2		This drug (also known as aldesleukin) has been used in the treatment of metastatic renal cell carcinoma. It is a very toxic drug of doubtful value. (Consult specialist literature for further information)
SEX HORMONES	Treatment with sex hormones or hormone antagonists plays an important part in the treatment of cancer affecting breast, prostate and endometrium. Hormones produce a temporary benefit to patients by suppressing the growth of cells which is, to some extent, hormone dependent. Side-effects greatly limit their use	

(*continued*)

Table 22.4 *(continued)*

Drug(s)	Mode of action	Dosage/clinical indications/side-effects/precautions
Androgens	See page 307	Androgens have a limited place in the treatment of metastatic breast cancer. Testosterone compound in an oily vehicle may be administered by slow IM injection 250 mg every 2 or 3 weeks. If hypercalcaemia develops treatment must be discontinued. As with all hormone therapy used in the treatment of cancer, the development of secondary sexual characteristics may be troublesome
Oestrogens	See page 307	Oestrogens such as diethylstilbestrol have been used in the treatment of prostate cancer. Owing to an unacceptable level of side-effects, e.g. gynaecomastia, fluid retention and risk of thrombosis, treatment with diethylstilbestrol has largely been superseded. Other oestrogens that may be used in the treatment of prostatic cancer are fosfestrol and ethinylestradiol
Progestogens	See page 307	Progestogens are second- or third-line treatments of breast, renal and endometrial cancers. Megestrol is given orally in doses ranging from 160 mg/day to 320 mg/day. Side-effects include weight gain due to appetite stimulation, and nausea. Deep-vein thrombosis and alopecia have been reported. Myelosuppression is not a problem. Medroxyprogesterone acetate is given orally or by deep IM injection. The dose is 0.4–1.5 g daily by mouth or 250 mg–1 g by injection. Side-effects include insomnia, fatigue, depression and headache. Skin reactions, nausea and indigestion occur at higher doses. Diabetic patients should be carefully observed because glucose tolerance is decreased
THALIDOMIDE	Is being evaluated in a number of conditions including myeloma. The action of the drug is not well understood but an immunomodulatory effect may be involved	

Dose determination

Many factors are involved in dosage determination, and it is the responsibility of the clinician to take all factors into account in arriving at the actual dosage and frequency of administration. All the above factors will be considered along with the following:

- patient's age, sex, body weight and other physical parameters, e.g. body surface area
- nutritional status
- full haematological profile
- renal and hepatic function
- neurological status
- pharmacokinetics of the drug.

Doses are determined according to generally well-defined regimens, being modified according to the factors outlined above. The main approaches are based on two parameters, i.e. body weight and surface area.

Dosage determination based on body weight

Many examples are given in the following pages. To take an example – melphalan – the dosage range in multiple myeloma is 150–300 micrograms per kg body weight daily, by mouth, for 4–6 days. The course is repeated after 4–8 weeks. Given that the patient has some degree of renal impairment, it may be decided to begin the course of therapy at the lower end of the dosage range. Blood counts will enable the effect of this dose to be monitored.

For a patient of body weight 68 kg the dose would be 150×68 micrograms per day for, say, 5 days: i.e. 10 200 micrograms, or $10\,200/1000\,\text{mg} \simeq 10\,\text{mg}$.

The number of 5 mg tablets to be administered each day is $10/5 = $ two tablets per day.

It is important to realise that the patient's 'true' body weight must be taken into account. In a patient suffering from fluid retention or obesity the actual weight on the scales should be treated with some caution since this is not generally a good indication of the patient's ability to metabolise the drug. Reference to standard height/weight tables may be required. The main factor to take into account is the patient's lean body mass.

Dosage determination based on body surface area (BSA)

This parameter is felt to be a more accurate indicator than body weight of the patient's ability to metabolise the drug. The patient's surface area is derived from tables. Given the patient's height (in cm) and body weight (in kg) the patient's body surface area can be determined from a nomogram (Fig. 22.3). Nomograms are available for both adults and children.

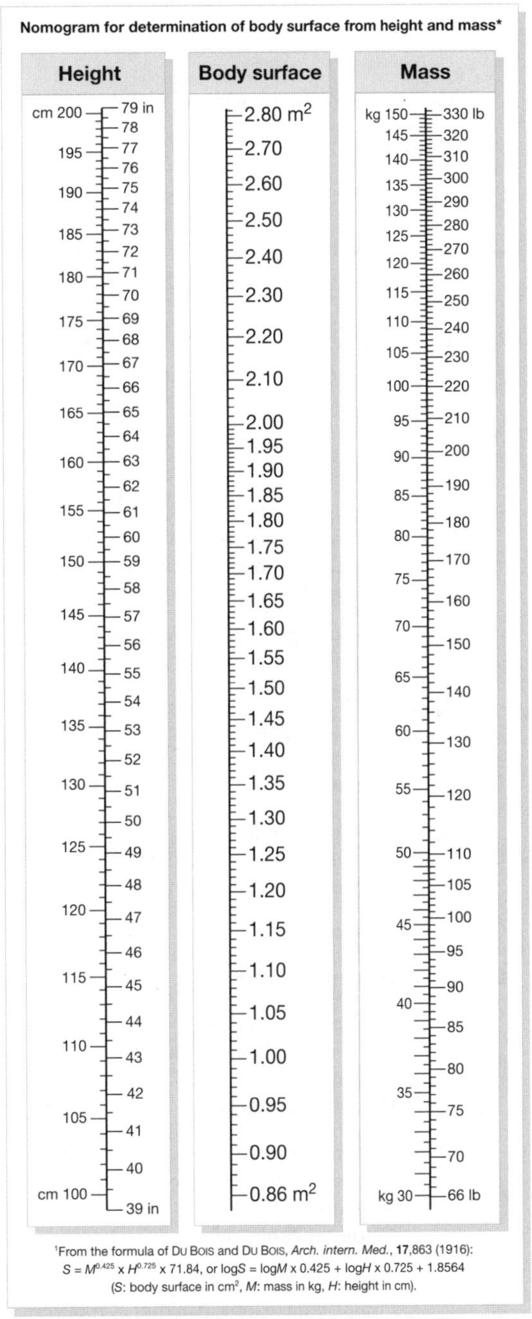

Figure 22.3 Nomogram (adult)*.

Prescribing

Prescribing cytotoxic drug therapy is more complex than the prescribing of more routine therapy. Great care must be taken to ensure that all personnel involved in the management of the patient have information that is

CHEMOTHERAPY PRESCRIPTION SHEET
REGIMEN: CISPLATIN single agent, 50mg/m^2

Cisplatin 50 mg/m^2 over 2 hours

PROTOCOL CHECKED BY: .... (Consultant) DATE:			
Cycle no.	Day number	Total no. of cycles	Interval between cycles
Weight	Height	Surface area	Max S.A.

Hb.	PLAT.	WCC.	NEUT.	UREA.	CREAT.	CrCl.

Note: 1. If urine output is less than 100 ml/hour, call Dr. to give IV Furosemide 10 mg.
2. IV fluids may be stopped 3 hours after cisplatin if patient can maintain oral intake of 1–2 litres for 6 hours after IV fluids discontinue.
3. Discharge supply of antiemetics should be started at 6 pm on day of chemotherapy

IF AN INFUSION DEVICE IS BEING USED PLEASE ENTER PUMP ID/MP No. ....

	Day/ Date/ Time	Fluid / Additive medicine	Volume / Dose	Route of Admin.	Duration of Admin.	Prepared by pharmacy: Sig.	Prepared by pharmacy: Date	Code no. Serial no. Batch no.	Start time	Given by
A		**Furosemide**	20 mg	Oral	Stat					
B		Sodium chloride 0.9% Potassium chloride 20 mmol Magnesium sulphate 8 mmol	1000 ml	IV	2 hours					
C		**Ondansetron**	8 mg	IV	Slow bolus					
D		**Dexamethasone**	8 mg	IV	Slow bolus					
E		Sodium chloride 0.9% Potassium chloride 10 mmol Mannitol 10 g **Cisplatin 25 mg/m^2**	450 ml	IV	1 hour					
F		Sodium chloride 0.9% Potassium chloride 10 mmol Mannitol 10 g **Cisplatin 25 mg/m^2**	450 ml	IV	1 hour					
G		Sodium chloride 0.9% Potassium chloride 20 mmol Magnesium sulphate 8 mmol	1000 ml	IV	2 hours					
H		Sodium chloride 0.9%	500 ml	IV	1 hour					

Doctors signature .... Date ....

Figure 22.4 Example of a pre-printed chemotherapy prescription sheet.

complete and accurate. Special prescription forms have been developed since it is not possible to provide all the necessary information on the standard form (Grampian Medicines Committee 2000).

A separate cytotoxic prescription should be used for ordering chemotherapy drugs from the pharmacy for each individual patient. Details of the patient's identity, diagnosis, height/weight/surface area, and blood count should be provided. The required regime, the names of the drugs included in the regime, the dose, route and method of administration, diluent and final volume should be entered and signed for by the prescribing doctor.

In clinical areas, chemotherapy regimens should be prescribed by consultants familiar with the use of cytotoxic medicines using a pre-printed prescription sheet (Fig. 22.4). A chemotherapy infusion administration record should be maintained throughout the infusion which reflects its ongoing progress in detail. Of particular importance are the infusion device number and which line is being used. The volume of fluid already infused and still to be infused should be checked after the first 15 minutes and hourly thereafter. The rate of the infusion and the expected time of completion should be recorded at each check.

Presentation

In view of the well-recognised hazards of manipulating cytotoxic drugs, their preparation for use should take place in a specially designated area within the pharmacy. This helps to ensure protection of staff, accuracy of compounding/reconstitution, and best presentation in a ready-to-use form, fully labelled with all the necessary details. Particular care is required in the labelling of the vinca alkaloid drugs, which must carry a warning that the drug is not for intrathecal use (see p. 79).

ROUTES OF ADMINISTRATION

Oral

Although cytotoxic drug therapy is very often given parenterally, there are nevertheless a number of effective oral cytotoxic preparations. These formulations are no less toxic in tablet or capsule form, and the same attention to care in their administration is required. In the interests of safety, tablets of cytotoxic medicines should be swallowed whole, and only in exceptional circumstances should they be crushed. Where nausea and vomiting are known side-effects an anti-emetic may need to be given in advance. Patients who are to take cytotoxic drugs while at home should be given clear written instructions in their use.

Subcutaneous and intramuscular

Because of the risk of damage to the tissues, only a few cytotoxic drugs are administered by these routes. Care should be taken to select an area with adequate subcutaneous/muscle tissue and to give the injection with a needle of the smallest possible calibre.

Intravenous

Absorption is more reliable by the intravenous route and, hence, it is the one most commonly used. Drugs with vesicant properties must always be given intravenously. The need for strict asepsis is paramount since chemotherapy patients will have some degree of immunosuppression.

A central venous catheter (e.g. Hickman catheter) may be used to provide long-term access to the patient's circulatory system, thus obviating the need for repeated venepuncture and injections, and avoiding damage to veins. It may be single, double or triple lumen. Either under general anaesthetic or under sedation and local anaesthetic, an incision is made just below the right clavicle and the cephalic vein isolated. A skin tunnel is then formed starting at a point between the nipple and the sternum. The catheter is drawn through the tunnel under X-ray control and inserted into the subclavian vein before reaching the cephalic vein and the superior vena cava where it is positioned at the entrance to the right atrium. Both veins are sutured. A Dacron cuff plugs the tunnel in the subcutaneous tissues which gradually become fibrosed, thus reducing the risk of ascending infection from the catheter exit point. A transparent dressing is applied and a cap placed on the protruding end. Patients and/or their families are taught to heparinise the line to keep it patent. This may be daily for the first 3 months and then twice weekly thereafter. A daily shower is encouraged. Patients should be encouraged to report any signs of discharge, pain or redness round the catheter or any movement of the catheter. The wound should be dressed and the cap renewed on a weekly basis. If the dressing becomes dislodged or there is evidence of infection, the dressing must be changed. A bacteriological swab should be taken if indicated.

SAFE HANDLING OF CYTOTOXIC DRUGS

The widespread use of cancer chemotherapeutic agents has led to an increased number of employees being exposed to potential contamination by them. The dangers which may be encountered fall into two categories. Certain cytotoxic drugs produce a local irritant effect, causing immediate damage to the skin and eyes. Others are, in addition, known to be mutagenic, carcinogenic and teratogenic agents. These long-term consequences resulting from absorption of substances via the skin, the lungs or the gastrointestinal tract warrant energetic implementation of policies by health authorities to reduce to the minimum, risks to their staff.

Personnel

Doctors, nurses and pharmacists involved in the handling of cytotoxic drugs should be instructed in the dangers, precautions, and techniques of administration. Training may be given by a suitably experienced senior member of medical, nursing or pharmacy staff and *only* those so trained should be responsible for the handling of these drugs. All personnel involved in the handling of cytotoxic drugs should be familiar with the written guidelines on the handling of cytotoxic drugs and be given a personal copy. A departmental register of those staff involved in such procedures should be maintained. In the event of an accident involving cytotoxic drugs, staff must report to their Head of Department. Such measures comply with the Code of Practice for COSHH Regulations. Staff, including those of childbearing potential, are not at risk when involved in the administration of cytotoxic drugs provided they adhere to the guidelines.

Reconstitution of cytotoxic drugs

The preparation of cytotoxic drugs should take place within the pharmacy department where a limited number of personnel working in this field are involved. A requisition for cytotoxic drugs in a ready-to-use form is made using a specialist prescription form for the purpose.

In exceptional circumstances, the reconstitution of injections may be necessary on the ward. This would only occur on the instruction of a senior member of specialist medical staff. Any manipulations involving cytotoxic drugs should be undertaken only in an area specifically designated by local policy for the purpose. The area must be one that is away from normal ward traffic and food areas. The windows and door should be kept closed but at the same time the room should be well ventilated. These areas should be equipped with a work top which has an impervious surface and intact edges. A sink and running water should be available in the room. A ready filled eye irrigation container should be available. Work should not be done at a position where draughts, mechanical ventilation or the air-conditioning system might convey aerosols or dusts to another occupied area. Drugs should be reconstituted using a safety pack supplied by the pharmacy department. A check on the calculation of the dose, concentration and volume of the drug(s) must be made by a doctor, pharmacist or registered nurse who has been suitably instructed in the subject. Drugs should be reconstituted on or over a plastic tray covered with absorbent material to contain any spillage and allow for ease of cleaning.

Protection against occupational exposure

Protection against exposure to cytotoxic drugs (or their metabolites) must be available for, and utilised by, all staff involved in the preparation of cytotoxic drugs. Protective clothing must be of the correct specification to ensure adequate protection of the skin and eyes, and to prevent inhalation of aerosolised drug particles. It should consist of:

- plastic apron; disposable
- gloves; these should be thick latex rubber, disposable except when preparing chlormethine (mustine) injections for which PVC gloves are required; they should provide a close fit with the sleeves; for long procedures, two pairs of gloves should be worn and should be changed every hour; gloves should be changed following spillage
- safety glasses; it is advisable to wear protective glasses or goggles complying with BS2092C which provide all-round protection, whether or not ordinary spectacles are worn; these should be washed thoroughly in soap and water after use
- face mask; a good-quality disposable surgical mask should be worn when reconstituting dry powder, especially if presented in an ampoule.

Every effort should be made to reduce aerosolisation. Ampoules, including those containing diluents, should be opened with care using a file if necessary and plastic ampoule breaker to avoid cuts and scratches. They should be held away from the face when being opened or drawn up from. Care should be taken when adding diluent to allow it to run slowly down the side of the ampoule. The exact volume of drug required should be drawn into a syringe and the remainder discarded or used immediately for another patient. Air from the syringe should be expelled into the empty ampoule over sterile cotton wool or a gauze swab. A new sheathed needle must be placed on the syringe before the final expulsion of air bubbles.

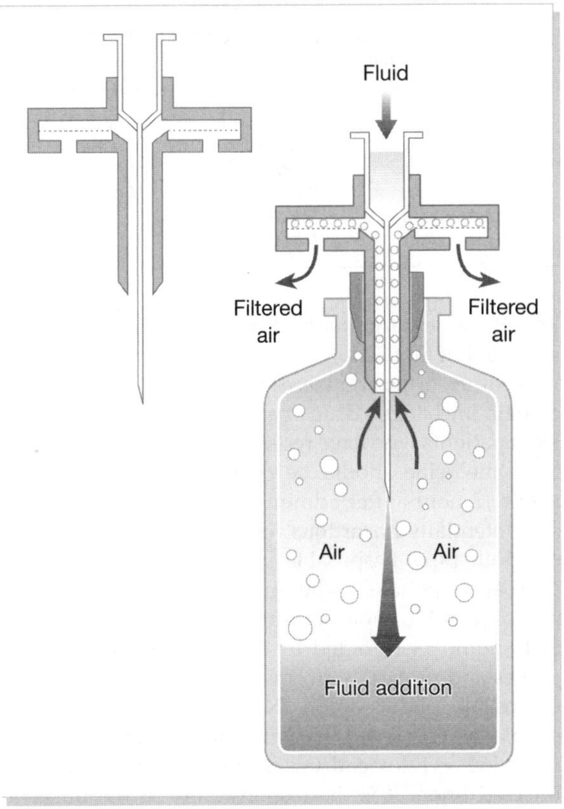

Figure 22.5 Special venting needle.

Drugs in powder form must be reconstituted with particular care as they may be released as a fine spray through the needle hole if excess pressure is produced in the vial. This may be avoided by removing an appropriate amount of air from the vial before injecting the diluting fluid or by the use of a special venting needle (Fig. 22.5).

Filled syringes should be suitably labelled and placed in a receiver ready for use. They should also carry a biohazard or cytotoxic drug warning label.

Disposal of surplus drugs and contaminated equipment

The use of disposable equipment is recommended whenever possible. Items of waste should be disposed of as follows:

- unused solution: seal ampoule or vial in a polythene bag and place bag in sharps container and send to pharmacy for destruction
- syringes, needles, empty ampoules, infusion sets: place in sharps container marked **cytotoxic material**
- masks, gloves, apron, foil trays, towels, swabs, infusion bags without administration set attached: seal in polythene bag and place in yellow incinerator bag.

All these items are incinerated at 1000°C.

Safety glasses should be washed thoroughly in soap and water, dried and hung up. The hands must be thoroughly washed on completion of any procedure involving cytotoxic drugs. Time-expired cytotoxic drugs should be returned to the pharmacy for disposal.

ADMINISTRATION OF CYTOTOXIC DRUGS

Very careful attention must be paid to the route of administration. While the use of an inappropriate route of administration is always hazardous, the consequences of using an incorrect route of administration for cytotoxic drugs can be catastrophic. Most notably, there have been tragic cases where a vinca alkaloid was given by the intrathecal route instead of intravenously. Most cytotoxic drugs are highly irritant to the tissues and, if extravasation occurs, local tissue damage and/or necrosis can occur. Most parenteral cytotoxic drugs are given intravenously either as a bolus into a freely running solution, or as an infusion. As with all parenteral administration the diluent used must be compatible with the drug and all expiry dates and storage instructions of reconstituted solutions observed. It is also important to ensure that the time taken to inject or infuse the drug is in accordance with the prescription. Intravenous infusions containing cytotoxic drugs should be controlled with the help of an infusion pump.

Parenteral administration

An assessment of the patient and a peripheral blood count are carried out prior to the administration of cytotoxic drugs to ensure that the patient is fit to withstand the treatment. Monitoring is also essential throughout the course of treatment. The patient's weight and height are measured in order to calculate the dose of drug(s) to be given. The calculation of the dose, volume and concentration should be checked and recorded.

Each syringe should be clearly labelled with the name and dose of the drug. The used vial or ampoule should be placed with the loaded syringe(s) in a receiver bearing the patient's name and/or prescription to allow a final check to be made.

Prior to administration of the drug, the prescription should be compared with the patient's name, the labelled syringes and the used ampoules/vials. When the person administering the drug is the one who prepared it, a check should be made by a second qualified person and recorded appropriately. For intramuscular and subcutaneous injections, two nurses must be involved, one of whom is registered, and the checking procedure followed in the standard way.

Particular care must be taken when assisting a doctor with the administration of drugs using the intrathecal route that the drug is intended for intrathecal use (see BNF).

In any event, it is particularly important to check that the correct patient is identified to receive the drug and that the correct route of administration is established. The prescription sheet must be signed by the person administering the chemotherapy.

Risks of contamination are still present during administration and therefore precautions should be continued. Gloves that provide protection for the donor from the cytotoxic drug must be worn.

The area round the injection site should be protected by an absorbent, disposable towel. A 'butterfly' needle is convenient when drugs which require a dilution intravenous infusion are being given. If there is any doubt about the siting of the needle, whether for infusion or direct bolus administration, the procedure should be abandoned and begun elsewhere.

Once an infusion of cytotoxic drugs has been established, responsibility rests with the nurse to observe the patient and provide continuing physical and emotional support. The point of entry of the needle into the vein should be observed frequently and any comments from the patient about the comfort of the area heeded. Leakage of the drug into the surrounding tissues, known as extravasation, may have disastrous consequences because of its irritant nature.

Any evidence of pain, burning or stinging at the injection site calls for an immediate assessment of the site. The doctor should be called at once and the infusion stopped. A ready-prepared pack for the first aid treatment of extravasation should be brought. The doctor will aspirate with the needle in place as much of the infiltrated drug as possible. Specialist advice should be sought to establish whether an antidote is available. Corticosteroids (to reduce inflammation), antihistamines and analgesics may require to be given. Cold compresses may also be ordered. Thereafter, frequent checking of the site will be required with careful documenting of progress until resolution occurs. Ideally, drugs liable to cause extravasation should be given through a central line, e.g. Hickman catheter. Cytotoxic drugs which are known to be particularly damaging on extravasation are listed in Box 22.2.

Box 22.2 Cytotoxic drugs which are particularly damaging on extravasation

Carmustine	Doxorubicin	Vinblastine
Chlormethine (mustine)	Epirubicin	Vincristine
Dacarbazine	Etoposide	Vindesine
Dactinomycin	Idarubicin	Vinorelbine
Daunorubicin	Melphalan	
	Mitomycin	

Vomitus, urine and faeces from treated patients may contain unchanged drug or active metabolites. Vomitus from patients who have received an oral dose of a cytotoxic medicine should be considered hazardous for up to 12 hours after administration; urine and faeces are potentially hazardous for up to 7 days following chemotherapy. Disposable utensils should always be used and care taken when placing them in the waste-disposal unit to avoid splashing the contents. Skin contact should be avoided by wearing disposable latex gloves and nurses' uniforms should be protected by a disposable plastic apron. Normal hygiene measures should be employed. Heavily soiled linen of patients receiving cytotoxic drugs should be dealt with as infected linen. It is the responsibility of the nurse in charge of the ward to advise all members of the nursing staff of those patients for whom these precautions must be taken.

Procedure in the event of an accident

Spillage of a cytotoxic drug onto intact skin

If any cytotoxic drug, apart from dacarbazine and melphalan, comes into contact with the skin, the affected area should be flushed with copious amounts of water.

If dacarbazine is spilled onto the skin, it should be washed off immediately with soap and water. In the case of melphalan, the contaminated skin should be treated with a *fresh* solution of sodium carbonate 3% w/v.

After skin contamination with methotrexate, if transient stinging occurs following washing with water, a bland cream, e.g. aqueous cream BP, should be applied to the affected area.

Spillage of a cytotoxic drug onto broken skin, into eyes or through needle penetration of the skin

If accidents involve cuts or needle penetration of the skin, the area should be washed with copious amounts of water.

If any cytotoxic drug enters the eye(s), the eye(s) should be irrigated thoroughly with sterile sodium chloride 0.9% solution.

In all such cases, the doctor and person in charge of the ward, department or clinic should be notified. The normal accident-reporting procedure should then be followed and a copy of the accident form sent to the Occupational Health Department.

Oral administration

Oral solid-dose forms of cytotoxic drugs constitute no risk to the handler if a few simple precautions are taken. If the patient has difficulty swallowing such preparations, advice should be sought from the pharmacy so that an alternative formulation can be provided. In general, tablets should neither be divided nor crushed, or capsules opened. All oral dosage forms should be dispensed and administered using a non-touch technique, if necessary wearing disposable gloves. If the outer coating of a tablet or capsule is intact there will generally be no hazard to the nurse. Disposable spoons and medicine measures should be used. A stainless steel triangle should be used when tablets require to be counted. It should be washed after use. In the event of contamination by free powder or the contents of a capsule, the same principles for dealing with spillage of parenteral drugs apply. To prevent inhalation of powder, it is essential to use a well-fitting face mask. For mopping up spilled powder, the disposable towel used should first be made damp. Disposal is by incineration.

MANAGEMENT OF SIDE-EFFECTS

The commonest adverse effects of cytotoxic drugs fall into four main categories:

- bone marrow suppression
- damage to the gastrointestinal mucosa
- damage to the skin and hair
- altered sexuality and fertility.

These effects reflect the areas of the body where normal cell turnover is greatest. *The severity of side-effects will depend on the drug(s) used and the dose given.*

Bone marrow suppression

Lowered resistance to infection

Immunity to infection is provided by the white blood cells. Because of their very rapid rate of turnover, the white blood cells are the ones most readily damaged by cytotoxic drugs. As treatment progresses and the white count falls, the patient's ability to combat infection lessens. Frequent monitoring of the white cell count assists the clinician in deciding whether the patient has sufficient white cells to withstand the next dose of treatment and still combat an infective attack. A white blood count of less than 5×10^9/litre significantly increases the risk of infection. Care is directed to minimising the risk of infection. Chemotherapy is likely to be withheld when the leucocyte count is less than 4×10^9/litre.

Decisions sometimes have to be made as to where and how best to nurse inpatients receiving cytotoxic therapy. In the early stages of treating acute leukaemia, for example, when the white count is still at a reasonable level, the patient may be nursed alongside other patients, and indeed this may be important to maintain the patient's morale. As treatment progresses, increasing levels of protection may be necessary. A single room, a laminar air flow unit and protective isolation nursing measures may have to be introduced depending on the white cell count.

Staff caring for an immunosuppressed patient should be free from colds and sore throats, and must not be involved if they have been in contact with viruses such as measles or chickenpox. Personal hygiene must be of the highest standard, especially hand hygiene. Strict aseptic technique must be employed while carrying out invasive procedures.

Recordings of the patient's temperature and pulse should be taken at least every 4 hours. Even a low-grade pyrexia must be reported. Regular inspection of the body for evidence of infection is essential. The commonest sites of local infection are the mouth, axillae, groins and perineum. Infections of lungs, gut and urinary tract produce signs and symptoms with which the nurse should be familiar. Observing, recording, reporting, taking laboratory samples and administering prescribed antibiotics are standard procedures. Fresh blood or a white cell transfusion may be ordered. Nursing care is directed towards keeping the risk of infection to an absolute minimum. An overwhelming infection can have fatal consequences. The dangers of infection cannot be overstated.

In addition to clinical care a high standard of food hygiene must be observed. Certain foods, e.g. those containing uncooked eggs/meat/fish, should be totally avoided.

Increased risk of bleeding

Platelets (thrombocytes) are essential for blood clotting. When the platelet level falls below 20×10^9/litre, the risk of spontaneous bleeding is significant. Although the patient's platelet count will be estimated at frequent intervals, it is also important for the nurse to observe for any signs of bleeding. This may range from overt bleeding, such as from an intravenous injection site or menorrhagia, to tiny petechial haemorrhages in the mouth or skin. More sinister is internal bleeding such as a subarachnoid haemorrhage or splenic bleed which may have fatal consequences. As a safeguard, chemotherapy is withheld when the platelet count falls below 100×10^9/litre.

Efforts must also be made to reduce the risk of bleeding. Injections should be kept to a minimum and restricted to the intravenous route. The risk of bleeding into a large and highly vascular area such as the buttock often makes intramuscular injections unacceptable. Mouthwashes are preferable to the trauma which a toothbrush may place on the gums. An electric razor should be used for shaving to reduce the risk of cuts to the skin. Blood pressure recordings are not taken in thrombocytopenic patients because the pressure caused by an inflated sphygmomanometer cuff may be enough to cause internal bleeding in the upper arm. Finally, care should be taken when handling and moving such patients to reduce the likelihood of bruising.

Platelet transfusions are given when the platelet count falls below 10×10^9/litre.

Anaemia

When the number of red blood cells or the haemoglobin is reduced, the patient becomes anaemic and will experience breathlessness on exertion, feel the cold and generally lack energy. The reduction in haemoglobin level is gradual and to an extent this allows the body to adapt. Everyday tasks can still be carried out but require greater effort. Although anaemia is not life-threatening and can be effectively treated with blood transfusions, patients do not feel at their best and may have less of a will to get better. Nursing care is directed towards providing comfort, assistance, reassurance and encouragement. Patients whose haemoglobin has dropped to 8 g/dL are likely to be transfused.

Damage to gastrointestinal mucosa

Nausea and vomiting

The severity of the symptoms of anorexia, nausea and vomiting are dependent on the drug(s) used, dose, frequency, route and regimen, and patients need to be reassured of this. Not all chemotherapy patients are sick. In some cases, however, vomiting has been so distressing that the patient has refused to accept a subsequent course of treatment. Cytotoxic drugs vary in their potential to cause nausea and vomiting (see Table 22.5). The aim is to try to prevent sickness occurring. Acute symptoms may be reduced in patients with a low risk of emesis by giving for example oral prochlorperazine or domperidone in advance. For patients at high risk of emesis, ondansetron and dexamethasone may be given intravenously at the start of treatment.

Table 22.5 Cytotoxic drugs known to be emetogenic

Risk of emesis	Example of cytotoxic
Mild	Etoposide Fluorouracil Methotrexate Vinca alkaloids
Moderate	Cyclophosphamide (intermediate and low doses) Doxorubicin Methotrexate (high doses) Mitoxantrone
High	Cisplatin Dacarbazine

Care should be taken in positioning the patient in a suitable part of the ward, giving consideration to the comfort of other patients. A supply of disposable sickness basins, towels, paper tissues and disposal bags should be made ready. Where appropriate, a container for dentures should be provided. A mouthwash and/or supply of cold water for rinsing the mouth after a bout of sickness should always be available. A call bell must always be to hand. Many patients appreciate the support of a nurse when they are being sick. Privacy is also essential. The patient is alarmed at this time and may be hampered by an intravenous infusion at least. By placing a hand across the patient's forehead, the nurse can provide a resistance against which to push, reducing the strain on the patient. The nurse can, with the other hand, help to support the sickness basin. Help is also often required to wipe the mouth and dispose of tissues. Sickness basins should be in plentiful supply so that the patient is not faced with a half-filled basin while waiting for the next wave of sickness to come. Used basins should be removed from the bedside immediately and measurements of volume recorded on a fluid balance chart. Repeated vomiting is exhausting for patients, and so, whenever possible, they should be given every assistance to try to sleep.

Patients troubled by nausea often find their own ways of minimising the problem. These include for example taking small amounts of food and fluid at frequent intervals and listening to relaxation tapes. There is some evidence to suggest that receiving chemotherapy sitting in a chair rather than lying in bed reduces the risk of vomiting. If the patient's condition permits, this is an option which can be offered. Care must be taken to ensure that the chair is comfortable and supportive, that the patient is not allowed to get cold and that the legs are supported if the patient is seated for prolonged periods. Acupressure wrist bands have proved a useful non-invasive method of controlling nausea and vomiting in some patients undergoing cytotoxic chemotherapy.

In some cases, past experience of vomiting following chemotherapy can lead to anticipatory nausea. The sight of the hospital, the ward, a particular member of staff, or the arrival of equipment at the bedside can, in themselves, make the patient feel very sick and can even provoke an attack of vomiting. In addition to anti-emetic therapy as described, lorazepam may be given to reduce anxiety.

Loss of appetite commonly accompanies treatment with cytotoxic drugs. In the short term, a reduced intake of food does no harm, and so, patients who decline a meal should not be badgered about it. Patients should, however, be encouraged to take some nourishment once the acute reaction has passed. To begin with, small amounts of what the patient chooses to take should be given at frequent intervals. Once the intake of very light foods/liquids can be tolerated, the process of increasing the volume and consistency should be a gradual one. Nutritional supplements tend to be rich and strongly flavoured, and so are difficult to tolerate in the early stages. They are better reserved for supplementing the diet once it is re-established. Finding foods and liquids which appeal to patients calls for some imagination on the part of the nurse. Involvement of the families is important here in providing patients with their favourite (often home-made) tasty items of food. Flexibility is essential so that patients may eat or drink at any time of the day or night as the fancy takes them. The involvement of the dietitian is of course vital in many cases so that patients' nutritional status can be successfully monitored and maintained.

Breakdown of oral mucosa

Very strict attention to oral hygiene is of the utmost importance in patients receiving cancer chemotherapy, especially methotrexate and corticosteroids. Guidance on mouth care should be given to patients at the outset and they should be encouraged to get into the habit of attending to this themselves, wherever this is possible. They should be taught to inspect the mouth regularly and to report any changes without delay, and to rinse the mouth with an effective mouthwash such as chlorhexidine gluconate. Where this is not possible, oral hygiene must be carried out by the nurse. Any suspect lesions should be swabbed for 'culture and sensitivity'. Treatment for clinically obvious thrush will be begun before laboratory results are received. Mouth pain may be relieved by using benzydamine hydrochloride oral rinse. Liquids which sting the mouth and hard foods should be avoided. Some patients like to suck crushed ice, chilled pineapple cubes, and lemon and glycerin swabs.

Constipation

The neurotoxic effect of vincristine can lead to severe constipation and may result in paralytic ileus. Preventive measures should therefore be taken at the start of treatment. These will include increased fibre in the diet and plenty of fluids.

Diarrhoea

Fluorouracil and doxorubicin may cause diarrhoea, necessitating the use of codeine phosphate or loperamide and the appropriate nursing measures such as a reduction in dietary fibre and an increase in fluid intake.

Damage to the skin and hair

Extravasation

Certain cytotoxic drugs are especially vesicant and if allowed to leak from the vein into the surrounding tissues can cause burning and necrosis which, in some cases, have resulted in skin grafting and amputation. The nurse plays a vital role in explaining, observing for and reporting this phenomenon. The management of extravasation is described on page 354.

Hair loss

Damage to the hair follicles reduces all hair growth on the body and makes the hair fall out. The term for this is alopecia or epilation. For both men and women this is a very distressing side-effect affecting body image, sexuality and self-confidence. Scalp-cooling techniques using gel packs may be used to reduce the concentration of drug in the capillaries of the scalp. The hair should always be groomed gently and, where it is clear that a wig will be required, arrangements should be made for it to be ordered while the colour, texture and style of the patient's hair are still apparent. The imaginative use of scarves and caps can help the patient through this period. Many patients, however, prefer to have no head covering at all and, particularly when at home, or in hospital where they feel safe, leave the head uncovered, especially when sleeping. The environment should be comfortably warm and free from draughts.

Altered sexuality and fertility

As well as alterations to body image in both males and females caused by chemotherapy, there may be a loss of sexual function and ability to reproduce. In the female, cytotoxic therapy may cause fibrosis of the ovary leading to amenorrhoea and sterility. The accompanying fall in oestrogen secretion may produce menopausal symptoms. In the male, there may be a total absence of sperm. Impotence and gynaecomastia may alter body image and reduce self-esteem. In both females and males, sterility may be temporary or permanent. Although women who have received chemotherapy have subsequently given birth to normal infants, genetic counselling should be given where pregnancy is desired by patients who have previously had chemotherapy because of the possible effects on the unborn child. For men who have received cancer chemotherapy, 'sperm banking' is a possibility. Suitable contraception is advised in particular situations. If nurses are to help patients to cope with sexual dysfunction caused by treatment, then they need to feel comfortable discussing the subject. Where this is not the case, the help of a trained counsellor may be required.

ROLE OF THE NURSE IN CANCER CHEMOTHERAPY

Nowhere in drug management is the nurse required to be more vigilant than in the care of the patient receiving cytotoxic drug therapy. She must also have a clear grasp of the principles of cytotoxic drug therapy and the likely effects the main drug groups will have on the patient. In this way she will know how to advise the patient, what to look out for and what action to take if required. She must act calmly, be available at those times when she is most required by the patient and take on the roles of teacher and counsellor. Extreme care is required in correctly identifying the patient and maintaining accurate records. With additional instruction, nurses are increasingly involved in the administration of parenteral chemotherapy. The skills required are of a technical nature and call for an understanding of how the various factors interact, e.g. rate of delivery, patient tolerance, etc.

Assessment of the patient

A full nursing assessment should be carried out, since the relationship between the nurse and the chemotherapy patient may last a considerable length of time. Special attention should be paid to the patients' understanding of the treatment planned for him, his attitude towards the treatment and his thoughts about the longer term. Measurements of weight and height are taken for use in calculating cytotoxic drug dosages. In patients with acute leukaemia, lymphoma or myeloma, a bone marrow aspiration or trephine biopsy will be carried out at intervals to review progress and calls for particular support from the nurse.

With each pulse of treatment and at the start of a new course, there must be a willingness to reassess the patient's condition, checking up on the development of infection or any other new symptoms of note. A review of the patient's psychological condition is equally important.

Support and encouragement

Patients require a careful explanation of their course of chemotherapy, how it is to be given, how it will work and what effects it is likely to have. The challenge for the nurse is to pitch the information at a level the individual patient can cope with. Patients should be gently told that they are to receive powerful drugs which may make them feel less well before they start to get better again. They should be discouraged from comparing themselves with neighbouring patients as no two patients react in an identical way. Realistic goals should be set in consultation with the patient. For example, the patient may be very anxious to continue working as much as possible throughout the treatment and this may demand some degree of flexibility on both sides. Patients often need to have information repeated, partly because they have a lot to assimilate and partly because they need the reassurance that treatment is progressing. They need to be reassured that someone will listen to their anxieties. Wherever possible, there should be continuity of nursing staff to ease communication and so that patients can build up a feeling of trust.

Patients spend a lot of time waiting. Most patients accept the fact that they need treatment and just want to get on with it. Waiting for blood results can be tedious. In some cases the treatment may have to be temporarily stopped because the white count is too low and this news can be received with disappointment and even anger. The nurse must allow for such reactions and provide the necessary support for both the patients and their families.

Chemotherapy patients have a lot to cope with. They may still be coming to terms with their diagnosis at the same time as trying to cope with treatment. They may also be trying to protect their families from the full impact of their condition and the treatment. Although they may be attending as outpatients, they may not be feeling very well. There may be issues that they want to discuss only with their carers in the expectation that they will understand. The ward or clinic becomes something of a 'haven' for them where, for example, hair loss, vomiting and malaise are accepted. Time must be found for the patient who needs to talk. As an active listener the nurse can gain much valuable information while at the same time helping the patient to off-load. Keeping a special record of how patients are feeling about their progress can be extremely helpful to all members of the healthcare team.

REFERENCE

Grampian Medicines Committee 2000 Policies and procedures relating to medicines in Grampian. Grampian Medicines Committee, Aberdeen

FURTHER READING

Armstrong A C, Eaton D 2001 Science, medicine and the future: cellular immunotherapy for cancer. British Medical Journal 323:1289–1293

Cohen M R, Anderson R W, Attilio R M et al 1996 Preventing medication errors in cancer chemotherapy. American Journal of Health-System Pharmacy 53:737–746

Chung-Faye G A, Kerr D G 2000 Innovative treatment for colon cancer. British Medical Journal 321:1397–1399

Curt G A 2001 Fatigue in cancer. British Medical Journal 322:1560

Donovan J L, Frankel S J 2001 Screening for prostate cancer in the UK. British Medical Journal 323:763–764

Eystein Lønning P 2001 Aromatase inhibitors and inactivators in breast cancer. British Medical Journal 323:880–881

Greenwald P 2002 Cancer chemoprevention. British Medical Journal 324:714–718

Grundy M (ed) 2000 Nursing in haematology oncology. Harcourt Health Sciences, Edinburgh

National Institute for Clinical Excellence (NICE) 2001 Guidance on the use of topotecan for the treatment of advanced ovarian cancer. NICE, London

Sjöström J, Bergh J 2001 How apoptosis is regulated and what goes wrong in cancer. British Medical Journal 322:1538–1539

CHAPTER CONTENTS

23

Drugs affecting the immune response

THE IMMUNE SYSTEM

The immune system is the body's defence against potentially harmful substances and microorganisms. Specific and non-specific mechanisms take part in the immunological response. The blood and lymphatic systems, bone marrow, thymus gland, liver and spleen interact to make this system effective. The bone marrow is responsible for the production of lymphocytes which are primed in the thymus gland (T lymphocytes) and possibly the bone marrow itself (B lymphocytes). These immunologically competent cells together with phagocytes (macrophages) circulate in the blood and lymphatic systems, liver and spleen, ready to react to an invasion by foreign substances (antigens).

Specific immune response

When a foreign substance (antigen) enters the body two different types of immunological response may occur (see Fig. 23.1).

Humoral immune response (antibody-mediated immunity)

On contact with the antigen, immunologically competent B lymphocytes change into plasma cells (effector cells). These plasma cells are capable of producing specific antibodies, the immunoglobulins. The antibody combines with the antigen (antigen–antibody reaction) and neutralises it, for example by coating bacteria to enhance their destruction by phagocytosis.

Another product of the primary contact of antigen with immunologically competent B lymphocytes is the memory cells. Memory cells are able to recognise the same antigen on a second contact, which results in a more rapid and sometimes more intense response. Plasma cells are formed much faster, which, in turn, results in a large amount of antibodies. The capability

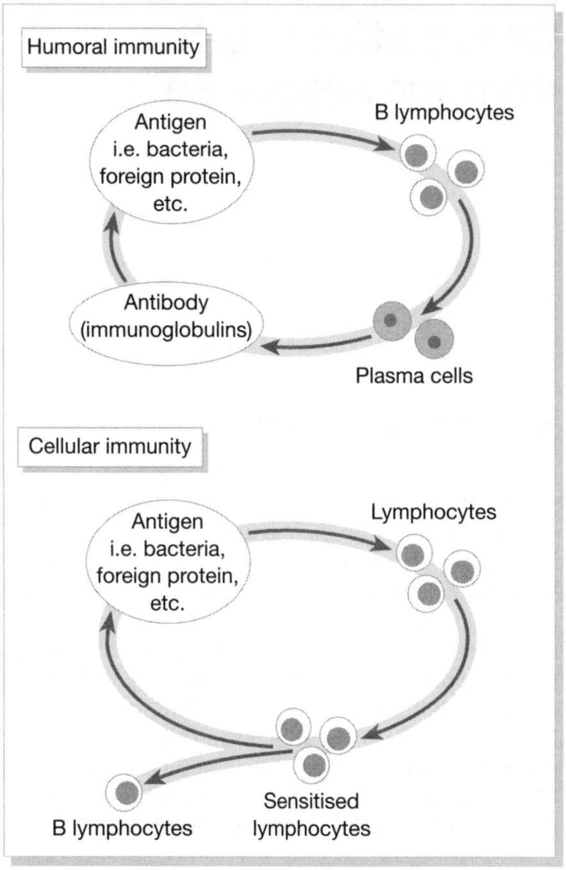

Figure 23.1 Humoral and cellular immunity.

of the memory cells to recognise specific antigens sometimes years after the primary contact forms the basis of active immunisation against bacteria and their toxins.

Cellular immune response (cell-mediated immunity)

Depending on the physicochemical properties of the antigen and its way of entry into the body, some antigens cause the production of sensitised lymphocytes, the T lymphocytes, which have antibody-like molecules on their surface (cell-bound antibody). The T lymphocytes are responsible for the specific cell-mediated immune response. On primary contact with the antigen they proliferate like the B lymphocytes and produce memory cells and effector cells. Unlike B lymphocytes, T lymphocytes produce different types of effector cells which directly take part in the immune reaction:

- cytotoxic effector cells (killer T cells) which can destroy other cells; this reaction to foreign cells is especially important in the rejection of transplanted organs
- T helper cells, which cooperate with the cytotoxic effector cells and also take part in the humoral immune response
- suppressor T cells, which can suppress the function of B lymphocytes and other T lymphocytes.

Non-specific immunity

Apart from the specific immune response, a number of non-specific antimicrobial mechanisms have been recognised. These non-specific factors often operate in conjunction with the specific immune response, which greatly increases the overall effectiveness. These non-specific mechanisms include:

- bactericidal lysozyme, which is present in tears and saliva
- phagocytosis: some leucocytes are able to ingest and kill bacteria
- acute inflammatory response to a foreign substance: release of histamine from sensitised mast-cells
- the non-specific antiviral agent interferon, which is a lymphokine produced by T cells in response to viral infections; interferon inhibits the intracellular viral replication (it also acts on the immune system by increasing the cytotoxic activity of T lymphocytes and inhibits the mitosis of tumour cells).

IMMUNISATION

Immunity can be induced, either actively or passively, against a variety of bacterial and viral agents.

Active immunisation

The objective of vaccination is to provide protection against certain infections such as diphtheria and tetanus. Active immunity is induced by injection of antigen in the form of inactivated or attenuated live organisms or their products (toxins). This stimulates the production of antibodies and a population of primed cells, which can expand rapidly on renewed contact with the antigen and inactivate the invading organism or its toxins. This means prevention or at least minimisation of the disease. Established disease cannot be treated by this method.

Active immunisation is used for the routine vaccination of babies and children, opportunistic vaccination of previously non-immunised adults and children, and for the vaccination of travellers going to specified areas and people at risk from infection through the nature of their work or their lifestyle. Vaccines are very effective when administered correctly. However, basic personal hygiene remains vitally important, especially for travellers.

Types of vaccines used for active immunisation

Live attenuated vaccines such as poliomyelitis, measles, mumps and rubella, tuberculosis (BCG), oral typhoid Ty21a and yellow fever vaccines contain strains of attenuated live organisms which, although non-pathogenic, are still capable of producing specific antibodies. Some live vaccines may contain small amounts of agents such as an antibiotic arising from the manufacturing process. Vaccines are listed in Table 23.1.

Inactivated vaccines (see Table 23.2). Bacterial and viral vaccines such as pertussis, typhoid and inactivated poliomyelitis (IPV) vaccines contain heat-killed or chemically inactivated organisms. Human diploid cell vaccines (HDCV) such as rabies and hepatitis A vaccines contain organisms cultured on human diploid cells and chemically inactivated. *Haemophilus influenzae* type b (Hib) vaccine, pneumococcal vaccine, influenza, hepatitis B and Vi polysaccharide typhoid vaccine contain immunising components of the organism.

Details of preparations used for vaccination and their storage are listed in Table 23.3.

Vaccines such as tetanus and diphtheria vaccine contain bacterial toxins inactivated by formaldehyde, to produce a toxoid.

Adsorbed vaccines such as diphtheria/tetanus/pertussis (DTP), and hepatitis B vaccine are inactivated vaccines adsorbed to an adjuvant such as aluminium phosphate or aluminium hydroxide. The adjuvant releases the antigen slowly and achieves a higher production of antibodies. An adsorbed low-dose diphtheria vaccine for adults is available either with or without tetanus. The low-dose diphtheria vaccine is sufficient to restore levels of immunity in previously immunised patients.

Combined vaccines such as measles/mumps/rubella (MMR), diphtheria/tetanus/pertussis (DTP), and diphtheria/tetanus (DT) vaccines are available to reduce the number of injections when immunising babies and children. The safety of MMR vaccine has been called into question. Advice from the Chief Medical Officers of the UK confirms the safety of this vaccine (see BNF) when used within accepted guidelines. The BNF gives detailed guidance on the vaccination schedules for infants/young children.

Duration of immunity

Injection with a vaccine does not provide immediate protection. There is usually an interval of a few days before the first antibodies appear. For live attenuated vaccines, with the exception of oral poliomyelitis vaccine (OPV) (three doses), a single dose is sufficient to produce enough antibodies to achieve durable immunity. An important additional effect of OPV is the establishment of local immunity in the intestine. OPV boosters are also recommended for pre-school children and school leavers. Rubella immunisation (live vaccine) is given to susceptible (non-immune) women of child-bearing age. Rubella is a cause of fetal damage, and pregnancy tests must be carried out before immunisation.

Inactivated vaccines produce a slow antibody or antitoxin response (primary response). Two injections may be needed to produce this effect. Further injections lead to an accelerated production of antibodies or antitoxins (secondary response) and therefore better protection. If the level of detectable antibody falls, a booster injection may be given to reinforce immunity. Immunity achieved in this way varies from months to years.

Routes of administration

Oral vaccines. Most vaccines are administered parenterally. Exceptions are OPV (see above) and oral typhoid vaccine (OTV). OTV contains live attenuated salmonella typhi (Ty21a). It is administered in capsule form.

Vaccines for injection. With the exception of BCG and oral vaccines, all vaccines should be given by deep subcutaneous or intramuscular injection. In infants, the anterolateral aspect of the thigh or upper arm is recommended. If the buttock is used, injection into the upper outer quadrant avoids the risk of sciatic nerve damage. Injection into fatty tissue of the buttock has been shown to reduce the efficacy of hepatitis B and rabies vaccine.

BCG vaccine is always given intradermally, except in infants and very young children; the percutaneous route by multiple puncture technique may be an acceptable alternative. In this case percutaneous BCG vaccine has to be used. The operator should stretch the skin between the thumb and forefinger of one hand, and with the other slowly insert the needle (size 25G), bevel upwards, for about 2 mm into the superficial layers of the dermis, almost parallel with the surface. A raised, blanched bleb showing the tips of the hair follicles is a sign that the injection has been made correctly. If this is not felt, and it is suspected that the needle is

Table 23.1 Live vaccines: clinical aspects

Live vaccine	Indication	Route	Dose	Intervals	Boosters	Specific contraindications	Comments
BCG	Contacts, active TB Immigrants from countries with high incidence of TB Healthcare staff All students Children 10–14 years Veterinary staff Prison staff Travellers	Intradermal	0.1 mL	Single	–	Generalised septic skin conditions	–
Measles/mumps/rubella	Routine immunisation children 12–15 months Risk group children	SC/IM	0.5 mL	Single	–	Allergy to egg	Safety of this vaccine has been endorsed by UK Chief Medical Officers
Oral poliomyelitis (OPV)	Routine immunisation of children	Oral	3 drops × 3	At intervals of 4 weeks	School entry, school leaving	–	Not with oral typhoid
	Travellers Health workers	Oral	3 drops × 3	At intervals of 4 weeks	10 years	–	Not with oral typhoid
Oral typhoid (OTV)	Laboratory workers Travellers > 6 years	Oral	1 cap × 3	Alternate days	Non-endemic areas, 3 doses annually	–	–
Rubella	Routine immunisation girls 10–14 years	SC/IM	0.5 mL	Single	–	–	–
	Non-immunised women	SC/IM	0.5 mL	Single	–	–	Avoid in early pregnancy
Smallpox	Laboratory workers who handle virus. See also comments	Central Public Health Laboratories/government policy					Global eradication of smallpox has been achieved but the threat of global bioterrorism is being taken seriously by governments. Stocks of the vaccine are being held under governmental control. (Concern has been expressed regarding the strain of virus that might be used in any attack)
Yellow fever	Laboratory workers	SC	0.5 mL	Single	10 years	Allergy to egg	–
	Travellers > 9 months	SC	0.5 mL	Single	10 years	Allergy to egg	Children < 9 months risk of encephalitis

Table 23.2 Inactivated vaccines: clinical aspects

Inactivated vaccine	Indication	Route	Dose	Intervals	Boosters	Specific contraindications	Comments
Cholera	Cholera vaccine is not required for international travel and is currently not available in the UK						
Diphtheria	Routine immunisation of children	SC/IM	0.5 mL × 3	At intervals of 4 weeks	School entry	–	Usually as DT or DPT
	Contacts of diphtheria cases – immunised	SC/IM	0.5 mL	Single	–	–	–
	– unimmunised	SC/IM	0.5 mL × 3	At monthly intervals	–	–	–
Diphtheria, tetanus and pertussis (DTP triple vaccine). A diphtheria and tetanus vaccine (DT) is available for use when immunisation against whooping cough is contraindicated	Routine immunisation of children	SC/IM	0.5 mL × 3	First dose at age 2 months followed by second dose after 4 weeks and third dose after another 4 weeks	A dose of DT is recommended at school entry at least 3 years from last dose of DPT	Where immunisation against whooping cough is contraindicated	Oral poliomyelitis vaccine may be given at the same time
Hepatitis A	Travellers	IM (deltoid)	1 mL × 2	2 weeks to 1 month	6–12 months	–	A combined hepatitis A and B vaccine is available for infants, children and adolescents from 1 year to 15 years who are at risk from both infections
	Occupational risk	IM (deltoid)	1 mL × 2	2 weeks to 1 month	6–12 months	–	–
Hepatitis B	Occupational risk	IM (deltoid)	1 mL × 3 (adult)	1 month and 6 months	–	–	–
	Cases of carrier contact	IM (deltoid) anterolateral thigh in infants	1 mL × 3 0.5 mL × 3 (0–12 years)	1 month and 6 months	–	–	–
	Lifestyle, e.g. parenteral drug abuser	IM (deltoid)	1 mL × 3 (adult)	1 month and 6 months	–	–	–
Haemophilus influenzae type b (Hib)	Primary immunisation of children up to 13 months	SC/IM	0.5 mL × 3	At monthly intervals	–	–	–
	Children 13–48 months	SC/IM	0.5 mL	Single	–	–	–
Influenza	Special risk conditions and/or environments	SC/IM	0.5 mL	Single (adult)	–	Allergy to egg; pregnancy	–
	Special risk conditions and/or environments	SC/IM	0.5 mL × 2	4–5 weeks (children 4–13 years)	–	Allergy to egg	–

(*continued*)

Table 23.2 *(continued)*

Inactivated vaccine	Indication	Route	Dose	Intervals	Boosters	Specific contraindications	Comments
Meningococcal group C conjugate	Children from 2 months. People up to and including 24 years old. Asplenic people	SC/IM	0.5 mL × 3	Monthly	–	–	Protects against group C disease only
Meningococcal plain polysaccharide A and C	Travellers to areas of the world where risks are higher than in the UK. Occupational risk and close contacts	SC/IM	0.5 mL	–	–	–	Infants respond less well than adults to this vaccine
Pertussis	Routine immunisation of children						See DTP vaccine
Pneumococcal (conjugate vaccine)	Asplenic people. Others at risk, e.g. people with heart/lung disease, diabetes mellitus. Suitable for children under 2 years	SC/IM	0.5 mL × 3	Monthly at 2, 3 and 4 months	After 2 years a single dose of polysaccharide vaccine is given	–	The polysaccharide vaccine is not suitable for children under 2 years of age
Rabies	Occupational risk	SC/IM	1 mL × 3	Day 0, 7, 28	–	–	Best response achieved by injection into deltoid regions
	Staff caring for a patient with rabies	Intradermal	0.1 mL into each limb (0.4 mL total)	Single	–	–	
	Travellers to remote areas	Intradermal	1 mL × 3	Day 0, 7, 28	–	–	–
	Post-exposure (not immunised)	SC/IM	1 mL × 6	Day 0, 3, 7, 14, 30, 90	–	–	Post-exposure treatment (not immunised) in combination with immunoglobulin
	Post-exposure (immunised)	IM	1 mL × 2	Day 0 and 3–7	–	–	–
Tetanus	Primary immunisation	SC/IM	0.5 mL × 3	At intervals of 4 weeks	School entry, school leaving	–	See DPT, DT
	Unimmunised adults	SC/IM	0.5 mL × 3	At intervals of 4 weeks	Injury 10 years after primary course	–	–
Typhoid	Occupational risk	SC/IM	0.5 mL × 2	4–6 weeks	3 years	Hypersensitivity to previous dose	–
	Travellers to areas with poor hygiene	SC/IM	0.5 mL × 2	4–6 weeks	3 years	Hypersensitivity to previous dose	–
	Travellers to areas with poor hygiene	SC/IM	0.25 mL (child >1 year)	Single	1 year	Hypersensitivity to previous dose	–

Table 23.3 Vaccines: preparation and storage

Vaccine	Type	Storage etc. • protect from light • never allow to freeze	Notes
Anthrax	Toxoid	2–8°C	Immunisation required only for workers at risk from exposure to the disease
Diphtheria	Toxoid	2–8°C Disposal at not less than 1100°C	Normally diphtheria vaccine is a component of triple vaccine (DPT)
Haemophilus influenzae type b (Hib)	Antigens conjugated with protein to improve antigenicity	2–8°C	Component of the primary course of childhood immunisation
Hepatitis A	Inactivated virus	2–8°C	Should not be mixed with other vaccines in same syringe
Hepatitis B	Hepatitis B surface antigen adsorbed onto aluminium hydroxide	2–8°C	Should be administered to members of risk groups, e.g. healthcare workers who have contact with patients' blood, tissues or blood-stained body fluids
Influenza	Highly purified virus strains which are most likely to be the cause of infection are used to prepare the vaccine	2–8°C	To be administered to risk groups, e.g. adults and children having chronic respiratory and/or heart disease, patients with a compromised immune system owing to a disease process or treatment but not if treatment includes high-dose corticosteroids. Immunisation not generally recommended as routine for fit young people or fit older people. Allergy to egg protein is a contraindication to the administration of this vaccine. The vaccine is normally offered to healthcare staff
Measles, mumps and rubella (MMR)	Live viruses of (attenuated) measles, mumps and rubella. Single antigen viruses are available	2–8°C	Vital part of the childhood vaccination programme. To be administered after first birthday and before school entry. Children with chronic conditions such as cystic fibrosis or kidney disease are at particular risk
Meningococcal	Purified, stabilised extract of the outer capsule of the organism (*Neisseria meningitidis*). Effective only against serogroup A and C organisms	2–8°C Reconstituted before use with the special diluent provided	Routine use not recommended. Should be administered to asplenic adults and children who may be travelling to an area where there is increased risk of infection due to group A organisms
Pertussis	Killed organisms (*Bordetella pertussis*) usually in combination with diphtheria and tetanus vaccines as DTP	2–8°C Test can be carried out to verify that the vaccine has not been frozen. Disposal at a temperature of not less than 1100°C	Public anxiety about safety and efficacy led to reduction in acceptance rates in the mid-1970s. This was followed by an epidemic. Public confidence returned and increased vaccination rates are now reflected in a great reduction in notifications. Specific recommendations are made regarding use of the vaccine in children with a history of convulsions. Research has shown that neurological complications after the disease are considerably more common than after vaccination
Pneumococcal	Polyvalent vaccine containing capsular polysaccharide from 23 types of pneumococcus	2–8°C Check before use that the vaccine is clear and colourless	Recommended for administration to all individuals over 2 years at risk from pneumococcal infection, e.g. asplenic patients, chronic heart disease, lung disease and diabetes mellitus

(*continued*)

Table 23.3 *(continued)*

Vaccine	Type	Storage etc. • protect from light • never allow to freeze	Notes
Poliomyelitis	Live oral polio vaccine (OPV). Inactivated polio vaccine (IPV) available where a live vaccine is contraindicated	SB vaccine 2–8°C Evans vaccine 0–4°C	OPV used in infants from 2 months of age. Vaccine strain virus may persist in the faeces for up to 6 weeks following ingestion. Suitable warnings to be given to parents/carers to observe strict personal hygiene. Contraindications to the use of OPV include patients who are immunocompromised
Rubella	Normally administered in MMR vaccine	2–8°C Use within 1 hour of reconstitution	
Tetanus	Toxoid and adsorbed tetanus vaccine. Available in combination with diphtheria and pertussis (DTP)	2–8°C Disposal at not less than 1100°C	Used for primary immunisation and in treatment of patients with tetanus-prone wounds, e.g. wounds contaminated with soil or manure. As with all ADR due to vaccine, yellow card reporting system should be used
Tuberculosis	BCG vaccine contains live attenuated bacteria derived from *Mycobacterium bovis*	2–8°C Reconstituted vaccine to be used within 4 hours	Special attention to be given to technique used for intradermal administration. Refer to Data Sheet Compendium. Immunisation with BCG vaccine follows tuberculin testing
Typhoid	Three vaccines available: 1. Whole-cell vaccine (heat-killed organisms) 2. Polysaccharide antigen 3. Oral typhoid vaccine (available as an enteric-coated capsule)	2–8°C The oral vaccine has the same storage requirements	Vaccines are not 100% effective
Varicella vaccine (chickenpox)	Available as a live, attenuated vaccine on a named-patient basis	2–8°C	For immunisation of immunocompromised patients, e.g. children with leukaemia or solid-organ transplants
Yellow fever	Live, attenuated organisms	2–8°C After reconstitution use within 1 hour	A single dose confers immunity that lasts for at least 10 years

too deep, it should be removed and re-instated before more vaccine is given. A bleb of 7 mm diameter is approximately equivalent to 0.1 mL injection. For BCG the site of injection is over the insertion of the left deltoid muscle; the tip of the shoulder must be avoided because of increased risk of keloid formations. For tuberculin sensitivity tests (Mantoux or Heaf), intradermal injections are given in the middle of the flexor surface of the forearm. This site should not be used for injecting vaccines. Rabies vaccine may be given intradermally if more than one person needs to be immunised or a rapid immunisation is required, e.g. staff caring for a patient with rabies. Subsequent doses of cholera and typhoid vaccines may also be given intradermally to minimise adverse reactions.

Contraindications

Contraindications apply to the administration of most vaccines. Some of these are outlined below. The current data sheet should always be consulted before the administration of a vaccine.

- Vaccination should be postponed if the patient suffers from an acute febrile illness; minor infections such as a cold are no reason to postpone immunisation.
- Severe local reactions, such as extensive redness and swelling, or general reactions, such as anaphylaxis, bronchospasm, general collapse, convulsions, etc. to previous vaccination.
- Vomiting and diarrhoea (OPV).
- Hypersensitivity to egg (influenza vaccine); anaphylactic reactions to egg (yellow fever, MMR, influenza vaccine). Hypersensitivity to egg is not a contraindication for the use of yellow fever and MMR vaccine. These vaccines have been prepared on chicken embryos or egg, and the egg protein might cause a reaction in allergic patients. However, a personal or family history of allergy is not a contraindication for the use of live vaccines in general.
- Live vaccines should not be given in pregnancy because of the theoretical possibility of harm to the fetus. After rubella injection, pregnancy should be avoided for 1 month after immunisation. Polio and yellow fever vaccination may be given if the risk of infection outweighs the possible risk associated with the vaccine.
- Two live vaccines may be given at different sites at the same time. OPV should not be used at the same time as oral typhoid vaccine.
- Immunoglobulins and live vaccines should be given 3 months apart because the antibodies in the immunoglobulin would inactivate the live vaccine; yellow fever vaccine may be given at the same time, because immunoglobulin prepared in the UK does not contain yellow fever antibodies (see passive immunisation).

Live vaccines must *never* be given to the following groups of patients:

- Patients on high-dose corticosteroids until 3 months after treatment has finished (children on lower-dose corticosteroids may receive a live vaccine after 2 weeks; children on low-dose alternate-day treatment may receive live vaccines; corticosteroid replacement therapy is not a contraindication).
- Immunocompromised patients either through illness or drug treatment; IPV should be used instead of OPV in household contacts of immunocompromised children because the vaccine could cause the disease in these children. After exposure to measles or chickenpox these patients should receive the appropriate immunoglobulin (see passive immunisation).
- Those with malignant conditions such as lymphoma, leukaemia, Hodgkin's disease.

Adverse reactions

Adverse reactions to vaccines are usually mild, and severe reactions are very rare. Since vaccines have become safer the risk associated with immunisation, particularly in children, is very much smaller than the risk of complications of the disease.

Most vaccines may produce mild local or systemic reactions such as redness and swelling at the injection site, raised temperature and screaming. Some vaccines such as measles vaccine may cause a mild form of the disease. Parents should be informed about possible adverse effects and advised on fever management after routine immunisation of their children.

Severe site reactions after BCG administration, such as large ulcers, abscesses and keloid formations, are due largely to the wrong immunisation technique (see Routes of administration).

After poliomyelitis immunisation there is a very rare occurrence of vaccine-related polio. Since the vaccine is excreted in the stool for up to 6 weeks after the immunisation the need for strict personal hygiene has to be stressed to household contacts of the vaccine, e.g. the importance of washing their hands after changing nappies.

Despite the rarity of severe adverse reactions, doctors and nurses always have to be prepared for an anaphylactic reaction after vaccination and must be familiar with the management of anaphylactic shock (see Ch. 13). All anaphylactic reactions should be reported to the Committee on Safety of Medicines using the yellow card scheme.

Tuberculosis: BCG (bacille Calmette–Guérin) immunisation

Vaccination against tuberculosis is discussed in greater detail because of the special tests and immunisation technique involved.

The incidence of tuberculosis declined 10-fold between 1948 and 1987. This decline ceased in 1987, since when small yearly increases have occurred. Incidence is higher in areas of deprivation and in groups at high risk, e.g. refugees. HIV is also a risk factor for tuberculosis.

Recommendations for immunisation

The following groups are recommended for immunisation with BCG, provided successful BCG immunisation has not previously been carried out, the tuberculin test is negative, and there are no other contraindications:

- routine immunisation for all children between the ages of 10 and 13, all students and persons requesting immunisation for themselves or their children
- high-risk groups such as healthcare staff, veterinary staff, contacts of cases with active respiratory tuberculosis
- immigrants from countries with a high prevalence of tuberculosis, their children and infants
- those intending to stay in Asia, Africa, Central or South America for more than a month.

For information on immunisation technique, contraindications and adverse reactions see page 369.

Immunisation reaction

Normally a local reaction develops at the injection site within 2–6 weeks; this consists of a small papule increasing in size for a few weeks up to 7 mm in width with scaling, crusting and occasional bruising. Occasionally a shallow ulcer develops; this should be exposed to the air. The lesion slowly subsides over a period of several months, leaving a small scar.

Use of BCG in bladder cancer

Intravesical BCG has been shown in numerous studies to be valuable in the treatment of superficial bladder cancer. The mechanism of action by which BCG inhibits tumour growth is at present unknown.

The tuberculin test

Before BCG immunisation a tuberculin skin test has to be carried out, except on babies under 3 months of age. A positive test implies immunity through past infection or immunisation. Therefore, test-positive people should not receive BCG. Those with a strongly positive test may have active disease and have to be referred.

Mantoux and Heaf tests are the only recommended techniques for tuberculin testing. Both tests use purified protein derivative (PPD), which is available in several strengths, as shown in Table 23.4.

The Mantoux test

The solution is injected intradermally on the flexor surface of the forearm at the junction of the upper third with the lower two-thirds. The results should be read 48–72 and up to 96 hours later. A positive result consists of a transverse induration of at least 5 mm diameter; 0–4 mm induration is negative; 5–14 mm is equivalent to a Heaf grade 2, and 15 mm or more, strongly positive (Heaf grade 3 or 4).

The multiple puncture test (Heaf test)

The Heaf test is carried out with a disposable head apparatus which does not require any disinfection as the standard reusable Heaf gun does. The use of the disposable head apparatus avoids the transfer of blood-borne infections such as hepatitis B and HIV, and is now the preferred method of Heaf testing.

The disposable heads attach by a magnet to a handle. Six standard steel needles are retained in a plastic base which is enclosed in an outer plastic case with holes corresponding to the needles. The needles protrude only after actuation and then remain protruding

Table 23.4 Tuberculin PPD

Strength (units/mL)	Dilution in PPD	Units in dose of 0.1 mL	Main use
100 000	–	10 000	Heaf (multiple puncture) test only
1000	1 in 100	100	For special diagnostic purposes only, e.g. low sensitivity
100	1 in 1000	10	Mantoux test (routine)
10	1 in 10 000	1	Mantoux test (special), TB suspects or hypersensitive to tuberculin

so that it is easy to detect and discard ones which have been fired. The heads are prepacked and sterile. There are three versions of the disposable head:

- white standard version for tuberculin testing in adults and children 2 years and over; the needles protrude 2 mm on firing
- blue for tuberculin testing of children under 2 years; needles protrude 1 mm
- red, containing 18 needles; it is used for giving BCG by the percutaneous multiple puncture technique and must never be used for Heaf testing.

Performing the Heaf test. The recommended site for testing is as for the Mantoux test. The correct disposable head has to be attached to the gun; tuberculin solution should be dropped from a syringe directly onto the skin at the testing site. The solution is then dispersed by the head of the gun, the gun pressed to the skin and fired. Excess tuberculin should be wiped off the skin, and six puncture marks observed. If the puncture marks are not present the test has not been carried out adequately. The results should be read ideally at 7 days, but can be read between 3 and 10 days.

The reaction is graded 0–4 according to the degree of induration produced:

Grade 0: no induration at the puncture sites
Grade 1: discrete induration at four or more needle sites
Grade 2: induration around each needle site merging with the next, forming a ring of induration but with a clear centre
Grade 3: the centre of the reaction becomes filled with induration to form one uniform circle of induration 5–10 mm wide
Grade 4: solid induration over 10 mm wide; vesiculation or ulceration may also occur.

Grades 0 and 1 are regarded as negative, and previously non-immunised individuals should receive BCG.

Grade 2 is positive, and no further immunisation is required.

Grades 3 and 4 are strongly positive and should be referred for further investigation.

Factors affecting the tuberculin test

The reaction to tuberculin protein may be suppressed by the following factors:

- glandular fever
- viral infections in general
- live viral vaccines
- Hodgkin's disease
- sarcoidosis
- corticosteroid therapy
- immunosuppressing diseases, including HIV.

Other factors which also affect the consistency of tuberculin testing include patient's age, skin thickness, tuberculin adsorption onto the surface of the syringe and tester/reader variation.

Immunisation of children

The immunisation of babies and children against infectious diseases such as diphtheria, pertussis, tetanus, measles, mumps, rubella and poliomyelitis has greatly reduced infant mortality and permanent physical and mental handicap caused by the illness. The introduction of the *Haemophilus influenzae* type b (Hib) vaccine in the 1970s was effective in children over 18 months of age. Subsequently vaccines with improved immunogenicity in children of less than 1 year were introduced.

The aim of the vaccination programme is to eliminate these diseases as far as possible from the population. For example, by giving rubella vaccine to young children it is intended to interrupt the circulation of rubella and thereby remove the risk of infection to non-immune pregnant women. Rubella immunisation of girls between the ages of 10 and 14 who previously have not received MMR vaccine, and non-immune women, continues to reduce the considerable risk to unborn babies. To achieve this aim a high uptake in child vaccinations is required. The BNF gives details of a schedule of vaccinations for children beginning with the first year of life up to school-leaving age.

Great concern has been expressed in the media and elsewhere about the safety of MMR vaccine. A study by Kaye et al (2001) provides evidence against a causal association between MMR vaccination and the risk of autism.

Risk groups

The risk groups are: HIV-positive, children with special conditions, people living in institutions such as old people's homes, occupational risk groups and travellers.

HIV-positive

HIV-positive patients are at increased risk from infectious diseases. Symptomatic and asymptomatic HIV-positive individuals can receive measles (or MMR), mumps, rubella, polio, whooping cough, diphtheria, tetanus, typhoid, hepatitis A and B, Hib vaccines and rabies vaccine as appropriate.

HIV-positive asymptomatic individuals may receive live polio vaccine, but polio virus may be excreted in the faeces for longer periods than is the case in normal persons. Contacts of recently immunised HIV-positive individuals should be advised to follow strict personal hygiene, especially after changing a nappy of an HIV-positive infant.

HIV-positive patients should *not* receive BCG, typhoid (oral) and yellow fever vaccines. Travellers intending to visit infected areas where a valid immunisation certificate is required should obtain a letter of exemption from their medical practitioner.

Vaccine efficacy may be reduced in HIV-positive individuals, and consideration should be given to the use of normal immunoglobulin after exposure to measles and to varicella-zoster immunoglobulin after exposure to chickenpox or herpes zoster.

Children and adults with special conditions

Some conditions, such as HIV (see above), asthma, chronic lung and congenital heart diseases, Down's syndrome, small-for-dates and prematurity, increase the risk from infectious diseases. Children with such conditions should be immunised as a matter of priority. Small-for-dates and premature babies should be immunised according to the recommended schedule like any other children. Apart from routine immunisations, children and adults at risk should also be immunised against influenza and pneumococcal infections.

Hepatitis B immunisation is recommended for haemophiliacs on regular blood transfusions and patients with renal failure, drug abusers, babies born to hepatitis B carrier mothers and certain occupational groups.

Children with neurological problems

Immunisation of children against whooping cough is recommended when they have established neurological problems such as cerebral palsy. In doubtful cases advice should be sought from a consultant paediatrician.

Children with a personal or family history of febrile convulsions and epilepsy should also receive the pertussis vaccine.

Children and adults living in institutions

Children in residential care, including those in nurseries and playgroups, are at special risk from measles and should be immunised, provided there are no contraindications.

Residents of nursing homes, old people's homes and other long-stay facilities where rapid spread after introduction of the infection may occur should be immunised against influenza.

Hepatitis B immunisation is recommended for staff and clients in residential accommodation, for those with a learning disability, and inmates of custodial institutions.

Occupational risk groups

Healthcare staff such as doctors and nurses, laboratory staff, veterinary staff, customs officers, prison staff, etc. may be at increased risk from infectious diseases such as hepatitis B, tuberculosis and rabies, etc. because of the nature of their work; they should be immunised.

Travellers

Travellers to areas where the risk of contracting an infectious disease is especially high, or the nature of travel presents a special risk, or a valid immunisation certificate such as for yellow fever and meningococcal meningitis is required, should be immunised. Advice on which immunisation is necessary for which country and on other measures for the prevention of diseases should be obtained from general medical practitioners well before travelling.

Apart from immunisation, the main measure for preventing diseases such as typhoid, cholera and hepatitis A in areas of poor hygiene and sanitation is strict personal, food and drink hygiene. Immunisation against cholera is not recommended (see BNF).

Hepatitis A vaccine is an alternative to immunoglobulin for those who need longer-term protection or who travel frequently to endemic areas. Immunoglobulin for protection against hepatitis A and strict personal, drink and food hygiene are still recommended for short-term and single holiday trips. In addition to appropriate immunisations, chemoprophylaxis will be required.

Passive immunisation

In this method of immunisation the appropriate antibody or antitoxin against the invading organism or toxin is injected. The antibodies are retrieved from immunised animals (antisera), e.g. diphtheria antitoxin, which is prepared in horses, or from immunised humans (immunoglobulins). The use of antisera has been widely replaced by the use of human immunoglobulins because of the serious side-effects associated with antisera, such as serum sickness and other allergic-type reactions. Reactions to human immunoglobulins are rare.

Types of human immunoglobulins

Non-specific polyvalent human immunoglobulin (normal human immunoglobulin) is produced from pooled plasma of a large group of donors, which contains antibodies currently prevalent in the population. Normal human immunoglobulin is used for:

- the protection of immunosuppressed children exposed to measles
- children under 12 months in whom there is a particular reason to avoid measles; immunisation with MMR vaccine should follow after a 3-month interval
- prophylaxis of infections following bone marrow transplantation
- protection of individuals against hepatitis A.

Normal human immunoglobulin is *not* recommended for the protection of previously non-immunised pregnant women exposed to *rubella*. If termination of pregnancy is not acceptable, it may be given to reduce the likelihood of a clinical attack, which may possibly reduce the risk for the fetus.

Immunisation with normal human immunoglobulin produces immediate protection which lasts for 4–6 weeks.

Specific immunoglobulin such as tetanus, hepatitis B, rabies and varicella-zoster immunoglobulin is produced from pooled blood of convalescent patients or recently immunised donors or donors who have a sufficient antibody titre.

Specific immunoglobulin is used for post-exposure treatment of previously unimmunised patients, usually in combination with the appropriate vaccine. Previously immunised patients need only a booster injection of the appropriate vaccine. Since varicella-zoster vaccine has no licence in the UK yet and is available only on a named basis for immunocompromised individuals, postexposure treatment for individuals at risk, such as pregnant chickenpox contacts and infants whose mothers develop chickenpox 1–4 weeks after the birth, receive only the immunoglobulin.

Treatment of the established disease with specific immunoglobulins is effective only if a high proliferation of the invading organism, especially viruses, or the bonding of toxins to body structure has not yet taken place. For example, in clinical tetanus a decrease of symptoms is only sometimes possible.

Anti-D (RhO) immunoglobulin is used to prevent a rhesus-negative mother forming antibodies to fetal rhesus-positive cells. It should be injected within 72 hours of birth or abortion to protect any subsequent child from haemolytic disease of the newborn.

Administration

Human immunoglobulins are administered intramuscularly because of the danger of aggregation and anaphylactic reactions if given intravenously. To produce intravenous preparations the immunoglobulin has to undergo specific treatment. Intravenous preparations, e.g. tetanus immunoglobulin for intravenous use, is indicated if a large amount of antibody or a quick rise of antibody titre is necessary, as in the case of clinical tetanus.

CONDITIONS TREATED WITH DRUGS AFFECTING THE IMMUNE SYSTEM

Intervention into this most important defence mechanism is justified only in certain circumstances. Risks and benefits of drug treatment have to be weighed up carefully. Treatment should be initiated only in a specialist unit under the supervision of an experienced physician. Drug treatment is indicated in the following conditions.

Organ transplantations

The immune system enables the body to distinguish between 'self' and 'non-self'. This causes the rejection of transplanted organs which are recognised as 'non-self' by the immune system of the recipient. Drugs which act by suppressing the immune response are vitally important in helping to prolong the life of a transplanted organ.

Autoimmune diseases

Sometimes the body's mechanism for preventing the recognition of 'self' components as antigen is disturbed and the system turns against itself: autoantibodies are produced. All diseases associated with the formation of autoantibodies are called autoimmune diseases. Major examples are:

- systemic lupus erythematosus
- scleroderma
- rheumatoid arthritis
- ulcerative colitis
- myasthenia gravis
- active chronic hepatitis
- chronic glomerulonephritis.

Some cancers

Examples include hairy cell leukaemia, certain lymphomas and solid tumours and Kaposi's sarcoma associated with AIDS (acquired immune deficiency syndrome). The treatment of these and other cancers is dealt with in more detail in Chapter 22. It is very important to recognise that treatment with immunosuppressive drugs greatly weakens the patient's defence mechanism. This fact must be taken into account when providing nursing care and planning treatment, e.g. every effort must be made to reduce the risk of infection to a minimum.

MAIN DRUG GROUPS

These drugs may be categorised as *immunosuppressants* and *immunomodulators*.

Immunosuppressants

Under this heading we consider the following:

- cytotoxic immunosuppressants
- corticosteroids
- ciclosporin
- other immunosuppressants.

Cytotoxic immunosuppressants

Azathioprine, the most commonly used drug in this group, is metabolised to 6-mercaptopurine, which suppresses cell-mediated immune reactions by preventing lymphocyte proliferation and function.

Usage. Azathioprine is used either alone or, more commonly, in combination with corticosteroids and/or other immunosuppressive agents in the management of renal and other organ transplantations, and autoimmune diseases, e.g. autoimmune haemolytic anaemia. The therapeutic effect may be evident only after a few weeks and may be corticosteroid-sparing, thereby reducing side-effects associated with high dosage and prolonged use of systemic corticosteroids.

Dosage and administration. Azathioprine is available as tablets and injection. Wherever possible oral administration is the preferred route of administration. The standard dose range in transplant rejection therapy is 1–4 mg/kg daily and 1–2.5 mg/kg daily for the treatment of autoimmune diseases. When the therapeutic effect is evident, doses should be reduced to the lowest effective level and should be maintained indefinitely in transplant patients because of the risk of organ rejection.

Elderly patients and patients with renal or hepatic impairment should receive doses at the lower end of the range.

Side-effects and cautions. Cytotoxic immunosuppressants are potentially dangerous drugs and have numerous side-effects. Careful monitoring and regular blood counts are required with dose adjustments if necessary. The most important side-effects are:

- marrow toxicity, which is dose-related and reversible
- hair loss, usually more significant in transplant patients
- increased susceptibility to viral, fungal and bacterial infections, usually more significant in transplant patients
- increased risk of neoplasia, particularly lymphomas
- gastrointestinal disturbances
- cholestatic hepatotoxicity, which requires an immediate withdrawal of the drug.

Azathioprine should be used with caution in patients with severe bone marrow depression; it should not be started in pregnancy owing to possible teratogenic effects. The decision to continue therapy in pregnancy must be very carefully considered.

Allopurinol inhibits the metabolism of azathioprine, thereby increasing its toxicity.

Azathioprine tablets should be taken after food to avoid gastrointestinal disturbances. The handling of azathioprine injections should follow the guidelines on the 'handling of cytotoxic drugs' (see p. 351). The contents of the vial should be reconstituted with Water for Injections to 15 mL. The solution is stable for 24 hours at room temperature (15–25°C). Any remaining solution should be discarded. Note should be made of any signs of infection, abnormal bleeding, jaundice, dark urine or clay-coloured stools. Patients should be advised about the importance of regular blood counts.

Corticosteroids

Corticosteroids (e.g. hydrocortisone and prednisolone) have multiple pharmacological properties (see Ch. 20). Corticosteroids are powerful immunosuppressants. They suppress the immune function of lymphocytes and interfere with both humoral and cell-mediated immune reactions. They are used to prevent organ transplant rejection, commonly in conjunction with other immunosuppressants. In autoimmune diseases they are used for their immunosuppressive and anti-inflammatory effects.

Ciclosporin

Ciclosporin is a cyclical polypeptide (a complex protein-like substance, derived from a soil fungus). It suppresses mainly cell-mediated immune reactions by inhibition of T lymphocyte proliferation. Ciclosporin is a potent immunosuppressive agent which prolongs the survival of allogeneic transplants involving skin, heart, kidney and other organs. Since the introduction of ciclosporin, the number of successful organ transplantations has increased significantly. It is virtually non-myelotoxic and can therefore be used for bone marrow transplantations. It has no cytotoxic actions. Oral ciclosporin is also used for the treatment of severe psoriasis which is unresponsive to other forms of treatment.

Dosage and administration. Ciclosporin is available as oral (capsule and solution) and parenteral preparations. Concentrate for infusion is used for initiation of therapy in organ and bone marrow transplantations usually 1 day before the operation and in the immediate follow-up period. Oral treatment should commence as soon as possible, depending on the patient's condition. The dosage for organ transplantations is initially 10–15 mg/kg daily, reduced over a period of months to a maintenance dose of 2–6 mg/kg daily. If corticosteroids are used at the same time, lower doses are used (consult specialist literature).

The dosage for bone marrow transplantations is initially 3–5 mg/kg daily by intravenous infusion followed by 12.5 mg/kg daily orally, which is slowly reduced after 12 months to zero or to a very low maintenance dose. Dosage levels are adjusted in the light of blood-level determinations.

Side-effects and precautions. The most important dose-related side-effect is its nephrotoxicity. Other side-effects are abnormalities in liver function, gum hypertrophy and gastric disturbances. Fluid retention, convulsions and hypertension occur more often in children than in adults. Ciclosporin should not be given in conjunction with other potentially nephrotoxic drugs such as aminoglycosides. Ketoconazole can increase the plasma concentration of ciclosporin.

The total daily dose may be given as a single dose or in two divided doses. Oral solutions may be taken with milk, fruit juice or cold chocolate drink to mask the taste (grapefruit juice should not be used). In order to ensure that the full dose is ingested the cup or glass should be rinsed. An improved formulation of ciclosporin (Neoral) is always taken in two divided doses.

Other immunosuppressants

A range of immunosuppressants is now available. These include mycophenolate mofetil, certain monoclonal antibodies and tacrolimus. Specialist literature should be consulted for details.

Interferons

Type I interferons (alfa and beta) are naturally occurring glycoproteins which have complex effects on the immune system and cell function. Type II interferons are characterised by gamma interferon.

Interferons have become more readily available in recent years owing to improved production methods involving biological engineering techniques.

Interferons are available only as injections to be administered subcutaneously, intramuscularly or directly into the lesions of Kaposi's sarcoma.

Interferon alfa is used in the treatment of hairy-cell leukaemia, chronic myelogenous leukaemia, AIDS-related Kaposi's sarcoma, hepatitis B and hepatitis C. Interferon alfa is also used as an adjunct in the treatment of malignant melanoma and for the maintenance of remission in myeloma.

Side-effects and cautions. The most frequently occurring side-effects are 'flu-like symptoms' which can be successfully treated with paracetamol. Interferon alfa also has a suppressive effect on the bone marrow which can lead to leucopenia and thrombocytopenia. Safety has not been established in children and therefore interferons are usually not recommended for use under the age of 18.

Interferon beta is used in the treatment of relapsing remitting multiple sclerosis. Multiple sclerosis is the commonest demyelinating disease of the nervous system and is the commonest cause of disability in young adults. Multiple sclerosis is thought to be caused by a combination of factors (including viral activity) which lead to an autoimmune destruction of the central nervous system myelin. Each of the interferons has been investigated as potential therapies in MS but interferon beta is the current choice based on clinical research findings. The mechanisms by which interferon beta produces therapeutic benefits are not well understood but could include the following actions: decrease in proliferation of T cells, restoration of T suppressor cell function and reduction in the secretion of interferon gamma which plays a role in the occurrence of spontaneous MS exacerbations. The use of interferon therapy in MS has been a significant cause of public debate on the non-availability of high-cost drug therapy within certain sectors of the NHS. Selection of MS patients for interferon therapy is generally done within agreed guidelines by consultant neurologists. Dosage levels are adjusted in the light of the patient's response. A dose of 0.25 mg (8 million units) is widely recommended.

NURSING THE IMMUNOSUPPRESSED PATIENT

The care of the immunosuppressed patient calls for an understanding, by everyone involved, of the potential dangers of being overwhelmed by infection with little or no resistance to fight it. It falls to the nurse in particular to provide as safe an environment as possible for the patient, and to observe for and act upon any signs or symptoms of infection as promptly as possible. There may be an assumption that most infections, with the help of modern medicines, are treatable and that no one is likely to die from infection. In the absence of a functioning immune system, the patient is at very great risk not only from bacterial invasion, but also from fungal and viral organisms.

The aspects of care which require special consideration, especially by nurses, may be considered under a number of headings.

Location/method of nursing. Patients who are immunosuppressed require to be isolated from microorganisms which will harm them. Protection is achieved by using a method of nursing known as protective isolation. The degree of immunosuppression will dictate the degree of protection required. The facilities available will also influence the situation. For some patients, it may be sufficient to nurse them in a single room within the ward. Others will require stricter control of the environment provided by either specially designed units with en suite facilities or a plastic isolator.

Environment. The patient's room should be kept scrupulously clean. Furniture, equipment and the floor should be wiped down daily using a detergent solution. Wherever possible, disposable cloths should be used. Mop heads should be laundered after use. Disposable equipment should be used wherever possible. Otherwise, equipment should be left in the room for the exclusive use of the patient. Flowers should be displayed outside the room since they or the water they are standing in are a potential source of infection.

Staff and visitors. Those coming into contact with the patient should not pose any risk of passing on infection. Staff suffering from a cold or sore throat, or who have any focus of infection such as an infected finger, should be temporarily employed elsewhere if not absent from duty. Numbers of visitors should be limited, and there should be a restriction on children visiting since there is an increased likelihood that they will have been in contact with viral infections such as measles or chickenpox which could prove fatal if acquired by the immunosuppressed patient.

Handwashing. Hands are considered to be the prime source of transfer of microorganisms. They should be thoroughly washed using an antiseptic cleansing solution such as chlorhexidine gluconate solution 20% before and after all clinical procedures. Procedures such as urinary catheterisation, catheter toilet, wound dressing, venepuncture, endotracheal suction, etc. must be carried out using a rigorous aseptic technique.

Food. Cooked food is safer than uncooked food. Fruit and vegetables should always be cooked, and salads avoided. Food in tins and sealed packets from reputable firms and within date are considered safe. Bottled water and canned or bottled juices may be used. Tap water should be boiled before using.

Observation. The nurse must be vigilant in observing the development of signs of infection at an early stage. Frequent and thorough inspection of areas likely to be the first focus of infection, such as the mouth, axillae, groins and anal area, should be made. Careful recordings of temperature and pulse should also be made. Any elevation of these vital signs should be reported at once. The development of any other significant features should be noted. For example, a productive cough may signal a chest infection; dysuria, a urinary tract infection; diarrhoea, gastroenteritis. Diagnostic tests such as a chest X-ray and bacteriological examination of appropriate body fluids will be ordered. Good observation, however, is in itself not enough. Careful documenting by each shift of nurses and prompt reporting are also essential.

Finally, it should not be forgotten that isolation can bring with it psychological difficulties, and so nurses must ensure that patients understand the need for such an arrangement and provide as much encouragement as possible.

STORAGE AND DISPOSAL OF VACCINES

Most vaccines have to be stored and transported under refrigeration at the recommended temperature (see Table 23.3). This means a cold chain should be maintained at all times by using insulated cooled containers for the transport of vaccines from one refrigerator to another. The potency of vaccines can be guaranteed only if they have been kept at the recommended temperatures. (Manufacturers' leaflets should be consulted.) For most vaccines, with the exception of OPV (0–4°C Evans), the recommended storage temperature is 2–8°C. OPV deteriorates very quickly and should not be allowed to remain at room temperature. As with all immunological preparations, the 'cold chain' must be maintained during transport and distribution.

Reconstituted vaccines must be used within the recommended period of time, usually between 1 and 4 hours, and safely discarded after an immunisation session.

Opened multidose containers of any vaccine have to be discarded after 1 hour for non-preservative-containing and 3 hours for preservative-containing vaccines, including OPV. Single-dose containers should be used where possible.

Unused vaccine and spent or partly spent vials should be disposed of, preferably by heat inactivation or incineration at 1100°C.

Spillage and contaminated waste should be dealt with by heat sterilisation or incineration at 1100°C.

REFERENCES

Kaye J A, del Mar Melero-Montes M, Jick H 2001 Mumps, measles and rubella vaccine and the incidence of autism recorded by general practitioners: a time trend analysis. British Medical Journal 322:460–463

FURTHER READING

Bong J J, Lansdown M 2002 Skin cancer in patients on long term immunosuppression. British Medical Journal 324:1344

Heller T 2001 How safe is MMR vaccine? British Medical Journal 323:838–839

NHS Executive 2002 Replacement chapter for immunisation against infectious disease 1996. DoH, London

Prasad K R, Lodge J P A 2001 Transplantation of the liver and pancreas. British Medical Journal 322:845–847

Salisbury D M, Begg N T (eds) 1996 Immunisation against infectious disease. Edward Jenner Bicentenary Edition. HMSO, London

Taylor B, Miller E 2002 Measles, mumps and rubella vaccination and bowel problems or developmental regression in children with autism: population study. British Medical Journal 324:393–396

CHAPTER CONTENTS

24 Nutrition and blood

NUTRITION AND VITAMINS

BACKGROUND

People who are ill can greatly benefit from well-managed nutritional support. Team working is the key to the success of this aspect of patient care. Within the nutritional support team, medical, surgical, nursing, dietetic and pharmaceutical skills must be available if patients are to receive high-standard, cost-effective therapy.

Malnutrition occurs in both the community and hospital settings. It occurs when an individual's nutrient intake falls below the metabolic requirements. The early detection of malnutrition is important because, if left untreated, it can severely compromise patient recovery.

The body has only limited reserves of immediately available energy and nitrogen sources. In the absence of adequate food ingestion, energy is derived from stores of glycogen in the liver, from muscle protein, and from fat in adipose tissue. However, glycogen stores are limited and are exhausted within the first 24 hours of starvation. Over the next few days muscle protein is broken down to provide glucose. In more prolonged starvation, fat is used to provide the energy source, and the brain adapts to utilise ketone bodies. When the fat stores have been utilised, accelerated protein breakdown resumes and leads eventually to death.

NUTRITIONAL SUPPORT

The aim of nutritional support is to arrest catabolism due to these losses and to restore the patient to a positive nitrogen balance. This can be accomplished by administering calories, nitrogen, fluid, electrolytes, vitamins and trace elements. Increasingly, the place of nutritional support is being recognised. Advances in the management of severe illness and trauma have meant that more patients survive the initial phase of their illness and require continuing supportive treatment. This involves the administration of appropriate fluids, electrolytes and nutritional requirements.

Protein

If nutrition is deficient, not only does the patient lose weight by the loss of skeletal muscle but also tissue repair and immune mechanisms are significantly inhibited as these processes require active cell turnover and therefore new protein formation. Amino acids are building blocks of protein. They can be divided into two groups: essential amino acids and non-essential amino acids. It is necessary that nutrition solutions contain a balanced content of essential amino acids and a broad spectrum of non-essential amino acids.

Energy

Energy is provided as carbohydrate or fat.

Electrolytes and trace elements

Sufficient quantities of electrolytes and trace elements must be given, not only for maintenance, but also to replace any significant losses. The action of each is summarised below:

- sodium
  - predominant cation in extracellular fluid
  - maintains integrity of cell membrane along with potassium
- potassium
  - major intracellular cation
  - required for transport of glucose across cell membrane
- calcium – continuous supply necessary to form and maintain skeleton, and to maintain homeostasis in nerve and muscle tissue
- magnesium – important factor in many enzyme reactions
- iron – required for haemoglobin synthesis
- copper – involved in release of iron from liver
- zinc – essential for many enzyme reactions
- cobalt – essential constituent of vitamin B_{12}
- manganese – involved in calcium and phosphorus metabolism
- iodine – required in synthesis of thyroid hormones
- fluoride – required for maintenance of skeleton
- chromium – deficiency leads to glucose intolerance.

Vitamins

All vitamins can be supplied by parenteral and enteral feeding regimens (see Table 24.1).

NUTRITIONAL ASSESSMENT

Nutritional support must be designed to suit the particular metabolic and nutritional needs of each individual. Careful assessment of the patient's nutritional state is required before the decision to use a particular product is made. This is normally carried out by the dietitian, who will obtain information from a variety of sources, including the patient, relatives, doctor and nursing staff. Close liaison between dietetic, medical and nursing staff is important.

ENTERAL NUTRITION

Identifying those requiring nutritional supplementation

There are many screening tools available to enable those patients who may benefit from nutritional supplementation to be identified. Most of these require the patient's current basal metabolic index (BMI) to be measured and also request that an estimation of the rate of weight loss is determined.

The BMI is calculated as the weight in kilograms over the height in metres squared, i.e.:

$$\text{BMI} = \frac{\text{Weight (kg)}}{\text{Height (m)}^2}$$

Weight categories may be classified in terms of range of BMI as follows:

- underweight $< 18\,\text{kg/m}^2$
- normal $18\text{–}24.9\,\text{kg/m}^2$
- overweight $25\text{–}29.9\,\text{kg/m}^2$
- obesity $30\text{–}39.9\,\text{kg/m}^2$
- extreme obesity $> 40\,\text{kg/m}^2$

In patients with a BMI $< 18\,\text{kg/m}^2$ urgent action is required to correct the under-nutrition.

Consideration must be given to the rate of unintentional weight loss; if it is > 6 kg in 12 months or > 3 kg in 3 months, action is required to stop loss of weight.

For patients who are experiencing major problems with food and fluids for more than 3 consecutive days, action is required if the patient is:

- leaving more than half of the meals provided
- unable to eat solid food or having physical feeding problems
- unable to retain or absorb food.

Before commencing supplements, it is important to assess and treat the underlying cause of weight loss. Poor appetite can be associated with fever, depression and recurrent infection. Treatment of these conditions should result in improvement in appetite and may not require a dietary supplement. Patients who have physical disabilities and/or swallowing problems may have their nutritional intake significantly improved by providing modified cutlery and crockery and/or altering the consistency of their food. In cases of acute malabsorption lasting 4 or more days, the cause should be identified and the dehydration corrected by advising adequate fluid intake.

Patients who may benefit from nutritional support through supplementation

Dietary supplementation is most appropriately used in patients:

- with malignancy
- before/after major surgery
- with malabsorptive conditions
- with degenerative conditions, e.g. multiple sclerosis, motor neurone disease, Huntington's disease

It is worth considering nutritional support for those with:

- pressure sores/leg ulcers
- swallowing difficulties
- dementia
- chronic medical/physical problems.

Advice that should be given at surgery/ward level

Prescribable supplements are not always appropriate as the first-line treatment for malnutrition. Patients should initially be encouraged to:

- Eat frequent small meals
- Have nourishing between-meal snacks
- Use full-fat milk enriched with 4 tablespoons skimmed milk powder/pint
- Add extra cream, sugar and butter to desserts, sauces and breakfast cereals
- Use Build Up or Complan as nourishing drinks between meals.

Increasing the energy and protein density of the diet through foods is much more acceptable from the patient's point of view.

Monitoring the patient

Once a patient has been identified as being 'nutritionally compromised', the first-line advice outlined above should be given. It is important that an individual's progress is reviewed to establish the success of first-line treatment. For some patients, modification of their normal diet and possibly the introduction of a non-prescribable product such as Build Up will be sufficient to reverse the nutritional decline. This conservative management of nutritional needs is likely to be supervised by nursing staff either at ward level or in the patient's home. The frequency of review and monitoring will be different in acute and primary care but it is important to highlight the need for further intervention. For some patients, commencement of a sip feed will be indicated.

If the nutritional problem persists, the patient should be commenced on an appropriate 1.5 kcal/mL dietary supplement, the choice depending on patient preference. Referral to the community or hospital dietitian should be considered.

All patients should be reviewed after being commenced on a sip feed. In primary care, this will usually be after 4 weeks or sooner if clinically thought necessary. In patients where there has been no improvement, the first-line advice should be reinforced and the patient commenced on an oral sip feed in addition to their fortified diet for 1 month. Most patients usually manage to drink one to two supplements/day in addition to ordinary foods.

In secondary care, this first review may be within 24–48 hours. Patients should be reviewed prior to discharge and only be discharged from hospital on a sip feed if it is clinically indicated. At this point, the patient's condition may have resolved and sip feeding can be stopped or continued for 7 days post-discharge and then reviewed in the community.

Once the nutritional problem appears to have resolved, sip feeds and fortified diet should be discontinued and patients should be encouraged to monitor their weight for 3 months. If problems recur then the supplements and fortified diet should recommence and this will become a new episode of care.

Type of supplements available

Prescribable supplements fall into three main groups.

Sip feeds. This group can be subdivided into complete supplements which contain all the essential nutrients (vitamins, minerals, energy and protein) and incomplete supplements which do not contain a full range of the essential nutrients. The energy content of the supplement varies. Some provide 1 kcal/mL while others contain 1.5 kcal/mL. Some nutritional supplements have higher fibre content. These products are often based on milk, fruit juice or yoghurt, and are available in several flavours. The majority of these products are lactose and gluten free and are suitable for patients with malabsorption, diarrhoea and known coeliac disease.

Single-nutrient supplements. The energy-only (carbohydrate) and protein supplements come in either powder or liquid form and are designed to be added to the patient's food and drink. The energy-only supplements are intended for patients with protein and fluid restrictions.

Other specialised products. A variety of specialised supplements are available such as semi-elemental feeds for use with patients who have malabsorption, products such as supplemented puddings for patients with swallowing difficulties, as well as the less-frequently used products specifically for patients with renal disease, liver failure or who are HIV positive. Dietetic advice is required before patients are commenced on these products.

Examples of prescribable supplements currently on the market are shown in Box 24.1.

Deciding which product to prescribe should be based on patient requirements and taste preference. Although it is possible to survive on some of the complete supplements in the absence of food, it is generally recommended that supplements are taken in addition to food and should not replace meals or snacks. Supplements used inappropriately can inhibit patients' ability to resume meeting their nutritional requirements from ordinary food.

Box 24.1 Prescribable supplements

Sip feeds
1 kcal/mL
Enrich
Ensure
Fresubin

1.25 kcal/mL
Provide Xtra

1.5 kcal/mL
Enrich Plus
Ensure Plus
Fortisip
Clininutren
Enlive
Fortijuce

Single nutrient supplements
Maxipro
Protifar
Vitapro
Polycose
Maxijul
Polycal
Calogen

Other specialised products
Calshake
Scandishake
Elemental 028

When to refer to a dietitian

Referral for dietary advice should occur when:

- the BMI is under 18 kg/m^2
- there is significant weight loss, illness or rapid unintentional weight loss; dietary supplements may be prescribed for patients with a BMI greater than 18 kg/m^2
- the patient has another medical condition requiring dietary intervention, e.g. diabetes, renal disease, malabsorption
- the patient's weight and/or intake continue to deteriorate.

The dietitian will complete a full nutritional assessment and recommend specific further treatment for the patient. The dietitian is able to assess the appropriateness of introducing an alternative supplement if there has been an intolerance/palatability problem.

Enteral tube feeding

People who cannot meet their nutritional or fluid requirements and who have a functioning small intestine (e.g. patients with neurological conditions or stroke; who have had head and neck surgery; who have had gut resection, or other GI disease) need to be fed using an alternative method. The most commonly used alternative methods are via a nasogastric, gastrostomy or jejunostomy tube. The decision as to the most suitable method for each individual patient is based on:

1. The *length of time* the patient is expected to require feeding by an alternative route. For short-term feeding, e.g. up to 2 weeks, the nasogastric route will be used.
2. The *functioning of the gastrointestinal tract*. The majority of patients will have a GI tract that is fully functional and long-term feeding will be required. The feeding route used will therefore be gastrostomy.

If the patient's stomach and duodenum need to be temporarily or permanently bypassed, jejunostomy is the required route.

Nasogastric tube feeding

A fine-bore nasogastric tube is used to facilitate this form of feeding. Since there is a wide range of systems available, it is advisable to seek the advice of the dietitian and nutrition nurse specialist.

The importance of ensuring correct positioning of a nasogastric tube cannot be overemphasised. Confirmation that the tube is not kinked and is in the stomach rather than in the oesophagus or lung must be made before starting a feed, using one of the following methods:

- aspirating the stomach contents and testing with pH indicating paper
- syringing a small amount of air down the tube and at the same time listening over the epigastrium with a stethoscope.

X-ray confirmation is time-consuming and costly, and so it is now used only for certain categories of patient, for example the unconscious, or where neither gastric position nor misplacement has been confirmed by the above two tests.

In the acutely ill or unconscious patient, it is important to establish that the stomach is emptying. This is an important precaution to take and can prevent potential hazards such as vomiting or gastric reflux which may lead to aspiration pneumonia. It is also important that the volume of feed given is increased gradually, particularly in patients who have received nothing via their gut for several days, in order to prevent gastrointestinal side-effects.

Regular aspiration of gastric contents is especially important for patients receiving intensive care, for the unconscious and for those on drug therapy which may interfere with absorption. Absorption can be assumed if there is little or no aspirate, abdominal distension or nausea and where bowel sounds are normal. Gastric emptying can be enhanced and gastric reflux minimised by raising the head of the bed while feeding.

A wide range of commercially made preparations to supplement the diet is available. For those totally unable to feed in the normal way, it is essential to use nutritionally complete foods of which there are a number. Nutritional supplements and nutritionally complete foods are classed as borderline substances approved for use in specific clinical conditions such as dysphagia, inflammatory bowel disease, malabsorption states and bowel fistulae. In spite of the name given to them, nutritionally complete foods may still not meet the patient's entire needs and additional vitamins and minerals may be required.

The availability of nutritional preparations, diverse in composition and nutrient ratios, permits the selection of a feed to meet the specific requirements of the patient. Manufactured polymeric feeds generally suit most tube-fed patients. Compared to hospital-made feeds, they are sterile until opened, their composition is known and constant, and they are more convenient.

To reduce the risk of bacterial contamination, correct preparation and storage of feeds are necessary. All individually prepared feeds should be refrigerated at 4°C until required for use. The feeds must be clearly labelled to indicate the date and time by which they must be used. To minimise the risk of growth of microorganisms, hospital-made feeds should be administered within 4–6 hours of hanging, and aseptically administered sterile feeds within 12–24 hours. Reservoirs and administration sets should be renewed once every 24 hours. Bacteriological testing of the feeds should also be carried out as per the local control of infection policy.

Tube feed regimen

Nausea and abdominal distension may be induced if the feed is administered too quickly. Continuous administration can minimise this problem, using either gravity drip or pump-assisted feeding. Continuous drip administration also minimises the risk of diarrhoea which may result from administering bolus feeds, particularly if the feed is hyperosmolar. Pump-assisted feeding will help patients who have some impairment of gastrointestinal function, as the flow rate can be controlled to meet their absorptive capacity, and this is the administration method of choice.

Whatever method of feeding is used, accurate entries should be made on the patient's fluid balance chart and a record kept of the patient's tolerance of the feed. Today's feed tolerance will influence tomorrow's feeding regimen. Doctors and nurses require access to details of the daily regimen, which has been worked out for each patient, including:

- a breakdown of energy, protein, electrolyte values, vitamins and minerals
- the total volume
- instructions regarding the volume of feed to be given per hour and how many hours in a 24-hour period the feed is to be administered.

Nurses have a considerable contribution to make to the care of the patient fed by tube. They are involved in:

- assisting in the assessment of the patient's nutritional state
- communicating with dietetic and medical staff
- storing feeds appropriately
- initiating and supervising the feed
- observing the patient, e.g. respiratory difficulty, tolerance of the feed
- providing the patient with encouragement
- keeping accurate records.

Diarrhoea is a complication of enteral feeding and may necessitate discontinuing the feed (after excluding drug therapy and infectious causes). There are some feeds on the market that are supplemented with soluble fibre, which has been advocated for the treatment of diarrhoea. The soluble fibre provides a substrate for colonic microflora to produce short-chain fatty acids. These fatty acids act in the ascending colon to promote absorption of water and sodium and therefore have a possible role in preventing diarrhoea.

Feeds with fructo-oligosaccharides or prebiotics that are undigested in the small intestine but pass to the colon where they are fermented also assist in preventing diarrhoea. Moreover, they selectively promote the growth of bifidobacteria and therefore reduce colonisation by *Escherichia coli* and *Clostridium difficile*. Examples of these feeds are Jevity Plus and Fresubin Isofibre.

Administration of medicines via enteral feeding tube

Enteral feeding tubes may be used as an alternative route for the administration of medicines. When prescribed by this route, medicines are administered in the form of a solution, suspension or emulsion. If the drug is not normally available in a liquid form, the pharmacist should be consulted for advice and assistance. It may be possible for a liquid form of the drug to be prepared in the pharmacy using a suitable formulation that takes account of the properties of the drug, such as stability in an aqueous form.

Crushing of tablets into the necessary fine powder cannot be achieved satisfactorily on the ward. If tablets are insufficiently powdered there is a risk of the tube being blocked with consequent risk of underdosage. It should be borne in mind that some solid-dose forms cannot be crushed, even to give a coarse powder. In some cases the crushing of a tablet may destroy the essential properties of the product.

Apart from using an oral liquid it may be acceptable to administer the injectable form of the drug via the enteral feeding tube. If this procedure is adopted, clear instruction must be given by the prescriber on the patient's drug prescription sheet. The pharmacist must first be consulted to ensure that the procedure is satisfactory and that there is no suitable alternative. Adding a medicine to a feed is not recommended as chemical or physical interaction may adversely affect the drug, the feed, or both. An unknown quantity of the drug may be lost if the food is altered or some is lost because of spillage or leakage from the delivery system.

The standard procedure for checking the position of the tube must be followed before administering medicines via the tube. To administer the medication, the tube is first clamped. The barrel of a suitably sized syringe is then attached. The medicine is poured into it and the clamp released. The medication is allowed to flow in by gravity. The tube is clamped again. Prior to and following the administration of each medication, a volume of water (20–30 mL) should be instilled. This will minimise the risk of tube blockage, and ensure that the medicine has passed through the tube and out into the stomach.

Administration of continuous nasogastric feeding using a fine-bore tube

For short-term feeding, e.g. up to 2 weeks, a fine-bore nasogastric tube is generally used. This procedure is outlined in Box 24.2.

Throughout the ongoing administration of the feed the nurse's responsibilities are as follows:

Checking the position of the tube

Prior to commencing each feed the position of the tube should be checked.

If the patient is restless or comatose, it is recommended that the tube position be checked more frequently.

Box 24.2 Administration of continuous nasogastric feeding using a fine-bore tube

Documentation
- Feed prescription sheet

The medicine
- Feed in feed container

The environment
- Patient seated or in bed; warmth, comfort, privacy (if preferred)

The nurse and the patient
- Patient identified; explanation given to patient

Technique
- Nurse ensures that hands are thoroughly washed before and after feed
- Feeding set connected to feed
- Feed run through to expel air
- Correct position of tube confirmed by:
  - auscultation
  - aspiration of stomach contents (turns pH indicating paper pink)
- Tube flushed with 20–30 mL water
- Feeding set connected to tube
- Flow and volume of feed regulated as per feed prescription
- Feed recorded

Hazards
- Aspiration pneumonia

If the tube starts to protrude, even as little as 1 cm, it should be removed and a fresh one passed. A partially removed tube must NEVER be pushed back down as there is a danger of the tube becoming kinked or entering the lungs.

Maintaining the flow of the feed

The flow rate should be checked hourly or more frequently as instructed.

If the rate of flow becomes sluggish, the tube and feeding set should be checked to ensure they are functioning properly:

If the fault is in the tube, it can be flushed through with lukewarm water.

If the fault is in the administration set, it should be disconnected and replaced.

Keeping the tube patent

Instil 20–30 mL water through the feeding tube between each feed container change, and before and after each dose of medication, to reduce the risk of occlusion caused by feed or build-up of drug deposits. When the feed is stopped (e.g. X-ray visit) and on completion of a feed, the tube must be flushed with 20–30 mL of water and plugged/capped. This will trap a column of water in the tube, reducing risk of blockage.

Minimising risk of infection

The feed container and feeding set should be changed at least once every 24 hours.

Keeping accurate records

The following records must be maintained:

- feed prescription
- fluid balance chart
- nursing care plan and progress notes.

Providing nursing care as required

- Assisting with the activities of living.
- Special attention to oral hygiene.

Reporting abnormalities

Gastrostomy/jejunostomy tube feeding

For longer-term feeding, either percutaneous endoscopic gastrostomy (PEG) or jejunostomy is the preferred option. The overall number of patients who have a gastrostomy has increased. The factors contributing to this increase include developments in healthcare technology, changes in clinical practice and growing numbers of elderly patients.

In the past, gastrostomies were usually placed surgically but this tended to restrict their availability. In the 1990s a percutaneous approach was performed which greatly simplified the technique, making it more accessible for a wider number of patients. Non-surgical gastrostomies may be placed radiologically or by endoscopy.

Assessment for gastrostomy feeding

All patients require to have their nutritional requirements fully assessed prior to being referred for a gastrostomy procedure. The decision to insert a gastrostomy tube is normally initiated in secondary care. The majority of patients then receive their continuing care in the primary care setting in either their own home, a nursing home or a community hospital.

Tube feeding system

All adults who have a gastrostomy tube in situ also require the following equipment:

- a feeding pump, with adaptor and battery charger
- supply of giving sets and possibly reservoirs
- pH indicating paper
- adhesive tape
- 50 mL syringes
- supply of feeding solutions.

Children may or may not use a feeding pump. It is often decided to bolus feed children in preference to using a pump-assisted regimen.

PARENTERAL NUTRITION

This method of nutritional support should be used only to prevent or correct malnutrition when no other route for the administration of nutrients is available. The intravenous route is the one referred to in this text. The vein used may be either a peripheral or a central one depending on the likely duration of the therapy.

Indications

The indications for parenteral nutrition are:

- preoperative – preparation of undernourished patients for surgery, chemotherapy or radiation therapy
- postoperative – when complications prevent a return to oral intake, e.g. prolonged postoperative ileus, sepsis or fistulae
- extensive burns, where nutritional requirements cannot be met enterally
- some patients with hepatic or renal failure
- where there is impairment of intestinal mobility and/or absorption of nutrients, e.g. chronic gastrointestinal tract disease – Crohn's disease, pancreatitis, short bowel syndrome

- prolonged coma/refusal to eat
- premature infants – where functional immaturity causes intestinal failure or difficulty in establishing oral or tube feeding.

Intravenous nutrition solutions

Protein is supplied by solutions of crystalline amino acids.

Glucose, which provides 16.8 kJ (4 kcal) per gram, is the best carbohydrate for intravenous use, but glucose solutions of high calorific value are hypertonic and must be infused via a central vein to provide rapid dilution. This minimises the risk of vein thrombosis which can occur if these hypertonic solutions are infused peripherally. Where glucose intolerance occurs, insulin may be required and blood glucose levels should be monitored.

Fat emulsion in the form of a lipid solution of, for example, Intralipid or Ivelip, may also be used as an energy source, providing 37.8 kJ (9 kcal) per gram. Lipid is also used as a source of essential fatty acids and a medium for giving fat-soluble vitamins. Lipid should not be used as the sole caloric source. The fat emulsion is hypotonic and can be infused by peripheral vein. In neonates the nutrients can be continuously infused along with fat emulsion via a peripheral vein. Peripheral vein feeding can be carried out in adults where fat emulsions are incorporated using the 3-litre bag, commonly named the 'Big Bag' system.

Electrolyte levels in intravenous solutions vary according to the individual requirements of the patient. Sodium, potassium, calcium, magnesium and phosphate are added to the nutrient solutions. Sodium acetate, a bicarbonate precursor, is incorporated to regulate the acid–base balance. It is necessary to incorporate trace elements into the intravenous admixture.

All vitamins can be supplied intravenously. Fat-soluble vitamins A, D, E and K are available in commercial preparations. Commercial water-soluble vitamin preparations for addition to intravenous nutrition solutions contain some or all of the following: ascorbic acid, thiamine, riboflavin, niacin, pyridoxine, pantothenic acid, vitamin B_{12} and folic acid.

Preparation of intravenous nutrition solutions

Standard total parenteral nutritional formulations may be acceptable for many patients because of the kidney's ability to maintain homeostasis. No single parenteral regimen would be ideal for all patients because of the wide variety of pathology and differing age groups, or for the same patient throughout. The composition of the solution requires to be determined from day to day by clinical and chemical monitoring. The patient's details are filled in by the prescriber along with the date, day of prescription, duration of prescription, volume of amino acids and glucose solutions, quantities of electrolytes and other additives.

The advantages of using a system where the intravenous nutrition is provided in a 3-litre bag are:

- risk of contamination by frequent changes of container and the use of airways and connections is minimised
- changing is required only once in 24 hours and therefore staff time is saved
- amino acids and calorie source are delivered simultaneously, thus spreading the dextrose load over 24 hours so that the incidence of glycosuria is reduced.

The intravenous admixtures should be prepared in the pharmacy as pharmaceutical calculations, drug stability incompatibilities, solubility and sterility are important factors. The ward preparation room is an unsuitable location for aseptic procedures, which are better carried out in the aseptic suite within the pharmacy department.

Amino acids, glucose solutions and lipids are combined in a 3-litre pack with additions of vitamins, electrolytes and other small volume components. Checks are made to ensure compatibility of the components.

Incompatibilities

It is essential that potential incompatibilities or the degradation rate of certain additive drugs in the presence of others are taken into consideration. Incompatibilities can usually be avoided or corrected. For example:

- insulin is unstable in the presence of bicarbonate
- insoluble carbonates may form if bicarbonate is added to calcium or magnesium; it is simpler to use a bicarbonate precursor such as sodium acetate
- vitamins are unstable in hypertonic intravenous solutions, especially in the presence of light.

The reaction can be slowed by using a freshly prepared solution and protecting it from bright light. It is essential that the solution be examined prior to setting up, and during the infusion, as precipitate may appear after a few hours. Pharmacists are aware that the fat emulsion may 'crack', especially if there are high levels of electrolytes, in particular calcium and magnesium, in the bag. If calcium and phosphate are present above a certain level, a precipitate of calcium phosphate may form, particularly if the solution has been stored in the refrigerator.

Intravenous nutrition and the administration system should not be used as a means of administering drugs. In addition to the risk of contamination, many chemical changes can occur. For example, penicillins are rapidly degraded in amino acid solutions, and tetracyclines form insoluble complexes with calcium and magnesium.

Administration of intravenous nutrition

Peripheral intravenous nutrition is suitable for patients requiring up to 7 days' intravenous nutrition. Long-term parenteral nutrition is administered through a central vein, preferably the superior vena cava. In both situations, the line must be inserted following strict skin cleansing and using an aseptic technique.

The care of both the central venous and the peripheral venous line used with intravenous nutrition should be meticulous. Responsibility for the care of the line is a combined one between medical and trained nursing staff, the overall aim being that no harm should come to the patient. The nurse's role is to explain to patients what is involved and to try to reassure them. It is essential therefore that the nurse is fully conversant with the procedure and associated care.

Complications of intravenous nutrition

The major complications associated with intravenous nutrition include:

- complications at line insertion
- sepsis
- line blockage
- air embolism
- phlebitis
- thrombosis
- metabolic complications associated with the nutrients
- mechanical problems
- psychological problems.

It is therefore important that protocols and procedures be designed to minimise the risk of such complications. Key factors in the prevention of complications are:

- meticulous aseptic handwashing
- strict attention to aseptic procedures
- adherence to hospital protocol for care
- staff who are:
  - knowledgeable
  - competent.

Care of the patient receiving intravenous nutrition

Patients receiving intravenous nutrition should be closely observed for the early detection of complications. Urinalysis should be performed every 4–6 hours to note the presence of glucose or ketone bodies. A 24-hour urine collection for measurement of urea level is used to estimate the nitrogen balance. The patient should be weighed regularly (e.g. twice weekly). Recordings of temperature and pulse are made every 4 hours, and the character of the respirations observed. Accurate recordings of the intake and output of fluid must be kept. Care must be taken to maintain accuracy of fluid recordings, especially on completion of one chart and the commencement of the next (e.g. at midnight). Regular checks should be made to ensure that the prescribed rate of infusion is being maintained and that sufficient volume of feed remains in the infusion pack. A volumetric pump is used so that the nurse is immediately alerted to occlusion of the line or the presence of an air embolus.

Transparent dressings allow for easy visualisation of the insertion site; any evidence of swelling, discoloration or pain should be reported at once.

No medications should be added to any part of the system nor should it be used for blood sampling or central venous pressure monitoring.

A special cover can be obtained for placing over the 3-litre bag to protect the feed from strong sunlight. Administration sets made of ultraviolet-absorbent material are also available.

The nurse has a vital role, not only in minimising the entry of microorganisms, but also in vigilant monitoring of the rate of the infusion. 3-litre bags must be used in conjunction with some form of infusion pump. This is not a substitute for frequent checking and, if necessary, making minor adjustments to the infusion rate. No attempt should be made to 'catch up' if the infusion is behind time.

The patient receiving nutritional support may be malnourished and/or debilitated to some degree. This patient requires much encouragement. General physical care increases in importance, including skin care, mouth care and exercise within the limitations of the infusion system and/or the patient's clinical condition. Bowel activity, which may be reduced, should be carefully noted.

Changing the infusion pack

Accurate identification of the patient is essential. Details on the pack must be compared carefully with the prescription. The infusion solution should be checked to ensure that it is not out of date, that the solution is free from precipitate and that there is no evidence of the bag having been damaged, rendering it unsterile.

Care is needed to connect up the new infusion bag as an aseptic procedure. This can be achieved by thorough handwashing and careful introduction of the administration set into the infusion pack. Utmost care should be taken to avoid perforating the bag. The administration set must be free of air bubbles before setting the rate controller and starting the infusion. A record of the new pack, batch number, and starting time is made and initialled by the nurse(s) involved. The volume of solution which has been administered is recorded on the patient's fluid balance chart.

The method and frequency of changing the administration set and the site dressing are important elements for the nurse to know but are beyond the scope of this book.

Intravenous nutrition at home

An increasing number of patients who have had, for example, small-bowel resection with resulting short bowel syndrome, require long-term intravenous nutrition. This may be carried out at home if it is anticipated that more than 3 months' intravenous nutrition will be required. Thorough training is given to the patient and spouse or parent, as appropriate. This will take 2–4 weeks. Nutritional requirements are supplied by the pharmacy in pre-assembled packs. Other stores/supplies are delivered every 4 weeks. An infusion pump, trolley, refrigerator and intravenous stand can be loaned by commercial companies who specialise in home-care delivery systems. The patient's home needs to have suitable facilities for the management of an aseptic infusion system at home, e.g. suitable worktop surface, adequate handwashing and storage facilities, telephone. If necessary, these requirements should be made available through the occupational therapy and social work departments.

The patient reports to hospital on a regular basis in order that checks can be carried out and, where necessary, the nutritional components altered. The patient must be supplied with a 24-hour contact in case there is a need for advice or emergency help. The general practitioner must be made aware of these developments and asked to be involved in shared care with the hospital consultant. Funding and finance are important issues, and should be organised prior to the final decision regarding a patient going home on intravenous nutrition.

Summary

Safe intravenous nutrition has been developed by doctors, pharmacists, biochemists, microbiologists, nurses and nutrition experts. The role of the nurse in this form of therapy (whether undertaken in a specialist centre or in the patient's own home) continues to increase. Ideally, a senior nurse with specific responsibility for nutrition patients is appointed. A high standard of nursing care, including assessment of the patient, meticulous levels of hygiene, close observation, accurate recording and prompt reporting, is of fundamental importance. Where care at this level is assured, the maximum benefit to the patient of this technique, which may be life-saving, is within reach.

VITAMINS

Vitamins are essential substances which are required in daily amounts ranging from micrograms to milligrams for growth, development and maintenance of the body. Many of them are involved in the control of the body's metabolic processes through participation in enzyme reactions. Others have additional roles as structural components of bone and in electrolyte balance. Vitamins are substances which are present in certain foods but which the human body is unable to manufacture.

A good mixed diet provides adequate amounts of vitamins, and some are also formed by bacteria in the colon so that vitamin supplements are normally unnecessary. Provided a sufficiency of vitamins is taken, which should be available in a good mixed diet, there is no advantage to be gained by taking further large doses of the various vitamins unless there is a form of malabsorption. Indeed further large doses may be harmful. Restricted diets or defective absorption or utilisation of food result in vitamin deficiencies which lead to a number of conditions requiring administration of appropriate vitamins. Other factors leading to vitamin deficiencies include anorexia and vomiting, gastrointestinal disease, liver damage and cancerous conditions. They can also arise in alcoholics and in the elderly on poor diets and also when natural demands for vitamins are increased in fevers, pregnancy, breast-feeding and metabolic disorders.

Vitamins present in food can be divided into two classes; the fat-soluble vitamins (including vitamins A, D, E and K) and the water-soluble vitamins (including vitamins B and C). Table 24.1 outlines the main features of these vitamins.

Table 24.1 Main features of vitamins

Vitamin	Sources	Function	Results of deficiency	Results of excess	Notes/clinical uses
A	Dairy products, e.g. milk, butter and cream. Also in fish liver oils. Can be formed in the body from carotene, a substance found in carrots, green vegetables and liver	Formation of rhodopsin, a pigment in some of the light-sensitive cells (rods) in the retina	Damage to skin and mucous membranes; corneal lesions; night blindness	Poisoning with vomiting and prostration, and over a longer period, painful swelling of bones. High levels may cause birth defects. Women who are, or may be pregnant should be advised not to take vitamin A supplements except on medical advice. They should not eat liver or liver products	Deficiency in UK is rare
B_1 (thiamine)	Egg, liver, wheatgerm and some vegetables	Essential for certain stages of carbohydrate metabolism			Deficiency may occur in chronic alcoholism and is best treated by parenteral administration of vitamins B and C. Recommended that: Use is restricted to essential IV injection is administered slowly (over 10 minutes) Facilities for treating anaphylaxis should be available Potentially serious allergic adverse reactions may occur during or shortly after administration
B_2 (riboflavine)	Same as vitamin B_1	Necessary for carbohydrate metabolism	Ulceration and infection of mucous membranes and skin		Deficiency only occurs with malnutrition
Nicotinamide	Animal and vegetable protein. Can be manufactured both by the body itself and by bacteria present in the gut		Pellagra		Deficiency rare except in general malnutrition
Pyridoxine		Necessary for metabolism of many amino acids	Peripheral neuropathy, convulsions and anaemia		Naturally occurring deficiency rare in Britain. An acute deficiency may be induced by treatment with the antituberculous drug, isoniazid, which reacts chemically with pyridoxine thus neutralising any of the vitamins present in the body. Pyridoxine used to treat deficiency and is used in prophylaxis

(*continued*)

Table 24.1 *(continued)*

Vitamin	Sources	Function	Results of deficiency	Results of excess	Notes/clinical uses
B_{12} (hydroxocobalamin)	See page 392				
C (ascorbic acid)	Fresh fruit and vegetables	Essential for development of collagen, cartilage and bone, and is concerned in haemoglobin formation and tissue repair	Scurvy – characterised by subcutaneous haemorrhage		Scurvy now rare but mild deficiency states may occur during pregnancy and in patients on restricted diets, particularly the elderly
D (calciferol)	Derived mostly from the diet, especially fish, eggs and liver. Can also be formed in the skin under the influence of sunlight	To promote the absorption of calcium from the intestine	Rickets in children, osteomalacia in adults	Very serious toxic effects – widespread calcification of tissues, particularly in the kidney, severe muscular weakness and abdominal pain	Requirements greatest in childhood and during pregnancy and lactation. Deficiency may arise in some ethnic minority groups who have a poor vitamin intake and cover their skin. In most cases, treatment with the natural dietary vitamin (D_2 calciferol) is adequate. The hypocalcaemia of hypoparathyroidism requires larger doses
E (tocopherol)	Wheat germ, soya-bean, lettuce and other green vegetables		In young children with congenital cholestasis, abnormally low concentrations may be associated with neuromuscular abnormalities		Available synthetically as tocopherols. Little evidence to suggest oral supplements are essential in adults even where there is fat malabsorption secondary to cholestasis. Neuromuscular abnormalities caused in children respond only to parenteral vitamin E
K	Green leafy vegetables. Also produced by bacteria in the intestine	Essential to assist manufacture, by the liver, of prothrombin and factor VII, needed for coagulation of blood	Haemorrhage, bruising		True deficiency rare as intestinal bacteria synthesise it in quantity. In newborn, intestinal bacteria are absent and therefore they are commonly given phytomenadione (vitamin K_1) by injection. In adults, deficiency is associated with fat malabsorption from pancreatic disease or obstructive jaundice. Replacement therapy is given in form of menadiol. Oral anticoagulants such as warfarin inhibit the use of vitamin K_1, thus preventing manufacture of essential clotting factors. Vitamin K may thus be used as an antidote to warfarin if need be

DRUG TREATMENT OF ANAEMIAS

BLOOD

Blood consists of a pale yellow fluid called plasma in which red cells, white cells and platelets are suspended. These cellular components all develop in the bone marrow. The blood fulfils a multitude of purposes, the chief functions being the transport of oxygen and nutritional materials to all the cells of the body and the removal of carbon dioxide and waste materials. Oxygen is carried by haemoglobin contained in the red cells, while carbon dioxide is transported partly in the plasma and partly in the red cells.

The main control mechanism ensuring the maintenance of a constant circulating red cell mass is provided by erythropoietin, which is produced by the kidney in response to anoxia and acts on the bone marrow to increase the rate of cell division, cell maturation and haemoglobin synthesis. Abnormality of any of these factors may give rise to anaemia. Excessive blood loss or destruction of blood cells may also lead to anaemia. Anaemia may therefore be defined as a reduction in the normal amount of red cells or haemoglobin or both. It is said to be present when the haemoglobin concentration is below the normal range for the age and sex of an individual. For adult males, the normal haemoglobin concentration is 130–170 g/litre; for females 120–155 g/litre. It is slightly lower in pregnancy.

THE ANAEMIAS

The types of anaemia most often encountered are iron-deficiency anaemia and megaloblastic anaemia.

Other conditions of the blood include anaemia associated with chronic renal failure, iron overload, aplastic anaemia and haemolytic anaemia.

IRON-DEFICIENCY ANAEMIA

Iron is absorbed as the ferrous salt in the duodenum and upper small intestine. It is carried to the bone marrow for the synthesis of haemoglobin. About 70% of the total body iron is present in erythrocyte haemoglobin. The remainder is stored in the liver, spleen and bone marrow. The absorption of iron is carefully regulated so that just enough is absorbed to make good any deficiency.

Iron is an essential constituent of haemoglobin. When red cells break down the iron is retained by the body and utilised in the formation of further haemoglobin. In health, the loss of iron from the body is 1–2 mg daily, which is replaced by absorption from a dietary intake of 10–20 mg. Iron is present in vegetables and meat, the concentration being higher in the latter. The main causes of iron-deficiency anaemia are:

- reduced iron stores at birth
- inadequate intake of iron
  - restricted diet
  - malnutrition
- increased requirements
  - pregnancy
  - breast-feeding
- chronic blood loss
  - profuse menstruation
  - disease of the gastrointestinal tract:
    hiatus hernia
    varices
    haemorrhoids
    ulceration
    colonic carcinoma
    bleeding
  - drug-induced:
    aspirin
    non-steroidal anti-inflammatory drugs
- malabsorption
  - coeliac disease
  - malabsorption syndrome.

Clinical features

The features of iron-deficiency anaemia include the general features common to all anaemias (Table 24.2).

The clinical features specific to iron-deficiency anaemia include glossitis, angular stomatitis and koilonychia.

Table 24.2 General features common to all anaemias

Feature	Cause
Fatigue	Lack of oxygen for internal respiration, hence lack of energy
Pallor of mucous membranes and skin	Reduced haemoglobin concentration
Dyspnoea on exertion	Exertion requires more oxygen, therefore more rapid passage through lungs required
Dizziness (fainting)	Reduced oxygen to brain
Feeling of cold	Reduced tissue respiration, therefore reduced production of heat
Palpitations/tachycardia	Compensatory attempt to increase oxygen level in tissues; may lead to cardiac failure
Exacerbation of angina	Angina caused by lack of oxygen to cardiac muscle; reduced oxygen-carrying capacity worsens the angina

Oral iron

Iron is usually given orally to correct a deficiency. The following formulations are available:

- ferrous salts in liquid and solid oral dose, including controlled release preparations
- formulations containing both ferrous sulphate and folic acid for use in pregnancy
- formulations containing vitamins and minerals in addition to ferrous sulphate.

The iron content of commonly used oral iron preparations is given in Table 24.3.

The daily dose of elemental iron should be 100–200 mg. The choice is dependent on efficacy, side-effects and cost.

Efficacy

Absorption of a soluble ferrous salt occurs in the upper part of the small intestine where the pH is lower; at higher pH levels, ferrous phosphates form which are not suitable. The efficacy of an iron preparation depends on how much of its iron content is released in this part of the gastrointestinal tract. Fluids and solid oral dose preparations are preferable to controlled-release preparations since the latter may release only a proportion of iron in the area where absorption takes place. Some inhibition of iron absorption can occur if it is taken with milk, tea or eggs.

Side-effects

Acceptability by the patient may be influenced by adverse effects. Gastrointestinal disturbances, including nausea, abdominal discomfort, diarrhoea or constipation may occur. The nausea may be reduced by taking the iron preparation after food. Patients should be advised of the possibility of these side-effects and also that iron causes discoloration of the stool. Where gastrointestinal disturbances occur with ferrous sulphate, the dose may be reduced or a change to ferrous gluconate or ferrous fumarate may help.

Table 24.3 Iron content of oral iron preparations

Iron salt	Amount	Ferrous iron content
Ferrous fumarate	210 mg	68 mg
Ferrous gluconate	300 mg	35 mg
Ferrous sulphate	300 mg	65 mg
Ferrous sulphate, dried	200 mg	65 mg

Cost

Controlled-release and liquid preparations are more expensive than simple tablet and capsule forms. Ferrous sulphate 200 mg (65 mg elemental iron) three times daily provides an effective dose which is relatively inexpensive.

Interactions

Iron salts should not be given with tetracyclines as the absorption of both drugs is impaired. Antacids and penicillin can also impair the absorption of iron.

Duration of treatment

The haemoglobin concentration should rise by about 100–200 mg/100 mL per day over 3–4 weeks. Treatment of iron deficiency should be continued for 3–4 months after the haemoglobin has returned to normal in order to replace depleted iron stores. Extra encouragement may have to be given to ensure that the patient completes the course of treatment. The underlying cause should have been treated as far as possible.

Parenteral iron therapy

When oral iron cannot be tolerated in any form, or there is malabsorption of iron, it may be necessary to give the iron by injection. Iron injections bypass the mechanism which controls the degree of iron absorption and the dose must be based on the actual iron deficiency as calculated from laboratory test results and the patient's ideal body weight. Iron sorbitol injection is given by *deep* intramuscular injection using the Z-track technique to prevent leakage along the needle track and subsequent staining of the skin (see p. 75). It can also cause severe arrhythmias and anaphylaxis in some patients. As a severe allergic reaction can take place, it is administered to a very limited group of patients, always in hospital and under very close supervision. There is no significant difference in the rate of haemoglobin response to injectable iron compared with oral iron, i.e. a rapid cure of anaemia cannot be effected by use of the injectable route. Iron dextrose and iron sucrose injections are also available. Both are given by slow intravenous injection or intravenous infusion.

MEGALOBLASTIC ANAEMIA

Both vitamin B_{12} and folate are necessary for the production of mature red blood cells. Vitamin B_{12} is present largely in meat; folate is found in both animal and plant foods. A deficiency of either will result in megaloblastic anaemia. In the normal person, a factor (the intrinsic factor) is produced by the stomach and is necessary for the absorption of vitamin B_{12} in the intestine. The main causes are:

- vitamin B_{12} deficiency:
  - malabsorption (due to disease, e.g. Crohn's or resection of the terminal ileum)
  - deficiency of intrinsic factor (as found in pernicious anaemia and after gastrectomy)
  - inactivation of vitamin B_{12} (by abnormal intestinal bacterial flora associated with anatomical abnormality of the small bowel)
  - veganism where there are low levels of available dietary vitamin B_{12}
- folate deficiency:
  - malabsorption (due to disease, e.g. coeliac disease, or resection of the jejunum)
  - increased demands (due to pregnancy and lactation, malignancy and chronic inflammatory diseases, and haemolytic diseases)
  - drugs (e.g. anticonvulsants, including phenytoin and phenobarbital; dihydroxyfolate reductase inhibitors, e.g. methotrexate, trimethoprim, pyrimethamine; H_2-receptor antagonists such as cimetidine or ranitidine, proton pump inhibitors, e.g. omeprazole)
  - inadequate intake of folate (due to dietary deficiency).

Pernicious anaemia

Pernicious anaemia is a particular form of anaemia in which the mature red cells are irregular in shape and size, and reduced in number. The cause of pernicious anaemia is an autoimmune gastritis which leads to a deficiency in the production of the so-called intrinsic factor, a protein normally secreted by the stomach, and essential for the satisfactory absorption of vitamin B_{12} in the terminal ileum. In addition to the megaloblastic anaemia, the deficiency of vitamin B_{12} leads to degenerative changes in the nervous system which, if untreated, ultimately render the patient immobile.

Clinical features

The megaloblastic anaemias present with the general features common to all anaemias (Table 24.2). In addition, the patient may have a red, raw, ulcerated tongue; a pale lemon-tinted skin (caused by haemolysis as the body recognises the cells as abnormal); and paraesthesiae. In very severe cases, ataxia and a spastic weakness of the legs develop – a condition known as subacute combined degeneration of the spinal cord.

The diagnosis of pernicious anaemia is confirmed by the Schilling test, a dual isotope test which confirms malabsorption of vitamin B_{12}. The test involves fasting the patient overnight, asking the patient to empty the bladder in the morning and discarding the urine. Two capsules of a short half-life radioactive vitamin B_{12} are given to the patient to swallow with as little water as possible and hydroxocobalamin 1 mg is given by intramuscular injection. The patient fasts for a further 2 hours. A 24-hour urine collection is obtained from the time the capsules and injection are given. It is essential that the collection is complete. In health, radioactive vitamin B_{12} would be absorbed into the gut and excess to requirements (15–40%) would be excreted in the urine. In pernicious anaemia, radioactive vitamin B_{12} is *not* absorbed and therefore passes in the stools instead of the urine (less than 3%).

There are two cobalamins available: hydroxocobalamin, which is highly bound by plasma proteins so that it is excreted slowly and thus its action prolonged; and cyanocobalamin, which is more rapidly excreted.

Hydroxocobalamin is the form of vitamin B_{12} used, as it is retained in the body longer than cyanocobalamin and therefore does not have to be given so frequently. Initial treatment is 0.25–1 mg by intramuscular injection on alternate days for 1–2 weeks then 250 micrograms weekly until blood counts are within normal range. A course of oral iron may be required to supply the increased number of mature red cells. Thereafter the maintenance dose is 1 mg every 3 months. Unless it is caused by dietary insufficiency, the lack of vitamin B_{12} in pernicious anaemia is permanent, and therefore replacement therapy must be parenteral and for life. Consequently, education of the patient/relative is important.

Treatment of other causes of B_{12} deficiency

Prophylactic B_{12} in the form of intramuscular hydroxocobalamin every 3 months should be given after total gastrectomy or total ileal resection and after partial gastrectomy if malabsorption is demonstrated. Prophylactic oral vitamin B_{12} (in the form of cyanocobalamin) at a dose of 50–150 micrograms daily between meals can be given to vegans.

Folate deficiency

Most causes of folate deficiency will yield to a course of treatment comprising 5 mg of folic acid by mouth daily for 4 months. A daily dose of 10 or 15 mg may be necessary where malabsorption occurs. Where megaloblastic anaemia is due to dihydroxyfolate reductase inhibitors, the conversion of folic acid to its active metabolites is inhibited. Folic acid will therefore not be effective; folinic acid may be used, 15 mg orally once daily.

Folate deficiency may occur in pregnancy with the possible development of neural tube defects. Prophylactic folic acid/iron combinations can be given. The level of folic acid in these preparations is insufficient to treat megaloblastic anaemia.

ANAEMIA ASSOCIATED WITH CHRONIC RENAL FAILURE

Erythropoietin is a hormone manufactured mainly by the kidney which is necessary for erythrocyte formation. If the kidneys fail, the level of erythropoietin in the blood falls with resulting anaemia. Epoetin is a genetically engineered human erythropoietin.

The commonest use of epoetin is in patients with anaemia of chronic renal failure, especially in patients on regular dialysis where it has been demonstrated to improve haemoglobin levels and quality of life, as well as reducing or abolishing red cell transfusion dependency for these patients. It is also licensed for the treatment of anaemia associated with cancer chemotherapy, especially platinum-based drug regimens and in myeloma.

Prescription would normally be initiated in a specialist hospital clinic setting and continued in primary care in accordance with an agreed form of shared-care protocol. The dosage depends on the exact preparation given and is usually administered subcutaneously; if necessary it can be given intravenously. Most patients can be trained in self-administration.

Side-effects. There is a dosage-dependent increase in blood pressure and therefore poorly controlled hypertension is an absolute contraindication. It requires immediate treatment and patients or relatives should be told to report headaches or confusion at once. Common side-effects include 'flu-like' symptoms with fever, myalgia and arthralgia. Darbepoetin is a derivative of epoetin which has a longer half-life and may be administered less frequently than epoetin.

IRON OVERLOAD

Iron overload may occur as a result of repeated blood transfusions to treat haemolytic anaemias. Desferrioxamine is used to reduce the iron level. It is a powerful iron-chelating agent which is given by subcutaneous infusion over 8–12 hours, three to seven times a week. The dose should reflect the degree of iron overload. For children starting therapy and who have low iron overload, the dose is usually between 20 and 50 mg/kg daily. Desferrioxamine is also used to treat acute toxicity usually seen in children who have swallowed iron tablets in mistake for sweets. The result of the ingestion of large quantities of iron tablets is severe necrotising gastritis with vomiting, haemorrhage and diarrhoea followed by circulatory collapse.

Iron excretion induced by desferrioxamine is enhanced by administration of ascorbic acid in a dose of 200 mg daily. It should be given separately from food as it also enhances iron absorption.

APLASTIC AND HAEMOLYTIC ANAEMIAS

Aplastic or hypoplastic anaemia is an uncommon disease which is caused by depression of the bone marrow. This may affect the formation and development of the red cells, neutrophils or platelets. In 50% of cases, no causative factors can be found; in the others, exposure to certain drugs/chemicals, ionising radiation or viruses may be linked. Anabolic steroids such as oxymetholone have been used to treat aplastic anaemia, but their effectiveness is unclear although they appear to benefit certain patients. A dose of 2–3 mg/kg is given daily for at least 3–6 months. Virilising effects are seen in females and in children.

Anaemias caused by excessive destruction of red blood cells in the spleen are termed haemolytic anaemias. They are due to either breakdown of red blood cells, which are defective (congenital haemolytic anaemias), or to the effects of poisons or infection (acquired haemolytic anaemias). It should be noted that haemolytic anaemias are uncommon among the indigenous population in the UK. Among the multiracial communities in some of the large inner cities, patients with haemolytic anaemia are encountered more frequently. Conditions such as sickle-cell anaemia and thalassaemia are associated with a haemolytic process. Where possible the underlying cause should be treated. Splenectomy may be necessary in some cases of haemolytic anaemia.

In either hypoplastic or haemolytic anaemia, red cell transfusions, platelet transfusions and antibiotics may be given as supportive therapy, and bone marrow transplantation may be considered in severe cases if the patient is under 40 and a compatible sibling donor is available.

Corticosteroids have an important part to play in the management of autoimmune haemolytic anaemias. Oral prednisolone is the first-line treatment for autoimmune haemolytic anaemia. This should only be prescribed in general practice after specialist advice and following confirmation of the diagnosis.

There are numerous secondary causes of autoimmune haemolytic anaemia, particularly lymphoproliferative disease, and any suspected case should be referred to a haematologist for investigation and follow-up.

Glucocorticoids quickly slow or stop haemolysis in two-thirds of patients. For severe disease, up to 60 mg of prednisolone can be given daily. Once haemoglobin stabilises, prednisolone may be tapered to 15–20 mg daily and continued for 2–3 months before tapering off entirely.

It is advisable to consider cover with H_2-antagonists to reduce gastric side-effects. For patients requiring long periods on steroid therapy, the prophylactic use of bisphosphonates to protect against steroid-induced osteoporosis is indicated.

The appearance of adverse effects is related to the duration of treatment and the dosage used. Gastrointestinal disturbances are common and, at daily doses of 15 mg and over, there is an increased risk of peptic ulceration. Salt and water retention may precipitate heart failure, particularly in the elderly. Steroid-induced hypokalaemia may require potassium supplementation.

With long-term treatment, features of Cushing's syndrome may develop, namely moon-face, bruising, hirsutism, impaired glucose tolerance, hypertension, acne, weight gain, osteoporosis and an increased susceptibility to infections. Mental disturbances can occur including any kind of mood change.

ANAEMIA IN PREGNANCY

Pregnancy increases the requirement for iron by approximately 2 mg daily, and a pregnant woman therefore needs 3–4 mg of iron per day. A normal diet contains 10–15 mg of iron.

There is no clear consensus on the use of supplementary iron in pregnancy. Pregnant women who are otherwise healthy do not need routine iron supplements. In women who are at risk of anaemia from previous menorrhagia or poor nutrition, prophylactic iron supplements should be recommended.

Folate supplements are in use for the increased demands of pregnancy. To avoid megaloblastic anaemia in late pregnancy, supplements are advised for those particularly at risk, e.g. with inadequate diet or for a twin pregnancy.

It has also been shown that administration of folate in the periconceptual period reduces the number of neural tube defects by 75%. For the prevention of a first occurrence of neural tube defects, 400 micrograms of folic acid is recommended daily before conception and then during the first trimester.

DRUGS USED IN NEUTROPENIA

Factors which stimulate the growth of white blood cells are used to reduce the risks of infection in patients where white blood cells have been depressed by cancer chemotherapy, bone marrow transplantation and treatments for HIV infection. Human granulocyte-colony stimulating factor (filgrastim and lenograstim) given by subcutaneous or intravenous injection stimulates the production of neutrophils. Human granulocyte–macrophage-colony stimulating factor (molgramcostim) also stimulates the production of white cells in the blood (granulocytes and monocytes). These factors are administered daily either by subcutaneous injection or intravenous infusion until the neutrophil count is in normal range, or for a maximum number of days depending on which product is being used for which condition.

FURTHER READING

Cannaby A-M, Evans L, Freeman A 2002 Nursing care of patients with nasogastric tubes. British Journal of Nursing 11(6):366–372

Manning E 2002 Management of vitamin and mineral deficiencies. Prescriber 13(3):43–64

Murphy A, Scott A 2000 Artificial nutritional support – what are the options. Hospital Pharmacist 7:146–153

Smith S, McCarthy H 1998 Guide to the investigation and treatment of anaemia. Prescriber 9(21):37–64

Smith S, McCarthy H 2000 Guide to the recommended use of drugs in anaemia. Prescriber 11(12):77–90

Thomson E C, Naysmith M R, Lindsay A 2000 Managing drug therapy in patients receiving enteral and parenteral nutrition. Hospital Pharmacist 7:153–163

CHAPTER CONTENTS

25

Drug treatment of musculoskeletal and joint diseases

ANATOMY AND PHYSIOLOGY

Movement of the bony framework results from the contraction of muscles at the joints. Although some joints (e.g. vertebral joints) have only slight movement caused by compression of cartilage, the majority of joints in the body (e.g. the hip joint) are freely movable as the result of the contraction of muscles surrounding them and are known as synovial joints (Fig. 25.1).

The characteristics common to all synovial joints are outlined in Table 25.1.

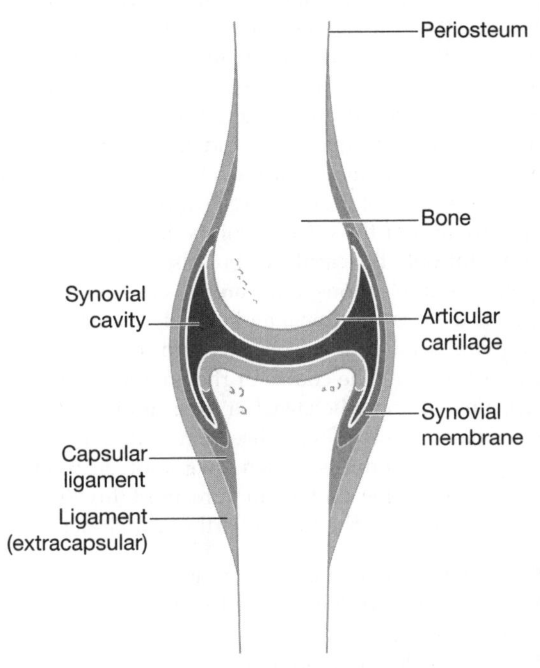

Figure 25.1 Synovial joint.

Table 25.1 Characteristics of a synovial joint	
Capsular ligament	A surrounding fibrous sleeve which joins the bones together, protects the joint without hindering movement
Articular cartilage	A smooth surface on the parts of the bones in contact, allowing free articulation of the joint
Synovial membrane	A layer of cells secreting a thick fluid known as synovial fluid, which lubricates the joint, holds the bones in close proximity to one another and provides nourishment for the structures within the joint cavity. As well as lining the capsule, synovial membrane covers the bony surfaces within the joint not covered by articular cartilage
Other structures	Many joints have ligaments continuous with the capsule which provide further stability Muscles or muscle tendons stretch across the joint Movement of bones occurs when the muscle contracts and thus shortens Joint structures and the muscles involved are supplied by both nerves and blood vessels

RHEUMATOID ARTHRITIS

Rheumatoid arthritis affects approximately 1% of the population and is more common in women than men. It is a chronic inflammatory autoimmune disease affecting the synovial membrane. It occurs most commonly between the ages of 40 and 60, but may afflict people of any age. In affected joints, the synovium becomes thickened, the amount of synovial fluid increases and the ligaments and tissues around the joint become inflamed, causing a build-up of pressure within the joint. Granulation tissue forms on the articular cartilages of the affected joints. In time this may erode not only the cartilages but also bone and even ligaments and tendons in the area. As the disease progresses there is additional and cumulative damage to the joints, leading to increasing deformity, pain and loss of function. The course of rheumatoid arthritis is variable and unpredictable, but for a significant number of patients it is a severe disease resulting in persistent pain and stiffness, progressive joint destruction, functional decline and premature mortality. Typical clinical features of rheumatoid arthritis include:

- joint pain, swelling and tenderness
- stiffness following inactivity (often worse in the morning)
- systemic 'flu'-like symptoms
- synovitis
- extra-articular features.

Another autoimmune inflammatory arthritic disease is ankylosing spondylitis, in which the sacroiliac and vertebral joints become ossified.

Management of rheumatoid arthritis

Curative treatment, though highly desirable, has yet to be achieved. At present the goals of management in rheumatoid arthritis are to relieve pain, stiffness and swelling, to prevent disease progression and deformities, to improve morbidity and function of joints and as far as possible to maintain the patient's normal lifestyle.

Drug treatment is only one element of the overall management, which should also involve a combination of interventions including exercise, physiotherapy, occupational therapy, education, emotional support and rest. The management plan can be individualised, based on considerations such as joint function, degree of disease activity, the patient's age, gender, occupation and response to previous therapy.

General measures

There are many general measures which can be used to help patients with rheumatoid arthritis. Education plays a vital role. Provision of information on the disease and its therapies gives patients a realistic outlook and allows them to be involved in therapeutic decisions. Education also emphasises the role of patients in controlling their own disease.

Because much of the pain and stiffness associated with rheumatoid arthritis comes from periarticular tissues, such as muscle and tendons, physiotherapists can advise on exercises and mobilisation techniques which can be tailored to the needs and capabilities of individual patients. Use of hydrotherapy may also help to improve mobility and general fitness as well as maintaining muscle bulk around the joints.

Occupational therapists can provide appliances and devices to help patients with the activities of daily living. These include, for example, support rails and adaptors for keys and taps. In addition to educating patients on their drug therapy, pharmacists can provide a range of devices which may assist compliance, such as Haleraids and wing caps on tablet bottles.

The role of the dietitian is also important. Some trials have suggested a consistent but modest benefit from the inclusion of fish oil, fish supplements or evening primrose oil in the diet. Various elimination diets have also been proposed. A diet which involves avoiding red meat, dairy products, fruit, herbs, additives and preservatives is popular with patients.

Joint replacement has been one of the greatest advances in the management of rheumatoid arthritis. Other surgical procedures that are beneficial include tendon transfers (manipulation to reduce deformity) and synovectomy (removal of the synovial membrane, which is often undertaken in patients with rheumatoid arthritis of the knee). Function may be greatly improved after tendon transfer, particularly in the hand. Although used less frequently, synovectomy can usefully debulk a synovial mass, resulting in reduced pain.

Treatment of rheumatoid arthritis

Rheumatoid arthritis should be treated as early as possible with disease-modifying antirheumatic drugs (DMARDs) to control symptoms and delay disease progression. All patients with persistent inflammatory joint disease of greater than 6–8 weeks' duration, already receiving simple analgesics and non-steroidal anti-inflammatory drugs (NSAIDs), should be considered for referral for specialist rheumatology opinion and DMARD therapy, preferably within 12 weeks. Early and sustained treatment with disease-modifying anti-rheumatic drugs slows erosive joint destruction and improves long-term disease outcome (see Table 25.2).

Mode of action. The precise mechanism of action of these drugs is unclear. All the DMARDs inhibit the release, or reduce the activity, of inflammatory cytokines. Activated T lymphocytes appear to be particularly important in this process and it is known that methotrexate and ciclosporin both inhibit T cells.

Use of DMARDs. Early DMARD therapy in rheumatoid arthritis is important to maintain function and reduce later disability. DMARD therapy should be sustained in inflammatory disease in order to maintain disease suppression. DMARD choice should take into account patient preference and existing co-morbidity. Patients should be counselled about the benefits and risks of specific DMARDs and should be provided with additional written information. Clear advice about monitoring of specific DMARDs should be available to the patient, GP and practice nurse. Good liaison between primary and secondary care is essential. Rheumatology nurse specialists have an important role in this aspect of care.

Sulfasalazine, methotrexate, intramuscular gold and penicillamine have a comparable clinical effect on disease activity but the first two are the current DMARDs of choice because of their more favourable efficacy and toxicity profiles. Hydroxychloroquine and auranofin (oral gold) are relatively weak DMARDs with a slower onset of action. Successive DMARDs are required for most patients in the medium to long term.

Tumour necrosis factor (TNF) blockade

DMARDs often produce only delayed, inadequate or temporary responses or troublesome unwanted effects. Drugs that block the effects of TNF offer a novel approach. TNF is a product of macrophages which acts on the immune system to induce the production of powerful pro-inflammatory mediators. Etanercept (twice weekly subcutaneous injections) and infliximab (given by infusion) are selective immunosuppressants which inhibit the activity of tumour necrosis factor. They are used for the treatment of highly active rheumatoid arthritis in adults who have failed to respond to at least two standard DMARDs. Etanercept or infliximab should be used under specialist supervision and withdrawn if there is no response after 3 months. Infliximab must be given concomitantly with methotrexate.

Analgesia

Analgesics in early rheumatoid arthritis are used as an adjunct to non-steroidal anti-inflammatory drugs (NSAIDs) and DMARDs. Paracetamol, codeine and combination medications containing paracetamol are effective in reducing pain in rheumatoid arthritis. Simple analgesics should be used in place of NSAIDs if possible and DMARDs should be introduced early to suppress disease activity.

Non-steroidal anti-inflammatory drugs

NSAIDs are effective and provide symptomatic relief of pain and stiffness without influencing the progression of rheumatoid arthritis. NSAIDs have anti-inflammatory, analgesic and antipyretic properties.

It is believed that NSAIDs produce their anti-inflammatory effect by inhibition of prostaglandin synthesis. There are over 20 different naturally occurring prostaglandins which are widely distributed throughout the body since they are synthesised by virtually every tissue. Prostaglandins are formed in the body by the enzymatic oxygenation of arachidonic acid and linoleic acid, the enzyme involved being cyclo-oxygenase (COX) (Fig. 25.2). Prostaglandins are very potent chemicals with a broad range of activities which include:

- inhibition of gastric acid secretion
- bronchial relaxation
- vasodilator and hypotensive activity, including control of blood flow through the renal medulla
- mediation of some aspects of inflammation
- contraction of the iris.

In rheumatoid arthritis it appears that control over the balanced production of prostaglandins is, to some

Table 25.2 DMARD profiles

Drug	Dose	Common minor side-effects	Rarer severe side-effects	Monitoring requirements	Advantages
Azathioprine	1–2.5 mg/kg per day	Nausea, hair loss	Leucopenia, sepsis, hypersensitivity reactions including malaise, dizziness, jaundice, rash – immediately withdraw	FBC, U and Es and LFTs weekly for first 4 weeks, then at least every 3 months	
Ciclosporin	2.5 mg/kg per day to a maximum of 4 mg/kg per day	Paraesthesia, tremor, fatigue, hypertrichosis, gingival hypertrophy	Hypertension, renal disease	Fortnightly U and Es, blood pressure and urinalysis for 2 months, then monthly thereafter. Use baseline creatinine to alter dose	
Hydroxychloroquine	Initially 400 mg daily in divided doses, maintenance 400 mg daily	GI disturbances, headache, rashes	Retinal toxicity	Assess renal and liver function before treatment	No blood monitoring required
Leflunomide	Initially 100 mg once daily for 3 days, then maintenance dose of 10–20 mg once daily	Alopecia, diarrhoea, nausea, rash	Leucopenia, thrombocytopenia hepatitis	FBC, U and Es, LFTs and blood pressure every 2 weeks for 6 months, then every 8 weeks. Exclude pregnancy before treatment, effective contraception essential during treatment	Therapeutic effect starts after 4–6 weeks and improvement may continue for a further 4–6 months
Methotrexate	7.5–20 mg once weekly	Nausea, diarrhoea, mouth ulcers, rash, abnormal LFTs, alopecia	Leucopenia/ thrombocytopenia pneumonitis, liver cirrhosis	FBC fortnightly for 23 weeks, then LFTs and plasma creatinine every 4–8 weeks	Rapid onset of action (6–10 weeks), can be given orally, IM or SC, weekly administration aids compliance
Penicillamine	125–750 mg once daily before food	Nausea, rashes, temporary loss of taste, reversible fall in platelet count	Proteinuria	FBC fortnightly until stable dose, then 4-weekly. Weekly urinalysis	
Sodium aurothiomalate	10 mg test dose to exclude hypersensitivity, then 50 mg weekly until signs of remission, then dose interval increased to weeks. Discontinue if no remission after 1 g	Mouth ulcers, rash	Thrombocytopenia/ leucopenia, proteinuria, colitis	FBC and urinalysis prior to each injection	
Sulfasalazine	Initially 500 mg daily, increasing in weekly steps of 500 mg to a maximum of 2–3 g daily in divided doses	Nausea, diarrhoea, headache, rashes, reversible oligospermia, staining soft contact lenses, abnormal LFTs	Leucopenia	FBC fortnightly, LFTs every 4 weeks for 12 weeks, then every 3–6 months	Rapid onset of action (8–12 weeks)

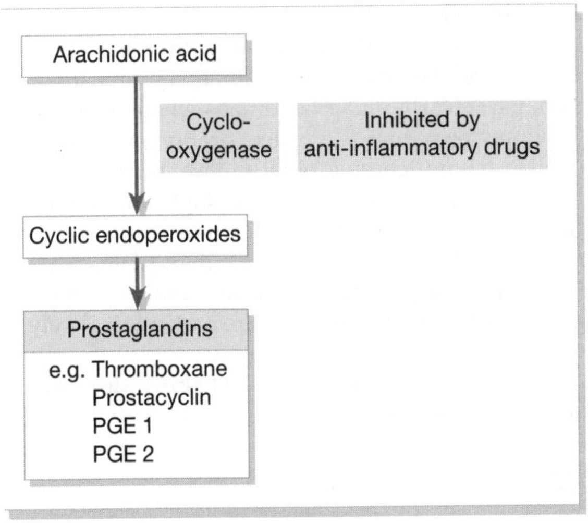

Figure 25.2 Formation of prostaglandins.

extent, lost and this results in excessive production of prostaglandins involved in inflammation. Administration of NSAIDs blocks the action of the enzyme cyclo-oxygenase, which effectively reduces the synthesis of prostaglandins. The therapeutic outcome is a reduction in pain, tenderness, swelling and temperature in the affected joints, decreased stiffness and increased joint movement.

Patient response to NSAIDs is highly variable, and therapeutic trials with several NSAIDs may be necessary to determine the best agent. It is estimated that 60% of patients will respond to any one NSAID. The drug should be changed after 1 week if there has been no response and an analgesic effect is the desired outcome or after 3 weeks if an anti-inflammatory effect is desired. Approximately 10% of patients will not find any NSAID beneficial.

There are over 20 NSAIDs available and Table 25.3 gives a selection of these. Ibuprofen is the most commonly used first-line agent as it combines good efficacy with fewer side-effects than other NSAIDs but its anti-inflammatory properties are weaker. Naproxen is also a good choice as it combines good efficacy with a low incidence of side-effects (but more than ibuprofen) and administration is only twice daily. Diclofenac has actions and side-effects similar to naproxen. Fenoprofen is as effective as naproxen, and flurbiprofen may be slightly more effective. Both are associated with slightly greater gastrointestinal side-effects than ibuprofen. Azapropazone produces a similar effect to naproxen but is associated with a high incidence of gastrointestinal side-effects. For this reason its use is restricted to rheumatoid arthritis, ankylosing spondylitis and acute gout where other NSAIDs have been tried and failed.

Table 25.3 NSAIDs: clinical aspects

NSAID	Plasma elimination half-life (hours)	Dosage
Acemetacin	4–5	60 mg twice daily
Azapropazone	12–14	600 mg twice daily; maximum dose in elderly: 300 mg twice daily (licensed only for rheumatoid arthritis, ankylosing spondylitis and acute gout where other therapies have failed)
Diclofenac	1–2	50 mg three times daily
Fenbufen	10–17	300 mg in the morning, 600 mg at bedtime
Fenoprofen	3	600 mg three times daily
Flurbiprofen	3–4	50 mg three times daily
Ibuprofen	2	400 mg four times daily
Indometacin	4–5	50 mg three times daily
Ketoprofen	2	100 mg twice daily
Mefenamic acid	2–4	500 mg three times daily
Nabumetone	24	1 g daily at bedtime
Naproxen	14	500 mg twice daily
Piroxicam	45	20 mg daily; maximum 14 days for acute musculoskeletal disorders
Sulindac	16	200 mg twice daily
Tiaprofenic acid	1.5–2	200 mg three times daily

Side-effects of NSAIDs. Toxicity is a major factor and side-effects are related to dose and duration of therapy. Common side-effects (especially in the elderly) are gastrointestinal toxicity, fluid retention and hypertension. Other less common but potentially serious side-effects are renal disease and hypersensitivity (including asthma). Uncommon and not usually serious side-effects are headaches, dizziness, tinnitus, rash (particularly with fenbufen) and abnormal LFTs (particularly with diclofenac).

Gastrointestinal toxicity

The use of NSAIDs is associated with gastrointestinal (GI) toxicity. The following side-effects occur to a varying extent with all preparations and all routes of administration:

- dyspepsia
- gastric erosions
- peptic ulceration

- small bowel inflammation and bleeding
- perforation
- haematemesis or melaena
- occult GI blood loss and anaemia.

The annual relative risk of mortality attributed to NSAID-related GI adverse effects is four times that for those not using NSAIDs. The rate of NSAID-related serious GI complications requiring hospitalisation has decreased in recent years. The reason for this is likely to be multifactorial. Intensive education programmes have alerted physicians and patients to the use of newer, less toxic NSAIDs and non-NSAID analgesics in populations at high risk. There has also been a much wider use of gastroprotective therapy (Box 25.1).

Risk factors for NSAID-associated gastroduodenal ulcers are list in Box 25.2.

It is important to note that the use of an enteric-coated, parenteral or rectal NSAID preparation is *not* protective. The systemic effects of NSAIDs are the predominant cause of damage.

Box 25.1 Summary of gastroprotective agents in rheumatoid arthritis

- Proton pump inhibitors (PPIs) – most effective
- Prostaglandin analogues – effective, but less well tolerated than PPIs and a problem in premenopausal women
- Histamine H_2-receptor antagonists – less effective than PPIs
- Mucosal protective agents (e.g. sucralfate) – less effective than PPIs

Box 25.2 Risk factors for NSAID-associated gastroduodenal ulcers

Definite risk factors
- Advanced age (*linear increase in risk*)
- History of ulcer
- Higher doses of NSAIDs
- Combination use of NSAIDs
- Concomitant use of corticosteroids
- Co-morbidity

Possible lifestyle factors
- Cigarette smoking
- Alcohol consumption

Every possible strategy should be employed to minimise risks of GI-related toxicity, e.g. smoking cessation and alcohol reduction.

If NSAID use is unavoidable, gastroprotective agents may be used, as summarised in Box 25.1

Renal toxicity

NSAID use is also associated with renal disease. Prostaglandins regulate and maintain intrarenal perfusion, particularly under conditions where renal blood flow may be reduced (e.g. dehydration or blood loss, cardiac failure, chronic renal failure, diuretic use or hypertension). By inhibiting prostaglandin synthesis under these conditions, NSAIDs may further impair intrarenal blood flow contributing to renal impairment (or overt renal failure), hyperkalaemia, oedema and hypertension. These problems are particularly likely in the elderly.

Strategies to minimise the risk of NSAID toxicity are summarised in Box 25.3.

COX-2 selective agents

NSAIDs act by direct inhibition of COX-1 and COX-2, via blockade of the COX enzyme site. The subsequent inhibition of prostaglandins reduces inflammation but also has collateral effects on platelet aggregation, renal homeostasis and gastric mucosal integrity. In an effort to reduce the side-effects of NSAIDs, particularly GI side-effects, agents have been developed that selectively block COX-2, with minimal effect on COX-1.

There are four COX-2 selective agents available: etodolac, meloxicam, celecoxib and rofecoxib. Etodolac and meloxicam inhibit COX-2 up to 50 times more than COX-1, and newer agents celecoxib and rofecoxib are even more COX-2 selective (see Table 25.4).

COX-2 selective agents are recommended for use in patients who are at high risk of developing GI side-effects but they are not recommended for routine

Box 25.3 Summary of strategies to minimise the risk of NSAID toxicity

- The lowest NSAID dose compatible with symptom relief should be prescribed.
- NSAIDs should be reduced and if possible withdrawn when a good response to DMARDs is achieved.
- Simple analgesics should be used in place of NSAIDs if possible and DMARDs should be introduced early to suppress disease activity.
- Only one NSAID should be prescribed at a time.
- Introduce gastroprotection in rheumatoid arthritis patients >65 years and in those with a past history of peptic ulcer.
- Consider intra-articular steroids, particularly when disease is localised.
- NSAIDs should be avoided in patients taking anticoagulants or corticosteroids.

Table 25.4 COX-2 selective agents

Drug	Dose
Etodolac	600 mg daily
Celecoxib	200–400 mg in divided doses
Meloxicam	7.5–15 mg daily
Rofecoxib	12.5–25 mg daily

use. Those at high risk are:

- patients over 65 years of age
- patients who are taking medicines known to increase the likelihood of upper GI side-effects (for example, corticosteroids and anticoagulants)
- patients with serious co-morbidities such as cardiovascular disease, renal or hepatic impairment, diabetes and hypertension
- patients requiring prolonged treatment with high doses of NSAIDs.

There is no justification for prescribing a COX-2 selective agent in combination with gastroprotective agents.

Aspirin and salicylates

Aspirin as an anti-inflammatory analgesic largely takes second place to NSAIDs. The required dose of aspirin for active inflammatory joint disease is at least 3.6 g daily. Gastrointestinal side-effects such as nausea, dyspepsia and gastrointestinal bleeding may occur with any dosage but anti-inflammatory doses are associated with a much higher incidence of side-effects.

Owing to an association with Reye's syndrome, aspirin-containing preparations should not be given to children under 16 years, unless specifically indicated, e.g. for juvenile arthritis.

Benorilate is a paracetamol–aspirin combination ester and may be useful in patients experiencing dyspepsia with other NSAIDs. Side-effects include tinnitus, dizziness and mental confusion.

Corticosteroids

Systemic corticosteroids have long been used in the management of rheumatoid arthritis and were the first drugs to result in reversibility of the disease. However, their place in therapy is still controversial.

Corticosteroids suppress cytokines and produce a rapid improvement in signs and symptoms of the disease. They have a potent anti-inflammatory effect. Unfortunately, the side-effects associated with long-term, high-dose therapy (for example osteoporosis, diabetes mellitus, hypertension and peptic ulceration) have severely limited the long-term role of corticosteroids in rheumatoid arthritis.

Place in therapy. Oral prednisolone can be used to provide temporary relief until a DMARD becomes effective or in patients with aggressive disease whose pain cannot be adequately controlled with a combination of DMARDs ('step-up' or 'step-down' approach). Once commenced, systemic corticosteroids can be difficult to withdraw, as the disease tends to flare with dose reductions.

In order to minimise side-effects, a daily maintenance dose of 7.5 mg of prednisolone, or less, given as a single dose in the morning, should be used.

Oral corticosteroids are not recommended for routine use as there is no sustained clinical or functional benefit and there is a high risk of toxicity with long-term use. The lowest possible dose of corticosteroid should be used for the shortest possible time. Oral corticosteroids should be withdrawn slowly to avoid rebound flare of symptoms. Patients should be warned of the risks of corticosteroids at the outset and issued with a steroid warning card. They should be monitored closely for side-effects such as diabetes, cataract and infection. There should be adequate prophylaxis and treatment of osteoporosis in patients taking oral corticosteroids.

Intra-articular steroid administration can effectively relieve pain, increase mobility and reduce deformity in one or more joints. Examples of drugs that are given via this route are methylprednisolone acetate, triamcinolone acetonide and triamcinolone hexacetonide. The duration of response to intra-articular steroids is variable and triamcinolone hexacetonide may produce the greatest response. The dose used is dependent upon the joint size. Methylprednisolone acetate 40 mg or triamcinolone hexacetonide 20 mg are suitable for use in large joints (for example, knees).

Intra-articular injections can be used for rapid and sometimes sustained symptomatic relief in target joints. Intra-articular injections to any one joint should not be given more than three times in 1 year. When intra-articular injections are being administered

- a sterile technique should be used
- patients should be advised to seek help if the joint fails to settle after injection.

OSTEOARTHRITIS

This is a degenerative non-inflammatory disease. Articular cartilage gradually becomes thinner because its replacement does not keep pace with its removal. Bone, formed at the margin of the articular cartilage, enlarges and may deform the affected joints and interfere with movement. Involvement of the knee, hip or other joints may become a major disability requiring surgical replacement.

Non-drug therapy

Patients who are overweight should be encouraged to lose weight so as to reduce stress on their joints and to increase their mobility. This strategy is particularly beneficial in patients with osteoarthritis of the knee.

Physiotherapists contribute significantly to management by advising on exercises tailored to the patient's needs, which can help to preserve the function of the joint as well as protect it from further damage.

Physiotherapy can also help patients regain muscle strength around weakened joints, improve the range of movement of affected joints and enhance general well-being. It is vital that patients are given a clear explanation of the nature of their disease, methods of management and likely prognosis as soon as osteoarthritis is diagnosed. This will help them to come to terms with the disease, understand how it will affect their life and how they can work with healthcare professionals to manage their condition. Providing social contact and access to telephone helplines allows patients to discuss their disease (with other patients, therapists and support groups) and share experiences, which can also effectively improve symptoms.

Drug therapy

Simple analgesics. Pain is the main reason why patients with osteoarthritis seek help from healthcare professionals. However, drug treatment is an adjunct and not a substitute for other types of treatment. As osteoarthritis has only a minor inflammatory component, paracetamol is now accepted as first-line therapy in uncomplicated osteoarthritis. It can be taken in a regular full dosage (up to 4 g daily) or on an 'as required' basis.

The effect of compound analgesics, which are commonly prescribed for osteoarthritis, is often disappointing as many contain subtherapeutic doses of opioids. However, preparations with a full dose of the opioid component often cause unwanted side-effects, such as constipation, especially in elderly patients. Analgesics such as co-proxamol are generally thought to be no more effective than paracetamol alone and are probably best avoided as they may be particularly hazardous in overdose.

Oral non-steroidal anti-inflammatory drugs (NSAIDs). Osteoarthritis is primarily a non-inflammatory disease. NSAIDs are frequently prescribed. NSAIDs should be reserved for patients whose symptoms are not controlled by other means or to manage acute exacerbations that are associated with inflammation.

Individual choice should be based on relative safety, patient acceptability and cost. Ibuprofen therefore should be used first-line because of its good safety profile and low cost. Secondly, not all NSAIDs are licensed to treat osteoarthritis. For example, because of its high level of side-effects, azapropazone is no longer licensed for osteoarthritis and meloxicam is only licensed for short-term treatment of acute exacerbations. Thirdly, the usefulness of NSAIDs is limited by their side-effects. These can be a particular problem in the elderly or in those with poor renal function. If it is absolutely essential to use an NSAID in an elderly patient or in a patient with a previous history of peptic ulceration, the concurrent administration of an H_2 antagonist, misoprostol or a proton pump inhibitor should always be considered.

In patients with renal insufficiency, NSAIDs should be avoided whenever possible or used in very low doses if the benefits are expected to outweigh the risks. In such cases, serum creatinine, urea and electrolytes must be monitored regularly.

Topical NSAIDs. A wide range of topical NSAIDs is available in a variety of formulations, such as gels, foams, creams, ointments and sprays. These products are promoted on the basis that they diffuse rapidly and directly into joints. This is claimed to result in high local and low plasma concentrations of the drug and theoretically gives a lower risk of systemic side-effects than oral NSAIDs.

GOUT

This is characterised by higher than normal levels of uric acid in the blood because of either overproduction or defective excretion by the kidneys. Uric acid is a waste product of the breakdown of cell nuclei and is produced in excess when there is large-scale cell destruction, e.g. following trauma, malignancy, treatment with cytotoxic drugs and starvation. The excess uric acid forms sodium urate crystals which are deposited in joints and tendons. Acute inflammation is due to substances released by phagocytes that have ingested the crystals. The joints most commonly affected are in the big toe, ankle, knee, wrist and elbow.

Clinical presentation

Acute gout often presents as a hot, red, swollen, exquisitely painful and tender joint. This may be associated with fever, leucocytosis (raised number of leucocytes) and raised erythrocyte sedimentation rate (ESR). Lower limbs are most commonly affected including the metatarsophalangeal joints (at the base of the toe), ankles and knees, but the wrist and small joints of the hand can also be affected. Ninety percent of initial attacks are monoarticular and most resolve spontaneously within a few days. Symptom-free intervals occur between attacks but subsequent attacks tend to be more severe, longer in duration and often involve additional joints.

Chronic tophaceous gout can develop after several years of acute attacks with progressive damage to cartilage, periarticular bony erosions evident on X-rays and deposition of tophi leading to disability. Tophi are amorphous deposits of uric acid and can appear either in association with acute gouty attacks or in a more chronic form. Tophi can develop in cartilage, synovium, bursae or tendon sheaths and are commoner in previously damaged joints.

There is an increasing tendency for the development of tophaceous gout in the elderly, particularly women on diuretics. The onset may be insidious without acute attacks and there may be confusion with osteoarthritis as it often affects the distal interphalangeal joints.

Treatment

The therapeutic approach to gout entails two phases. Firstly, the elimination of pain and joint inflammation. Secondly, the reduction of blood uric acid levels to normal and the resorption of tophaceous deposits. Acute attacks of gout are usually treated with NSAIDs such as diclofenac, indometacin, ketoprofen, naproxen, piroxicam or sulindac (see Table 25.3). The use of azapropazone should be restricted to patients in whom less-toxic drugs have become ineffective, but is contraindicated in patients with a known history of peptic ulcer disease. A beneficial effect can be observed within hours of ingesting an NSAID but an attack may take several days to resolve completely. Severe pain intensity may warrant concurrent use of analgesics such as paracetamol or codeine.

Colchicine is probably as effective as NSAIDs. Its therapeutic effect is due to immobilising polymorphonuclear leucocytes arriving at the acutely inflamed joint so that they enter the joint in fewer numbers, resulting in less phagocytosis of urate crystals and release of lysosomal enzymes into the joint. 1 mg of colchicine is given initially followed by 500 micrograms every 2–3 hours until relief of pain is obtained, or vomiting or diarrhoea occurs, or until a total dose of 6 mg has been reached. The course should not be repeated within 3 days.

Most common side-effects are nausea, vomiting and abdominal pain. The use of colchicine is limited by the development of toxicity at higher doses but it is of value in patients with heart failure since, unlike NSAIDs, it does not induce fluid retention. Moreover, it can be given to patients receiving anticoagulants.

Long-term control of gout

Patients who are obese should be encouraged to lose weight and those who overindulge in alcohol should be encouraged to consider the risks. This is on the basis that there is a good correlation between the level of uric acid and body weight and also excessive alcohol intake since alcohol stimulates purine synthesis in the liver which breaks down to form uric acid. Long-term management and prophylaxis of gout can be achieved in two ways:

- blocking the production of uric acid by the administration of a xanthine-oxidase inhibitor such as allopurinol
- increasing the excretion of uric acid by the administration of a uricosuric drug such as probenecid or sulfinpyrazone.

Frequent recurrence of acute attacks of gout may call for the initiation of long-term ('interval') treatment. For long-term control of gout the formation of uric acid from purines may be reduced with the xanthine-oxidase inhibitor allopurinol, or the uricosuric drug sulfinpyrazone may be used to increase the excretion of uric acid in the urine (see Table 25.5). Treatment should be continued indefinitely to prevent further attacks of gout by correcting the hyperuricaemia. These drugs should never be started during an acute attack. The initiation

Table 25.5 Drugs used to treat gout

Drug	Dose	Side-effects
Allopurinol	Initially 100 mg daily after food. Maintenance (mild conditions) 100–200 mg daily; in moderately severe conditions 300–600 mg daily; in severe conditions 600–900 mg daily	Rashes – withdraw therapy; if rash mild, reintroduce cautiously but discontinue immediately if recurrence
Sulfinpyrazone	Initially 100–200 mg daily with food, increasing over 2–3 weeks to 600 mg daily until serum uric acid levels normal, then reduced to maintenance dose of 200–300 mg daily	GI disturbances occasionally, allergic skin reactions

of treatment may precipitate an acute attack and therefore colchicine or an anti-inflammatory analgesic should be used as a prophylactic and continued for at least 1 month after the hyperuricaemia has been corrected (usually about 3 months of prophylaxis). However, if an acute attack develops during treatment, then the treatment should continue at the same dosage and the acute attack should be treated in its own right.

Allopurinol is a well-tolerated drug which is widely used. It is especially useful in patients with renal impairment or urate stones where uricosuric drugs cannot be used; it is *not* indicated for the treatment of asymptomatic hyperuricaemia. It is usually given once daily, since the active metabolite of allopurinol has a long half-life, but doses over 300 mg daily should be divided. It may occasionally cause rashes.

Sulfinpyrazone can be used instead of allopurinol or in conjunction with it in cases that are resistant to treatment.

Drugs causing hyperuricaemia and gout

Certain drugs can precipitate an attack of gout:

- Thiazide and loop diuretics can precipitate an attack of gout by inhibiting the tubular secretion of uric acid.
- Aspirin in low doses inhibits the tubular secretion of uric acid.
- Cytotoxic drugs causing a high rate of cell kill may increase purine production with a consequent increase in the production of uric acid which may result in an acute attack of gout.

MYASTHENIA GRAVIS

Neuromuscular transmission depends on the release of acetylcholine from the nerve terminal. This is followed by an interaction between the neurotransmitter acetylcholine and receptor sites on the postsynaptic membrane. This results in an action potential being triggered, leading to muscle contraction.

Myasthenia gravis is an acquired autoimmune disorder involving the production of antibodies to the acetylcholine receptors at the neuromuscular junction. Acetylcholine is therefore blocked at nerve endings and this leads to muscle weakness affecting more commonly the external ocular muscles causing ptosis (drooping of the eyelid) and diplopia (double vision), the bulbar muscles causing dysphagia (difficulty in swallowing) or indistinct speech and occasionally aphasia (inability to speak). Neck and shoulder muscles may also be affected such that patients have difficulty holding up the head and raising the arms. Limb muscles may be affected and movement restricted. These symptoms may be exacerbated by emotional disturbances, strenuous exercise and pregnancy. The condition has a remitting and relapsing course.

Test for myasthenia gravis

Acetylcholine is broken down by the enzyme acetylcholinesterase. If acetylcholinesterase is inhibited, the concentration of acetylcholine at the motor end-plate rises and its action is potentiated. Inhibition of acetylcholinesterase results in an increase in the concentration of acetylcholine at the neuromuscular junction, thus overcoming the reduction in functioning receptors. Edrophonium chloride is an acetylcholinesterase inhibitor (anticholinesterase) with a very short duration of action and is used to test for the presence of myasthenia gravis where antibody assays are not available or the titre is normal. In patients with muscle weakness when fatigued, a raised serum titre of antibody to acetylcholine receptors (present in about 85% of cases) establishes a firm diagnosis. For more immediate diagnosis and in seronegative tests an intravenous edrophonium chloride test can be done.

A test dose of edrophonium chloride 2 mg intravenously is given, followed 30–60 seconds later (if no adverse drug reaction has occurred) by 8 mg. A positive response, defined as improvement in strength (e.g. recovery of ptosis, increased limb strength or increased vital capacity) will occur within 20–30 seconds of injection and subside after about 3 minutes.

Muscarinic side-effects of anticholinesterases include increased sweating, salivary and gastric secretion, increased gastrointestinal and uterine motility and bradycardia. Adverse effects such as severe bradycardia and cholinergic crisis leading to respiratory arrest occur occasionally. Severe cholinergic reactions can be countered by injection of atropine sulphate, which should always be available. It is recommended that resuscitation equipment is also available and to premedicate with atropine sulphate 0.6 mg intravenously. Edrophonium chloride can also be used to determine over- or under-treatment. In patients overtreated with anticholinesterases, administration will have no effect or it will intensify symptoms. In contrast, undertreated patients will show a transient improvement in muscle power.

Treatment

Anticholinesterases are first-line treatment for myasthenia gravis and provide symptomatic relief. They are of greatest benefit in patients with mild symptoms, often completely correcting weakness in those cases and improving the strength of those moderately affected. Neostigmine can be given orally or by subcutaneous or intramuscular injection and has a maximum duration of action of 4 hours. It has pronounced muscarinic effects (including increased salivation and colic) and may need to be given up to every 2 hours. Pyridostigmine is less powerful and has a slower onset of action but a longer duration of action than neostigmine. It also has less muscarinic side-effects and is therefore the treatment of choice. The usual starting dose of pyridostigmine is 30–60 mg every 4–6 hours. The maximum daily dose is 720 mg. Distigmine has the longest action but the danger of a cholinergic crisis caused by an accumulation of the drug is greater than with shorter-acting drugs.

Adverse effects of these drugs (colic, diarrhoea) can usually be controlled by propantheline 15 mg three times a day and 30 mg at night. Excessive dosages should be avoided because they may impair neuromuscular transmission and precipitate cholinergic crisis. This is due to flooding the neuromuscular junction with acetylcholine, resulting in continual stimulation of postsynaptic acetylcholine receptors. The membrane is not allowed to repolarise, and this results in a depolarising block. In patients taking a high dosage of an anticholinesterase, cholinergic toxicity can be distinguished from myasthenic crisis by the presence of hypersalivation, lacrimation, increased sweating, vomiting and miosis.

SKELETAL MUSCLE RELAXANTS

Patients with various disorders of the musculoskeletal system and of the central nervous system suffer from muscle spasm. This spasm may produce pain and deformity. Treatment with drugs is generally only moderately effective. The drugs used in the treatment of muscle spasticity are diazepam, baclofen, dantrolene and tizanidine. Diazepam has some antispasmodic effect but sedation can be a problem, particularly on higher doses. Baclofen acts at the spinal level similarly to diazepam. Adverse effects such as sedation and hypotonia can be limiting. Dantrolene acts directly on skeletal muscle. It is used in severe spasticity, multiple sclerosis, spinal cord injury and stroke. Dosage should be increased slowly but if no benefit has been obtained after about 6 weeks the drug should be withdrawn. Drowsiness may be a problem if the patient has to drive or operate machinery. Tizanidine is an alpha$_2$-adrenoceptor agonist indicated for spasticity associated with multiple sclerosis or spinal cord injury.

FURTHER READING

Akil M, Amos R S 1995 Rheumatoid arthritis – clinical features and diagnosis. British Medical Journal 310: 587–590

[Anonymous] 2001 Etanercept and infliximab for rheumatoid arthritis. Drug and Therapeutics Bulletin 39: 49–52

Geba G P, Weaver A L, Polis A B et al (2002) Efficacy of rofecoxib, celecoxib and acetaminophen in osteoarthritis of the knee. JAMA 287:64–71

Gibson T 2001 Successful management of acute and chronic gout. Prescriber 12:107–113

Harris A 1996 Management of myasthenia gravis. Pharmacy in Practice 6(9):350–351

National Institute for Clinical Excellence (NICE) 2001 Guidance on the use of cyclo-oxygenase (COX) II selective inhibitors, celecoxib, rofecoxib, meloxicam and etodolac for osteoarthritis and rheumatoid arthritis. Technology Appraisal Guidance – No 27. NICE, London

Parkinson S, Alldred A 2002 Drug regimens for rheumatoid arthritis. Hospital Pharmacist 9:11–15

Platt P 2001 The future of rheumatoid arthritis management. Future Prescriber 2:6–9

Snaith M L 1995 Gout, hyperuricaemia and crystal arthritis. British Medical Journal 310:521–524

Starey N 2001 NSAIDs in the treatment of osteoarthritis. Evidence Based Medicine in Practice:3–9

Wood J 1999 Gout and its management. Pharmaceutical Journal 262:808–811

CHAPTER CONTENTS

26

Drug treatment of eye conditions

ANATOMY AND PHYSIOLOGY

The eye is a spherical organ situated in the orbital cavity whose bony walls and fat help to protect it from damage. The visible part of the eye is only a proportion of the whole, so that the eye is best considered in vertical cross-section viewed from the side (see Fig. 26.1).

The walls are in three layers. The outermost layer is a fibrous coat consisting of the sclera (the white of the eye) covering all but the anterior part of the eye, which is transparent and known as the cornea.

In the middle is a vascular layer which, like the sclera, covers the posterior five-sixths of the eye and is known as the choroid. The anterior sixth comprises the ciliary body, an essential part of the process of accommodation of the eye, and the iris, the pigmented muscular structure which gives the eye its colour and serves, through autonomic nervous stimulation, to control the amount of light entering the eye.

In the centre of the eye is the eyeball which consists of an anterior and a posterior segment separated by the lens. The anterior segment is in turn made up of an anterior chamber and posterior chamber separated by the iris. Both chambers contain a transparent fluid, known as aqueous humour, secreted by the ciliary glands. Aqueous humour circulates from the posterior chamber through the pupil into the anterior chamber and back to the general circulation via the trabecular meshwork and then the canal of Schlemm. In health, the intraocular pressure of fluid remains fairly constant. The remaining larger posterior segment of the eyeball is known as the vitreous body and is filled with a transparent, jelly-like substance which, along with the aqueous fluid, helps keep the shape of the eye.

The eye is protected by accessory organs which include the eyebrows, eyelids and eyelashes, and the lacrimal apparatus.

The lacrimal apparatus (see Fig. 26.2) is essential for the flow of tears. Tears are composed of water, salts and

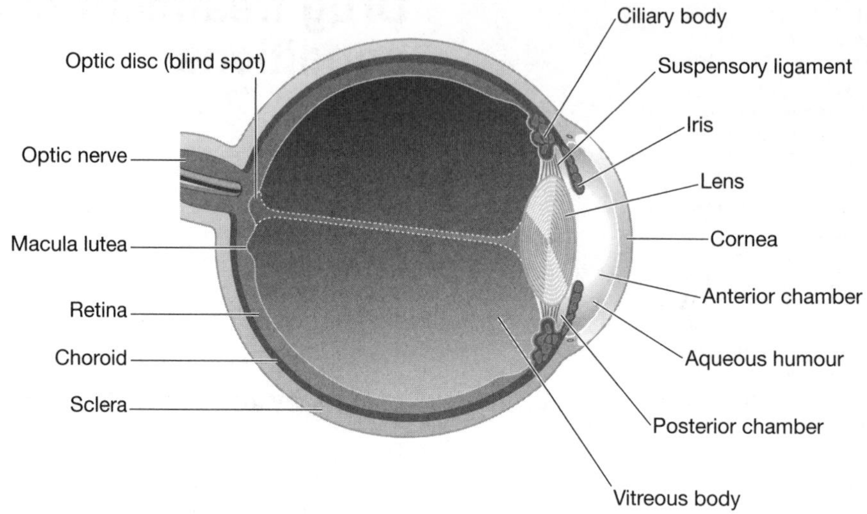

Figure 26.1 The eye.

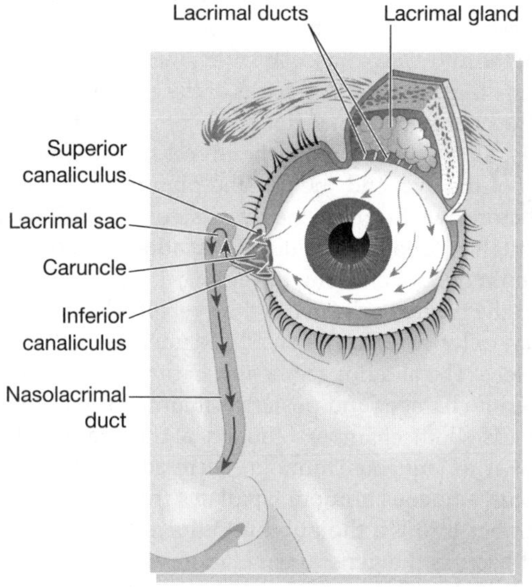

Figure 26.2 The lacrimal apparatus. (From Waugh A, Grant A 2001 Ross and Wilson Anatomy and physiology in health and illness, 9th edn. Churchill Livingstone, Edinburgh.)

a bactericidal enzyme, lysozyme. Added to this fluid are oily secretions from the Meibomian glands. These combined fluids serve to protect the eye in several ways:

- the constant washing of the fluid over the cornea, through blinking, removes grit
- the lysozyme helps to prevent microbial infection
- the oily nature of the fluid helps to keep the conjunctiva from drying up.

COMMON EYE CONDITIONS

- Red eye (including glaucomas)
- Eyelid disorders
- Lacrimal disorders.

Red eye

Patients often present with a red eye. This rather obvious sign should be fully investigated to ensure that any very serious condition (e.g. glaucoma) does not go undetected. Causes of red eye include:

- conjunctivitis – bacterial or viral
- corneal ulceration due to microbial infection
- episcleritis and scleritis
- acute closed-angle glaucoma
- foreign body in the eye.

Eyelid disorders

Lumps. It is important to ensure that any lumps on the eyelid are carefully investigated to exclude serious conditions such as basal-cell carcinoma. Commonly presenting conditions are chalazion (Meibomian cyst) and stye – a local infection of a lash follicle.

Drooping of the eyelid (ptosis). This condition may indicate the presence of a serious disease such as myasthenia gravis or a condition that may arise due to the ageing process.

Children who present with a drooping eyelid must be very fully investigated by a specialist as this may indicate a serious condition.

Patients with thyroid disease sometimes develop proptosis which may require surgery. If fulminant disease threatens a patient's vision, high doses of corticosteroids, or emergency radiotherapy, may save the patient's sight.

Facial palsy may cause symptoms of ocular exposure. Exposure keratitis may result and this can lead to blindness. The use of lubricants in reversible cases will protect the eye in the short term. Surgery is indicated in some cases. A gold weight may be implanted in the upper eyelid to facilitate closure.

Inflammatory eyelid disorders

These include the following:

Blepharitis. This is a chronic condition in which the patient complains of sore eyelids. Styes often accompany blepharitis, and the lid margins are inflamed and crusted. The condition may be present in patients suffering from an inflammatory skin disease such as eczema.

Acute inflammatory conditions of the eyelids must be taken as indicating a potentially serious condition which could result in loss of sight or the spread of a life-threatening infection.

Orbital cellulitis. This may result from the spread of infection from sinuses. Urgent specialist treatment is required in such cases.

Allergy. Allergic reactions can occur as a result of contact with a wide range of allergenic materials from plant or animal sources. Cosmetics may also cause allergic reactions.

Viral infections. Infections due to the herpes simplex or herpes zoster virus can result in a vesicular rash on the eyelid.

Lacrimal disorders

Excessive tear production

Some patients may experience a watering eye owing to blockage of the lacrimal sac or nasolacrimal duct. Surgery may be indicated to resolve this problem.

Dry eye syndrome

This is a more common condition, especially in older patients. Patients with this condition suffer considerable discomfort which is due to a deficiency of either aqueous humour or the mucin component of the tear film. It is often associated with rheumatoid arthritis (Sjögren's syndrome) and autoimmune diseases such as pemphigoid. Certain drugs may be a cause of dry eye syndrome (see p. 226).

EYE INJURIES

Eye injuries can result from a number of causes, notably foreign bodies, blunt injury, or chemical damage. Injuries arising from the use of metal tools on glass, stone or metal can result in penetrating injuries to the eye. Chemical damage to the eye must be treated with copious amounts of a suitable irrigating fluid (Dunne et al 1991) such as sterile sodium chloride solution 0.9% or sterile water. In emergency situations, freshly drawn tap water may have to be used. Eye injuries due to chemicals of alkaline reaction, such as lime, need to be treated very urgently because alkalis have a penetrating action on ocular tissue, causing iritis and cataract formation.

PRE- AND POSTOPERATIVE TREATMENT

Local eye treatment, both pre- and post-surgery, will depend on the condition being treated and the surgical procedures used. The main agents used are mydriatics (Table 26.1), anti-infective agents (Tables 26.2–26.4), anti-inflammatory drugs (Table 26.5) and certain specialised drugs (Table 26.6). Single-use containers must be used to reduce the likelihood of infection. If these are not available, a container should be reserved for the specific use of a named patient. It should be noted that many eye drop formulations contain preservatives and other adjuncts. These may cause sensitivity reactions.

MEDICAL CONDITIONS AND THE EYE

Many serious medical conditions have ocular symptoms. Examination of the eye may lead to the diagnosis of a serious general condition, e.g. diabetes mellitus, rheumatoid disease or hypertension. Systemic treatment is indicated in these conditions, the details of which are given in relevant chapters.

GLAUCOMA

Glaucoma is the commonest cause of blindness in the world. It is characterised by a raised intraocular pressure (IOP) which leads to cupping and degeneration of the optic disc, impairment of optic nerve head function and nerve fibre-type visual field loss. If the condition is

Table 26.1 Mydriatics and cycloplegics (antimuscarinics)

Drug	Form/dose	Actions/indications	Contraindications/side-effects/nursing points
Atropine	1% eye drops and eye ointment	Long-acting (7 days) antimuscarinic. Dilates pupil and paralyses ciliary muscle	As with other eye drops, there are risks of systemic absorption resulting in dry mouth, etc. Patients at extremes of age are more likely to suffer side-effects than are other patients. Mydriatics may precipitate acute closed-angle glaucoma
Cyclopentolate	Eye drops 0.5% and 1%	Used for producing cycloplegia for refraction in young children. Effect lasts for up to 24 hours. Also used for relieving pain from pupillary spasm in eye injuries	Contraindications similar to those of other drugs in this class
Homatropine	Eye drops 1%	Similar to cyclopentolate	
Tropicamide	Eye drops 0.5% and 1%	Similar to cyclopentolate. Very short-acting mydriatic (3 hours)	

Table 26.2 Anti-infective agents – antibacterials

Drug	Form/dose	Actions/indications	Contraindications/side-effects/nursing points
Chloramphenicol	Eye drops 0.5%, 2 drops every 3 hours or more frequently; eye ointment 1%	Used for both treatment and prevention of bacterial infections, e.g. conjunctivitis. Eye ointment useful for application at night (long action). Valuable to prevent secondary bacterial infection in viral conjunctivitis	As with all eye drops there is a possibility of transient stinging on application. The risk of aplastic anaemia from absorption on long-term use is not well founded
Ciprofloxacin	Eye drops 0.3%	Antibacterial in corneal ulceration	Must be used intensively throughout the day and night (see BNF for details). May cause localised itching and burning, and bitter taste due to systemic absorption
Framycetin (also available with hydrocortisone 0.5% where an anti-inflammatory action is required)	Drops 0.5%; eye ointment 0.5%; ophthalmic powder 500 mg for subconjunctival infection	Bacterial infections, e.g. conjunctivitis	Most antibacterial agents are applied several times daily depending on clinical need. All locally applied anti-infective agents have the potential to cause sensitivity reactions. Antibacterial agents combined with corticosteroids should not be applied where viral infections are present – or suspected – since local defence mechanisms will be compromised
Gentamicin	Drops 0.3%	Bacterial infections; a broad-spectrum agent	Has poor ocular penetration and potential toxicity. These problems limit its use

Note. Other antibacterial eye preparations available include chlortetracycline (ointment), ciprofloxacin (drops) and polymixin in various combinations. Propamidine is a non-antibiotic preparation used in the treatment of acanthamoeba keratitis (see BNF for details).

Table 26.3 Anti-infective drugs – antifungals

Drug	Form/dose	Actions/indications	Contraindications/side-effects/nursing points
Natamycin	Applied locally as a 5% suspension*	Fungal corneal ulcers can arise as a result of the inappropriate use of topical corticosteroids	The treatment of fungal infections of the eye is highly specialised and requires highly skilled diagnosis and treatment. The preparations marked with an asterisk are only available from specialist units and are not available commercially
Nystatin Ketoconazole	100 000 units/mL*	Fungal corneal ulcers and keratomycosis	

Table 26.4 Anti-infective drugs – antivirals

Drug	Form/dose	Actions/indications	Contraindications/side-effects/nursing points
Aciclovir	Eye ointment 3%, five times daily	Herpes simplex infections and herpes simplex keratitis	Treatment must be continued 3 days after healing
Fomivirsen	Intravitreal injection. In newly diagnosed disease, 165 micrograms in 0.025 mL, given weekly for 3 weeks, followed by 165 micrograms every 2 weeks. (See BNF for treatment of previously treated disease)	Cytomegalovirus (CMV) retinitis in patients with AIDS	Side-effects can be a reason for suspending therapy. Local irritation and inflammation, visual disturbances, cataract and IOP increase are potential major problems
Ganciclovir	Slow-release ocular implant, inserted surgically	To treat sight-threatening CMV retinitis in AIDS patients. Topical treatment does not replace systemic therapy	

Table 26.5 Anti-inflammatory drugs

Drug	Form/dose	Actions/indications	Contraindications/side-effects/nursing points
Corticosteroids			
Betamethasone (other topical corticosteroids are available, see BNF)	0.1% every 1–2 hours for acute phase. Reduce frequency and use eye ointment 0.1% at night	Indicated for the short-term treatment of inflammatory conditions such as uveitis and scleritis. Also used postoperatively to reduce inflammation	Expert supervision of topical corticosteroid therapy is required since the dangers from topical therapy are significant. Steroid glaucoma may result and undiagnosed herpes simplex infection may be aggravated, leading to loss of vision or even of the eye. As in other conditions, therapy with corticosteroids can produce great benefits for patients, but the dangers and side-effects must be guarded against by all concerned with the patient's care
Other anti-inflammatory drugs			
Antazoline	Drops: antazoline 0.5% with xylometazoline 0.05%; apply four times daily	Allergic conjunctivitis	To be avoided in patients with cardiac disease, hypertension, etc. because of possible systemic absorption. Avoid in closed-angle glaucoma
Nedocromil sodium	Drops 2%; apply four times daily	Allergic conjunctivitis and vernal keratoconjunctivitis	Transient burning and stinging

Other products are available for the treatment of seasonal allergic conjunctivitis, e.g. azelastine and related drugs (see BNF for details).

untreated, defects in the field of vision enlarge, leading to visual loss. Normal IOP is 16 mmHg ± 3 mmHg. A pressure of 21 mmHg (measured by tonometer) or higher may represent a pathological condition and requires treatment. High IOP causes compression of the microcirculation of the optic disc, resulting in ischaemia, the extent of which will depend on the IOP and vascularity/blood supply of the optic disc. Some eyes can withstand an IOP of 30 mmHg or more without damage owing to the presence of a good blood supply to the optic disc. In other eyes a pressure of less than 21 mmHg can cause visual impairment. IOP is maintained as a result of balance between inflow and outflow of aqueous humour, which is secreted constantly by the ciliary body. The aqueous humour circulates around the lens before passing through the pupil into the anterior chamber. Aqueous humour leaves the eye through the angle of this chamber by filtering through the trabecular meshwork and is returned to the general circulation via the canal of Schlemm. In addition to raised IOP, other risk factors for developing glaucoma include age, race and family history. These factors must all be taken into account when diagnosing the condition.

Table 26.6 Drugs used in association with ophthalmic surgery

Drug	Presentation	Uses/notes
Acetylcholine	1% irrigation	Surgical procedures which require rapid and complete miosis
Antimetabolites of mitomycin	Local application or subconjunctival injection	To prevent scar formation following surgery (consult specialist literature)
Apraclonidine	0.5% eye drops 1% eye drops	Short-term treatment of chronic glaucoma Control of IOP postoperative situations
Diclofenac sodium	0.1% eye drops (single-dose units)	Inhibition of intraoperative miosis during surgery for cataract. Also has anti-inflammatory and pain-relieving properties
Fluorescein sodium	1% or 2% single-dose containers	For the detection of lesions and foreign bodies. Single-use containers are essential to reduce the risk of infection
Flurbiprofen sodium	0.03% eye drops in polyvinyl alcohol 1.4%	Similar uses to diclofenac sodium. Reduction of inflammation postoperatively
Ketorolac trometamol	0.5% eye drops	As for flurbiprofen sodium
Rose bengal	1% eye drops. Single-use containers	Similar use to fluorescein, but more expensive
Sodium chloride	As normal saline or as a component of Balanced Salt Solution (BNF)	For irrigation during surgery

An increased IOP can result from an increased production of aqueous humour or from impaired drainage. In clinical practice most cases of glaucoma arise from poor drainage of the aqueous humour from the anterior chamber. This is believed to result from a progressive degenerative process in the trabecular meshwork and the endothelium of the canal of Schlemm.

Types of glaucoma

Glaucomas can be divided into two main categories, namely, primary open-angle glaucoma (POAG) and acute closed-angle glaucoma (ACAG).

Primary open-angle glaucoma

This is the most common form. Patients may not notice the gradual visual loss taking place, presenting only when serious damage has occurred. Hereditary factors are involved, and diabetics and very short-sighted people are especially at risk of developing this condition. Prevalence increases in the over-80 age group to 10%. Screening is advisable in certain situations, e.g. older people and children of affected patients. Treatment of POAG is summarised in Tables 26.7–26.9. Latanoprost (a prostaglandin) is used to treat POAG as a once-daily eye drop. This costly product is reserved for use in patients where first-line treatments are inappropriate. The drug acts by increasing uveoscleral outflow. Patients should be monitored for changes in eye pigmentation.

Brimonidine, a selective, second-generation alpha$_2$-adrenoceptor agonist reduces IOP by reducing aqueous humour production and enhancing uveoscleral outflow. Since this drug has no clinically significant effect on the heart or lungs it may be a suitable alternative to beta-blockers.

Carbonic anhydrase inhibitors act on the form of the enzyme found in the ciliary epithelium, reducing the production of aqueous humour.

Primary acute closed-angle glaucoma

In this condition the affected eye is hard, red and painful, and the presentation is acute. The distinction between open-angle glaucoma and closed-angle glaucoma is made on the basis of the appearance of the anterior chamber angle on ocular examination. In this form of glaucoma, drainage of the aqueous humour is blocked by the iris. Intraocular pressure builds up very quickly, vision becomes blurred and there is headache, sickness and ocular pain. Older and long-sighted people are more at risk than younger people of developing this condition.

POAG and ACAG are separate entities which require different management. ACAG requires urgent intervention. Initially, IOP is reduced medically, followed by surgery to prevent recurrence. In both cases, the aim of treatment is to reduce IOP and maintain the reduction. Common glaucomatous conditions are compared and summarised in Table 26.10.

Secondary glaucomas

These conditions result from developmental abnormalities and acquired defects. A detailed discussion of

Table 26.7 Treatment of glaucoma (POAG) with beta-blockers

Drug	Form/dose	Actions/indications	Contraindications/side-effects/nursing points
Betaxolol	Drops 0.5%, twice daily; also available as a suspension	These drugs reduce the secretion of aqueous humour by blocking beta-adrenoceptors in the iris and ciliary body and are used in the treatment of chronic open-angle glaucoma. Long-term treatment is indicated with these drugs so as to achieve prolonged reduction of IOP	History of cardiovascular disease, asthma. Systemic absorption can occur causing beta-blockade. Patient should be encouraged to shut the eyes for several minutes, or the punctum should be occluded. These eye drops may cause bronchospasm and cough due to systemic absorption. This may be of particular concern in older patients. Betaxolol is the only selective $beta_1$-blocker but may still cause problems in susceptible patients
Carteolol	Drops 1% and 2%, twice daily		
Levobunolol	Drops 0.5% once or twice daily		
Metipranolol	Drops 0.1% twice daily		
Timolol	Drops 0.25% and 0.5% twice daily. Also available as a 0.25% gel-forming solution for a longer action, daily		

Table 26.8 Treatment of glaucoma (POAG) with parasympathomimetics and sympathomimetics

Drug	Form/dose	Actions/indications	Contraindications/side-effects/nursing points
Parasympathomimetics			
Carbachol	Drops 3%, up to four times daily	Acts in a manner similar to that of pilocarpine	History of cardiovascular disease. Systemic absorption can occur. Sweating, colic, bronchospasm and hypersalivation can occur (see also p. 146)
Pilocarpine	Drops 0.5–4%, three to six times daily. Also available as an ophthalmic gel 4%	Reduces the pupil size and opens up the trabecular meshwork. It is a miotic. All of these drugs are used in the treatment of POAG; combinations of these drugs may be used	Pilocarpine should not be used if there is inflammation since vision can be adversely affected
Sympathomimetics			
Adrenaline (epinephrine)	Drops 0.5% or 1%, once/twice daily	Indicated in the treatment of open-angle glaucoma; causes increase in outflow of aqueous humour and dilates the pupil	Not used for the treatment of ACAG. Cardiovascular problems due to systemic absorption. Stinging and redness of the eye
Brimonidine	Drops 0.2%	Used to treat POAG in patients where beta-blockers are contraindicated or as an adjunct treatment to beta-blockers	Cardiovascular complications may arise in patients with cardiac problems
Dipivefrine	Drops 0.1%, twice daily	A pro-drug which is converted into the active drug (adrenaline (epinephrine)) in the eye	As for adrenaline (epinephrine), but may be less of a problem owing to the pro-drug action
Guanethidine	Drops 5%, once/twice daily	Guanethidine and combination of guanethidine and adrenaline (epinephrine) have actions/indications similar to those of adrenaline (epinephrine)	Use with caution in patients with cardiovascular disease; long-term use may cause conjunctival fibrosis
Guanethidine and adrenaline (epinephrine)	Drops 1% guanethidine and 0.2% adrenaline (epinephrine) *or* 3% guanethidine and 0.5% adrenaline (epinephrine), once/twice daily		

these conditions is beyond the scope of this text. The developmental abnormalities that can result in glaucoma include inborn errors of metabolism and certain skeletal, cardiovascular and ocular changes that occur in conditions such as Marfan's syndrome. Acquired defects that may result in glaucoma include ocular inflammatory conditions, degenerative conditions, tumours, trauma and postoperative complications. Drug treatment, especially local application of potent corticosteroids (betamethasone and dexamethasone), can cause glaucoma of the chronic open-angle type. Any drug which dilates the pupil may result in acute

Table 26.9 Treatment of glaucomas with carbonic anhydrase inhibitors

Drug	Form/dose	Actions/indications	Contraindications/side-effects/nursing points
Acetazolamide	250 mg tablets or sustained-release capsules 0.25–1 g daily individual doses (injection also available)	Acetazolamide inhibits carbonic anhydrase. This enzyme regulates bicarbonate production. Bicarbonate anions balance sodium cations involved in aqueous humour secretions. Mainly used in the treatment of ACAG to reduce IOP prior to surgery	Acetazolamide may induce a mild acidosis. It is contraindicated in idiopathic renal hyperchloraemic acidosis. The drug is also contraindicated in conditions associated with electrolyte level disturbances, e.g. Addison's disease. Careful monitoring of fluid and electrolyte state is required in long-term therapy. Periodic blood cell counts are advisable. Patients should be advised to report any unusual skin rashes. The appearance of significant side-effects should be reported at once. It may be necessary to terminate treatment. Not recommended for long-term use
Brinzolamide	Eye drops 10 mg/mL two to three times daily	Used alone or with beta-blockers in raised IOP and open-angle glaucoma	Local irritation, taste disturbance and significant systemic effects (see specialist literature)
Dorzolamide	2% drops applied three times daily if used alone. In combination with timolol 0.5%, twice-daily applications required	Reduces IOP in POAG. A topical carbonic anhydrase inhibitor. Treatment of POAG where beta-blockers alone are inadequate	Severe renal impairment, hyperchloraemic acidosis, pregnancy and breast-feeding

Table 26.10 Primary glaucomas – a comparison

Primary open-angle glaucoma (POAG) or chronic simple glaucoma	Acute closed-angle glaucoma (ACAG) or primary angle-closure glaucoma
• In this condition, the angle of the anterior chamber is open • Incidence rises with age, onset insidious • Equally common in both sexes • More common in Afro-Caribbean population than in Caucasians • Predisposing factors include high myopia asymmetric intraocular pressure, and non-ocular diseases such as diabetes mellitus and hypothyroidism • Caused by obstruction to the outflow of aqueous humour through the trabecular meshwork • Intraocular pressure (IOP) rises above the normal range of 10–21 mmHg • Raised IOP damages retinal nerve cells (anoxia caused by compression of blood vessels) • Loss of visual field results	• In this condition, the angle of the anterior chamber is closed • Incidence rises with age • Female to male ratio 4 : 1 • Acute rise in IOP to 70–80 mmHg. Hard, painful red-eye • Peripheral iris obstructs angle of anterior chamber (structurally predisposed eyes are where anterior chamber is narrow) • Causes include mature cataract, dilatation of pupil by dim light or drugs • Symptoms include pain, blurred vision, nausea and vomiting • Emergency treatment of this condition is essential
Treatment. Drugs are used which cause reduction of formation of aqueous humour/increase outflow of aqueous humour • Drugs reducing aqueous humour formation – beta-blockers, carbonic anhydrase inhibitors and selective adrenergic agonists • Drugs increasing outflow – parasympathomimetics and prostaglandins • Sympathomimetics have a dual action (see Table 26.8) • Latanoprost (or bimatoprost) (prostaglandin analogues) may be used where other drugs are inappropriate. This drug may cause changes in eye coloration. Monitoring is essential The aims of treatment should be a 20–30% reduction of IOP at which damage occurred	*Treatment.* Medical reduction of IOP followed by iridectomy • Acetazolamide (IV) used perioperatively (side-effects/dosage levels require careful monitoring and preclude the use of this drug for chronic management except as a last resort). Mannitol by IV infusion may also be used to reduce IOP • Parasympathomimetics may be used after IOP has been lowered • A beta-blocker may be preferred because the miotic effect of pilocarpine may result in the formation of posterior synechiae • Since the other eye is at risk of developing ACAG, appropriate topical medication will be required (pilocarpine or a beta-blocker) (see Tables 26.7 and 26.8)

closed-angle glaucoma. Patients with narrow angles only are at risk of developing this dangerous condition. Both local and systemic drugs can cause acute closed-angle glaucoma in susceptible patients. Atropine (parasympathetic blocking drug) and phenylephrine (sympathomimetic) are potential causes of acute closed-angle glaucoma. Systemically administered drugs which have an antimuscarinic (parasympathetic blocking)

Table 26.11 Local anaesthetics

Drug	Form/dose	Actions/indications	Contraindications/side-effects/nursing points
Lidocaine (lignocaine)	Drops 4% with fluorescein 0.25%	Local anaesthetic with staining agent to help in the diagnosis of ocular lesions. The dye (fluorescein) is taken up by the damaged tissue	
Oxybuprocaine	Drops 0.4%	Local anaesthetic	
Proxymetacaine	Drops 0.5%	Local anaesthetic	Causes less stinging than other agents and is useful for children
Tetracaine (amethocaine)	Drops 0.5% and 1%	Local anaesthetic	Local sensitivity reaction to the drug or preservative used in the eye drops may occur

Table 26.12 Preparations for tear deficiency

Drug	Form/dose	Actions/indications	Contraindications/side-effects/nursing points
Acetylcysteine and hypromellose	Drops 5%/0.35%; apply four times daily	This product provides lubrication, and the acetylcysteine has a mucolytic action which is useful where accumulations of mucus occur	As with other eye conditions, appropriate eye hygiene must be carried out to reduce discomfort from crusting on the eyelid margins
Hypromellose	Drops 0.3%, used hourly if necessary (a range of products is available)	Lubricant in tear deficiency	Frequent applications needed. Inpatients may prefer self-administration of these drops where this can be arranged. The choice of a particular preparation will be determined by acceptability to the patient
Paraffins	Liquid or with yellow soft paraffin	Lubricant in recurrent corneal epithelial erosion	Cause visual disturbance. Best used before sleep
Polyvinyl alcohol (PVA)	Drops 1.4%	Lubricant in tear deficiency	Mucomimetic action. May provide a longer period of relief from symptoms than is provided by hypromellose
Povidone	Drops 5%	Lubricant in tear deficiency	

action or side-effects can precipitate closed-angle glaucoma. The main groups of drugs that can cause problems (especially in older people) are:

- antidepressant drugs of the tricyclic group, e.g. amitriptyline
- anti-Parkinson's disease drugs, e.g. trihexyphenidyl (benzhexol)
- atropine-like drugs
- pseudoephedrine, which may be present in cough medicines or decongestant preparations.

TREATMENT OF INFECTIONS OF THE EYE

Many infections of the eye are amenable to treatment with topical antimicrobial agents. Wherever possible the drugs used are those which are not used to treat systemic infections so as to reduce the risk of resistance developing. In severe infections it may be necessary to use supporting systemic therapy. Tables 26.2 and 26.3 provide summaries of the main topical anti-infective agents. Acanthamoeba keratitis may arise from poor contact lens hygiene. Treatment requires intensive therapy managed by a specialist.

LOCAL ANAESTHETICS (see also p. 446)

Local anaesthetics (see Table 26.11) are applied to the eye to relieve pain following injury or to reduce discomfort prior to ophthalmological procedures. Hypersensitivity may occur and stinging on application may be a problem.

TREATMENT OF TEAR DEFICIENCY

Tear deficiency (see Table 26.12) produces a very troublesome 'dry eye' condition leading to sore, uncomfortable, 'gritty' eyes. The condition can be alleviated by the regular use of water-based lubricant eye drops, or simple eye ointment for use at night.

TREATMENT OF INFLAMMATORY EYE CONDITIONS

The local application of corticosteroids to the eye is potentially hazardous (see p. 413). The anti-inflammatory action is, however, very valuable. Local application of corticosteroids in cases of undiagnosed infection (e.g. herpes simplex viral infection) can lead to a rapid worsening of the condition, which may even cause the loss of an eye. Anti-inflammatory drugs are detailed in Table 26.5.

MYDRIATICS AND CYCLOPLEGICS

These drugs (see Table 26.1) dilate the pupil and paralyse ciliary muscles. The main uses of these drugs are pre- and postoperatively and in diagnostic procedures (e.g. refraction). The pain due to certain eye injuries (e.g. corneal abrasion) can be relieved by the application of homatropine eye drops. Adverse effects are briefly described in Table 26.1. Many eye drops contain very toxic drugs and should be safely stored when not in use.

BLEPHAROSPASM

Botulinum toxin, produced by the bacterium *Clostridium botulinum* type A, is one of the most powerful neurotoxins known. It can be fatal in severe untreated cases of botulinum food poisoning. The toxin paralyses muscles by blocking the release of acetylcholine from the presynaptic neurones. The effect is irreversible and remains until new nerve end-plates form.

A standardised preparation of the toxin (botulinum A toxin–haemagglutinin complex) is licensed for the treatment of blepharospasm and hemifacial spasm. The potency of the product is expressed in units. The toxin's muscle-weakening action is exploited therapeutically in some dystonias (involuntary muscle spasms), the injection being indicated for blepharospasm and hemifacial spasm. Sufferers typically have uncontrollable blinking spasms in both eyes, symptoms usually starting insidiously in the 50–70 age group. Spasms become more frequent and severe, with both eyes clamping shut, resulting in many patients effectively being blind. Botulinum A toxin injection (120 units per affected eye) reduces the intensity of the spasm in 2–5 days. Further injections (into the medial and lateral orbicularis oculi of the lower lid) are required every 8 weeks. There is no evidence that repeat treatment leads to resistance. However, there are adverse effects, blurred vision, local pain, swelling, ptosis, dry eye and photophobia. In view of the nature of the side-effects it is vitally important to counsel the patient before the treatment is administered.

The toxin has been used to treat children with cerebral palsy (Crouchman 1997). When combined with physiotherapy, injections of the toxin into specific muscle groups have produced improved mobility.

ADMINISTRATION OF EYE PREPARATIONS

The eye is a delicate and vital structure which protects itself in several ways. The immediacy of the blink reflex is evidence of the protective response made to the slightest threat to the eye. An ophthalmic procedure, be it the application of eye drops or of ointment, is approached against this background. Despite the fact that many patients may tolerate more painful procedures with equanimity, procedures involving the eye can cause particular anxiety. Ophthalmic treatment calls for a manner which conveys confidence to patients, helping to ensure that they are relaxed before, during and after the procedure. As with all procedures, a clear explanation is given to patients to gain their cooperation.

Risks of infection must be guarded against by washing the hands with a suitable antiseptic cleansing solution before and after each procedure. If there is a discharge from the eye or evidence of old ointment, it may be necessary to swab the eye first. A damaged eye is particularly susceptible to infection, so that, whenever possible, a single-use presentation (e.g. of an eye drop) is used. This is especially important when a suspected corneal abrasion is being examined using fluorescein. Where single-dose units are not available, or when larger volumes are required, a separate multidose container should be used for each patient. Care must be taken not to contaminate the dropper or nozzle of eye preparations. Patients who have undergone surgery as an outpatient and have evidence of a recent ocular infection should be given a fresh supply of eye drops after the operation, a separate bottle being supplied for each eye if both require treatment.

When applying eye medication the standard procedures for administering and recording medicines are followed. All containers should be labelled with the patient's name and the date of opening. The label on the eye preparation should be compared with the prescription. The special points to note are:

- the name of the medication, the strength (usually expressed as a percentage)
- the amount
- which eye is to be treated, if not both
- the time
- the frequency of administration
- that the preparation is 'in date'.

As with other forms of medication, eye drops may be administered once only (including preoperatively), or on a regular basis. Intensive treatment may also be indicated such as in the case of an infection. In order to convey all the necessary information a specially designed prescription sheet is required (Fig. 26.3). This should enable prescriptions to be written for non-standard intervals, regular intervals and on a once-only basis.

In order that the medication is administered safely and effectively, it is important to position the patient suitably. The head requires to be tilted back and maintained in a steady position so that the risk of damaging the eye by contact with the equipment in use is minimised. To achieve this, the patient should be lying or else sitting, in which case the head should be supported by a pillow or the back of the chair. Where possible the nurse should work from the affected side so as to be close to the working area and in greater control of the procedure.

As always, safety aspects should be considered. Good lighting is essential for carrying out procedures on delicate structures such as the eye. Light should be from above and behind the nurse. With photophobic patients, consideration must be given to light reaching them, otherwise they may be unable to open their eyes. Movements of the hand should be gentle and controlled. Gloves are not worn, as the disposable type are seldom close fitting and therefore in danger of causing damage if they are allowed to touch the sensitive corneal surface of the eye. In all cases, the nurse must be alert to any sign of adverse reaction to a drug used locally in the eye. This may take the form of a worsening of inflammation or spread of inflammation to surrounding skin.

In the event of the wrong preparation having been administered or the wrong eye being treated, the doctor must be notified *at once* so that any corrective action may be ordered without delay.

Teaching patients to administer eye medications

Nurses play an important role in teaching patients to master the technique of self-administration of eye medications. Compliance and independence will be more readily achieved where the patient is provided with motivation and encouragement.

When teaching a patient to administer an eye medication the special points to emphasise are:

- the need to wash the hands thoroughly first
- the need to avoid contamination
- the importance of using only the prescribed medications.

Because of the systemic toxicity of many ophthalmic drugs it is especially important that all eye preparations are kept out of the reach of children. Similarly, safe disposal of any remainder when treatment is discontinued, or the container changed, is essential.

Patients may be helped to select for themselves a suitable position in which to administer the medication. To instil eye drops, some patients find lying flat and feeling for the lower lid is a successful method with gravity assisting. This may be inconvenient or impossible for others and they may prefer to work in front of an up-standing mirror, although coordination of the hand and eye may take time to master by this method. Self-application of an eye ointment and removal or insertion of a contact lens or artificial eye are best performed in front of a mirror.

Compliance aids

A number of patients experience problems using eye drops owing to difficulty in aiming the drops and squeezing the plastic bottle (Winfield et al 1991). Aids to the instillation of eye drops are available which assist patients to use their eye drops in accordance with the prescriber's directions. The type of aid needed will depend on the patient's particular needs. If the patient has difficulty in aiming the bottle, an Easidrop or Autodrop should be considered. These devices are designed to help the patient to position the dropper to expel a drop. Squeezing the bottle can be a particular problem for older patients whose grip strength may be reduced. For patients who have difficulty in both aiming and squeezing the bottle, the Opticare device (Fig. 26.4) or Autosqueeze may be useful. Whichever device is selected the patient should be given guidance and instruction in its use. In some circumstances it may be appropriate for the patient to use the selected device in the ward for a period prior to discharge so as to help ensure continuity of treatment. The use of a compliance aid often helps the patient gain benefit from the treatment and at the same time achieve greater independence. There is also potential to achieve better use of resources if the number of visits by a district nurse to instil eye drops can be reduced.

Eye drops

Eye drops are sterile aqueous solutions or suspensions, presented in multiple application dropper bottles which may be of glass fitted with a removable glass dropper and teat. An alternative presentation is a flexible plastic container with orifice through which drops are expelled

OPHTHALMIC PRESCRIPTION AND RECORDING SHEET

Arrangement of sections

Page 1	Intensive treatment (illustrated)
Page 2, 3	Regular prescriptions (and pages 5 and 6 on continuation sheet)
Page 4 (top)	Prescriptions at non-standard intervals e.g. Pre-op preparation Intensive dilatation or Intensive pilocarpine
Page 4 (bottom)	Once Only prescriptions e.g. Sub-conjunctival injections

Instructions for use

1. No eye medication must be given unless prescribed on this sheet.
2. Each prescription must be signed by a doctor.
3. Administration times should be indicated by the prescriber by circling the appropriate time.
4. The nurses must record the administration of the medicine by entering their initials in the appropriate boxes.
5. To discontinue a prescription the doctor must draw a line through the complete entry, enter the date in the discontinued/stop date column and initial.

INTENSIVE TREATMENT All Doses 1-2 Drops

DATE	FORM/MEDICINE/STRENGTH (Block Letters)	EYE	SIGNATURE	DISCONTINUED	
				DATE	INITIALS

	TIMES OF ADMINISTRATION—Please Circle																							COMMENTS
DATE	01	02	03	04	05	06	07	08	09	10	11	12	13	14	15	16	17	18	19	20	21	22	23	24	

DATE	FORM/MEDICINE/STRENGTH (Block Letters)	EYE	SIGNATURE	DISCONTINUED	
				DATE	INITIALS

	TIMES OF ADMINISTRATION—Please Circle																							COMMENTS
DATE	01	02	03	04	05	06	07	08	09	10	11	12	13	14	15	16	17	18	19	20	21	22	23	24	

WARD	HOSP	SURNAME	FORENAME	AGE	UNIT NUMBER	CONSULTANT	KNOWN DRUG/MEDICINE SENSITIVITY	
							1	2

Figure 26.3 Ophthalmic prescription and recording sheet.

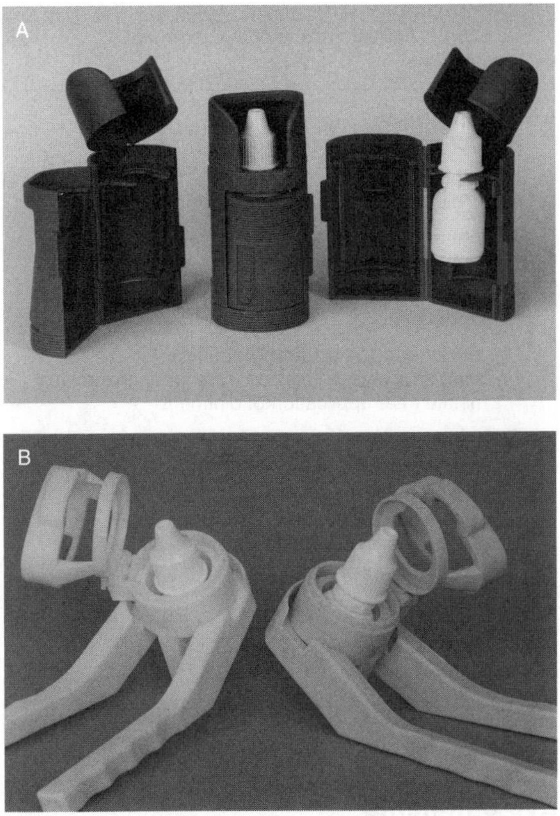

Figure 26.4 A. Opticare device. B. Opticare for arthritic patients.

with pressure of the fingers. Both types of container are used by individual patients in the community. Although eye drops in multiple application containers contain preservatives there is always a risk of contamination in use. A multiple application container should be used for not more than 4 weeks, after which the original container should be rejected and a new container started. In some formulations a shorter 'life' may be indicated on the label.

Single-application containers should always be used in surgical procedures because of the increased risk of infection. Solutions presented in this way do not contain preservatives and so a new single-use unit should be used for each application. Both single-application and multiple-application packs should have tamper-evident closures and packaging.

The question of the number of drops which can be instilled into the eye requires clarification. One drop from an eye dropper is 50 microlitres (μL) and will overload the average conjunctival sac which has a capacity of 25 μL (Lessar & Fiscella 1985). To overcome this, where more than one drop of the same preparation is to be instilled (or another preparation used) an interval of 5–10 minutes should elapse before instilling the second drop. This may present difficulties in ophthalmology units where a considerable number of patients may be receiving several different forms of drops in succession. If there is a high rate of tear secretion, aqueous solutions will be quickly diluted or eliminated from the eye into the nasolacrimal duct, thus becoming unavailable for ophthalmic absorption but available for systemic absorption. This may result in systemic side-effects (e.g. dry mouth with atropine). Some practitioners recommend pressure over the punctum after administration as a means of restricting tear flow into the duct. The frequency of instillation of drops varies and will depend on, for example, the degree of infection or inflammation. In the treatment of acute glaucoma, a very intensive regimen of instillation is followed initially which is then gradually reduced in frequency to hourly, continuing until the intraocular pressure is controlled and the pupil pinpoint.

Every effort is made to avoid causing irritation to the eye. Drops used straight from the refrigerator cause discomfort for the patient. If eye drops have been refrigerated, sufficient time should be allowed for the drops to attain room temperature before use. A drop instilled from a height greater that 2.5 cm directly onto the cornea will cause stinging. Any irritation caused by faulty technique will result in increased tear secretion with consequent loss of therapeutic benefit owing to a dilution effect. In addition, the patient will often react by squeezing the lids in an accentuated blink reflex, expelling the solution between the lids or down the nasolacrimal duct.

If, after the instillation of drops, the patient complains of irritation of the skin or a feeling of heat and tightness, an allergic reaction should be suspected and the doctor informed.

Instillation of eye drops (see Fig. 26.5)

Where the eyes are sticky, this procedure is preceded by bathing the eyes using sterile 0.9% sodium chloride solution. There is some debate about the aspect of the eye into which drops should be instilled. Since the tears pass from lacrimal glands situated on the lateral aspect of each eye across the eyeball before draining into the nasolacrimal duct, it would seem logical to instil drops into the outer aspect of the lower fornix so that they are washed across with the tears, allowing time to take effect before draining into the nasolacrimal passage. Besides, the lower fornix is part of the conjunctiva and is less sensitive than the cornea. However, some authorities advocate using the middle or the inner

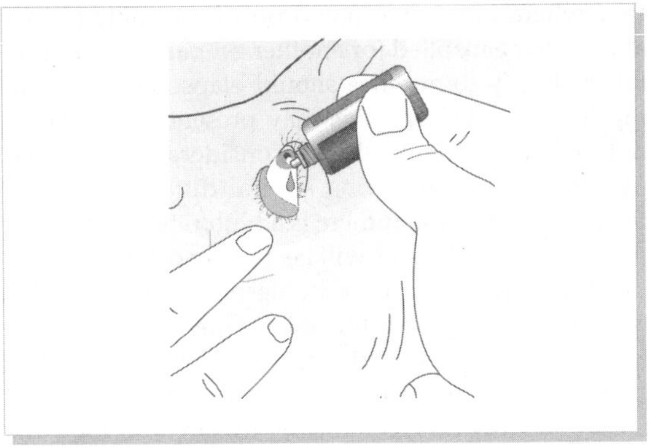

Figure 26.5 Instillation of eye drops.

Box 26.1 Administration of eye drops

Documentation
- Prescription and recording sheet

The medicine
- Eye drops in accordance with prescription and at room temperature
- Eye drops 'in date'

The environment
- Well-lit location with no 'through traffic'

The nurse and the patient (general)
- Identification of patient and comparison with prescription
- Cooperation and relaxation of patient achieved by careful explanation and gentle approach
- Patient discouraged from rubbing eye/reassurance given that blurring of vision is normal and will soon pass
- General comfort of patient on completion of procedure

The nurse and patient (specific)
- Encouragement to open eye and look upwards

Technique (general)
- Patient's head supported/nurse working from patient's affected side
- Hand hygiene before and after each treatment and before treating the eye

Technique (specific)
- Eversion of lower eyelid
- Adequate warning to patient prior to actual instillation
- Instillation from correct height
- Extreme care to avoid touching any part of the eye
- Immediate replacement of cap if multiple-application bottle in use
- Excess medication mopped from cheek

Hazards
- Physical trauma
- Infection
- Systemic absorption

Special features
- Self-medication with or without compliance aid

Box 26.2 Administration of eye ointment (see Fig. 26.6)

Documentation
- As for instillation of eye drops

The medicine
- Eye ointment in accordance with prescription

The environment
- As for eye drops

The nurse and the patient (general)
- As for eye drops

The nurse and the patient (specific)
- Patient encouraged to close eyes for approximately 1 minute after application of ointment

Technique (general)
- As for eye drops

Technique (specific)
- Nozzle held 2.5 cm above patient; ointment squeezed along lower lid from inner canthus outwards

Hazards
- Physical trauma
- Infection

aspect. The method which can be achieved by nurse and/or patient may be the deciding factor (Box 26.1).

Eye ointments

In addition to the more commonly used eye drops many ophthalmic drugs are available as eye ointments. Eye ointments are essentially dispersions of the active ingredient in a sterile bland base, such as soft paraffin, polyethylene glycol or a specially formulated gel. Useful properties of eye ointments include:

- duration of action longer than that of eye drops
- an emollient soothing action
- ease of application
- long shelf-life.

Eye ointments soften crusts, thus preventing adherence of eyelids and eyelashes when the patient is asleep. However, there may be some interference with vision owing to the smearing of the cornea with the ointment base (Box 26.2).

Rodding

This procedure is done to prevent formation of adhesions between the eyelid and the eyeball which can arise as the result of chemical burns of the conjunctiva. In the first few days after injury the procedure is likely to be uncomfortable and a local anaesthetic such as 0.5% tetracaine (amethocaine) eye drops is instilled in advance.

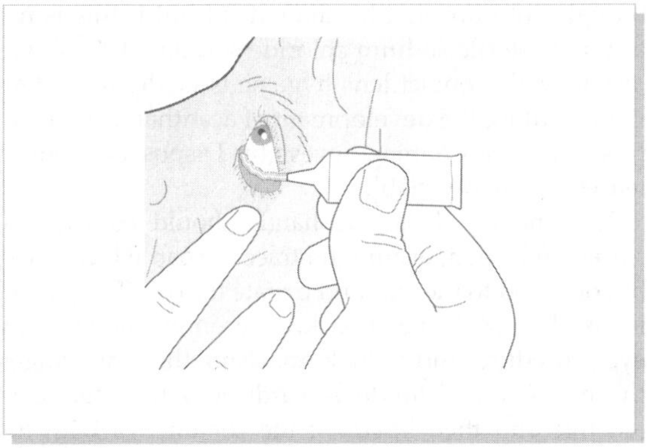

Figure 26.6 Administration of eye ointment.

Box 26.3 Eye bathing

Documentation
- Nursing care plan

The medicine
- Sterile 0.9% sodium chloride solution

The environment
- As for instillation of eye drops
- Tray or trolley cleaned, pack and solution prepared as for surgical dressing

The nurse and the patient
- As for eye drops

Technique (general)
- As for eye drops

Technique (specific)
- Uninflamed, uninfected or operated eye bathed first
- Upper lid bathed with patient looking down; lower lid with patient looking up
- Sterile technique
- Each eye swabbed from inner canthus out to prevent infection of the punctum, the lacrimal apparatus or the other eye
- Each swab used once and discarded
- Dry wool never used as it may leave wisps attached to the eyelashes; swabs always well rung out

Hazards
- Physical trauma
- Infection

Sterile petroleum jelly is used to lubricate the rod in most cases, although sometimes an antibiotic ointment may be prescribed. By passing the rod under the upper eyelid then moving it from side to side, exerting slight pressure outwards, any adhesions are broken down and a film of grease is left between the two surfaces.

Cleansing the eye

The eye may be cleansed by bathing and irrigating.

Box 26.4 Irrigation of the eye

Documentation
- Dependent on condition being treated – nursing care plan or standard prescribing and recording sheet

The medicine
- Sterile sodium chloride 0.9% solution (sachet, plastic bag or prefilled disposable undine) or special irrigation solution
- As prescribed at body temperature

The environment
- As for eye bathing

The nurse and the patient
- As for eye drops

Technique (general)
- As for eye drops

Technique (specific)
- Sterile technique
- Patient holding receiver firmly against appropriate cheek with head tilted slightly towards receiver
- Patient allowed to become accustomed to temperature of solution by pouring a little over cheek first
- Eyelids held apart using thumb and forefinger
- Solution directed in steady stream over eyeball from inner canthus outwards
- Patient asked to move eyeball up, down and from side to side so that entire eye is cleansed
- Eyelids and cheek left dry
- Eyepad applied if instructed

Hazards
- Physical trauma
- Infection

Eye bathing

This procedure (Box 26.3) may be used to soothe the eye(s) and to remove crusts from the eyelid(s).

Irrigation of the eye

This procedure (Box 26.4) is carried out mostly in accident and emergency departments and occupational health centres for the emergency removal of irritant chemicals. The volume and nature of the irrigation solution and the equipment used is dependent on the agent which has caused the injury.

CARE OF AN ARTIFICIAL EYE

Patients who have had enucleation of an eye performed and have been fitted with a temporary shell or prosthesis, should have the prosthesis removed twice a day, or according to the surgeon's preference, to allow it and the socket to be cleaned with sterile normal saline. The prospect of this activity calls for some degree of fortitude but the nurse's mind will quickly be concentrated on the technique involved and on the great need to provide the patient with encouragement.

At first, patients are likely to be understandably tense and frightened that the procedure will be painful. They should be warned that they will feel the presence of something in the socket but there will be no pain. About 3–4 days following the operation, the prosthesis is replaced with an artificial eye.

After a few days, when it is felt that patients are ready to look at themselves in a mirror, and when they feel they want to become involved in the care of their eye, the nurse must be prepared to spend time with them. Patients may be taught to carry out eye toilet in front of a bathroom mirror. Until they becomes fully confident, a towel may be placed in the washhand basin to protect the artificial eye from damage should it slip through the fingers. By the time patients are discharged, they should be quite confident with the procedure. When the socket is completely healed, patients will be able to rinse the artificial eye under running water and come to no harm.

When a patient with an artificial eye requires to have the eye stored for any length of time, for example during surgery, it should be placed in a container of 0.9% sodium chloride solution so that it does not dry out and become rough.

CONTACT LENSES

Because of the increased use of contact lenses and the very discreet nature of many of them, nurses must make a conscious effort to ask patients whether they wear contact lenses or to observe whether they are in use. This should be done on the patient's admission to hospital. Lenses should be removed for safekeeping before any general anaesthetic. They should also be removed prior to any eye procedure to prevent irritation and so as not to be spoiled, unless medical advice has been given to the contrary. Great care must be taken in storing them since they are easily damaged, and are both costly and inconvenient to replace. They are normally kept in a specially supplied contact lens case, although in an emergency a suitable alternative such as a universal container may have to be found. The container should be labelled with the patient's name, ward and unit number and stored in a safe place.

Handling of lenses should be kept to a minimum and they should not be allowed to dry out because of the danger of cracking. Lens solution is normally brought into hospital by the patient but if this is not available sterile sodium chloride solution 0.9% serves just as well. Contact lens hygiene is vitally important in preventing the development of acanthamoeba keratitis which can damage eyesight. Disposable contact lenses are also available.

To remove a lens, the hands should be washed, rinsed and dried, leaving no trace of soap which could be conveyed to the lens and irritate the eye. The patient is asked to tilt the head back, as recommended for any eye procedure, and to look up. Using the index finger, the lens is gently slid downwards onto the bulbar conjunctiva and then lifted off the conjunctiva with the thumb and index finger. The utmost care is required not to drop a lens as it may then be very difficult to find.

Drugs and contact lenses

Consideration needs to be given to contact lenses and the concurrent administration of medicines. Some patients find that inserting contact lenses is painful and so they may be prescribed local anaesthetic eye drops to instil in advance. It is now well recognised that soft, hydrogel lenses can absorb drugs and preservatives in certain preparations instilled into the eye, leading to toxic reactions. Coloured eye drops such as rose bengal will stain soft contact lenses permanently. Rifampicin, used in the treatment of tuberculosis, and sulfasalazine colour body secretions, including the tears, an orange-red – leading to pigmentation of the contact lens. In certain conditions, however, the water absorption property of the lens can be used to advantage; a soft hydrophilic lens may be inserted to avoid repeated instillation of drugs such as pilocarpine in the treatment of glaucoma. Unless medically contraindicated, soft lenses are better removed during the period the patient is receiving treatment. Hard lenses are not affected in this way.

Adverse effects from many drugs taken systemically can occur. A number of drugs cause a reduction in tear secretion causing blurred vision (e.g. antihistamines, antimuscarinics, phenothiazines, some beta-blockers, diuretics and tricyclic antidepressants). Oral contraceptives may also cause ocular complications.

Drugs which reduce blinking such as anxiolytics, hypnotics, antihistamines and muscle relaxants can affect contact lens wear. Drugs which increase tear secretion include ephedrine and hydralazine and they too can cause eye problems in those who wear contact lenses. Contact lens wearers may also experience ophthalmic discomfort in association with taking drugs such as isotretinoin, primidone and aspirin.

REFERENCES

Crouchman M 1997 Toxin can relieve spasticity in CB. GP Medicine October 17

Dunne A et al 1991 Eye irrigation – practice procedures and problems. Hospital Pharmacy Practice 1:219–226

Lessar T S, Fiscella R G 1985 Antimicrobial drug delivery to the eye. Drug Intelligence and Clinical Pharmacy 19:642–654

Winfield A J, Williams A, Jessiman D et al 1991 Assisting patients with their eyedrops: 1. Identifying the problems. British Journal of Pharmaceutical Practice 13:10–14

FURTHER READING

Bateman D N, Clark R, Azuara-Blanco A et al 2001 The impact of new drugs on management of glaucoma in Scotland: observational study. British Medical Journal 323:1401–1402

Dunne A, Winfield A J, Williams A et al 1991 Eye irrigation – practice, procedures and problems. Hospital Pharmacy Practice (October): 1–4

Editorial 2001 New guidance on the use of eye preparations. Pharmaceutical Journal 267:307

Fraser S, Bunce C, Wormald R et al 2001 Deprivational late presentation of glaucoma: case–control study. British Medical Journal 322:639–643

Khaw P T 1997 Glaucoma. Prescriber's Journal 37:34–45

Kulshrestha M 2002 Guide to the treatments for glaucoma. Prescriber 13:78–86

Levin S, Migdal C 2001 Current management of open-angle glaucoma. Prescriber 12:61–71

Rene C et al 1996 Rationale behind the choice of topical beta-blockers in glaucoma. Pharmaceutical Journal 256:276–277

Royal College of Ophthalmologists 2001 Guidelines for the management of ocular hypertension and primary open-angle glaucoma. Royal College of Ophthalmologists, London

Williams A, Winfield A J 1990 Topical medication for eye patients. Nursing Times 86(27):42–43

CHAPTER CONTENTS

27

Drug treatment of ear, nose and oropharynx

This chapter is concerned mainly with the topical (local) use of medicines.

DRUG TREATMENT OF DISORDERS OF THE EAR

Anatomy and physiology

Sound waves reaching the auricle are channelled through the external auditory canal to the tympanic membrane (eardrum), which vibrates in response. These vibrations are transmitted through the ossicles to the cochlea, which converts them into impulses for transmission by the auditory nerve to the brain (Fig. 27.1). There are three main parts to the ear:

- outer ear – auricle and external auditory canal
- middle ear – tympanic membrane and ossicles
- inner ear – cochlea and vestibular labyrinth.

Common conditions

Each part of the ear may be affected by disease. The outer ear may be affected by skin conditions such as eczema, dermatitis and boils, with itching and pain as the presenting symptoms. Inflammation of the external auditory canal is known as *otitis externa*. Wax, secreted by cells in the external auditory canal, may cause some loss of hearing where production is excessive. The ciliated epithelial cells which line the middle ear secrete mucus. *Otitis media* with effusion ('glue ear') is a condition where the middle ear becomes congested with mucus. Where the mucosa becomes infected, resulting in pus formation, the resulting painful condition is known as acute otitis media. Occasionally, pressure build-up will cause the tympanic membrane to rupture; this results in pressure release and subsidence of pain. Repeated episodes of infection with recurrent discharge of pus may lead to persistent

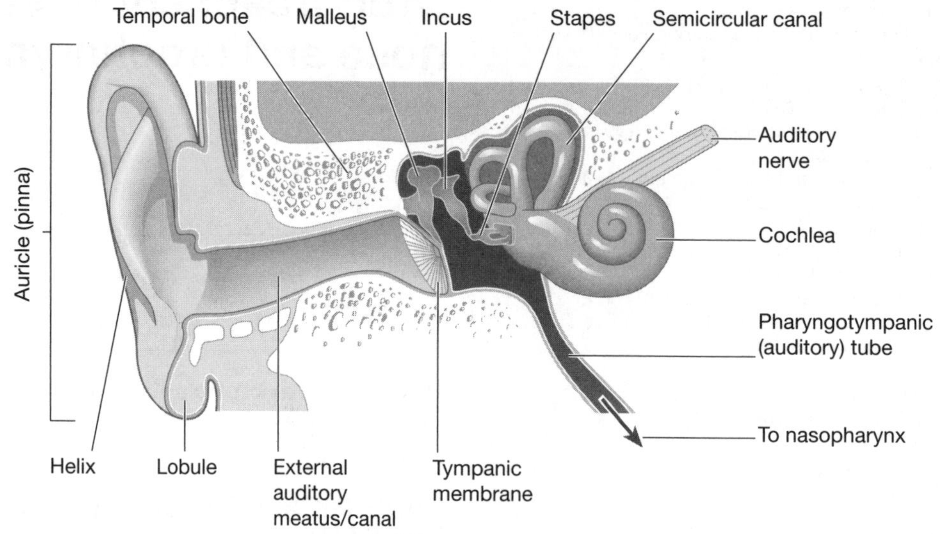

Figure 27.1 The ear. (From Waugh A, Grant A 2001 Ross and Wilson Anatomy and physiology in health and illness, 9th edn. Churchill Livingstone, Edinburgh.)

Table 27.1 Treatment of common forms of otitis

Condition	Main features	Treatment
Otitis externa (OE)	Inflammation of meatal skin, associated with infection and/or eczema. Itching and pain without hearing loss. Predisposing factors include loss of self-cleaning epithelium. Over-enthusiastic cleaning of the ears may be a contributing factor	Exclude chronic otitis media before initiating treatment. Aural toilet, astringent ear drops, e.g. aluminium acetate, antimicrobial agents may be indicated depending on swab/culture. If eczematous condition is present, topical steroids may be required
Otitis media (OM)	Hearing impairment, earache – due to inflammation/ infection	See OME/AOM/COM
Otitis media with effusion (OME)	Hearing impairment, earache – associated with behavioural problems in children 2–7 years. As with AOM, worse in water	Observation, pain relief and antibiotics, simple analgesics for pain in acute conditions. Surgery required in order to achieve resolution of the condition
Acute otitis media (AOM)	Earache, discharge, hearing impairment, tympanic membrane inflamed, fever, lymphadenopathy. Occurs from first year of life onwards. Referral for specialist advice is needed in cases of acute pain/neurological involvement	Local treatment with antibiotic ear drops is of no value. The aim is to avoid progression to COM. Oral antimicrobial agents are widely used. A pragmatic approach is adopted, choice of antibiotic depending on pathogen present. Oral amoxicillin is the first choice. Antibiotic resistance is a growing problem. Prophylactic antibiotics may be needed if AOM is recurrent
Chronic otitis media (COM)	History of childhood ear problems, recurrent discharge, hearing problems. If neurological symptoms occur (e.g. vertigo), urgent referral to specialist. The condition occurs in approximately 5% of the adult UK population. It should be noted that there are linkages between the above conditions	Aural toilet to remove debris, e.g. keratin and necrotic bone. Antibiotic treatment, depending on sensitivity of organisms

rupturing of the tympanic membrane and the condition known as chronic otitis media. Conditions affecting the inner ear are dealt with in Chapter 18. In the investigation of all significant ear problems, suitable hearing tests should be carried out. In addition, it is vitally important to exclude serious underlying conditions.

The main features and treatment of otitis externa and the various forms of otitis media are outlined in Table 27.1

Treatment of otitis media (OM)

Key elements of treatment of all forms of OM are aural toilet, exclusion of complicating factors and the need to ensure that an acute condition does not become chronic. Aminoglycoside antibiotics may be used in resistant cases, even if the eardrum is perforated. The risk of ototoxicity arising from the infected pus is greater than the risk of side-effects from the antibiotic.

Although antibiotics are widely used to treat OM, the role of these agents has been questioned. The evidence to show that any improved outcome is achieved with antibiotic therapy is sparse. Infecting organisms are commonly *Streptococcus pneumoniae*, *Haemophilus influenzae*, staphylococci and streptococci.

ADMINISTRATION OF EAR (AND NOSE) PREPARATIONS

Procedures relating to disorders of the ear and nose involving the use of drugs follow somewhat similar lines. As always, the standard procedure for prescribing and recording medications must be followed. To prevent cross-infection, the hands should be washed before and after each procedure and each patient should have a separate medicine container. When checking ear and nose preparations against the prescription, special note should be made of the strength of the medication and, for example, the number of drops to be instilled and whether both ears/nostrils are to be treated. Explanation of the procedure is important in order to gain the patient's cooperation so that the medication is allowed to take maximum effect with minimal discomfort. Correct positioning of the patient helps to minimise discomfort and ensure penetration of the medication to the part where it is intended to take effect. Ear and nose procedures are usually carried out with the nurse working at the side being treated. Before instilling ear or nose drops, instructions may be given by the doctor to mop the ear canal or nasal passage using a cotton-tipped applicator for better penetration of the medication. Care should be taken when patients have a history of epistaxis. Because of the delicate membranous structures involved it is important to administer such preparations at a suitable temperature. Ear drops should be used in the temperature range between room and body temperature. If ear drops are instilled from a bottle recently stored in a refrigerator they may cause a mild vertigo. Nasal drops should be allowed to reach room temperature prior to instillation if previously stored in the refrigerator.

Box 27.1 Instillation of ear drops

Documentation
- Standard prescribing and recording sheet

The medicine
- Prescribed ear drops
- Separate bottle for each patient
- At room temperature, at least

The nurse and the patient
- Patient identified
- Patient given explanation
- Patient assisted as necessary into position either sitting with head tilted to one side OR lying on side with ear to be treated uppermost
- Patient's clothing protected
- Patient made comfortable

Technique
- If instructed, external auditory meatus gently mopped with cotton-tipped applicator
- Hand hygiene before and after actual instillation of drops
- Bottle shaken if it contains a suspension and required amount drawn into dropper
- Cartilaginous part of pinna gently pulled up and back (for a child, down and back)
- Drops instilled in external canal without allowing dropper to come into contact with ear
- Gentle massage applied over tragus to help work in drops
- Patient encouraged to maintain position for several minutes to allow drops to reach eardrum
- Cotton wool ball lightly placed in external meatus if necessary
- Excess medication wiped away

Patients may be helped to feel more secure throughout the procedure if they are given an absorbent tissue to hold. If, for any reason, they have to rise quickly, the tissue may be used to mop excess medication which would otherwise run out of the ear or nose. For patients receiving ear drops who are unable to maintain the required position, a wisp of cotton wool may be *gently* placed in the ear canal to ensure that the drops remain in contact with the epithelium. The prescribed volume of ear drops may range from two to four drops. On every occasion it is important to check that the top of the glass dropper is not chipped or cracked. Patients using any of these preparations at home should be reminded to use only a preparation intended for themselves, keep it away from children, and safely discard the container and any remaining medication at the end of the course of treatment (Boxes 27.1 and 27.3).

Ear drops

Ear drops are solutions or suspensions of active ingredient(s) in water, propylene glycol or other suitable vehicle.

Ear ointments

Ear ointments have properties similar to those of ointments in general. Some *eye* ointments may also be prescribed for ear conditions. The customary way of introducing an ointment into the ear is to insert ribbon gauze which has been impregnated with the ointment. The wick is left in for 24 hours. Oral analgesics may be required prior to removal of the wick each day.

Removal of ear wax

It is sometimes possible to loosen small amounts of ear wax using wax-softening drops alone. Syringing with warm water using an ear syringe or an electronic pulsed water unit (Box 27.2) is carried out to remove plugs of wax which block the ear causing discomfort and deafness, or when closer inspection of the eardrum is required. Syringing is preceded for several days by a course of wax-softening drops such as olive or almond oil or sodium bicarbonate ear drops. Some proprietary preparations contain an organic solvent which may cause sensitisation and should be used only where oil or sodium bicarbonate ear drops have failed. Because of the potential danger of perforating the tympanic membrane, the ear is examined by a doctor or practice nurse using an otoscope before syringing takes place.

Box 27.2 Syringing the ear

The medicine
- Tap water at body temperature (38C)

The environment
- Usually GP's clinic/surgery by practice or district nurse

The nurse and the patient
- Hand hygiene before and after procedure
- Patient given clear explanation of what is involved
- Patient informed that there may be some discomfort
- Privacy, warmth, comfort
- Patient seated in upright chair with towel over appropriate shoulder
- Patient asked to hold receiver against neck just below ear to be treated

Technique
- Syringe filled with water or pulsed water unit primed and air expelled
- Pinna pulled up and back
- Fluid directed along roof of auditory canal without undue force but at a steady rate
- Content of returned fluid observed
- Procedure repeated until all wax removed
- Meatus inspected periodically using otoscope to check that wax has been removed and ear has not been damaged
- Patient's understanding checked as he may not have heard
- External auditory meatus gently but thoroughly mopped dry

Hazards
- Infection of the middle ear resulting from rupture of the tympanic membrane
- Otitis externa

DRUG TREATMENT OF DISORDERS OF THE NOSE

Anatomy and physiology

The nasal passages are lined by a highly vascular mucous membrane covered with ciliated epithelium which warms and moistens the entering air and traps a certain amount of dust. When the mucous membrane is congested or inflamed there is considerable resistance to inflow, and breathing through the nose is correspondingly difficult.

Common conditions and their treatment

Nasal allergy

Examples of nasal allergy include hay fever and allergic rhinitis. Sodium cromoglicate inhibits the release of chemical mediators such as histamine from mast cells. It is these mediators which, when released in response to exposure to an allergen, cause an allergic reaction. Sodium cromoglicate is used prophylactically, and treatment should be commenced several weeks before the hay fever season commences and continued on a regular basis.

In severe rhinitis, administration of a corticosteroid such as beclometasone (in a spray form) directly into the nose decreases inflammation and oedema of the nasal mucosa. Corticosteroids (as a spray) should not be administered in the presence of nasal infection. The possibility of systemic absorption of corticosteroids must always be considered. Systemic corticosteroids may be required in short courses for severe conditions. Oral antihistamines may also be required. Azelastine is an antihistamine available for use as a nasal spray.

In cases where there are severe associated symptoms, e.g. allergic conjunctivitis, supplementary medication may be required.

Nasal congestion

Congestion occurs in vasomotor rhinitis, nasal polyps and the common cold. Most decongestants are sympathomimetic drugs which cause vasoconstriction of the mucosal blood vessels and provide relief of congestion. The most significant adverse reaction is rebound nasal congestion if treatment is prolonged. Ephedrine nasal drops should be used for no more than 5–7 days to avoid rebound congestion. Xylometazoline (nasal drops or spray) is much longer-acting than ephedrine but more likely to cause rebound nasal congestion.

Ipratropium nasal spray (an antimuscarinic agent) is used to treat watery rhinorrhoea (see also p. 211).

Sinusitis

Acute sinusitis frequently follows a viral upper respiratory tract infection. It is caused by inadequate ventilation and drainage in the paranasal sinuses. Bacterial infection may develop if the sinuses are blocked with mucus. Facial pain and headache are common and may be associated with nasal congestion and post-nasal drip. A broad-spectrum antibiotic (co-amoxiclav) and a topical decongestant spray are valuable. Steam inhalations and analgesics will provide symptomatic relief.

Nasal infection

Local antibiotics have little place in the treatment of nasal infections but a cream containing chlorhexidine 0.1% and neomycin sulphate 0.5% is applied locally in the treatment of staphylococcal infections and prophylaxis against nasal carriage of staphylococci.

Intranasal chlorhexidine has been reported to cause anaphylactic circulatory arrest when applied to mucous membranes. In cases where a reaction is possible, careful history-taking is essential. If in doubt, chlorhexidine must be avoided in susceptible patients (Chisholm et al 1997). A nasal ointment containing mupirocin is available for hospital use in the eradication of nasal carriage of MRSA.

Epistaxis (nosebleed)

Epistaxis may result from a variety of causes including disordered clotting mechanisms. Persistent epistaxis requires full investigation. Packing, surgery and/or cautery may be required in some instances.

Nasal packs may be used to control severe epistaxis and as a rule are inserted by the doctor. The patient understandably is often very alarmed by the blood loss and requires a nurse to stay with, and reassure, him. Diazepam may be given orally and may be continued until the acute episode is over and the pack is removed. The insertion of a pack into the nasal cavity is done with the patient sitting up with clothing suitably protected. Using a suitable size of nasal speculum, the doctor, with the aid of forceps, inserts sterile half-inch (1 cm) ribbon gauze which has been impregnated with bismuth iodoform paraffin paste (BIPP). Alternatively, a Brighton catheter or a Foley catheter may be inserted into the nose and inflated to stop the bleeding. Patients appreciate a mouthwash after a nosebleed and may get rid of clots from the back of the throat by gargling. It is often advisable to administer an oral analgesic prior to removal of a nasal pack which, with drying, becomes painful to remove. To begin with, only half of the packing should be gently pulled out to see what happens. If there is no bleeding, the remainder can be removed but if the first stage has caused bleeding, the remainder of the pack should be left in place and a further attempt made later.

ADMINISTRATION OF NOSE PREPARATIONS (see also p. 432)

Nasal preparations

Nasal preparations usually take the form of nasal drops (Box 27.3). Instead of instilling drops, they may be sprayed into the patient's nose in powder form using a nasal insufflator. A nasal spray is also available which is inserted into the anterior nares. The container is squeezed two or three times to instil the medication. The effect, however, is very transient since the cilia lining the nasal cavities remove the drug in about 20 minutes. The nasal mucosa is utilised as a route for the administration of certain medications.

DRUG TREATMENT OF OROPHARYNGEAL DISORDERS

Anatomy and physiology

The oropharynx consists of the oral cavity within which there are the gums, teeth, hard palate, soft palate and uvula, tonsils and tongue. The oral cavity is lined throughout with mucous membrane containing small mucus-secreting glands. Three pairs of salivary glands,

Box 27.3 Instillation of nasal drops

Documentation
- Standard prescribing and recording sheet

The medicine
- Nasal drops as prescribed

The nurse and the patient
- Patient identified
- Explanation given to patient
- Patient assisted into supine position with head hyperextended (if not contraindicated), e.g. with head over edge of bed or with pillow under shoulders
- Patient left comfortable on completion of procedure

Technique
- Hand hygiene before and after instillation of drop
- Patient assisted if necessary to close off one nostril at a time and drop(s) inserted in the other without touching any part of the nose with the dropper
- Patient encouraged to sniff liquid into back of nose or, if unable, to maintain position for about 1 minute
- Patient instructed not to blow nose; patient offered bowl into which excess drops collected can be spat out

namely, parotid, submandibular and sublingual, also pour their secretions into the mouth. These combined secretions make up saliva which contains water, mucus, mineral salts and salivary amylase. Approximately 1.5 litres of saliva flow through the mouth in 24 hours; its purpose is to lubricate the oral cavity, initiate the digestion of starches and assist with chewing, swallowing and speaking. The output of saliva is increased by the sight of food, eating and drinking, brushing the teeth, and movement of the jaws.

The lining of a healthy mouth is moist and pink. The teeth are free from caries, the papillae on the tongue are visible and the lips intact. There is no discomfort or odour.

Common conditions and their treatment

Careful assessment and investigation of all oral lesions is essential since the lesion may be an indication of the presence of a serious underlying medical condition. Patients with long-standing oral lesions that do not respond to standard treatments should be investigated using microbiological, biochemical, haematological and immunological tests. Biopsy may be required in order to eliminate malignant disease.

There are many causes of oral ulceration; infection, trauma, blood disorder, gastrointestinal disease, nutritional deficiency, and drug therapy causing immunodeficiency such as cancer chemotherapy all predispose to a breakdown of the oral mucosa. Treatment of the underlying condition should resolve the oral problem. Aphthous ulcers are very painful, non-specific mouth ulcerations which are difficult to treat. Good oral hygiene is an essential part of the treatment of all oral lesions.

Sore throat

Sore throat caused by bacteria or (more usually) viruses is a common condition. It is often very difficult to identify the cause. Unless the sore throat is associated with respiratory distress (when hospital admission is called for), simple management methods are appropriate. Salt water gargles, paracetamol or a soothing lozenge may be helpful. Compound analgesics and NSAIDs are not recommended. Oral rinses containing an anti-inflammatory drug (benzydamine) may be worthwhile. The cause(s) of recurrent sore throat should be investigated in detail. Failure of previous therapy may be a cause (owing to inadequate therapy and/or non-compliance). Antibiotic therapy (penicillin V 500 mg four times daily for 10 days) may be required if the presence of beta-haemolytic streptococcus is confirmed. The use of antibiotics to prevent the complications of streptococcal pharyngitis (rheumatic fever or acute glomerular nephritis) is not supported by the evidence (SIGN, 1999). Surgery (tonsillectomy) is normally only carried out following assessment of the patient (against defined criteria) over a 6-month period. Long-term treatment with certain drugs (see p. 135) may be a cause of a persistent sore throat. This cause should always be eliminated by careful investigations including the patient's detailed drug history.

Acute tonsillitis

The condition presents with sore throat, often with pain on swallowing, pyrexia and upper respiratory infection, possibly associated with otalgia. Children are most commonly affected. Difficulties may arise in determining whether the infecting organism is bacterial or viral. On examination, the tonsils are engorged with or without purulent discharge, with localised lymph node enlargement. Treatment is designed to alleviate symptoms. Antibiotic therapy should not be delayed until the results of a swab have been obtained. Oral penicillin V (or erythromycin in penicillin-sensitive persons) is the first line of treatment. Ampicillin should be avoided since in cases of glandular fever an erythematous rash will develop. If first-line antibiotics fail, a cephalosporin

Table 27.2 Some drugs used for the treatment of aphthous ulcers

Drug	Notes
Benzydamine hydrochloride	Used as a mouthwash or solution spray to relieve pain and inflammation
Hydrocortisone lozenges (2.5 mg)	Held in the mouth as near as possible to the ulcer to reduce inflammation
Tetracycline	May be of benefit in the form of a mouthwash
Triamcinolone dental paste	A specially formulated paste designed to adhere to mucous membranes; contains a potent corticosteroid; care should be taken to treat any concomitant infection that may be present

or co-amoxiclav may be required. Increased fluid intake, analgesia or a suitable oral rinse will be helpful. Glandular fever (infectious mononucleosis) is associated with very swollen tonsils often covered with a dirty yellow membrane. Management of glandular fever is directed towards alleviating symptoms. Antipyretics and analgesics will be needed.

Oral ulceration and inflammation

Hexetidine solution 0.1% w/v has antibacterial and antiprotozoal activity. It is used in the treatment of gingivitis and pharyngitis, and for oral hygiene generally. The solution (15 mL) should normally be used undiluted although some patients may find the taste rather unpleasant. It should be used two to three times daily.

Hydrogen peroxide solution 6% (20 vols) is an oxidising agent which, when in contact with organic matter, effervesces releasing oxygen; this has some mechanical cleansing action. This solution is particularly useful in dealing with anaerobic organisms which cause acute gingivitis or where the tongue is so heavily furred that other solutions are rendered ineffective. To minimise the likelihood of local irritation, 15 mL is diluted with a cartonful of warm water. The mouth should be rinsed for 2–3 minutes two to three times per day.

Aphthous ulcers. These are difficult to treat because of the problem of maintaining an adequate concentration of drug in contact with the lesions. Table 27.2 gives some drugs which may be prescribed.

Oropharyngeal infection

Mild oral lesions are treated with a salicylate-containing gel but this is not suitable for prolonged use in children owing to the possibility of absorption of salicylate leading to adverse reactions. Tetracycline mouthwash may be helpful in treating severe herpetic infections of the mouth. The mouthwash is prepared by mixing the contents of a capsule with a small amount of water immediately before use. The resulting solution is held in the mouth for 2–3 minutes, three or four times a day. The solution should not be swallowed.

Fungal infections

Fungal infections of the mouth, principally candidiasis (thrush), are especially likely to arise in patients who are debilitated or immunosuppressed. The commonest groups affected are the very young, the elderly and those receiving a course of broad-spectrum antibiotic, cytotoxic medication, or intensive chemotherapy for AIDS.

Nystatin (suspension or pastilles) is commonly used to treat oral candidiasis. The medication should be retained in the mouth for as long as possible to ensure maximum effect. Patients will need to be given guidance on the best way to use the particular product and the need to avoid eating or drinking for a short time after treatment.

Amphotericin, in the form of suspension (or lozenges), is an alternative antifungal agent especially where the infecting organism is resistant to nystatin. Miconazole is an antifungal agent with a wide spectrum of activity against pathogenic fungi and some Gram-positive bacteria. An oral gel is available containing 125 mg in 5 mL. The gel is retained in the mouth in contact with the lesion for as long as possible.

Denture hygiene. When candidal infection has been diagnosed, the care of a patient's dentures becomes a particularly important part of oral hygiene. First, the dentures should be removed and left to dry for 8 hours. They should then be immersed in sodium hypochlorite or chlorhexidine gluconate 0.2% (if denture made of chrome cobalt) overnight and rinsed well before being reused. This should be repeated twice weekly. If possible, the patient should stop using the dentures for 2 weeks. Miconazole, either in the form of an oral gel or a denture lacquer, may be prescribed for application to the surface of the denture as part of the overall care and treatment of oral candidiasis.

Viral infections

Viral infections of the mouth include herpetic stomatitis. Vesicles form in the mouth and these break down to give ulcers. The treatment of choice for herpes simplex virus infections of the skin near the mouth is aciclovir cream 5%. This product is available over the counter for the treatment of cold sores. Treatment also includes a soft diet with good fluid intake. Good oral hygiene is essential. Supplementary treatment with antibiotics, antifungal agents and analgesics may be required.

Tongue lesions

Black hairy tongue and furred tongue are treated with a combination of oral hygiene and appropriate therapy where a specific underlying condition can be identified.

Oral leukoplakia is caused by the Epstein–Barr virus and presents as white plaques on the tongue. Biopsy of the mucous membrane reveals pre-cancerous changes. It can occur in smokers and where there has been long-standing infection such as chronic candidiasis and tertiary syphilis. It can also occur in AIDS patients. Treatment of the underlying cause generally resolves the condition.

Other oral lesions

- Blisters due to pemphigus vulgaris
- Benign mucous membrane pemphigoid
- Oral manifestations of lichen planus
- Erythema multiforme (may be caused by a drug reaction)
- Angina bullosa haemorrhagica.

Treatment of the above conditions involves oral hygiene, topical corticosteroids, local antiseptics and analgesics, and in the case of erythema multiforme a course of oral/systemic corticosteroids may be required.

- Gingivitis may arise because of poor oral hygiene but may present as acute necrotising ulcerative gingivitis which requires antimicrobial therapy (metronidazole).
- Squamous cell papilloma. These benign lesions are caused by the human papilloma virus. Treatment is surgical excision to prevent recurrence.

Malignant disease

Oral cancer is rare, but suspicious presentations (long-standing ulceration/white patches) should be referred for specialist investigation and treatment.

CARE OF THE MOUTH IN SPECIAL SITUATIONS

Reduced salivary flow

Dry mouth (xerostomia) can cause considerable discomfort. It may result from a reduction in salivary flow such as occurs with:

- certain drugs, e.g. antispasmodics and tricyclic antidepressants or drugs having antimuscarinic side-effects
- radiotherapy to the head and neck
- infection of a salivary gland
- inflammation of the mouth or throat
- dental or oral surgery.

Local and systemic treatments are available. Artificial saliva products containing electrolytes and gelling agents at neutral pH are available as a spray, lozenge or pastille.

Pilocarpine (a muscarinic drug) is administered as a tablet (5 mg) in cases of salivary gland malfunction following radiotherapy for head and neck cancers. The contraindications and side-effects are very significant, as would be expected from a potent muscarinic drug (see p. 145).

In general, lozenges, sprays, etc. have little proven therapeutic benefit but do offer some comfort when required. Boiled sweets or chewing gum may be just as helpful.

Lowered resistance to infection

In situations where patients are receiving chemotherapy or radiotherapy, or are immunosuppressed for any other reason, a broad-spectrum antimicrobial such as chlorhexidine gluconate 0.2% may be used prophylactically in the form of a mouthwash. Patients may choose from a variety of flavours. The solution (10 mL, four or five times per day) should be held in the mouth for 1 minute before being expelled. In view of possible incompatibility, 30 minutes should be allowed to elapse before using toothpaste. The patient should be warned that the solution may cause brown staining of the teeth. On completion of treatment, staining can be removed by a dentist. Stained fillings may have to be replaced.

Post-tonsillectomy

Mouthwashes are administered after tonsillectomy to remove blood clots from the throat. Using the mouthwash as a gargle may help to clear the throat by mechanical action. The solutions used in this situation are intended to:

- detach blood clots and debris (hydrogen peroxide solution)
- ease pain using local analgesic (benzydamine hydrochloride solution)
- treat or prevent infection (povidone-iodine solution)
- cleanse and refresh (thymol mouthwash solution).

Post-radiation inflammation of the throat

Patients receiving radiotherapy to the head and neck, or chest can suffer from an extremely sore throat. This may be soothed without aggravating the existing reaction by using sodium bicarbonate solution or povidone-iodine solution as a mouthwash or gargle.

ORAL HYGIENE

The need to carry out oral hygiene in one form or another to rid the mouth of debris is part of everyday living. When illness presents, the need for oral hygiene is much greater. For example, with anorexia, vomiting, constipation, pyrexia, dehydration and fatigue, the tongue and the teeth become dry and coated, and if left uncared for result in a foul taste, bad smell and the development of oral sepsis.

Where fluid intake has to be restricted, the mouth quickly becomes dry, as it does when a patient is mouth-breathing or receiving continuous oxygen therapy. Patients who are immunosuppressed, as the result of a disease such as leukaemia or treatment such as radiation or cytotoxic drugs, are prone to mouth infections. The cells of the oral mucosa and salivary glands divide at a moderately rapid rate. Anticancer treatments aimed at rapidly replicating malignant cells are unfortunately not sufficiently selective and so the mouth is often adversely affected. Diuretics, psychotropics and insulin, as well as sympathomimetic and parasympathomimetic agents, all alter salivary function. Antibiotics may encourage opportunistic bacteria to flourish in the mouth by reducing the resident flora. The many situations regarded as 'high risk' for developing some form of discomfort of the mouth are evidence of how important this procedure is for nurses.

Some patients can be left to attend to this aspect of their care, some simply need to be prompted or given encouragement. Other patients are capable of carrying out the procedure for themselves but may need assistance in gathering together the necessary equipment. Many patients are wholly dependent on the nurse to meet every need. The purpose is to remove, and prevent the build-up of, plaque, to stimulate the flow of saliva and reduce the risk of complications such as candidal infection and parotitis. The three direct methods employed are:

- brushing the teeth with toothpaste and water
- rinsing the mouth with mouthwash solution
- swabbing the mouth (Box 27.4).

Box 27.4 Swabbing the mouth

The medicine
- Mouthwash solution tablets
- Soft paraffin

The environment
- Privacy, warmth, comfort

The nurse and the patient
- Patient given explanation, if appropriate, of what is involved
- Patient assisted, if necessary, into position which allows ease of access

The technique
- Nurse ensures that hands are socially clean before and after procedure
- Patient's dentures removed if appropriate
- Mouth examined using spatula and torch to identify area requiring greatest attention, e.g. tongue
- Solution prepared
- Excess solution squeezed from each swab before use
- Oral cavity gently and systematically wiped from inside using mouthwash solution
- Each swab used for one wipe only and then discarded
- Mouth re-inspected
- Soft paraffin applied sparingly to lips if indicated
- Dentures thoroughly brushed before being replaced
- Discarded material carefully disposed of
- Patient made comfortable
- Observations noted on nursing records

Hazards
- Infected mouth
- Spread of infection to other patients
- Inhalation of swab or solution by unconscious patient

Wherever possible, patients should be encouraged to brush their teeth in the usual way or have their teeth brushed for them. Research has shown that use of a toothbrush is the most effective method for cleaning the teeth and removing plaque (Howarth 1977). A brush may also be used to deal with the problem of a heavily coated tongue and in edentulous patients for cleaning the gums and cheeks also. The act of cleaning one's teeth is an important and beneficial part of any programme of rehabilitation for disabled patients. Stroke patients, for example, can be helped to regain independence and to overcome a lack of awareness which many of them have of one side of the face. Patients with a reduced platelet count whose gums are very liable to bleed are nevertheless also encouraged to use a toothbrush although it must be a soft one.

Alternatively, an electric toothbrush may be used since the brushes rotate and are less traumatic than a conventional toothbrush.

Mouthwashes are easier for patients to manage when they feel weak and unwell. Swabbing with the finger or a foam stick, though not a pleasant procedure for the patient, is essential for those who are acutely ill, unconscious or in the terminal stages of illness. This approach needs to be gentle yet effective. The airway of the unconscious or semiconscious patient must be protected at all times. Because of the danger of inhalation, any excess of the solution used for cleaning the mouth should be wrung out of the swab before use. Man-made woven swabs are less inclined to fray and are therefore safer. Care must be taken to ensure that the sponge of an applicator is not retained in the mouth by accident. With conscious patients, the tongue and roof of the mouth should be touched carefully so as not to make the patient 'gag'. Although oral hygiene is not a sterile procedure, sterile disposable equipment is used for each patient to prevent cross-infection. Gloves are worn by nurses for their own protection, and care should be taken to dispose of soiled materials safely. Ideally, food debris should be removed from the teeth after each meal. Patients appreciate being given the opportunity to rinse dentures after meals. It should be remembered that many patients do not like to be seen without their dentures and so privacy should be provided. Very ill patients will require to have the mouth cleaned at least every 2 hours. Whichever method is applied the aims of oral care are the same, i.e. to cleanse and moisten the mucosa.

There are further ways of helping to keep the mouth of conscious patients clean and moist. Apart from encouraging and facilitating nasal breathing, imaginative ideas of suitable food and drinks, if permitted, may be put into practice. Flavoured ice lollies, chips of ice, boiled sweets or chewing gum may help. Fruit juices, especially those containing lemon, stimulate the flow of saliva and are cleansing and refreshing but may cause the mouth or lips to sting if the mucosa is irritated or broken.

In summary, the role of the nurse in oral hygiene is:

- to assess the state of the patient's mouth
- to select the appropriate method of oral hygiene for the patient
- to estimate the amount of assistance the patient requires with the procedure
- to assist the patient with oral hygiene as required
- to observe, report and record details of the condition of the patient's mouth
- to teach aspects of oral hygiene to patients and relatives.

As with other fundamental nursing procedures, most patients are highly appreciative of the care given to make the mouth feel more comfortable. The contribution mouth care can make to improving the appetite and boosting morale cannot be overemphasised. It is a nursing responsibility to ensure that oral hygiene is accorded the high priority it so often warrants.

Special measures taken to keep a patient's mouth clean and comfortable are generally required only for as long as the patient is acutely ill. As the patient's general state of health improves there is usually a corresponding improvement in the condition of the mouth.

PREPARATIONS USED IN GENERAL CARE OF THE MOUTH

The preparation selected for use will depend on local guidelines as contained in a nursing formulary or laid down in some other way, although it cannot be overemphasised that the frequency and standard of mouth care are every bit as important as the individual mouthwash solutions used. The properties of two commonly used preparations are described below.

Thymol

Mouthwash solution tablets. One tablet dissolved in 125 ml (one paper carton) of water yields an aromatic, pleasant-tasting alkaline solution containing thymol, which has mild antimicrobial and deodorant properties.

Compound thymol glycerin. This product, when diluted with three times its volume of water, yields a solution with similar properties to that produced by dissolving a mouthwash solution tablet. Both solutions are used to freshen the mouth and for mechanical cleansing. Most patients with a sore mouth appreciate the soothing properties of warm mouthwashes. However, some patients, especially if they are pyrexial, welcome the refreshing effect of a cold mouthwash.

Care must be taken to avoid microbial contamination of thymol mouthwashes by rejecting any unused solution on completion of the procedure. Thymol, in the concentrations normally present in mouthwash solutions, is only a very weak antimicrobial agent. If solutions become contaminated, bacterial growth can occur with consequent risk of infection, especially in immunosuppressed patients.

REFERENCES

Chisholm D G, Calder I, Peterson D et al 1997 Drug points: intranasal chlorhexidine resulting in anaphylactic circulatory arrest. British Medical Journal 315:785

Howarth H 1977 Mouth care procedures for the very ill. Nursing Times 73:354–355

Scottish Intercollegiate Guidelines Network (SIGN) 1999 Management of sore throat and indications for tonsillectomy. Publication No. 34. SIGN, Edinburgh

FURTHER READING

[Anonymous] 2001 Nurse-led upper respiratory tract infection clinic: Part I triage of sore throats and hoarseness. Primary Care Pharmacist: 22–28

Heals D 1993 A key to wellbeing. Oral hygiene in patients with advanced cancer. Professional Nurse 8(6):391–398

Little P, Gould C 2001. Pragmatic randomised controlled trial of two prescribing strategies for childhood acute otitis media. British Medical Journal 322:336–342

Ludman H 1988 ABC of ear nose and throat. British Medical Association, London

Peate I 1993 Nurse-administered oral hygiene in the hospitalised patient. British Journal of Nursing 2(9):459–462

Roos K, Håkansson E G, Holm S 2001 Effect of recolonisation with 'interfering' α streptococci on recurrences of acute and secretory otitis media in children: randomised placebo controlled trial. British Medical Journal 322:210–212

Torrance C 1990 Oral hygiene. Surgical Nurse 3(4):16–20

CHAPTER CONTENTS

28

Drug treatment of skin disorders

INTRODUCTION

The skin can be described as the body's largest organ (other than the lungs) in terms of surface area. The skin provides a waterproof surface and retains essential fluids. It acts as a barrier against infections and is a major controller of body temperature, the heat of the body being regulated by the blood vessels and sweating. It protects underlying organs from physical, chemical and other injuries. The nerve endings in the skin serve as a relay between external influences and internal organs. The skin acts as an organ of expression, betraying the innermost feelings – anxiety by sweating, anger by a red flush and fear by pallor. It is an important store for water, containing 18–20% of the total water content of the body, which is distributed mainly in the dermis. This percentage decreases with age.

ANATOMY AND PHYSIOLOGY

For practical purposes the skin can be considered in three areas (Fig. 28.1):

- epidermis
- dermis
- accessory organs, e.g. sweat glands, sebaceous glands, the nails and the hair follicles.

Epidermis

The outermost layer of the skin is the epidermis. The epidermis itself has five layers. From the inside out, they are:

- the stratum basale where active columnar cells (keratinocytes) divide
- the stratum spinosum which consists of several layers of irregularly shaped cells
- the stratum granulosum where granules are visible in the cells' cytoplasm

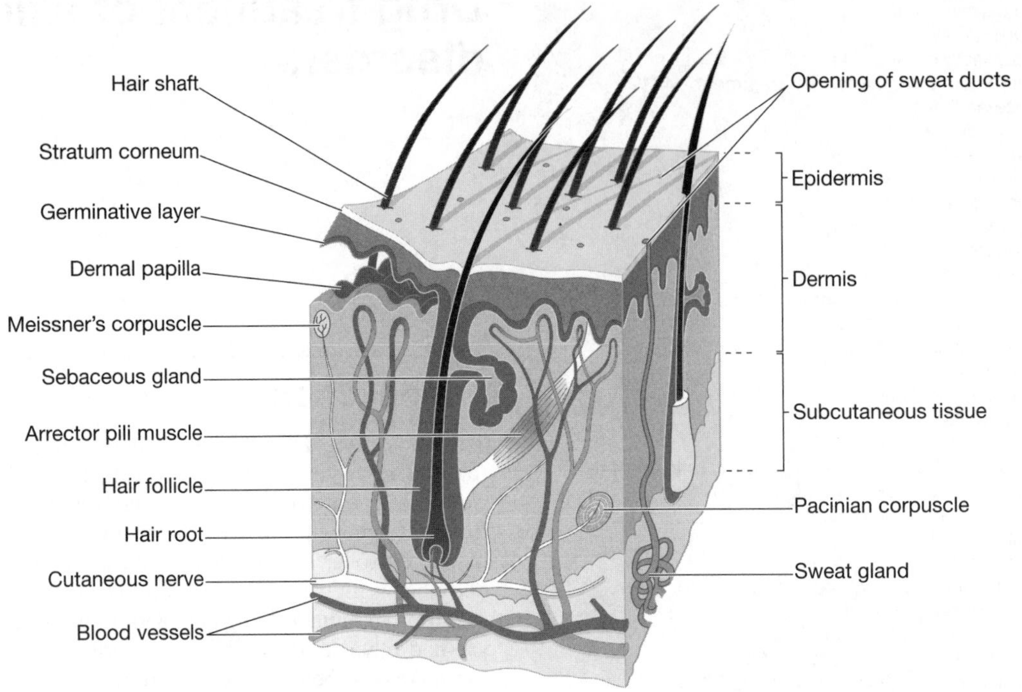

Figure 28.1 Anatomy of the skin.

- the stratum lucidum – a layer of living cells which contains a translucent compound from which keratin is formed; this layer is only present in the palms of the hands and soles of the feet
- the stratum corneum – a horny layer of thin, flat, non-nucleated cells which have become keratinised, i.e. where the protoplasm has been replaced by keratin, a protein which toughens the epidermis and renders it waterproof. The surface of the skin is composed of dead cells which are constantly being rubbed off.

Within the epidermis, a continuous synchronised process takes place in which the cells of the stratum corneum that flake off are replaced at the same rate by new cells generated in the stratum basale. The process repeats itself as the new cells migrate through the epidermal layers, gradually changing in shape and size and in turn reaching the surface where they are shed.

Specialised cells, known as melanocytes, are to be found in the basal layer. They are responsible for the production of melanin, a protective pigment released following exposure to sunlight.

Dermis

The dermis is thicker than the epidermis and consists of two layers of fibrous connective tissue (collagen) which support the epidermis and give it its elasticity. The papillary layer lies next to the epidermis and as its name implies is made up of papillae – tiny projections containing capillaries which nourish the epidermis and nerve endings responsible for the reflex action in response to painful stimuli. The reticular layer consists of a thick mesh of collagen fibres which make the skin strong and flexible. Blood vessels, nerves and fatty tissue are also present and it is throughout this layer that the sweat glands, sebaceous glands and hair follicles are located.

Accessory organs

Sweat glands

Millions of tiny sweat glands are located in the dermis all over the body. There are two types of sweat gland.

Exocrine glands are the commoner type and are mostly concentrated in the palms, soles and forehead. They become active when the body temperature rises through exercise, a hot environment or emotional stress. They promote cooling by evaporation of their secretion on the skin's surface. Apocrine glands are found in the axillary, anal, genital and mammary areas of the body. Sweat is produced by these glands under the influence of the sympathetic nervous system when emotionally stressed and at times of sexual arousal.

Sebaceous glands

Sebaceous glands are situated in the dermis. Their function is to produce sebum, an oil containing fatty acids, cholesterol and substances toxic to bacteria. Sebum is discharged through the sebaceous duct into the hair follicle, moving along the shaft of the hair to the skin surface keeping both the skin and the hair soft. The glands are located all over the body, except the palms and soles, in close association with body hair.

Nails

The nails are keratininsed epidermal cells which have a horny texture and serve to protect the fingers and toes. A nail consists of:

- a body which is the exposed part – it is an extension of the germinative area of the epidermis and is composed of a greatly thickened stratum lucidum; the area beneath the nail body is highly vascular
- the lunula (moon-shaped) under which are the epithelial cells
- the cuticle, a fold at the base and sides of the nail
- the nail root whose cells dictate the rate of nail growth.

Hair

A hair behaves in a similar way to a nail in that it is formed by a group of cells at its base which multiply and push forward to the surface of the skin where it is ultimately shed or removed. The base of each hair, referred to as the bulb, is situated in the dermis. A pointed projection of the dermis protruding into the hair bulb is known as the papilla. The papilla nourishes the cells of the hair follicle housing the hair root. The root is the part beneath the surface of the skin; the shaft is the visible part. By the time the hair follicle reaches the surface, its cells have become hard and keratinised.

COMMON CONDITIONS AND THEIR TREATMENT

Eczema

Eczema is recognised by a characteristic inflammatory reaction in the skin caused by a number of factors, either internal, external or a combination of these. Internal (constitutional) factors are thought to underlie a number of different types of endogenous eczema. For those forms of eczema associated with external factors (exogenous) the term dermatitis still tends to be used. Lawton's classification of eczema (Hughes & Van Onselen 2001) is given in Box 28.1.

Eczema may be further subdivided into acute, subacute and chronic forms. Where there is an acute reaction, the clinical features include erythema and small vesicles that break down causing weeping, oedema and scaling. In subacute eczema, features of both acute and chronic eczema are in evidence. The skin is red and thickened as the result of inflammation and scratching to relieve the associated itch. Many patients are very troubled by itching. The scratching is often followed by serious local damage, leading to lichen simplex, a leathery patch in an accessible area of the patient's skin. In chronic eczema, the same features are present although they are less pronounced, but there is more thickening and scaling. Pigmentation may be increased.

Endogenous eczema

Atopic eczema

This form of eczema commonly arises in infancy. There is a hereditary tendency to develop immediate allergic reactions with inflammation, intense itch and excoriation especially on the face and skin creases. It is strongly

Box 28.1 Classification of eczema

Exogenous
- Contact irritant
- Contact allergic
- Photosensitive

Endogenous
- Atopic eczema
- Seborrhoeic
- Discoid
- Gravitational
- Pompholyx

Unclassified
- Asteatotic
- Lichen simplex
- Juvenile plantar dermatosis

linked with a history (personal or close family) of other atopic diseases such as asthma and hay fever.

Exogenous eczema

Contact dermatitis

This form of skin disease is associated with exposure to an irritant or an allergen. Contact irritant dermatitis is more common than the allergic form. Contact with highly toxic substances such as acids may result in an acute irritant dermatitis. Repeat exposure to certain less toxic substances such as detergents may also lead to an irritant dermatitis although it may take longer to appear. Contact irritant dermatitis is more prevalent among people in certain occupations such as hairdressing and nursing. The hands are most commonly affected. On first exposure to an offending allergen, susceptible individuals are unaware of an immune response developing. It is only on subsequent exposure to the allergen that there is an eczematous reaction at the point of contact. Contact allergic dermatitis arises in susceptible individuals who have a hypersensitivity to certain materials (e.g. rubber), metals (e.g. nickel), perfumes (e.g. in soap), etc.

Treatment

Eczema and dermatitis are treated similarly, but it is especially important in cases of dermatitis to avoid or remove the causative agent (e.g. cosmetic, household cleaner). Treatment with bland emollients is often helpful (allowing patient choice). Creams for direct application are easy to use and provide welcome relief from itching. Emollient bath additives are useful in many cases of dry skin. The use of topical corticosteroids, starting with a mild product, then moving to a moderate product depending on response, provides symptom control. Overuse of corticosteroids must be avoided. Alternating emollients with corticosteroids may be a useful strategy.

Coal tar preparations have a limited place in the treatment of chronic atopic eczema. Poor acceptance by the patient and possible long-term side-effects have curtailed their use. Ichthammol has properties similar to those of coal tar but is milder in action.

In situations where allergy and/or infection are present, oral antihistamines or antibiotics will be required. The use of gamolenic acid in atopic eczema is not based on firm evidence of therapeutic benefit. Seborrhoeic eczema of the scalp is treated by shampoos containing coal tar or selenium, or a specially formulated corticosteroid scalp preparation in the form of a mousse. The preferred treatment is a shampoo containing ketoconazole, an antifungal agent.

Psoriasis

Psoriasis is a chronic skin disorder characterised by circumscribed red plaques covered by thick, dry, silvery adherent scales which make the skin itchy and unsightly. It occurs when there is an excessive production of epidermal cells and the shedding of old skin cells remains normal, resulting in the characteristic lesions of psoriasis. It may occur at any age and can appear in any area of the body although lesions more frequently arise on bony prominences such as the elbows, knees and sacral area. The scalp is another common site. There are numerous types of psoriasis whose names reflect such aspects as the appearance of the skin; the location of the plaques; the presence of papules or pustules; whether it is of an acute or chronic form; and localised or generalised. The cause of this condition is not known but genetic factors and trigger factors such as stress may be involved.

Treatment

Topical and oral therapies are available, many of which require specialist advice. For mild conditions, an emollient may be useful to minimise scaling. This will seldom provide adequate relief but can be helpful when plaque thickness has been reduced by other therapies. Salicylic acid (2% ointment) has keratolytic properties but care should be taken, especially with stronger products, to control the amounts applied in order to avoid absorption leading to systemic toxicity (see p. 450).

Coal tar preparations have anti-inflammatory and antiscaling properties. Choice of product will depend on the site of the plaques and the preference of the patient. Dithranol is a more potent agent than coal tar. The use of dithranol requires expert management by both prescriber and nurse. Dithranol acts by combining with deoxyribonucleic acid, resulting in the inhibition of nucleoprotein synthesis and so diminishing cellular proliferation. Short-contact applications of 1 hour are effective, the strength of dithranol depending on the patient's condition within a range of 0.15–2%, often incorporated in Lassar's paste. Dithranol can cause severe skin irritation and, for this reason, it must be used strictly in accordance with the prescription. It must be applied only to psoriatic plaques (protecting surrounding skin) commencing with a low concentration and gradually increasing this to an optimum concentration which produces a therapeutic effect without irritation. Dithranol stains skin purple-brown but this fades in 2 or 3 weeks. It is essential for nurses to wear gloves and avoid all contact, especially with the eyes, when applying dithranol preparations. Hands should be thoroughly washed after use.

A range of strengths of dithranol is available in cream formulations, which are easier to apply than stiff pastes. Contact time will depend on the strength of active ingredient, e.g. 0.1% overnight contact, 1–2% maximum of 1 hour. A novel dermal delivery system for dithranol presents dithranol (1 or 3%) in a special cream. The dithranol is incorporated in a protective 'sandwich' which maintains the stability of dithranol. Contact time is 30 minutes.

Topical corticosteroid creams have a limited place in the treatment of plaque psoriasis. Skin atrophy can result and render the condition intractable to treatment. A mild or moderate corticosteroid may be used in the flexures. Potent corticosteroids may be used on the scalp in the short term.

Calcipotriol (a derivative of vitamin D) is used topically for mild to moderate plaque psoriasis. A scalp preparation is available. Unlike dithranol, it is easy to use and is non-staining. Tacalcitol is used once daily for similar conditions.

For more severe psoriasis not responding to topical treatments, oral treatments may be required. Acitretin (a vitamin A derivative) is an oral retinoid, available only in hospital, which should be prescribed only by or under the supervision of a consultant dermatologist; 25–30 mg is administered daily for 2–4 weeks, then adjusted according to response. This will usually be in the range of 25–50 mg daily for a further 6–8 weeks; however, a higher dose and longer treatment time may be needed. Side-effects include dryness and cracking of the lips, pruritus and nosebleeds. Acitretin is teratogenic, and contraceptive measures in women who may become pregnant should be commenced at least 1 month before treatment initiation and continued for at least 2 years following cessation of the drug. Tazarotene is a retinoid available as a gel formulation for the treatment of mild to moderate plaque psoriasis affecting up to 10% of skin area.

Oral treatment of severe resistant psoriasis with ciclosporin may be used under close specialist supervision. Side-effects and contraindications may be severe. Dosage is initially 2.5 mg/kg daily in two divided doses, gradually increasing to 5 mg/kg per day. Treatment is discontinued if no improvement is seen in 6 weeks.

Another drug is methotrexate used in severe, uncontrolled, resistant cases, under hospital supervision, for its antimitotic activity. It is a folic acid antagonist which inhibits cellular proliferation. In view of the toxicity of this drug it is very important to monitor the patient's response and to adjust the dose accordingly.

Photochemotherapy involves the use of an oral photosensitising agent (a psoralen) (P) and exposure to ultraviolet A light (UVA). The treatment, known as PUVA, is used for both initial treatment and maintenance therapy. Long-term dangers of this form of therapy are not yet confirmed.

Appropriate treatment of psoriasis improves the appearance of the skin. However, because drugs cannot cure the underlying cause of the disorder, psoriasis tends to recur.

Psoriasis in all its forms can have a very damaging psychological impact on patients. Full support, counselling and advice are essential, as is compliance by the patient.

The main approaches used in the treatment of psoriasis are summarised in Box 28.2.

Acne

Acne vulgaris is a common condition affecting mainly adolescents but it can occur later in life. It is caused by excess production of sebum by the sebaceous glands leading to a blockage of hair follicles by skin debris and hardened sebum. Acne normally affects the skin on the face and neck, and less frequently the back and chest.

Acne may be classified as follows:

- mild
  - papules (inflamed spots)
  - pustules (raised, pus-filled spots with a white centre)
  - comedones (blackheads – dark, owing to the effect of oxygen on sebum)
- moderate – more extensive papules and pustules with possible scarring
- severe – many papules and pustules with significant scarring.

Box 28.2 Summary of treatment options for psoriasis

Topical
- Keratolytics
- Coal tar
- Dithranol
- Steroids
- Vitamin D analogues
- Phototherapy – ultraviolet B (UVB)

Systemic
- PUVA – psoralens and ultraviolet A
- Retinoids
- Methotrexate
- Ciclosporin

Treatment

Treatments available include topical and oral preparations. Topical products are intended to remove follicular plugs and reduce skin bacterial flora. Benzoyl peroxide alone or in combination with an antimicrobial agent is widely used. Such products have both a keratolytic and antimicrobial action. Irritation of the skin commonly occurs but will normally subside. Azelaic acid (20% cream) has similar actions to benzoyl peroxide. Gels containing nicotinamide (4%) have an anti-inflammatory effect which may be valuable in mild to moderate inflammatory acne.

Tretinoin reduces sebum production. When applied to the skin it produces an erythematous reaction, and skin peeling may occur after application for several days. Topical preparations of erythromycin, tetracycline or clindamycin are useful in patients with mild to moderately severe acne. A combination product of an antibiotic and retinoid is available for topical use. Topical corticosteroids should not be used for acne.

Topical retinoids (forms of vitamin A) have anticomedogenic properties, both locally and systemically. Creams and gels of both tretinoin and isotretinoin are available. Redness of the skin and peeling may occur, which should settle in time. Contact with mucous membranes and eyes must be avoided. Both topical and oral retinoids are contraindicated in pregnancy and eczema.

If acne is severe, a course of oral tetracycline or erythromycin may be prescribed – 250 mg three times daily before meals for 1–4 weeks then reduced to twice daily until improvement occurs. Several months' treatment or even longer may be required. Resistance to commonly used antibiotics is common. Female patients must stop tetracycline if they become pregnant because this drug is deposited in developing teeth and bones. If the treatments described above are unsuccessful, isotretinoin, an oral drug, may be prescribed. This has an action which is similar, but more powerful, to that of tretinoin. It is a hospital-only preparation and should be prescribed only by or under the supervision of a hospital consultant. Side-effects include dry lips, nosebleeds and some loss of hair. Isotretinoin is teratogenic and must not be given to pregnant women. Contraceptive measures in women who may become pregnant must be effective and must last for 1 month after completion of treatment. Broad-spectrum antibiotic treatment can compromise the effectiveness of combined oral contraceptives. This is thought to be due to the effect of the antibiotic on the gut flora which is responsible for recycling ethinylestradiol from the large bowel. Suitable guidance must be given to patients on contraception.

Rosacea

Rosacea is a form of acne but, unlike acne vulgaris, it is not comedonal. As with acne vulgaris, the condition, characterised by facial flushing, causes considerable distress to those affected. The condition can develop if not treated, leading to persistent facial erythema and inflammatory episodes with swelling, pustules and papules.

The causes of this disorder are poorly understood but ultraviolet light, extremes of temperature and certain foods/drink are thought to act as triggers. Emotional stress can exacerbate the condition.

Treatment

Antibiotic treatment is used to reduce inflammation. In mild cases, topical metronidazole (cream) is commonly used. For more severe rosacea, an oral antibiotic such as oxytetracycline (500 mg twice daily) or tetracycline (500 mg twice daily) may be added. Where these drugs are contraindicated as in renal impairment doxycycline (100 mg daily) may be used instead. In severe cases, minocycline (100 mg daily) may be further added. Where there is resistance to antibiotics or there are persistent clinical features, oral tretinoin may be prescribed. Laser therapy may be required for the treatment of telangiectasia.

As well as complying with the prescribed treatment, patients can assist by avoiding or reducing their intake of spicy foods, chocolate, hot drinks, alcohol, etc. An effective, non-irritant sunscreen should be used to prevent a worsening of the condition. Redness may be effectively disguised with the assistance of a camouflage cream.

Pediculosis

Contrary to popular belief, head lice (*Pediculus humanus capitis*) are not confined to dirty long hair. In fact they flourish on both clean and dirty hair (both short and long) and are passed from person to person when one head is in prolonged contact with another. They are not caused by bad hygiene. Often adults will be involved in the passing on of the infestation. The head louse would appear to have a preference for the blood of children. The reason for this is not understood. As boys get older they are much less susceptible to infestation than are girls. Mixing at home, at school or while playing increases the risk to all children. There is never a single case of head lice.

Lice are born, live and die on the host, leaving the head only to transfer to a similar environment. They spend their time feeding off the scalp and reproducing.

The eggs laid are glued to the base of a strand of hair and are well camouflaged as they change in colour to match the skin. Once the eggs incubate, each hatches to produce a louse which, left untreated, will eventually sap the host's strength and leave the person generally unwell. The empty shells remain firmly glued as the hair continues to grow and they change to a pure white colour distracting attention from any new live eggs which are always laid at the base of a hair. It is the white shell left behind that is called a nit.

Treatment

It is essential that the correct diagnosis is reached by a healthcare professional before treatment is begun. A living, moving louse must be found to confirm the diagnosis. Detection of live lice is by 'wet combing.' The most successful formulations for treating lice are lotions, liquids and cream rinse formulations, which stay on the head long enough to kill eggs as well as lice. Lotions, being of an alcohol base, are unsuitable for young children or those with asthma or eczema, in which case liquids and cream rinses must suffice. Shampoos are not recommended as the contact time is inadequate.

In order to prevent resistance developing, a mosaic approach is currently recommended whereby if, out of three possible treatment options, the first one fails, treatment moves to the second option and so on to the third (Aston et al 1998). The insecticides available are malathion (liquid, lotion and cream rinse), permethrin (cream rinse), phenothrin (liquid, lotion and mousse), and carbaryl (liquid and lotion). Malathion is an organophosphate which should not be used more than once a week and for not more than 3 consecutive weeks. Carbaryl is considered a potential human carcinogen and is a prescription-only medicine. Whichever course of treatment is selected, two applications of insecticide should be made, 7 days apart. The head should be thoroughly checked 2–3 days after the final application, using a plastic detection comb.

When applying a lotion or liquid to the head it is important to use enough of it (at least 50 mL per application; more if the hair is thick). It should also be remembered that it is the scalp that has to be treated rather than the hair. The hair should be parted while it is still dry and the lotion sprinkled into the parting until the whole scalp has been moistened, taking care to avoid contact with the eyes. The scalp is massaged gently, paying particular attention to the back of the head and to the areas behind the ears. The hair may then be combed and should be allowed to dry naturally. The application is removed 12 hours later using ordinary shampoo.

If one member of a family is affected, the whole family must be treated to make certain that they are all free from infestation. Classmates should be treated similarly. Mothers should be advised to make a regular check on their children's heads and to encourage combing of the hair especially at bedtime.

Nurses in the community, at school and in hospital should exercise diplomacy when dealing with affected patients or explaining the condition to a child's mother. While not wanting to create offence or embarrassment, the nurse, as a health educator, must ensure that this particular problem is not allowed to go unchecked.

Scabies

Sarcoptes scabiei is the mite responsible for the parasitic infection, scabies. The mite burrows into the outer layers of the skin especially of the flexures where, after fertilisation, the female lays its eggs. An intensely pruritic rash caused by an allergy to the mite's excretions develops 2–6 weeks after initial infection along with a widespread rash. Scabies is a contagious disease most commonly seen in children, teenagers and those living in institutions.

Treatment

The diagnosis of scabies is confirmed by identification of the mite with the naked eye or with the assistance of a magnifying glass, or by sending skin scrapings for laboratory analysis.

Treatment involves the application of a scabicide to cool, dry skin. Formerly, it was recommended that treatment be applied after a hot bath and in a warm environment but it has been found that this may increase absorption of the medication through the skin and reduce its efficacy (National Prescribing Centre 1999). Malathion 0.5% aqueous solution or permethrin 5% cream may be used. The treatment should be applied to the whole body from the neck down and left on the skin for 8 hours (permethrin) and 24 hours (malathion). In children under the age of 2 and in cases where treatment has failed, the head should also be treated. The infected patient (with or without symptoms), all members of the patient's household and anyone who has had skin to skin contact within the last 2 months should be treated at the same time.

Pruritus

Pruritus or itching is considered to be due to the stimulation of the subepidermal nerve plexuses by proteolytic enzymes which are released from the epidermis as a result of either primary irritation or allergic sensitisation reactions.

Pruritus may be localised or generalised. Itching in localised parts of the body is often the result of local causes. Itching around the anus may be the result of threadworm infestation in children or from haemorrhoids. Genital pruritus in women (pruritus vulvae) may be caused by vaginal infections such as *Trichomonas vaginalis* or, in older women, by hormone deficiency. It may be the result of a skin condition or a systemic disorder. Itching is a common symptom of many skin disorders including:

- eczema
- psoriasis
- lichen planus
- urticaria
- body lice
- scabies
- fungal infection.

It can also be an important feature of systemic disorders such as:

- blood disorders, e.g. haemachromatosis, polycythaemia, lymphomas
- endocrine disorders, e.g. diabetes
- liver disease, e.g. obstructive jaundice
- renal disease, e.g. chronic renal failure.

Drug hypersensitivity may also cause severe itching.

Treatment

Although scratching may provide temporary relief, it often exacerbates the condition by increasing inflammation. Assessment of the patient with pruritus involves first establishing the underlying cause so that appropriate therapy can be initiated. Where local applications are to be used for symptomatic relief the patient's history must be checked for previous allergy and the skin inspected for signs of excessive dryness, cracking, weeping or broken areas. The patient must be given instruction on the correct method of application and advice to refrain from scratching or rubbing – which damages the epidermis and creates a vicious circle of lesion, more scratching and further damage.

A number of types of medication are used for the relief of skin irritation. Itching from dry skin is often soothed by a simple emollient. For mild itching arising from sunburn, urticaria or insect bites, a cooling lotion such as calamine, with the possible addition of menthol, may be helpful. The menthol, however, may give rise to hypersensitivity reactions in some patients. Crotamiton (10%) in a cream or lotion form may be useful in some cases of pruritus. Doxepin (see p. 241) is available as a cream (5%) for use in pruritus of eczema. Because of the possibility of systemic side-effects, the cream should be applied thinly not exceeding 3 g per application. Oral antihistamines should be used in allergic rashes. Chlorphenamine (chlorpheniramine) is an inexpensive antihistamine which is short-acting and mildly sedating. Where the irritation prevents sleep, a sedating antihistamine taken at night promotes sleep as well as relieving itching. Terfenadine, which acts longer than chlorphenamine (chlorpheniramine), does not cause sedation. Cardiovascular problems have been reported with terfenadine, notably arrhythmias. It is important to avoid potentially dangerous drug interactions – for example, with drugs liable to cause electrolyte imbalance. Terfenadine is a prescription-only medicine. The sedating oral antihistamine alimemazine may be useful in some cases.

The risk of using preparations for pruritus other than simple emollient and soothing preparations is that prolonged or heavy use may cause skin irritation, resulting in aggravation of the itching. Since itching can be a symptom of many underlying conditions, treatment should be reviewed after a week.

SKIN PREPARATIONS

Diseases of the skin are treated by both topical (local) and systemic therapy. A wide range of products is now available ranging from relatively simple emollients to sophisticated formulations containing potent drugs such as corticosteroids.

Emollients and barrier preparations

Emollients are used where a moisturising type of product is likely to be beneficial. They soothe and hydrate the skin and are indicated for dry scaling disorders. Frequent application is required since their effects are short-lived. They are useful in various dermatological conditions such as dry eczematous disorders and, to a lesser extent, psoriasis. A wide range of emollient preparations is available. The choice of product will depend on consideration of the patient's condition, the patient's preference and clinical experience.

Both aqueous cream and emulsifying ointment have emollient properties and either may be used for hand-washing or in the bath as a soap substitute to prevent the drying effect of soap on the skin. Several proprietary emulsions are available for use in the bath as 'all-over' emollients. Patients should be warned that the bath will be slippery.

Emollients are available for use in conditions such as ichthyosis, traumatic dermatitis, dry eczema, certain types of psoriasis and also where movement of a joint is impaired by dryness or cracking of the overlying skin. Aqueous cream which contains emulsifying ointment 30% in water is a light emollient. White soft paraffin (white petroleum jelly); emulsifying ointment which contains emulsifying wax 30%, white soft paraffin 50% and liquid paraffin 20%; and liquid and white soft paraffin ointment (50/50) are more greasy. E45 cream contains light liquid paraffin 12.6% and white soft paraffin 14.5% as well as hypoallergenic lanolin. Lanolin may cause sensitisation in some patients. This should be suspected if an eczematous reaction occurs at the site of application.

Barrier creams are used to provide protection against repeated hydration and irritation which can result in napkin rash, intertrigo, pressure sores and problems in areas surrounding stomata. Zinc and castor oil ointment is an effective yet inexpensive emollient and barrier preparation with mild astringent properties. However, there is no substitute for diligent nursing care. For example, with napkin rash, a local dermatitis, the first-line of treatment is to ensure frequent napkin changes and that plastic pants are not too tight nor have rough edges which chafe the skin. Rashes may clear when left exposed to the air and an emollient may be helpful. Barrier creams often contain water-repellent substances such as dimeticone or other silicones but it is doubtful whether these water-repellent creams are any more effective than traditional compound zinc ointments.

Topical corticosteroids

Topical corticosteroids are used for the treatment of a wide variety of inflammatory conditions of the skin other than those due to an infection. Corticosteroids suppress various factors causing inflammation but they are not curative since the underlying cause of the inflammation is not affected. When treatment is discontinued the condition may recur.

The choice of a topical corticosteroid must be made with care. In most cases a mild corticosteroid is used at the start of treatment. Rule of thumb is to use the minimum amount of the lowest potency corticosteroid (see p. 450). If a patient ceases to respond to a particular corticosteroid, another of similar potency may be tried before resorting to a more potent corticosteroid. Topical corticosteroid preparations are categorised into four groups according to potency (Box 28.3).

Adequate use of emollients may reduce the need for large quantities of steroids. Where large areas are to be covered by steroids the nurse or patient should wear gloves and the preparation should be applied sparingly. Application of excessive quantities of external corticosteroid preparations can result in undesirable local and systemic side-effects. The more potent the preparation, the more care is required as absorption through the skin can cause pituitary adrenal suppression. The body's immune system is suppressed, thus increasing the risk of infection. Absorption is greatest from areas of thin skin and raw surfaces, and the effect is increased by occlusion. Very potent steroids should be used only for short periods. Local side-effects of topical corticosteroids include:

- thinning of the skin, sometimes resulting in stretch marks which may be permanent
- fine blood vessels under the skin surface possibly becoming prominent and resulting in a red rash if the vessels become damaged (telangiectasia); because the skin on the face is especially vulnerable to such damage, topical steroids are not usually prescribed for use on the face
- increased hair growth
- a possible temporary reduction in pigmentation at the site of application
- acne at the site of application in some patients
- delayed wound healing.

Children and, in particular, babies are especially susceptible to side-effects due to increased absorption owing to their thinner skin and greater proportion of surface area relative to weight. Potent and very potent steroids should not be used for children. If a mild corticosteroid such as hydrocortisone is prescribed for treating eczema, care should be taken because napkins and plastic pants act as an occlusive dressing and increase

Box 28.3 Topical corticosteroids grouped according to potency

Mild
Hydrocortisone 1%

Moderately potent
Alclometasone dipropionate 0.05%
Clobetasone butyrate 0.05%

Potent
Beclometasone dipropionate 0.025%
Betamethasone 0.1%
Diflucortolone valerate 0.1%
Fluocinolone acetonide 0.025%
Hydrocortisone butyrate 0.1%

Very potent
Clobetasol propionate 0.05%
Halcinonide 0.1%

absorption. The BNF provides guidance on the amounts to be prescribed taking into account the weekly quantities that should be applied when treating adult patients.

Some proprietary topical corticosteroid preparations contain antibiotics or other antibacterial agents. These may be prescribed where infection complicates the underlying condition. Even given the problems associated with corticosteroids, there can be no doubt that patients do derive great benefit from these drugs. It should be noted that preparations containing hydrocortisone (up to 1%) are available over the counter for the treatment of dermatitis, insect bite reactions and mild to moderate eczema. Pharmacists provide advice on the use of these products to ensure appropriate use.

Topical antimicrobials

Antibacterial, antifungal and antiviral preparations are used for skin infections that are not too deeply seated and are therefore amenable to local therapy. Topical antimicrobial therapy should be carefully managed and avoided if at all possible owing to local sensitisation reactions. The problem of bacterial resistance is of major concern, and it follows that the antimicrobial agents used topically should ideally not be the same as those agents used systemically. Table 28.1 summarises the main drugs used together with indications and precautions.

Disinfectants

Chemical disinfectants play a limited role in helping to achieve the control of infection in both hospital and community practice. The limitations of disinfectants are well known. Poor range of activity and effectiveness, toxicity, inconvenience and high cost all contribute to the declining use of these agents. In order to reduce the risk of cross-infection, single-use sachets should be used whenever possible. In addition, the availability of a wide range of sterile disposable equipment, improved physical sterilisation methods and

Table 28.1 Topical antimicrobial agents

Drug/product	Indications	Notes/side-effects/precautions
Antibacterial agents		
Mupirocin 2% ointment	Gram-positive infections	Unrelated to any other antibiotics. Not suitable for pseudomonal infection. Not to be used for longer than 10 days to reduce risk of resistance developing. Avoid use in hospitals
Neomycin 0.5% cream	Bacterial infections	Not to be used to treat large areas as it may be absorbed and cause ototoxicity. Not used systemically. Care in patients at extremes of age and in renal impairment
Silver sulfadiazine 1% cream	Prophylaxis and treatment of burns	Compound of silver and a sulphonamide. Contraindicated in pregnancy, and breast-feeding. Itching, rashes and argyria have been reported
Antifungal agents		
A wide range of drugs is available. Some examples are: Benzoic acid compound ointment Clotrimazole Econazole Ketoconazole Miconazole Terbinafine Tioconazole	Fungal skin infections	Valuable antifungal drugs but may cause local irritation, allergic reactions and stinging. These drugs are available as creams, gels, ointments, dusting powders and shampoos. Choice of product will depend on nature and site of the infection
Antiviral preparations		
Aciclovir (5%) and penciclovir (1%) available as creams	Labial and genital herpes simplex infections. Systemic therapy needed for more deep-seated infections	Apply five times daily at first sign of attack. Penciclovir is applied every 2 hours during waking hours for 4 days
Formaldehyde Glutaraldehyde Podophyllum resin Podophyllotoxin (the active component of the resin)	Plantar warts Persistent warts Genital warts	All of these drugs are potent agents which must be prescribed and used with great care so as to avoid adverse reactions in both patients and healthcare staff Salicylic acid (a keratolytic) may be combined with podophyllum resin for the treatment of plantar warts

cleaning techniques have further reduced the need for chemical disinfectants. Disinfectants have a limited place in wound management procedures (see p. 458) and in the preparation of skin prior to surgery. Alcoholic solutions (70% v/v) alone, or containing chlorhexidine 0.5% w/v, are often used for such purposes. Chlorhexidine combined with a cleansing agent may be used if the patient's skin is contaminated. Hand preparation prior to surgical procedures is carried out using a detergent/chlorhexidine combination and a suitably thorough technique. Alcoholic chlorhexidine solution may be useful as a hand rub after washing but this will not achieve decontamination of unwashed skin. A handwash containing povidone-iodine is an alternative to chlorhexidine, but iodine may cause sensitisation in some individuals.

Hard surfaces may be treated with ethyl or isopropyl alcohol (70% v/v) in a suitable form (spray or swab). Glutaraldehyde solution has a place in the disinfection of surgical equipment that cannot be heat-treated. However, special precautions must be taken to avoid contamination of the environment with fumes of the product.

Sunscreens

Sunlight is composed of a spectrum of wavelengths of electromagnetic radiation. Of these, ultraviolet radiation can be particularly harmful to the skin. People vary widely in their sensitivity to ultraviolet radiation. Fair-skinned people have least tolerance and burn easily, whereas people with darker skin can withstand exposure for longer periods without noticeable harm. In addition, ultraviolet radiation may be harmful in certain diseases, e.g. lupus erythematosus and rosacea. Certain drugs such as chlorpromazine, demeclocycline and amiodarone can increase the skin's sensitivity to sunlight and in all these cases protection will be required even for short periods of exposure.

Sunscreens contain substances such as ethylhexyl *p*-methoxycinnamate, titanium dioxide, zinc oxide, avobenzone and aminobenzoic acid, which absorb UVB (medium wavelength solar ultraviolet radiation) and, in this way, provide protection. A range of sunscreens is available, graded according to the degree of protection – the sun protection factor (SPF). This figure indicates the amount of ultraviolet radiation which will be absorbed – the higher the SPF, the greater the degree of protection. For skin protection in dermatological conditions, an SPF of 15 or more is required. For maximum benefit, the sunscreens must be applied frequently. They are applied before sunbathing to prevent erythema while allowing the skin to tan. People with fair skin should start with a sunscreen with a higher SPF. As the skin tans, a low SPF may suffice. Because sunscreens generally filter out only UVB, patients with sensitive skin should spend as little time as possible exposed to sunlight, even if they are using a sunscreen. Prolonged exposure of skin to strong sunlight increases the long-term risk of skin cancer, due to the damaging effects of UVA (long wavelength solar ultraviolet radiation) to which most sunscreens provide only limited protection.

Shampoos

Dandruff (*pityriasis capitis*) is the condition where the accumulation of dead cells on the scalp results in flaky scaling. Regular washing with a mild shampoo several times a week may be sufficient to keep the scalp free of dandruff. However, many people find that a medicated shampoo is required. Shampoos containing tar extracts may be useful as they soften the dead scales and make them easier to remove. Shampoos containing pyrithione zinc reduce the formation of dandruff by slowing the growth of skin scales and have the advantage of not having to be prescribed. The use of selenium sulphide-containing shampoos is no more beneficial than non-medicated shampoos. Where dandruff is severe and unresponsive to these treatments, ketoconazole shampoo, alone or in conjunction with weak corticosteroid gels or lotions applied to the scalp, may be helpful. Cradle cap in infants is treated with olive oil or arachis oil before shampooing.

Antiperspirants

Hyperhidrosis (overproduction of sweat) may be a localised or a more generalised problem. A generalised problem condition can be treated with an antimuscarinic but side-effects (see p. 258) may limit the use of this form of treatment. Localised hyperhidrosis may respond to treatment with a paint containing 20% w/v aluminium chloride in alcohol. The paint is applied overnight to the area affected following careful cleaning and drying. In very resistant cases surgery may be required to remove areas of maximum sweat production. Botulinum A toxin (see p. 418) by local injection may be useful in intractable cases.

Problems associated with skin preparations

Table 28.2 indicates some of the potential problems of using certain dermatological preparations. The list should not be regarded as fully comprehensive but it does identify the major problem areas likely to be encountered by nurses.

Table 28.2 Problems associated with some dermatological preparations

Problem	Ingredient causing problem	Methods of risk reduction/precautions
Absorption – systemic	Azelaic acid; corticosteroids (especially potent agents); neomycin; salicylic acid; terbinafine	Avoid contact by using disposable gloves or applicator if available. Wash hands after use (nurse and patient). Occlusive dressings increase absorption – use only when/as prescribed. Discontinue breast-feeding owing to risks
Eye irritancy	Aluminium chloride; benzoyl peroxide; carbaryl; dithranol; podophyllum resin; sulphur	Never use on face. Patient should be warned not to rub eyes when (or after) using product. Wash hands after use
Flammable products	Alcohol (especially in high concentrations); collodions; ether	Should never be used near naked flame, electric heaters or other ignition sources
Granuloma	Talc in dusting powders	Avoid contact with broken skin/body cavities
Infection	Many dermatological preparations, especially those containing a high percentage of water and/or prepared by dilution of a proprietary product. Preservative system may be inadequate	All dermatological products should be used with care to avoid contamination/cross-infection. Observe expiry dates/conditions of storage. Single-use packs should be used for preservative-free products. Particular care is needed where large areas of broken skin are involved
Irritancy of respiratory tract	Dusting powders; pressurised aerosol	Take care to avoid inhalation, especially in sensitive subjects
Photosensitivity	Antihistamines; coal tar; tretinoin	Patient should be warned to avoid exposure to strong sunlight
Sensitisation reactions	Antihistamines; local anaesthetics; neomycin	Be alert to this possibility. Use of product may have to be discontinued
Skin/fair hair	Clioquinol; coal tar products; dithranol	Patient should be warned in advance about possible discoloration of skin and/or hair
Skin irritancy	Dithranol; formaldehyde; malathion; podophyllum resin; sulphur; tioconazole	Should be applied only to those areas to be treated. Normal skin may be protected by a bland agent, e.g. soft paraffin. Confine application to lesions
Staining of personal linen and the patient's bath	Coal tar products; dithranol; potassium permanganate	Patient should be warned in advance. Particular items of 'old' linen may be advisable when these products are in use

TOPICAL THERAPY IN SKIN DISORDERS

Skin diseases affect 20–33% of the population at any one time, and typically GPs spend at least 10% of their working time dealing with these diseases (All Party Parliamentary Group on Skin 1997). This workload also impacts on other healthcare professionals, especially nurses. Much needed improvements in services to patients suffering from skin diseases can be achieved not only by improving the structure of provision for them but also by developing the role of nurse specialists.

It is important to recognise that many systemic diseases manifest at least one of their diagnostic features in the skin (Table 28.3). Moreover, the skin acts as a barometer for the general health of the body and this should not be forgotten when treating specific skin diseases.

Table 28.3 Skin manifestations of systemic diseases

Systemic disease	Skin manifestation(s)
Chronic obstructive airways disease	Dusky hue or bright pink
Chronic renal failure	Yellow-brown; uraemic frost
Congestive cardiac failure	Cyanosed; oedematous
Diabetic coma	Dry, smelling of acetone
Hypertension	May be highly coloured
Hypoglycaemia	Profusely sweating
Iron-deficiency anaemia	Pale
Myxoedema	Dry; coarse
Obstructive jaundice	Deep yellow, itching
Pernicious anaemia	Pale lemon-tinted
Thyrotoxicosis	Warm; moist
Viral diseases of childhood	Characteristic rashes; itching

The comfort of the patient

Treatment of the skin, whether carried out at the bedside or in a treatment room, calls for consideration of a number of factors. First and foremost, privacy must be provided and maintained, and every effort must be made to ensure that the dignity of the patient is preserved. The room should be adequately ventilated but free of draughts.

When caring for patients with a disorder of the skin the nurse should ensure that the environment is conducive to good communication. Here, an individualised approach to the patient is of paramount importance. The management of patients with an apparently similar condition should play no part. Only in a one-to-one situation can there be a satisfactory exchange of views leading to better understanding. The chances of patients maintaining compliance with the treatment prescribed will be greatly increased if they are helped by the nurse to understand the rationale behind it.

Irrespective of the treatment being followed, all patients with skin conditions need to be cared for with real sensitivity. Feelings of shame, disgust and fear have for long troubled patients with skin diseases, often forcing them to hide from the gaze of others. To some extent, this situation has been perpetuated by the attitude of health professionals towards these patients. Sadly, staff may make patients with skin conditions feel 'unclean' by isolating them unnecessarily in single rooms and adopting overprotective measures while treating them. In time, the patient may respond with antisocial behaviour which, in turn, may affect the attitudes of others until what can only be described as a 'leper complex' develops. Unless it is absolutely necessary to do otherwise, these patients should be shown the same consideration afforded to all other patients. Trust and confidence need to be restored by adopting an open and optimistic outlook. This in itself has a beneficial 'therapeutic' effect.

Assessment

There is no substitute for identifying the cause of the problem and tackling it at source. Since two people suffering from the same condition will rarely present in an identical way it is essential that a thorough assessment is made by examination and questioning. Both visual (often using a hand lens) and tactile examination will be required. Temperature, tension and sensitivity of the skin may be ascertained by careful touching of the affected part(s) using a disposable plastic glove as appropriate. Where it is suspected that a skin condition is due to a reaction to an irritant or allergen, systematic questioning may help to identify the cause, as will carefully managed patch testing.

Treatment selection

Selection of a product by either doctor or nurse requires care since the choice is very wide indeed. The BNF alone contains several hundred different topical applications. In addition, specially formulated products can be prescribed for patients whose needs cannot be met by an 'off the shelf' formulation. In this case the range of products available is as wide as the prescriber's imagination.

Many skin conditions require the attention of a consultant dermatologist (or other clinician) who will prescribe the treatment. Products containing antibiotic, corticosteroid or other potent drugs, come into this category since the use of these agents is accompanied by certain risks. Symptoms may be masked by the use of corticosteroids, and the use of certain antibiotics is associated with sensitisation reactions. Otherwise, dermatological preparations are prescribable by nurses suitably qualified to select the appropriate product from the Nurse Prescribers' Formulary or according to a Patient Group Direction.

In hospital practice, nurses who have had additional training may prescribe limited treatment for a skin problem from a formulary of nursing care products (e.g. to cleanse; to moisturise; to soothe) under the control of a Patient Group Direction. In primary care, suitably trained community staff may do likewise using the Nurse Prescribers' Formulary (e.g. pediculosis; scabies; wound management). In the future, those who have been trained to prescribe from an extended Nurse Prescribers' Formulary will be able to prescribe also a whole range of treatments for minor ailments of the skin (e.g. acne; atopic dermatitis; contact dermatitis; chronic skin ulcers) and injuries (e.g. abrasions; bites – animal and human; burns and scalds; and minor lacerations).

Prescribing of topical preparations

Topical preparations which contain a specific drug should be regarded in exactly the same way as any other medicine. It follows therefore that prescribing, administration and recording of such products should be in accordance with established policies and procedures for medicines management.

Special prescription sheets are required for the prescribing of topical preparations in hospital as it is necessary to incorporate a greater amount of information than the standard inpatient prescription sheet allows. The prescription should include:

- date of the prescription
- name of the preparation; a specially made up formula may consist of several different substances which should be listed
- formulation and its strength; where necessary, details such as aqueous or oily should be given; it is better, where possible, to describe the strength as a percentage; ratios (e.g. 1:9) can be misleading
- quantity to be applied; this may be difficult to quantify; sparingly, liberally, 1 cm or 'a worm' are expressions which may be used; the most commonly used instruction

given is 'as sparingly as possible' (see also p. 447)

- site(s) for application; these should be described specifically (e.g. 'all active areas', 'wherever the skin is dry'); vague expressions such as 'all over' should be avoided
- dressings and bandages to be used; the size of each should be appropriate to the size of the patient's lesion
- number of times of administration; this should span a 24-hour period and should be divided evenly throughout the patient's waking day
- doctor's signature.

Prescribing systemic therapy for dermatological conditions is carried out in the same way as all other systemic prescribing.

Formulation of topical preparations

Several different pharmaceutical preparations (ointments, lotions, etc.) are available, each of which has distinctive physical characteristics quite apart from the nature of the active ingredient. In some instances products are used solely for their physical properties, e.g. emollients, barrier preparations and sunscreens. Although a detailed discussion of formulation aspects is outside the scope of this book, certain important principles are emphasised below since they have practical implications for the nurse. Typically, a pharmaceutical product intended for topical application will have some, or all, of the following components.

Active ingredient(s)

The concentration of the active ingredient(s) will normally be expressed as a percentage weight in weight, e.g. 1% w/w hydrocortisone cream.

Vehicle

The overall characteristics of the product will depend on the vehicle chosen. The vehicle may be aqueous, non-aqueous, liquid or semi-solid depending on the properties required and nature of the active ingredient. Penetration of the active ingredient into the skin is influenced by the properties of the vehicle and nature of the condition being treated. The make-up of the vehicle used in proprietary preparations varies greatly. In order to help trace the source of a local reaction to a product it may be necessary to seek information on all the components of the product in order that the source of the problem can be identified.

Antimicrobial preservative agent

The risk of microbial contamination of topical products, especially those containing a high proportion of water, during their use is significant and so it is essential, unless the product is a single-use pack, to include an antimicrobial agent.

Emulsifying/suspending agent

These are required to give a product physical stability, e.g. an emulsifying agent stabilises oil-in-water preparations, and a suspending agent is necessary when insoluble powders of high density are included in a liquid preparation.

Other additives

For example, a buffering agent may be included to give a preparation with a pH approximating to that of normal skin.

Topical preparations and their use

The terms 'cream', 'ointment', 'lotion', etc., are precise but may not always be used correctly. Care should be taken to determine the actual properties of the product, which may not always be reflected by the name.

Creams

Creams are normally oil-in-water emulsions which, since water is the continuous phase, are easily removed, even from hairy areas, by normal cleansing procedures. The evaporation of the water present in the cream produces a useful cooling effect. Drainage from a lesion is facilitated because creams absorb exudates. Drugs normally incorporated into creams include corticosteroids, antibacterials and antifungal agents. Good penetration of the active ingredient into the skin is achieved and may be enhanced because of the presence of a surfactant (emulsifying agent) in the cream. Creams also have a softening effect on thickened tissues.

Although creams normally contain an antimicrobial preservative, they should be used with great care to avoid microbial contamination since the antimicrobial agents available for incorporation into creams have a limited spectrum of activity. The antimicrobial agent (and/or active ingredient) may cause skin sensitivity in some patients. Creams are more cosmetically acceptable than ointments especially when applied to the face, as they disappear when rubbed into the skin.

Ointments

It is very important to distinguish between ointments and creams because the two products have different properties. Ointments are normally greasy anhydrous preparations which do not mix with water and therefore should not be applied to exuding lesions. They are occlusive and encourage hydration. Ointments are more difficult than creams to remove from the skin. Soft paraffins are widely used in ointment bases, incorporating liquid paraffin to achieve the required consistency. Ointments soften crusts but are generally not suitable for application to hairy areas. They are particularly useful for application to dry scaly areas.

Being non-aqueous, antimicrobial agents are only occasionally required to be included in ointments and so there is less risk of sensitisation from this source than with creams. However, lanolin (wool fat) and derivatives are sometimes included in ointments and may cause contact sensitivity.

Other preparations

Products are also available that combine the properties of both ointments and creams. Such formulations are described as ambiphilic. The formulation is a stable emulsion system with a uniform distribution of fat and water.

Application of creams and ointments. As already stated, ointments and creams generally have different properties and the indications for their use relate to these. However, the guidance given above is not inflexible. A most important aspect is to use a preparation which is acceptable to the patient. These products should be applied as sparingly as possible to affected part(s). If applying a prescribed product, the prescriber's instructions must be complied with. Creams and ointments are best applied in the same way as make-up. Small dots of the product are placed at suitable intervals over the area to be treated. Using the tip of the index finger and/or second finger for small areas and the palm of the hand for larger areas, the cream should be spread evenly as far as it will go within the area to be treated. Plain lint or gauze dressings may be required to cover areas to which creams and ointments have been applied.

Pastes

These preparations are essentially similar to ointments but contain a high proportion of powders, have a very stiff consistency, and will adhere to lesions at body temperature. Pastes also have protective properties. Lassar's paste, for example, contains 24% by weight of zinc oxide and 24% by weight of starch with 50% white soft paraffin and 2% salicylic acid.

Application of pastes. Pastes should be applied only to specific lesions, e.g. in psoriasis, and not to the surrounding skin. Where a paste contains a highly active ingredient (e.g. dithranol), it will be necessary to protect the skin adjacent to the lesion with a bland product such as yellow soft paraffin. If the paste is soft enough (temperature will obviously influence the consistency of the product), it may be applied with the finger(s) of a gloved hand. Pastes which cannot be applied in this way may be applied with a wooden spatula. Pastes will seldom require to be covered with a dressing, except where it is necessary to protect the patient's linen from staining by the active ingredient. They are not popular with patients as they are messy and difficult to apply.

Paste bandages

A range of bandages is available which are impregnated with a zinc oxide paste combined with either coal tar, calamine, ichthammol or hydrocortisone. Paste bandages are used for the treatment of conditions such as eczema, leg ulcers and chronic dermatitis.

Dusting powders

Dusting powders are of two main types, medicated and non-medicated. All dusting powders have a basis of starch (absorbent) and talc (lubricant). Non-medicated powders are used in general nursing care to reduce friction and absorb moisture between folds of skin. The skin should be clean and well dried before each application. Excessive use should be avoided since 'caking' in folds of skin may result – causing local irritation or trauma.

Medicated powders have a limited place in the active treatment of skin diseases since it is generally not possible to achieve a satisfactory concentration of active ingredient at the site of the lesion for any length of time. Dusting powders containing suitable active ingredients are mainly used in prophylaxis (e.g. the prevention of athlete's foot, or the prevention of neonatal staphylococcal cross-infection). Dusting powders containing antibiotics are occasionally used in the treatment of superficial bacterial infections such as impetigo when the powder will tend to stick to the lesions.

Lotions

Lotions are normally simple formulations containing active ingredients in an aqueous solution or suspension.

Occasionally oily lotions are used, but such preparations have properties very different from those of a lotion with an aqueous base since they are water-in-oil emulsions. Lotions with an aqueous base are used in weeping eruptions where they cool and dry the skin by evaporation. In very acute conditions, lotions are used to relieve superficial inflammation and assist in the removal of crusts. When even the presence of fine solid particles cannot be tolerated by the patient, lotions which are simple solutions are used until the most acute phase of the condition has passed. Then lotions containing powders in suspension can be used. The cooling properties of a lotion may be enhanced by the addition of alcohol to the vehicle but this may cause stinging. (Excessive cooling due to the use of lotions must be avoided, especially in the elderly.)

Lotions may be useful for the application of a drug to a hairy area of the body where the use of a greasy ointment or stiff paste would be inappropriate or impracticable. In very acute conditions, lotions may be applied as wet dressings using lint or other closely-woven fabric. As with all dressings, care should be taken on removal to avoid damaging the epithelium. Any dressings that have dried out should be thoroughly wetted with the lotion before being carefully removed. Lotions may also be applied to small lesions using cotton wool, or to larger areas using a suitable flat brush.

Paints

Paints are solutions of the active drug in a suitable solvent, such as water, alcohol or a mixture of solvents, depending on the nature of the active ingredient. Application to the skin is normally by means of a brush.

Pressurised aerosols

Pressurised aerosols are widely available for the application of drugs to the skin in conditions such as superficial bacterial infections. Protective applications can also be applied in this way. It is important to use the product in accordance with the manufacturer's recommendations, and to ensure safe disposal of the empty canister. Pressurised aerosols are convenient to use, and confer the advantages of a 'non-touch' technique, but are relatively expensive.

Nail varnishes

A varnish formulation containing an antifungal agent is available for the treatment of fungal infections of the nails. The varnish ensures prolonged contact of the antifungal agent with the infected tissue.

Skin cleansing procedures

Skin cleansing

Before applying a topical preparation, the skin should be clean. To prevent accumulation, previous applications to the skin should be removed. This is especially important where drugs such as corticosteroids are involved. In order to remove creams, paints, powders or lotions, the patient, or the site, should be bathed using simple soaps and warm water. (Perfumed toilet soap should be avoided.) Pastes, ointments and certain paints are best removed with cotton wool soaked in liquid paraffin or olive oil.

Bathing

With increasing changes in the skin towards dryness after about the age of 35, the tendency should be towards a reduction in the frequency in bathing. Soaking in a hot bath makes the skin dry owing to loss of natural oils and causes epidermal cells to shrink on drying. Any itching of the skin is increased. A conscious effort should be made to adjust routine and not to overwash patients, particularly elderly people and those patients whose skin is noticeably dry. Nurses are well placed to make an assessment of the patient's skin and decide on the care required.

Patients with skin conditions should be advised to resist the temptation to use any cosmetic bath additives. Detergents or antiseptics may cause the patient further problems and should be avoided. To occlude the skin and thus prevent drying by evaporation, liquid paraffin or olive oil may be used. An emollient such as emulsifying ointment may be added to the bath water. This also acts as a mild occlusive and helps to retain moisture in the skin. An oily bath is obviously exceedingly dangerous and therefore it is vitally important that the patient is forewarned of the risk of slipping. The nurse should make a careful judgement as to whether the patient can be safely left to get out of the bath unaided. In any case, the bath should be emptied before the patient climbs out. A secure bath mat should be made available. After using an emollient, the bath needs careful cleaning. It should be filled full with hot water and have a suitable detergent added – having first ensured that there are no patients in the vicinity who may mistakenly think that the bath has been filled for their use. The bath is then allowed to empty and as it does so, the water should be agitated and the sides cleaned to remove all traces of the emollient.

Scalp treatment

Shampoos may be used for cleaning or for treatment purposes. Triethanolamine lauryl sulphate 40% forms the basis of some shampoos. It has no additives and is the least irritant. It is therefore useful as a simple cleansing agent for the scalp. Psoriasis of the scalp may be treated with either a tar-based or a desquamative shampoo. Antiseptic shampoos are available for the infected scalp.

Precautions have to be taken to protect the eyes and face from contact with shampoos used as treatment. The patient should be warned to keep the eyes closed throughout the procedure. With gloved hands, two applications are made – the first, a thorough wash to cleanse the scalp; the second, active treatment. Between applications and at the finish, the shampoo should be rinsed out of the hair. The hair is dried with a hair-dryer as soon as possible. Some scalp applications are flammable and when using such products patients should be warned not to dry the hair near a naked flame.

Application of topical preparations

(Box 28.4)

Topical preparations should not be applied to normal skin as this wastes time, wastes the product and may do harm. Generally speaking, if the condition is acute then the frequency of the treatment and the strength of the active ingredient(s) may be increased – rather than increasing the amount applied. It is only the active ingredient(s) in contact with the affected skin which is going to aid healing – not the layers on top. 'A little can do a lot of good, a lot can do a lot of harm' is a maxim worth remembering.

Box 28.4 Application of topical preparations

Documentation
- Special prescription sheet for topical medicines

The medicine
- Creams, ointments, pastes, dusting powders, lotions
- Paints as prescribed

The environment
- Such as to ensure privacy
- Adequately ventilated but free of draughts

The nurse and the patient
- Patient identified
- Explanation given to patient
- Willingness of nurse to listen to what patient wants to say
- Patient given realistic encouragement

Technique
- Hand hygiene before and after administration
- Polythene gloves worn by nurse
- Preparations applied gently and sparingly
- Dressing kept to minimum size necessary

Hazards
- Irritation of the skin
- Infection from contaminated containers

Patients' response to treatment

Inpatients undergoing treatment for a skin condition should be given the opportunity at least every 48 hours to express how they feel their condition is responding, and the comments should be recorded in the patient's progress report. In order to gain an account which truly reflects the patient's view of his progress, the nurse must be prepared, as far as possible, to listen to him when he chooses to raise the subject. The opportunity will often arise during a treatment session. It is not sufficient for the nurse to express her view of progress being made. Whatever the nurse observes about the patient himself, or his skin, it is important to record what the patient says – even if it is simply that he is feeling better or worse.

Patient compliance

Skin conditions are frequently of a chronic or recurring nature which often necessitates teaching patients and/or relatives how to continue treatment. Advice given may include appropriate skin cleansing and the method of application as well as any special precautions such as skin protection and protection of personal linen. Teaching should be realistic and helpful if a reasonable degree of compliance is to be assured. There would be little point in asking a patient to apply a tar preparation before going out in an evening because of its antisocial effect. To most patients, a large unsightly dressing would be equally unacceptable. For the application of an ointment, some disabled patients may find a long-handled ointment applicator of assistance in reaching inaccessible parts of the body. Where there is a degree of difficulty in applying skin preparations, in the absence of a capable family member, it is essential to arrange for the treatment to be carried out by the district nurse.

Safety and storage

In hospitals, topical applications must be kept in a locked cupboard set aside for external preparations, careful attention being paid to expiry dates. To prevent cross-infection, patients should be supplied with individually dispensed skin applications. Where this is not possible, a quantity of the preparation should be removed from its container with a spatula. If more of the preparation is required, a new spatula should be used. Since rolling up a collapsible tube to expel the contents may obliterate the label it is preferable to squeeze the tube progressively along its entire length.

Hazards

Nurses should be aware of the potential hazards inherent in treating skin conditions. Moreover, they should take the opportunity given to them to set a good example to the patient when carrying out treatments. The precautions to be taken are as follows:

- Skin preparations should be applied in accordance with the prescription.
- Polythene gloves should be worn when applying any preparation to the skin (unless a spatula or brush is being used) so that the nurse does not risk absorbing the active ingredients.
- Creams, especially those prepared by dilution of a primary product, may support bacterial growth and should therefore be used with care to avoid contamination. All creams will bear an expiry date after which the preparation should not be used.

Topical corticosteroids. Although these products are very effective the risks of inappropriate use are very significant (see p. 447). Application must always be in accordance with the prescription. Nurses applying topical corticosteroids should take precautions to prevent contamination of the product and the possibility of absorption of the active ingredient. Patients will need guidance on the amounts to be used. The fingertip unit (FTU) (Long et al 1998) is a useful method of providing guidance to patients (see BNF).

WOUND MANAGEMENT

Introduction

A wound can be described as any break in the continuity of the skin resulting from physical, mechanical or thermal damage or that develops as a result of the presence of an underlying medical condition (Thomas 1990). Irrespective of the type of wound being treated, the overriding objective is to promote healing and prevent infection. Patients who are poor risks for good wound healing include those with a poor nutritional status, uncontrolled diabetes or obesity; the heavy smoker; those of advanced age; and those receiving cytotoxic therapy and/or corticosteroids in combination with surgery. Some of these patients may need additional supportive therapy such as enteral or parenteral nutrition. Patients in hospital rather than at home are at increased risk of developing infection because of exposure to pathogenic microorganisms, many of which have become resistant to antibiotics. While it is not possible to eliminate this risk totally, it can be minimised. Broad principles of wound management are applicable in all settings, although the precise management of a wound will depend on the clinical assessment by the individual practitioner. Many trusts have established written guidelines for the treatment of wounds and it is essential that nurses are aware of these and follow the recommendations made. An understanding of the underlying physiological processes is essential if treatment is to be both efficient and effective.

Physiology

Several physiological processes take place during the healing of any wound.

Haemostasis

The first step the body takes in response to injury is to try to reduce excessive blood loss. This is achieved in several ways. The damaged blood vessel attracts platelets to try to 'plug the hole'. The blood vessel also constricts, thus reducing blood flow to the damaged area. Inflammatory exudate containing plasma, antibodies and white blood cells is released through the now more permeable capillary walls and infiltrates the tissues surrounding the wound.

Inflammation

An inflammatory response follows, caused mainly by histamine released by the mast cells. Since histamine causes blood vessels to dilate, there then develop heat and redness. Swelling and pain result from the action of histamine on the blood vessel walls, increasing their permeability.

Cell migration

Macrophages move towards the site of the wound and their first role is to fend off invading bacteria, which they do by phagocytosis. Microorganisms and necrotic tissue are ingested by the macrophages; this causes the macrophages to die, and, in the process, leads to dirty yellowish debris known as slough.

Cell proliferation

Immature fibroblasts migrate to the site of the wound, and new blood vessels start to grow into the wound

Table 28.4 Classification of wounds according to appearance

Appearance	Significance	Comments
Red	Granulation tissue	Caused by establishment of new blood vessels. Precedes epithelialisation
Pinky-white	Epithelialisation	Care is needed to distinguish epithelialisation from slough formation
Yellowish	Slough	Caused by accumulation of dead cells
Brown or black	Necrosis	Caused by death of tissue
Localised heat, swelling, redness, tenderness, pus, foul odour	Clinical infection	Inflammatory response

space. A network of vessels develops in which the fibroblasts divide. The deep red, new tissue is known as *granulation tissue.*

Cell maturation

Epidermal cells then migrate across the granulation tissue to cover the wound. The stage of healing which involves the maturation of the dermis and the production of collagen is known as *epithelialisation*. Once the skin barrier is finally restored, complete wound healing can be said to have been achieved.

Assessment of the wound

An assessment must be carried out before any specific local treatment is instituted and before the choice of a suitable dressing is made. Assessing a wound involves careful examination of its appearance in order to establish the physiological stage the wound has reached (see Table 28.4). Other features including the size and form of the wound as well as the presence of pain and the patient's general condition should be considered (see Box 28.5). Having arrived at a clinical description of the wound, based on the above classification, any local treatment can be considered and a suitable dressing selected.

Types of wound

Incised wounds

In surgery, the aim is to create a wound that will heal by first intention. Adequate preoperative skin preparation, aseptic operative conditions and appropriate postoperative wound management are fundamental requirements.

Box 28.5 Wound assessment

Wound assessment should include:

- **Location** of wound
- **Cause** of wound, relevant illnesses, nutritional status
- **Form:**
  - superficial break
  - sinus
  - cavity
- **Aetiology:**
  - venous/arterial leg ulcer
  - pressure sore*
  - dehisced wound
  - diabetic foot ulcer
  - burns
- **Tissue type:**
  - granulating
  - epithelialising
  - sloughy
  - necrotic
  - clinically infected
- **Size:**
  - length
  - width
  - depth
  - area
- **Exudate:**
  - low
  - medium
  - heavy
- **Pain assessment**
- **General skin condition**

*Calculate pressure sore risk assessment score (National Prescribing Centre 1999).

Local and systemic factors may delay wound healing, increasing the likelihood of scarring.

Chronic wounds

There are great similarities in the principles of managing 'difficult' wounds. In many trusts, local guidelines have been devised in an effort to promote principles of good practice, a systematic approach and multidisciplinary working. In each case, assessment of both the patient and the wound is essential. Careful handling of the part, the use of an aseptic technique and relief of pressure always apply. Selection of an appropriate product or dressing calls for an understanding of the physiological processes involved. Healing can take place only if the patient is adequately nourished and hydrated. Documentation of what has been observed and the actions taken must be carried out. Where no improvement occurs, there must be a willingness to reassess the wound and review the approach being taken.

Leg ulcers. There are many possible causes of leg ulcers, including varicose veins, deep-vein thrombosis, atherosclerosis, diabetes mellitus and rheumatoid arthritis. The majority of leg ulcers have a vascular aetiology – either venous, arterial, or a mixture of the two. Most leg ulcers are venous and are caused by a failure of the valves in the veins. The remainder are arterial or mixed in origin. They are caused by a blockage in one of the smaller arteries causing a lack of blood flow to the area leading to ischaemia and tissue breakdown.

Compression bandaging is commonly used in the treatment of venous leg ulceration reducing pain and oedema and greatly improving the quality of life. Before the application of any compression system, however, an accurate assessment of the patient and the wound, including estimation of the ankle brachial pressure index (ABPI), should be carried out to exclude arterial disease. The ABPI is established using the Doppler ultrasound test. The lower the ABPI is, the greater the severity of lower limb peripheral arterial disease. Compression bandaging is used in the treatment of venous ulcers to assist venous return. It would be totally contraindicated in the management of an arterial ulcer.

Pressure sores. Decubitus ulcers are generally caused by the sustained application of surface pressure over a bony prominence which inhibits capillary blood flow to the skin and underlying tissue. They may also arise as a result of friction, shearing forces or moisture. Risk is further increased when the patient is:

- elderly
- obese
- immobile
- a smoker
- poorly nourished
- sensorily deprived (e.g. paralysis, diabetes).

Careful assessment of the patient and the sore is essential. A variety of scales, e.g. Waterlow, Norton, have been devised to assist the assessment process. Treating the cause is as important as treating the sore. For example, changing position, meeting nutritional requirements and controlling incontinence are vital. A vast range of mattresses and cushions is available to provide comfort and prevent sores from getting worse.

Burn injuries. The cause of a burn may be thermal, chemical or electrical. First aid may involve resuscitative measures, including replacement of lost fluid. The burn should be cooled and then covered using, for example, cling-film. On arrival at hospital, tetanus protection and analgesia will be required. Assessment of the burn surface area guides the physician in terms of fluid and electrolyte loss.

Wound infection and possible septicaemia are a major threat to the burns patient. Warmed sodium chloride solution 0.9% is used to irrigate the burned area. Non-adherent dressings are essential in order to minimise pain and to avoid removing granulating tissue. Additional dressings are required to absorb the exudate from the wound.

Local wound treatments

Two methods are in general use for cleansing wounds – swabbing and irrigation. Swabbing, unless carried out very gently, can damage the wound tissue and may simply redistribute microorganisms in the area of the wound (Morison 1992). This suggests that cleansing should be omitted unless there are clear indications for it to be carried out. Wounds which are obviously contaminated or where there is heavy exudate, crusting or slough require to be irrigated. There is a problem associated with irrigation in that sufficient pressure is needed to remove the debris without at the same time damaging the tissues.

The first-choice solution for wounds that have minimal contamination is either sterile water or physiological saline (Morison 1989). Water is thought to damage tissues, resulting in pain, whereas the use of a physiological solution minimises this risk. If an antiseptic is indicated, care must be taken in balancing bactericidal efficacy against possible damage to healthy tissue. The physical action of the fluid may be what is beneficial rather than any antibacterial activity.

An unconventional method of treating sloughy, necrotic wounds, reintroduced in the 1990s, is the use of sterile larvae (maggots). When applied to devitalised tissue, the maggots secrete powerful proteases that liquefy the slough, which they then suck up. Treatment is confined to the area of slough. After 2–3 days, by which time the maggots have tripled in size, they are washed off with sodium chloride 0.9% solution. With concerns over the increasing incidence of antibiotic resistant bacteria, this form of treatment is of considerable interest.

A range of local treatments is available. These are summarised in Table 28.5. It is emphasised that these products should be used only where clinically indicated.

Surgical dressings

The purpose of a surgical dressing is generally to stem bleeding, absorb exudate and/or provide protection so that healing may be allowed to take place. The ideal wound dressing may be considered in terms of the wound, the patient and the dressing itself.

As far as the wound is concerned (Morgan 1994) the dressing should be:

- of good absorbency, removing excess exudate without allowing 'strike through' to the surface of the dressing
- able to maintain optimal conditions for wound healing, including high humidity at the wound–dressing interface, high thermal insulation properties, and gaseous exchange
- impermeable to microorganisms
- able to provide physical protection for the wound
- free from toxic substances and shedding fibres
- removable without causing damage to the newly formed tissues.

Table 28.5 Local wound treatments and their main indications

Product	Main indications
Aserbine cream	Desloughing agent
Chlorhexidine solutions	Skin disinfectant. The very dilute solutions often used have little antibacterial action. May be combined with cetrimide which provides detergency
Hydrogen peroxide 10 volumes	Wound cleansing and deodorising agent. Not to be used in cavity wounds and ulcers. Very limited antibacterial effect
Povidone-iodine spray	Slow-release iodine preparation. Wide antibacterial spectrum
Sodium chloride solution 0.9%	General cleansing of skin and wounds
Sterile larvae (maggots)	Debridement of wounds that are sloughy, necrotic, infected and malodorous
Varidase Topical powder	Streptokinase–streptodornase used for sloughing ulcers

As far as the patient is concerned, the dressing should be:

- comfortable, offering effective pain relief and providing a feeling of confidence and sense of security
- non-allergenic.

The dressing itself should be:

- in a sterile presentation, preferably a unit pack
- conveniently packaged for ease of removal in aseptic procedures
- compatible with commonly used medicaments
- made so as to allow observation of the wound, and should be radiotranslucent
- economical in use
- easily disposable.

No single product has all the above properties or is suitable for all wound types or at all stages of healing, although dressings developed in the last 25 years combine many of the highly desirable properties listed. Nurses require not only to know what wound care products are available but also to have an understanding of how each of them works.

Classification of dressings

Dressings can be classified under a number of headings but it is unlikely that one classification system will meet all the needs of the nurse. In Table 28.6, dressings are classified broadly according to the materials used in their manufacture. This classification includes an indication of the main properties of the materials.

The work of Winter (1962, 1971) and Bucknell (1984) gave great impetus to the development of surgical

Table 28.6 Classification of dressings

Material	Example(s)	Main properties/comments
Alginates (derived from certain seaweeds)	Kaltostat, Sorbsan	Gel-forming on wound surface; haemostatic; simple alginate sheets may require absorbent backing
Foams	Allevyn, Lyofoam	Presented as a foam sheet with a special wound contact surface
Hydrocolloids	Comfeel, Granuflex, Tegasorb	Gel-forming in contact with wound (gel maintains moist environment at wound surface)
Hydrogels	Geliperm, Sterigel	Provide moist environment which encourages wound healing. Do not provide high absorptive properties. Available as an amorphous form or as a sheet dressing. Very costly for routine use
Vapour-permeable films and membranes	Mepore, Opsite, Tegaderm	Such films protect wound from bacterial contamination and are semipermeable to allow passage of water vapour, thus preventing maceration of wound
Polysaccharides	Debrisan, Iodosorb	Available as beads; draw up tissue exudate. Should be renewed before beads are saturated
Textiles (cotton)	Cotton wool, gauze	Absorptive properties. Do not have any interactive properties

dressings which may be described as interactive. Such dressings, the gels and gel-forming products, interact with the wound to create a 'microclimate' that encourages wound healing. In contrast, the simple woven textiles have no beneficial interactive properties. In the future it is likely that dressings containing biological agents that stimulate the wound-healing process will be developed. According to Miller et al (1995), as cited by Harding et al (2002), the only dressings that correct abnormalities in the healing of chronic wounds are those that contain hyaluronic acid.

Alginates. Alginate dressings are manufactured from a variety of seaweeds which, when they come into contact with blood or exudate, turn into a hydrophilic gel and are thus highly absorbent. Kaltostat may be used in a wide range of heavily exuding wounds, bleeding or non-bleeding. Sorbsan has similar properties.

Foams. Foam dressings are suitable for exuding wounds. There are two types in use. A foam is produced by a chemical reaction. The foam forms to occupy the wound cavity and is both absorbent and non-adherent. Lyofoam is a polyurethane foam sheet one side of which has been heated to form a hydrophilic surface. It creates a moist environment which encourages wound healing and has significant absorptive properties.

Hydrogels. These novel materials contain 96% water. The material is given strength and flexibility by a polymer, polyacrylamide. Geliperm is an example of such material. This interactive dressing provides a moist environment which encourages wound healing. The dressings are very comfortable for the patient and easy to remove. The availability of hydrocolloid dressings and the high cost have limited the use of hydrogel dressings.

Hydrocolloids. Hydrocolloid dressings contain cellulose derivatives which, when they come into contact with the wound, liquefy to produce a pus-like fluid. Examples include Granuflex and Comfeel. As the dressing absorbs moisture from the wound, debridement takes place which may temporarily increase the size of the wound but then allows healing to take place. Although no secondary dressing is necessary, it is important to ensure that the dressing extends at least 2 cm beyond the edge of the wound. In this form of dressing the liquefying process of itself produces a very strong odour, about which the patient should be warned. A bath or shower is still possible since the dressing is waterproof.

Vapour-permeable films and dressings. These synthetic polymer dressings have the advantage of being waterproof, transparent and comfortable. They therefore maintain a moist environment, permit easy observation of the wound and may be used in many sites. Their most appropriate use is for dressing surgical wounds, catheter insertion sites and superficial burns or pressure sores. The heavy exudate associated with leg ulcers and deep pressure sores precludes their use for deep wounds. Examples include Opsite and Bioclusive.

Polysaccharides. Polysaccharides (synthetic sugars) are used in the form of beads, pastes or granules. Debrisan and Iodosorb are examples of bead dressings, which, when placed in contact with a wound, rapidly draw the exudate into the beads, which swell to form a gel.

Dressings require to be changed before the beads become fully saturated, e.g. once or twice a day. They are suitable only for sloughy, exuding wounds. Care must be taken not to spill Debrisan beads on the floor as they are very slippery.

Textiles. Simple absorbent pads such as lint, gauze, and gauze and cotton tissue provide protection, keep wounds warm and are of good absorbency. However, they may adhere to the wound surface and shed fibres into the wound. Microbiological protection is limited. Structured dressing pads which have an outer sleeve of non-adherent material, possess properties similar to those of the various simple absorbent pads but they are generally easier to remove. Some contain a layer of activated charcoal which is useful for deodorising malodorous wounds and ulcers. Tulle dressings are of open weave and are often impregnated with soft paraffin or polyethylene glycol. These are especially suitable in the management of abrasions and superficial burns because of their non-adherent property. They may be impregnated with chlorhexidine or framycetin for an antimicrobial effect.

Selection of a suitable dressing

The challenge for health professionals is to select a dressing or combination of dressings which will suit a particular wound and the stage reached in the healing process. The use of a dressing selector (Table 28.7) may be of assistance. The choice of dressing should be recorded in the patient's notes to ensure continuity of care and assist in the evaluation of treatment.

Prevention of wound infection

The more disturbance, albeit well intentioned, of a wound, the greater the likelihood of introducing infection and healing being delayed. Consequently, dressings should be left in place for as long as possible (Morgan 1994). Apart from achieving high standards of asepsis

Table 28.7 Example of a dressing selector

Wound type	Dressing	Notes
EPITHELIALISING WOUND		
Low exudate	Semipermeable non-adherent dressing or a hydrocolloid	Avoid unnecessary disturbance
Medium to high exudate	Hydrocolloid sheet or alginate sheet	Change every 3 days or earlier if leaking
CLEAN/GRANULATING WOUND		
Shallow – low to moderate exudate	Hydrocolloid sheet or foam sheet dressing	Leave in place for at least 5 days or change earlier if leaking
Cavity, large – low to moderate exudate	Hydrocolloid paste or amorphous hydrogel, with a secondary dressing of either a hydrocolloid sheet or a semipermeable film	Leave in place for at least 5 days or change earlier if leaking
Shallow – moderate to high exudate	Alginate sheet with an absorbent secondary dressing	Change secondary dressing daily, primary every 3 days
Deep or flask-shaped wound – moderate to high exudate	Alginate cavity filling with an absorbent secondary dressing	Change secondary dressing daily, primary every 3 days
Note: Overgranulating wound: use a foam dressing or alternatively use double-layered Granuflex		
WOUNDS WITH SLOUGHY/NECROTIC TISSUE		
Small and superficial	Hydrogel sheet dressing with occlusive backing left in place, unless obvious infection, or hydrocolloid	Leave dressing for at least 3 days. Reclassify at regular intervals. Change daily if obvious signs of infection
Extensive or large deep cavity	Amorphous hydrogel with a secondary dressing of a semipermeable film or a hydrocolloid dressing	Leave 3–5 days or change earlier if leaking. Daily if infection present
INFECTED WOUNDS		
Small and superficial	Antibacterial dressing Amorphous hydrogel with a secondary dressing of a semipermeable film	Short-term use for superficial infections Systemic antibiotics should be used only following laboratory confirmation of infection and sensitivities
If moderate/excessive exudate present	Alginate dressing	For multiresistant organisms (e.g. MRSA etc.) seek advice from infection control team
MALODOROUS WOUNDS		
Moist wounds	Charcoal dressing	Can be used when excess exudate is present
Fungating lesions	Metrotop gel	Fungating malodorous tumours and malodorous gravitational and decubitus ulcers

For further information on types of dressing or on wound management in general, contact your tissue viability/infection control nurse or your pharmacist.

during actual wound care procedures, however, certain preoperative measures are taken to prevent (or reduce the likelihood of) wound infection. Intensive preoperative skin preparation using a well-defined regimen may be commenced 3 days prior to orthopaedic, cardiac, or other forms of surgery, where the infection risk is great and/or where the consequences of infection are especially dangerous for the patient. Such measures will also reduce the possibility of infection becoming established in underlying tissues.

Various forms of systemic therapy may also be used to prevent postoperative wound infection. A course of antibiotic or other form of antimicrobial therapy may be given. Gut irrigation procedures with a solution of antibiotics have also been used preoperatively.

Tissue engineering

Human dermal replacement therapy, developed through advanced tissue engineering, is being used in the treatment of diabetic foot ulcers. The process involves implanting a human-derived dermis made by fibroblast cells and comprising the constituents of healthy human dermis, namely collagen, extracellular matrix proteins and growth factors. Once implanted, the graft stimulates epithelialisation and enhances the healing process. The implications of this revolutionary form of treatment for diabetics and those who provide for them are far-reaching. There is the potential for healing which is more rapid than that achieved by conventional therapy, and a reduction in surgical procedures such as amputation.

The development of proteinase inhibitors, gene therapy, vascular endothelial growth factor and embryonic stem cells as possible means of healing chronic ulcers is the subject of research.

REFERENCES

All Party Parliamentary Group on Skin 1997 An investigation into the adequacy of service provision and treatments for patients with skin diseases in the UK. All Party Parliamentary Group on Skin, London

Aston R, Duggal H et al 1998 Head lice: a report for consultants in communicable disease control (CCDCs). Public Health Medicine Environmental Group Executive Committee

Bucknell T E 1984 Factors affecting wound healing. In: Bucknell T E, Ellis H (eds) Wound healing for surgeons. Baillière Tindall, London, pp 42–74

Harding K G, Morris H L, Patel G K 2002 Healing chronic wounds. British Medical Journal 324:160–163

Hughes E, Van Onselen J (eds) 2001 Dermatology nursing: a practical guide. Churchill Livingstone, Edinburgh

Long C C, Mills C M, Finlay A Y 1998 A practical guide to topical therapy in children. British Journal of Dermatology 138:293–296

Morgan D A 1994 Formulary of wound management products, 6th edn. Euromed Communications, Surrey

Morison M J 1989 Wound cleansing: which solution. Professional Nurse 4(5):220–225

Morison M J 1992 A colour guide to the nursing management of wounds. Wolfe, London

National Prescribing Centre 1999 Modern wound management dressings. Prescribing Nurse Bulletin 1(2):6

Thomas S 1990 Wound management and dressings. The Pharmaceutical Press, London

Winter G D 1962 Formation of the scab and rate of epithelialisation of superficial wounds in the skin of the young domestic pig. Nature 193:293–294

Winter G D 1971 Healing of skin wounds and the influence of dressing on the repair process. In: Harkiss K J (ed) Surgical dressings and wound healing. Crosby and Lockwood, London

FURTHER READING

Barneston R St C, Rogers M 2002 Childhood atopic eczema. British Medical Journal 324:1376–1379

Bellingham C 2001 Proper use of topical corticosteroids. Pharmaceutical Journal 267:377

Cunliffe B 2001 Acne. Pharmaceutical Journal 267:749–752

Harding K G, Morris H L, Patel G K 2002 Healing chronic wounds. British Medical Journal 324:160–163

Kelly C J G, Ogilvie A 2001 Raised cortisol excretion rate in urine and contamination by topical steroids. British Medical Journal 322:594

National Prescribing Centre 1999 Using topical corticosteroids in general practice. MeReC Bulletin 10(6): 21–24

Naumann N, Lowe N J 2001 Botulinum toxin type A in the treatment of bilateral primary axillary hyperhydrosis: randomised, parallel group, double blind, placebo controlled trial. British Medical Journal 323:596–598

Williams H 2002 New treatments for atopic dermatitis. British Medical Journal 324:1533–1534

CHAPTER CONTENTS

29

Anaesthetic agents

INTRODUCTION

Detailed knowledge of individual anaesthetic drugs is necessary only for nurses working in the operating theatre or intensive therapy unit. However, all surgical ward nurses should have an appreciation of what constitutes a modern anaesthetic. Most important of all is an understanding of the drugs used in the pre- and post-anaesthetic management of the surgical patient.

Despite the technological complexity of modern anaesthetic practice, the exact mechanism of general anaesthesia has yet to be elucidated. The fact that compounds as diverse as inorganic gases, ethers and steroids can produce general anaesthesia suggests that their action is non-specific. In contrast, the mode of action of local anaesthetic drugs is well understood: transmission of peripheral nerve impulses is blocked by the reversible 'plugging' of sodium channels, preventing membrane depolarisation.

Both *induction* and *maintenance* of anaesthesia can be achieved by drugs given intravenously or by inhalation. Inhalation agents work by diffusing from the alveoli into the blood flowing through the lungs. In adults, induction is usually by the intravenous route and maintenance by inhalation. The intravenous dose depends on factors such as the patient's age, weight and general health. Babies and young children are often anaesthetised by breathing inhalational agents because it can be difficult to find a vein suitable for cannulation. The needle-phobic adult can be offered inhalational induction with sevoflurane, which is smooth, rapid and not unpleasant. Once the patient is asleep, anaesthesia is usually maintained by a mixture of anaesthetic gases in oxygen.

Depending on the nature of the operation, a patient may either breathe spontaneously, or have the lungs mechanically ventilated while paralysed with a muscle relaxant (or *neuromuscular blocking*) drug.

PREOPERATIVE MEDICATION

In the days of ether and chloroform, premedication was essential. Ether caused profuse salivation and tracheobronchial secretions, and therefore atropine was used routinely as a drying agent. In contrast, chloroform predisposed the patient to dangerous cardiac arrhythmias, and heavy sedation was indicated to minimise the risk.

Sedative drugs are no substitute for explanation and reassurance by nursing staff. However, a benzodiazepine such as temazepam or lorazepam given orally helps patients to relax before going to theatre. Children are sometimes prescribed alimemazine (Vallergan) syrup. The introduction of EMLA cream has allowed pain-free needle insertion. EMLA stands for 'eutectic mixture of local anaesthetic'; it is a white cream containing two local anaesthetic ingredients, lidocaine (lignocaine) and prilocaine. An hour before venepuncture, it is applied to the back of the hand and covered by an occlusive dressing to facilitate penetration into nerve endings in the epidermis. Tetracaine (amethocaine) gel (Ametop) works more quickly but often causes redness of the skin.

Many patients undergoing surgery will be taking medicines for conditions unrelated to their operation. Abrupt discontinuation can have adverse effects. For example, stopping beta-blockers (which slow the heart) can cause rebound arrhythmias and myocardial ischaemia or infarction. The nurse will be guided by the anaesthetist, and should be prepared to administer certain drugs (particularly heart and blood pressure medication) as usual, with sips of water, even if the patient is 'nil by mouth'. On the other hand, oral hypoglycaemic agents should never be given to a fasting patient. Insulin will be administered with dextrose by intravenous infusion. The anaesthetist may prescribe additional medication such as a nitrate patch (e.g. Transiderm-Nitro) for a patient with angina. Patients with asthma should have their salbutamol (or equivalent) inhalers available for use prior to induction of anaesthesia.

Patients who are pregnant or who have a hiatus hernia are at increased risk of inhaling gastric contents, which can cause a fatal pneumonitis. A histamine type 2 receptor antagonist such as ranitidine is given before caesarean section to stop gastric acid secretion. Immediately before induction of anaesthesia, 30 mL 0.3 molar sodium citrate solution is given by mouth to increase the pH of the stomach contents.

INHALATIONAL AGENTS

Nitrous oxide entered medical practice in the 1840s and its use is widespread. However, the 'ideal' inhalational agent has yet to be developed; the features of such an agent are given in Box 29.1.

Box 29.1 Desirable features of an 'ideal' inhalational agent

- It should not form flammable mixtures with oxygen or other agents.
- The vapour should not be unpleasant to inhale.
- The drug should be insoluble in the bloodstream, allowing rapid induction and elimination.
- The drug should be free of organ-specific toxic effects, e.g. renal or hepatic failure, and should not undergo metabolism in the body.
- Depression of the cardiovascular and respiratory systems should be minimal.
- The drug should possess analgesic properties.

Nitrous oxide is supplied in blue cylinders. It is a weak anaesthetic, and has to be administered with at least 30% oxygen. On the anaesthetic machine in the operating theatre, nitrous oxide and oxygen are directed to *vaporisers*, which are filled with potent liquid anaesthetic. Halothane, enflurane, isoflurane, desflurane and sevoflurane are the five agents currently available in the UK. The depth of anaesthesia is varied by altering the concentration of vapour carried by the oxygen and nitrous oxide. A 50/50 mixture of oxygen and nitrous oxide is marketed as Entonox and Equanox. The cylinders have a blue body with a blue and white shoulder. The gas is carried by ambulances for use in emergency situations and is used for analgesia during labour and for short potentially painful procedures such as dressing changes. Some patients feel little effect from breathing the gas, yet others may lose consciousness. Therefore, the mask should always be applied by the patient. Should loss of consciousness occur, the mask will fall away.

INTRAVENOUS AGENTS

Intravenous anaesthesia became established in the 1920s. Again, the 'ideal' agent does not exist, but its features are shown in Box 29.2.

Thiopental, a barbiturate, is still used after half a century, although it has been largely superseded by propofol (Diprivan). Propofol allows a clearer-headed recovery with less nausea or vomiting. In addition, anaesthesia can be maintained by continuous infusion, since recovery is rapid, even after prolonged administration for total intravenous anaesthesia (TIVA). Midazolam (Hypnovel) is an intravenous benzodiazepine used mainly to provide sedation for endoscopies. Flumazenil (Anexate) is a specific benzodiazepine

Box 29.2 Desirable features of an 'ideal' intravenous agent

- The drug should not cause pain on injection.
- Induction of anaesthesia should be rapid and smooth.
- Return of consciousness should also be rapid with no hangover, nausea, vomiting, or unpleasant dreams.
- Depression of the cardiovascular and respiratory systems should be minimal.
- Serious adverse reactions should be extremely rare.

antagonist which reverses its effect. Ketamine increases heart rate and blood pressure, and is favoured for the shocked patient. It is used in military surgery, and for emergency procedures outside hospital such as amputation of a trapped limb. It is rarely used unsupplemented in hospital because recovery is associated with unpleasant dreams and hallucinations, which are minimised if the patient is disturbed as little as possible in the recovery period.

MUSCLE RELAXANTS

Muscle relaxant drugs are used to paralyse a patient's muscles to allow passage of a tracheal tube, to maintain relaxation of the body's muscles for abdominal surgery, and to facilitate artificial ventilation. Suxamethonium chloride (Anectine formerly Scoline) is a particularly short-acting drug. It has a common, unique side-effect: pains in muscles not usually associated with strain after exercise, for example, between the scapulae. The complaint is commonest in the muscular young patient who is up and about soon after the operation. A rarer problem is a genetic deficiency of the enzyme needed to break down the drug and terminate its action. A patient scheduled for a short procedure might have to be kept asleep with the lungs mechanically ventilated for a number of hours until the drug effect wears off. This complication is often called 'Scoline apnoea'. There are a number of other muscle relaxant drugs (Box 29.3) which differ in their onset and duration of action.

ANALGESICS

Opioids are naturally occurring and synthetic drugs which produce morphine-like effects. They act on receptors found in the brain and spinal cord. Short-acting synthetic opioids such as fentanyl, alfentanil and remifentanil are commonly used as components of the anaesthetic. Longer-acting drugs tend to be used for

Box 29.3 Non-depolarising muscle relaxants

Atracurium
Cisatracurium
Mivacurium
Pancuronium
Rocuronium
Vecuronium

Box 29.4 Side-effects of opioids

- Respiratory depression
- Nausea and vomiting
- Dysphoria and hallucinations
- Cough suppression
- Constipation
- Pupillary constriction

postoperative analgesia. There is little to choose between equipotent doses of different opioids; morphine is the reference by which all newer drugs may be judged in terms of analgesic efficacy and side-effects. Box 29.4 lists the side-effects common to all opioids. The potential for causing slowing of breathing and respiratory arrest is by far the most important.

Postoperative analgesia has traditionally been prescribed as a fixed-dose intramuscular injection of opioid, to be given no more frequently than 4-hourly. This regimen is unsatisfactory because it does not allow for patients' enormous differences in analgesic requirements after the same operation. Some patients are reticent about asking for analgesia because of fear of the injection, demonstrating apparent failure to cope, or developing addiction. Moreover, drugs given intramuscularly are not well absorbed when patients are cold after lengthy surgery and skeletal muscle is poorly perfused. If injections are repeated in an attempt to control pain, there is a risk of absorption of dangerously large amounts when the patient warms up.

A major advance in the management of postoperative pain has been the development of patient-controlled analgesia (PCA). In response to pressing a button, the patient receives boluses of opioid by the *intravenous* route. The key to understanding PCA is the 'lock-out interval'; this is the period after a bolus during which any further attempts by the patient to receive opioid will be turned down by the machine. A PCA system might initially be set to deliver a 1 mg bolus of morphine with a lock-out interval of 5 minutes. Since there are 12 × 5 minutes in an hour, the patient would be able to receive a maximum of 12 × 1 mg, i.e. 12 mg per hour.

Box 29.5 Contraindications to NSAIDs

- Renal impairment, dehydration or hypovolaemia
- Bleeding abnormalities or risk of postoperative bleeding
- History of peptic ulcer or gastrointestinal bleeding
- Asthma known to be worsened by aspirin or NSAIDs

Were this to prove inadequate, the anaesthetist would administer a further loading dose and increase the bolus setting. The safety of PCA relies on *only* the patient pressing the button. Dihydrocodeine 60 mg 4-hourly (maximum 240 mg/24 h) is an effective oral opioid for the patient being weaned from intravenous morphine.

Patients' pain, degree of sedation and respiratory rate should be evaluated and recorded as routinely as pulse and blood pressure. Wherever opioids are administered, naloxone (Narcan), which is a specific antagonist, should be immediately available.

Non-steroidal anti-inflammatory drugs (NSAIDs) work by inhibiting enzymes involved in mediating pain from damaged tissue. Diclofenac (Voltarol) and ketorolac (Toradol) are related to aspirin. Their advantage is that there is no risk of respiratory depression. They can be given *in addition to* opioids, improving the quality of postoperative analgesia and reducing the required dose of opioid with its concomitant side-effects. However, there are important contraindications (Box 29.5).

Diclofenac (Voltarol) suppositories are well absorbed. The rectal route avoids the potentially serious complications of intramuscular injection: nerve damage and abscess formation. Regular doses of paracetamol 1 g (orally or rectally, 6-hourly) can be given *in addition* to an NSAID. Both paracetamol and NSAIDs have an 'opioid-sparing' effect, i.e. they reduce the requirement for morphine.

ANTI-EMETICS

Nausea and vomiting are frequent minor complications of surgery and anaesthesia. A number of factors contribute to its likelihood (Box 29.6).

Table 29.1 lists examples of anti-emetic agents and their respective modes of action. Ondansetron is the most effective, although more expensive than the others. It is therefore usually prescribed as a 'second-line' drug.

LOCAL ANAESTHETICS

Local anaesthetics (Box 29.7) work by blocking conduction of nerve impulses conveying pain. The various agents have different durations of action and toxicity. They can be injected anywhere from the site of the incision (local infiltration) to the cerebrospinal fluid (spinal block). Local anaesthetics can contribute to analgesia following most operations. If catheters are inserted close to nerves running from the area of the operation (e.g. brachial plexus for hand surgery) analgesia can be maintained for as long as is necessary by topping up with local anaesthetic when pain returns. Bupivacaine (Marcain) acts longer than lidocaine (lignocaine), although it is more toxic in overdose. There is less risk of CNS or cardiac toxicity after inadvertent intravascular injection of levobupivacaine compared with bupivacaine. Epidurals are increasingly being used for postoperative analgesia following major abdominal, vascular and thoracic surgery. Drugs are injected via a catheter to bathe the nerves outside the spinal cord. Side-effects

Box 29.6 Factors contributing to postoperative nausea and vomiting

- The age of the patient (twice as likely in children) and sex (women have higher incidence, greatest in weeks 3 and 4 of the menstrual cycle)
- History of motion sickness or vomiting after previous anaesthetic
- Whether anti-emetics are given during anaesthesia
- Which anaesthetics/analgesics are used (opioids increase the incidence)
- Type of operation (e.g. laparoscopy, squint, or middle ear surgery have high incidence)
- Adequacy of postoperative analgesia

Table 29.1 Anti-emetic agents and their actions

Agent	Action
Cyclizine (Valoid)	Antihistamine
Hyoscine (Scopolamine)	Anticholinergic
Metoclopramide (Maxolon)	Dopamine antagonist (benzamide)
Ondansetron (Zofran)	5-HT_3 antagonist
Prochlorperazine (Stemetil)	Dopamine antagonist (phenothiazine)

Box 29.7 Local anaesthetics

Lidocaine (lignocaine) (Xylocaine)
Prilocaine (Citanest)
Bupivacaine (Marcain)
Levobupivacaine (Chirocaine)
Ropivacaine (Naropin)

of epidurals include hypotension (due to block of sympathetic nerves and treatable with ephedrine), urinary retention and block of motor nerves causing inability to move the legs. The doses necessary for epidural use can be reduced by mixing the local anaesthetic with opioid. Prilocaine (Citanest), the least toxic local anaesthetic, is used for Bier's block. This is a technique which facilitates hand or forearm surgery (a common procedure is reduction of a Colles' fracture). The arm is held up in order to drain its blood and a tourniquet is inflated. Local anaesthetic is then injected into a vein on the back of the hand. It is crucial that the tourniquet is not released for at least 20 minutes, in order to prevent a large toxic dose of local anaesthetic entering the circulation. The symptoms and signs of local anaesthetic toxicity relate to the drug reaching the brain and heart by either excessive absorption into the bloodstream or inadvertent injection into a blood vessel (Box 29.8).

Treatment of local anaesthetic toxicity

The *immediate* treatment is to call for help, clear the airway and administer 100% oxygen. Ventilation must be started at once if the patient has stopped breathing. With effective oxygenation, cardiac arrest ought not to occur. However, if a patient develops intractable ventricular fibrillation following bupivacaine, bretylium tosylate (5–10 mg/kg) might be effective in restoring normal rhythm.

Box 29.8 Symptoms and signs of local anaesthetic toxicity

Symptoms
- Numbness of tongue or lips
- Light-headedness
- Tinnitus
- Anxiety

Signs
- Slurring of speech
- Drowsiness
- Convulsions
- Cardiorespiratory arrest

FURTHER READING

Cox F 1999 Systematic review of ondansetron for the prevention and treatment of postoperative nausea and vomiting in adults. British Journal of Theatre Nursing 9(12):556–566

Dawson L, Brockbank K, Carr E C J et al 1999 Improving patients' postoperative sleep: a randomised control study comparing subcutaneous with intravenous patient-controlled analgesia. Journal of Advanced Nursing 30(4):875–881

Duncan K, Pozehl B 2000 Effects of performance feedback on patient pain outcomes. Clinical Nursing Research 9(4):379–401

Gunta K, Lewis C, Nuccio S 2000 Prevention and management of postoperative nausea and vomiting. Orthopaedic Nursing 19(2):39–48

Slowikowski R D, Flaherty S A 2000 Epidural analgesia for postoperative orthopaedic pain. Orthopaedic Nursing 19(1):23–33

CHAPTER CONTENTS

30 Palliative care

INTRODUCTION

Where there is advanced disease with no curative treatment, emphasis must be placed on the palliation of symptoms so as to allow the best possible quality of life for patients and their family (WHO 1990). Inpatient hospice care and domiciliary nursing services are provided by charitable organisations such as Macmillan Cancer Relief and Marie Curie Cancer Care, often in association with health authorities, whose staff are specially trained in palliative care.

Palliative care requires multidisciplinary effort. Its essential components are:

- symptom control
- effective communication
- rehabilitation
- continuity of care
- support in bereavement
- education
- research (O'Neill & Fallon 1997).

In palliative care, dying is considered to be a normal process. It is neither hastened nor postponed. Relief from pain and other distressing symptoms is of prime importance. Physical, psychological, social and spiritual aspects of care are integrated to allow the patient to live as actively as possible. Support for the family is provided during the patient's illness and in their own bereavement.

PAIN

Although palliative care is made up of several different but complementary elements, the effective relief of pain is perhaps the major challenge facing clinical staff. The treatment of acute and chronic pain resulting from relatively uncomplicated conditions presents few problems. (Specific pain relief regimens are dealt with in the text where appropriate.) In contrast, the relief of chronic

Table 30.1 Products used for the relief of pain

Product groups	Examples	Availability
Non-opioids	Aspirin	Tablets
	Paracetamol	Tablets, suppositories
	NSAIDs	Tablets, injections, suppositories, local applications
	Nefopam	Tablets, injection
Weak opioids – limited place in treatment of mild/moderate pain	Co-proxamol	Tablets
	Dihydrocodeine	Tablets, injection
Strong opioids (long-acting)	Buprenorphine*	Tablets, injection
	Morphine	Tablets, oral solution, injection, suppositories
	Diamorphine	Tablets, injection
	Hydromorphone	Normal-release and controlled-release capsules
	Phenazocine	Tablets, injection, suppositories
	Oxycodone	Suppositories
	Fentanyl	Transdermal patch
Strong opioids (short-acting) – not recommended in palliative care	Dextromoramide	Tablets, suppositories
	Dipipanone	Tablets (in combination with cyclizine)
	Pethidine	Tablets, injection
	Pentazocine*	Capsules, injection, suppositories

*Antagonistic effects if used in combination with other opioids and therefore best avoided.
A number of combination products are also available, e.g. paracetamol with a small dose of codeine. Soluble tablets are also available in a number of instances.

pain in, for example, inoperable cancer requires a high degree of specialist skill. Chronic pain presents in many ways and seldom arises from clearly defined anatomical sites. Multiple pains are often reported by patients with advanced malignant disease. In addition to having pain, the patient may feel depressed and demoralised. Sleep may be prevented. The pain may 'spill over' and affect the patient's family and friends. Just as the presentation of pain can vary, so too can the causes of pain and the sites involved. The treatment chosen will be greatly influenced by the nature of the pain.

As with any treatment programme, it is vitally important to take a careful history and to recognise that the patient will have the expectation of becoming pain-free without reduction in mental alertness. The patient's previous experience may result in fear due to the expectation of pain. Tensions may result which can greatly increase the patient's pain and associated problems. Opportunity should be given to talk over worries and fears. A basic principle is to seek to anticipate crises and avoid having to resort to injections if at all possible. A wide range of products is available for the relief of pain. This reflects the great variation in the presentation and severity of pain. Table 30.1 indicates the range of commonly used products.

Assessment of pain

The basis of successful palliative care is assessment. At an appropriate time and without tiring the patient, details of how the illness began and how the patient and the patient's family have coped with it, should be established.

Assisting the patient in the completion of some form of pain assessment tool can help to identify the location of the pain, when it arises and its exact nature. The effect of medication or any other activity which helps, as well as those things that make the pain worse, can be recorded. The severity and the nature of the pain can vary and so it is essential that these are continually reviewed and, where necessary, modifications made to the treatment regimen.

Treatment of pain

The management of pain in malignant disease and palliative care is underpinned by the World Health Organization's analgesic ladder (WHO 1990). The steps of the ladder represent the severity of the pain and the level of drug therapy required. The choice of therapy thus depends on the severity of the pain. Mild pain is treated with a *non-opioid* analgesic drug such as aspirin or paracetamol in therapeutic dosages at regular intervals (see Table 30.2). If pain persists or worsens after the maximum recommended dosage has been reached, a *weak opioid* such as co-proxamol or dihydrocodeine is added so that both drugs are being given on a regular basis (see Table 30.3). If this does not relieve the pain, a *strong opioid* such as morphine sulphate or diamorphine is substituted for the weak

Table 30.2 Non-opioids

Drug	Adult dose/route	Notes
Aspirin	300–900 mg orally every 4–6 hours. Maximum daily dose 4 g	Common ingredient of many proprietary preparations patients may buy. Careful drug history may reveal multiple analgesic use. Gastric irritation may be a problem – should be given after food, and antacids may be prescribed. Soluble forms may be more acceptable to the patient. Risk of drug interactions. Bronchospasm and skin reactions have been reported in hypersensitive patients. Often given in combination with codeine in co-codaprin tablets. Enteric-coated tablets available
Paracetamol	500 mg–1 g orally every 4–6 hours. Maximum total daily dose 4 g	Liver damage is a major concern following overdosage (see p. 139). Available in various forms, including a paediatric elixir and suppository. Doses for children must be carefully assessed
Nefopam	60 mg orally three times daily. Can increase to 90 mg. 20 mg IM every 6 hours	Dose should be reduced to 30 mg in elderly patients
Naproxen	500 mg twice-daily *after food*	See page 401
Ibuprofen	400 mg orally, 8-hourly with or after food	NSAID of choice for treatment of pain associated with inflammation. Diclofenac is a more potent alternative
Diclofenac	75–150 mg orally, 8-hourly, after food, 75–150 mg PR daily in divided doses, 75 mg IM up to twice daily	As with all oral NSAIDs, monitor for signs of gastric irritation

Table 30.3 Weak opioids

Drug	Adult dose/route	Notes
Co-proxamol	2 tablets every 4–6 hours. Maximum 8 tablets in 24 hours	Used for moderate pain – alone or in combination with a non-opioid analgesic
Dihydrocodeine	30–60 mg 4-hourly	

Table 30.4 Strong opioids

Drug	Adult dose/route	Notes
Morphine sulphate	See Table 30.5	Drug of choice
Diamorphine	Approximately one-third of dose of oral morphine	Highly soluble; small-volume injection
Fentanyl	Initial dose '25' patch replaced after 72 hours; otherwise dose based on previous 24-hour opioid requirement	Used for chronic intractable pain Available as 25, 50, 70, 100 microgram/hour strengths
Hydromorphone	1.3 mg oral 4-hourly	Alternative to morphine
Oxycodone	10 mg oral twice a day. Maximum 200 mg twice a day	Alternative to morphine

opioid (see Table 30.4). If a particular drug fails to relieve the patient's pain, it should be replaced by one from a higher step up the ladder and not simply changed to another of the same.

At each step of the ladder, adjuvant therapy in the form of drugs such as corticosteroids, antidepressants, anxiolytics and phenothiazines which enhance the effect of analgesics, or radiotherapy may or may not be used.

Strong opioid analgesics

Extensive experience has shown that strong opioids are the most valuable drugs in achieving pain relief for many cancer patients with severe pain. Morphine remains the drug of choice for many reasons which are summarised in Box 30.1. The advantages obtained by using morphine far outweigh the disadvantages, some of which are more imagined than real. One notable benefit of morphine is that, as well as being highly effective in relieving pain, it confers a state of mental detachment (see Box 30.1).

The overall aim of treatment is to keep the patient pain-free and alert by keeping the plasma concentration of drug *continually* within the patient's own effective zone. This is achieved by *regular* administration of the selected dose of the chosen strong opioid. The determination of dose will depend on the patient's previous history of analgesic use, and renal function, as outlined in Table 30.5.

Dosage levels. It may be necessary to increase the dose by titration to the patient's pain. Sequential increments will be required depending on current dosage, as indicated in Table 30.6.

Box 30.1 Advantages and disadvantages of morphine

Advantages
- Highly effective in reasonable dose
- Active orally
- Wide range of presentations available, e.g. oral solutions, tablets (including slow-release tablets), injection and suppositories
- Widely available
- Relatively inexpensive
- Side-effects manageable
- Extensive literature/research findings

Disadvantages
- Controlled drug – record keeping
- Causes constipation
- 'Morphine myths'. There are still concerns in the minds of some clinicians that morphine causes respiratory depression, addiction, tolerance and euphoria. As a result, it may be considered as a drug of 'last resort'. In fact, these perceived problems are seldom seen where morphine (and other strong opioids) are used in the treatment of cancer pain.

Strong opioids may be increased stepwise. There is no general limit as to how much the patient can take. However, where there is renal impairment care should be taken to avoid accumulation of the morphine metabolite M6G (morphine-6-glucuronide).

Dosage intervals. Regular administration (4-hourly) is essential to ensure continuous relief of pain. Modified-release preparations provide relief when given at 12-hourly or daily intervals. Careful adjustment of dosage can help to ensure that the patient has the benefit of a pain-free, undisturbed night's sleep.

Administration. Whenever possible, the oral route should be used since it allows the patient to maintain some degree of analgesia control and is preferable to the pain caused by injections into an often emaciated patient. Oral morphine is prepared as a solution, suspension, tablets and capsules.

Vomiting or dysphagia may make it impossible, however, to administer opioids by mouth, and/or the patient may be too weak or drowsy to cope safely with this method. Acute breakthrough pain is another indication for changing to another method. A summary of non-oral routes of administration of opioids is given in Table 30.7.

In the last few days or hours of life, alternatives to the oral route will often have to be considered. Where there is no choice but to give a strong opioid parenterally, the subcutaneous route is preferred since it is the least painful method. Diamorphine is very often chosen in preference to morphine because a very small quantity of diluent is required to reconstitute the

Table 30.6 Dosage increments of morphine

Morphine dosage (4-hourly)	Dosage increment
5 mg, 7.5 mg	2.5 mg
10 mg	5 mg
20 mg	10 mg
30 mg	15 mg
60 mg	30 mg

Table 30.5 Determination of morphine dose

Patient's analgesic history	Dose of morphine (oral)
Previously controlled on non-opioid	5 mg* morphine every 4 hours
Previously controlled on weak opioid	10 mg* morphine every 4 hours
Previously on other strong opioids	Equivalent dose of morphine, e.g. the conversion factor for pethidine is 0.125, i.e. 100 mg pethidine = 12.5 mg morphine. If the pain was poorly controlled, the equivalent morphine dose should be increased by 50%
Poor renal function	Doses given (see * above) should be reduced by 50%
Poor hepatic function	Severe hepatic failure has an effect on morphine metabolism but it is rare to need to reduce the dose of morphine on this account

powder formulation. The use of an ambulatory pump allows continuous subcutaneous infusion treatment to be delivered and a steady concentration of analgesia to be achieved without the need for repeated injections.

Breakthrough pain arising while the patient is receiving either morphine or diamorphine, should be treated with one-sixth of the total daily dose of the drug in use, as required.

Side-effects of opioids. The common adverse effects of opioid drugs are dry mouth, constipation, sedation, and nausea and vomiting.

Although the mechanism is unclear, there is a clear association between the use of morphine and dryness of the mouth (White et al 1989). A supply of quenching drinks, pieces of soft fruit, boiled sweets, ice cubes, etc. is needed to provide ongoing relief. Oral hygiene is of paramount importance.

Opioid analgesia is notorious for its constipating effect, and so in almost every case laxatives should be prescribed prophylactically and to be given regularly. As the disease progresses and the dose of opioid has to be increased, the dose of laxative should also be increased.

Patients should be warned about drowsiness, which is always particularly evident at the outset of treatment or following an increase in dose but does not normally persist after the first few doses.

Nausea in particular may be anticipated, and a centrally acting anti-emetic such as haloperidol may be given at bedtime. Nausea is an initial side-effect and usually resolves after a few days.

Cautions. There are a number of cautions, including hypotension, asthma, prostatic hypertrophy, and hepatic and renal impairment but these should not be a deterrent to the use of morphine in terminal illness.

Adjuvant drug therapy. Opioid drugs are, in some patients, ineffective in dealing with particular types of pain, and more specific treatment may be required. Table 30.8 outlines some of the drugs used as adjuncts.

Table 30.7 Non-oral routes for opioids

Route	Notes
Intravenous or intramuscular	Suitable where relief of pain can be achieved by 4-hourly injections. Greater frequency than this is not acceptable. Diamorphine is more soluble than morphine and the dose can be given in a smaller volume of water. Diamorphine can be combined with certain drugs, e.g. levomepromazine (methotrimeprazine)
Rectal	Morphine can be given rectally in doses similar to oral doses. The rectal route may not be acceptable to some patients
Intrathecal	Combination of low-dose strong opioid and bupivacaine can be given intrathecally. This treatment is suitable for ambulant patients, but spinal catheter care requires special skills
Transdermal	Fentanyl is available as skin patches. Transdermal systems are expensive and have a slow onset of action. Careful conversion from oral morphine is necessary to achieve equivalent dose

Table 30.8 Drugs used as adjuncts for control of pain

Drug	Adult dose	Indications/notes
Amitriptyline	25–75 mg at night orally	Useful in pain of neuropathic origin. Anticholinergic side-effects may cause problems in higher doses
Carbamezepine	100–200 mg every 6–8 hours orally, increasing if necessary to 1.2 g daily in divided doses	Similar indications to amitriptyline. Side-effects include GI disturbances and visual disturbances. If necessary, blood level monitoring can be used as a basis for dosage adjustment
Dexamethasone	Up to 8 mg twice daily by mouth. Dose should be reduced to lowest level that will control symptoms	Particularly useful for relieving pain by reducing inflammation which may cause nerve compression or raised intracranial pressure. Other benefits of dexamethasone include appetite stimulation. Major side-effects associated with corticosteroids may occur
Hyoscine butylbromide	20–60 mg by subcutaneous infusion over 24 hours	Smooth muscle spasm in bowel or ureter
Baclofen	10 mg every 8 hours, increasing slowly up to 100 mg daily; given after food	Spasm of skeletal muscle. Side-effects may be troublesome. These include sedation, drowsiness, nausea, ataxia, headaches and tremor
Dantrolene	25 mg daily	May be worthwhile alternative to baclofen where this drug is poorly tolerated
Diazepam	2–15 mg daily	Higher dose may be too sedating

A variety of other forms of therapy are used to relieve pain, promote relaxation and enhance well-being in the terminally ill patient. Treatment which may be used to complement drug therapy includes transcutaneous electrical nerve stimulation, nerve block, progressive muscle relaxation and body massage.

Use of syringe drivers in palliative care

Analgesics in palliative medicine with or without accompanying agents such as anti-emetics, sedatives or anticholinergics are commonly administered by the subcutaneous, epidural or intrathecal route using a syringe driver, set at a fixed rate normally measured in millimetres per hour (see also p. 86). This method of administration is indicated when the patient has difficulty in swallowing, is vomiting, has an intestinal obstruction or has diarrhoea affecting absorption. It may be used when the patient is semiconscious or unconscious.

Ambulant patients are not restricted since the device is lightweight and may be carried and concealed in a holster. It is especially useful in palliative care as it reduces the need for repeated injections and provides a steady-state concentration of drug in the plasma.

Care must be taken to observe for and respond to any signs of inflammation at the infusion site which would be painful and interfere with absorption of the medication.

When setting up a syringe driver, the same care is needed as with the administration of any medication. The drug(s) should be drawn up in a small amount of diluent as prescribed, using a 20 mL syringe. Water for Injections is normally used as there is less likelihood of precipitation, although a few drugs (e.g. ketamine, ketorolac, octreotide) must be diluted with sodium chloride 0.9% solution. Using the appropriate diluent is important in reducing the risk of incompatibility and inflammation at the chosen site. Further diluent is drawn up, measured against a ruler with a millimetre scale and then used to prime the tubing. Details of the contents of the syringe should be entered on the additive label, which is then attached to the syringe (and not the driver). Great care must be taken to place the syringe safely in the driver with the actuator release button moved into place. The rate should be carefully checked.

The needle is inserted at an angle of 45° into the anterior aspect of the upper arm or thigh or into the anterior chest or abdominal wall. While the infusion is in progress, 4-hourly assessment of the patient's pain should be carried out. At the same time, the infusion site should be checked for signs of inflammation or leakage and the syringe and tubing checked for cloudiness of contents. Checks should be made and recorded of the rate setting and the volume of fluid remaining. The number of millimetres of content should tally with the length expected. Unless there are problems, the site may last for up to 1 week.

As with all infusion devices, care must be taken to handle the equipment carefully. It should not be allowed to get wet and the progress of the plunger must not be impeded in any way. The driver may be encased in a plastic bag while the patient is bathing/ showering.

Box 30.2 Compatible combinations of drugs and diamorphine

Diamorphine + metoclopramide + dexamethasone
Diamorphine + midazolam + hyoscine hydrobromide
Diamorphine + metoclopramide + midazolam
Diamorphine + cyclizine* + hyoscine hydrobromide
Diamorphine + levomepromazine* (methotrimeprazine) + hyoscine hydrobromide

*May cause irritation at injection site.

Preparations given via syringe driver

Diamorphine is the opioid of choice for subcutaneous injection (see p. 73) and, if required for more than 24 hours, for subcutaneous infusion also. If the patient has been receiving oral morphine, the equivalent dose of diamorphine is calculated as one-third of the morphine dose.

Only certain drugs may be mixed with diamorphine and only in certain combinations (see Box 30.2). At times, two syringe drivers may be needed.

SYMPTOMS OTHER THAN PAIN

While pain relief is the cornerstone of care in terminal illness, it is vitally important not to neglect other symptoms that may trouble the patient. Indeed, the alleviation of symptoms such as anxiety and depression can raise the pain threshold enabling the amount of analgesia to be reduced. An outline of drugs used to relieve these other symptoms is given in Table 30.9.

GI symptoms

Nausea and vomiting

Nausea is a distressing symptom at any time whether or not the patient vomits. In turn, it leads to loss of appetite and loss of weight.

Table 30.9 Symptom relief in palliative care

Symptom	Drug	Dose/route/frequency	Notes
GASTROINTESTINAL TRACT			
Nausea/vomiting	Dexamethasone	8–16 mg oral or injection daily for 5 days, then 4–6 mg daily	Reduces intracranial pressure
	Cyclizine	50 mg oral 8-hourly	Used if nausea and vomiting caused by bowel obstruction or raised intracranial pressure
	Metoclopramide	10 mg oral 6-hourly	Used when nausea and vomiting caused by GI disorders, cytotoxics or radiotherapy
	Domperidone	10–20 mg oral 6-hourly	Used in functional dyspepsia and where nausea and vomiting caused by cytotoxics or radiotherapy
	Mebeverine hydrochloride	135 mg oral 8-hourly	Useful in treating colic
	Hyoscine butylbromide	20–60 mg SC in 24 hours	Useful in treating colic
	Dicycloverine (dicyclomine)	10–20 mg oral 8-hourly	Useful in treating colic
	Haloperidol	1.5 mg oral once or twice daily	Used if nausea and vomiting is caused by e.g. hypercalcaemia, renal failure
	or		
	Prochlorperazine	20 mg oral, then 10 mg after 2 hours, then 5–10 mg every 8–12 hours	Reduces intestinal secretions
	Levopromazine (methotrimeprazine)	6.25–25 mg oral every 4–8 hours	Powerful, broad-spectrum anti-emetic
	Ondansetron	4 mg oral twice daily	Used for treatment-induced emesis
Anorexia	Prednisolone	15–30 mg oral daily	
	Dexamethasone	2–4 mg oral daily	
	Metoclopramide	10–20 mg oral before meals	Useful where fullness or heartburn is the problem
Constipation relief	Glycerin suppository	One, once only	Stool softener and mild irritant
	Phosphate enema	One, once only	Useful where lower colon and rectum contain soft faeces
	If unsuccessful Arachis oil enema	One, once only, at night	Given as retention enema (foot of bed elevated) to soften faeces impacted higher up. Stimulant laxative may be given next morning
	Sodium citrate micro-enema	One, once only	Small volume (5 mL) stimulant
			Alternatively, manual evacuation done under sedative/analgesia cover
Prevention of constipation	Dantron suspension capsules	 10 mL oral at night 1–2 oral at night	Stimulant laxative and stool softener. Should be started whenever opioid analgesia prescribed
	Docusate sodium (capsules or solution)	Up to 500 mg oral daily in divided doses	Stimulant laxative and stool softener
	Senna tablets	2–4 at night	Stimulant laxative
Diarrhoea	Loperamide	4 mg initially, then 2 mg oral after each loose stool up to 16 mg daily	Antimotility effect
	Codeine phosphate	30 mg oral every 6–8 hours	Antimotility effect
Dysphagia	Mucaine	10 mL hourly *or* 15 minutes before meals	Local anaesthetic
	Dexamethasone	8 mg	Corticosteroid used temporarily to shrink tumour if causing obstruction

(*continued*)

Table 30.9 *(continued)*

Symptom	Drug	Dose/route/frequency	Notes
Hiccup	Chlorpromazine	10–25 mg oral every 6–8 hours	May be used for intractable hiccup. Warn patient of sedative effect
	or		
	Haloperidol	1.5 mL oral 8-hourly	Dose adjusted according to response
	Metoclopramide, dimeticone	10 mg oral or IM 8-hourly	Alone or added to an antacid to relieve flatulence
	Peppermint water	20 mL as required	Relieves colic and distension
	Granulated sugar	One or two heaped teaspoonfuls as required	Eaten as the granules
	Baclofen	10 mg oral or IM every 6–8 hours	Used for intractable hiccup
	or		
	Nifedipine	20 mg oral 12-hourly	Used for intractable hiccup
Mouth problems	Chlorhexidine gluconate mouthwash 0.2%	10 mL for 1 minute twice daily	Cleansing
	Povidone-iodine mouthwash 1%	10 mL for 30 seconds up to four times daily	Cleansing
	Vitamin C effervescent	1 g tablet broken on tongue	Cleansing
	Nystatin suspension	200 000 units (2 mL) 4-hourly. Lozenges available	Antifungal – prevention of candida
	Nystatin suspension	500 000 units (5 mL) 4-hourly for 5 days	Antifungal course for immunocompromised patient
	Fluconazole	500 mg oral daily	Dentures also require to be treated
	Aciclovir	200 mg oral five times daily. Cream also available	Antiviral – treatment of herpes simplex
	Choline salicylate gel	Applied 3-hourly	Topical analgesic
	Benzocaine compound lozenges	To suck	Potent local anaesthetic. Available direct from manufacturer
	Glandosane oral spray	As required	Artificial saliva; flavoured
RESPIRATORY TRACT			
Dyspnoea	*If airways reversibility*		
	Salbutamol	2.5–5 mg via nebuliser 4-hourly	Salbutamol and ipratropium may be nebulised together
	Ipratropium	250–500 micrograms via nebuliser 4-hourly	
	otherwise		
	Morphine sulphate (injection)	5 mg/mL with 4 mL sodium chloride 0.9% solution via nebuliser over 10 minutes	Alternatively, diamorphine hydrochloride may be used via nebuliser. If already on morphine, dose should be increased 20–50%
	Need for anxiolytic		
	Diazepam	2–5 mg oral 8-hourly	
	or		
	Lorazepam	1–4 mg SL daily	Sublingual route used for rapid onset
	Acute severe dyspnoea		
	Midazolam	2.5–5 mg by slow IV injection (over 3–5 minutes) followed by lorazepam as above	
	Bronchospasm or partial obstruction		
	Dexamethasone	4–8 mg oral daily	
Intractable cough	Simple linctus	5 mL oral 4-hourly	
	or		
	Codeine linctus	10 mL oral 4-hourly	
	or		

(*continued*)

Table 30.9 *(continued)*

Symptom	Drug	Dose/route/frequency	Notes
	Morphine solution	2.5–5 mg oral 4-hourly	If already on morphine, increase dose by 20–30%. May be too sedating
	Bupivacaine (injection)	5 mL (0.25%) via nebuliser 4-hourly	May block cough receptors and paralyse gag reflex
	Dexamethasone	Up to 16 mg oral daily in divided doses (last dose no later than 18.00 (6 p.m.)	Especially useful in relief of cough caused by pleural, pericardial or diaphragmatic irritation
	Hyoscine hydrobromide	400–600 micrograms SC every 2–4 hours (or even half-hourly) *or* 600 micrograms–2.4 mg by SC infusion in 24 hours	Used to treat excessive respiratory secretions
	or		
	Hyoscine butylbromide	20–60 mg in 24 hours	Fewer central side-effects
SKIN			
Pruritus	Emulsifying wax 3% in water		Soap substitute
	Aqueous cream	Apply frequently as required	Emollient; soap substitute
	Chlorphenamine (chlorpheniramine)	4–8 mg oral three times a day	Antihistamines with sedating effect help the patient to get a night's sleep
	Promethazine	25–30 mg oral at night	
	Cetirizine	10 mg oral daily	Non-sedating antihistamine. Available as a liquid
	or		
	Fexofenidine	180 mg oral daily	Non-sedating antihistamine
	or		
	Stanozol	5–10 mg oral daily	Anabolic steroid
Sweating	Any agent with an anticholinergic effect		
CENTRAL NERVOUS SYSTEM			
Insomnia	Temazepam	10–40 mg oral at bedtime	Short-acting hypnotic with little hangover effect
Anxiety	Haloperidol	1–3 mg oral 8-hourly	
	Chlorpromazine	25–50 mg oral 8-hourly	Causes more sedation
	Diazepam	2 mg oral 8-hourly	
Confusion	Haloperidol	1–3 mg oral 8-hourly	
	or		
	Chlorpromazine *alternatively*	25–50 mg oral 8-hourly	More sedating than haloperidol
	Levomepromazine (methotrimeprazine)	50–200 mg by SC infusion in 24 hours	Used for severe restlessness
	or		
	Haloperidol	5–30 mg by SC infusion in 24 hours	
	Extreme restlessness Midazolam	20–40 mg by SC infusion in 24 hours	Sedative and antiepileptic
Depression	Amitryptiline	25–100 mg oral at night	
	Clomipramine	25–100 mg oral at night	
	Sertraline	50–150 mg oral daily	
	Venlafaxine	75–150 mg oral daily	

Careful assessment is needed to elicit any underlying cause which may be treatable – such as hypercalcaemia, oropharyngeal thrush, constipation or urinary tract infection. Prescription sheets should be examined to identify any medicine which could be the source of the problem. Nausea is an acknowledged side-effect of morphine. Changes in presentation (e.g. rectal, or by injection instead of oral) may help. Where nausea and vomiting persist, there is no alternative but to prescribe an anti-emetic. The choice is made on the basis of cause and the site of action of the specific anti-emetic. Since there may be more than one cause of nausea and vomiting, more than one anti-emetic may be required.

Anorexia

Often no reason can be found for loss of appetite in terminal illness. If an underlying cause can be found it should be treated. Causes range from a dry mouth, ill-fitting dentures and oral thrush to drug treatment, chemotherapy/radiotherapy and hypercalcaemia. Meals should be small and light, consist of what the patient fancies and be served when the patient asks for something to eat. Some patients may like and benefit from an aperitif in the form of sherry, whisky or brandy. There may be a place for the use of appropriate nutritional adjuncts on the advice of the dietitian. Relatives understandably are disappointed and distressed when the patient has no interest in food and so they may need encouragement of a different sort at this time.

Constipation

Difficulty in moving the bowels is common in cases of advanced cancer and is a major cause of anxiety and discomfort. As always, it is essential to carry out a thorough assessment before embarking on treatment. This may include a rectal examination to establish whether the rectum is full. Note should be taken of any faecal smearing suggestive of overflow. Faecal impaction can lead to many other problems including urinary retention, overflow, restlessness, confusion and falls, each one leading to the next. Evidence of intestinal obstruction should be reported at once and any measures to relieve constipation withheld until the patient has been examined by a doctor.

Drug treatment is the commonest cause of constipation, especially where opioids such as morphine or codeine-containing substances are being used. In terminal illness, laxatives should be begun along with opioid treatment, or for anyone receiving antimuscarinics. As the opioids are increased, so too should be the dose of laxative.

The choice of laxative and dose should be tailored to each patient's needs. Most patients will benefit from a faecal softener with a peristaltic stimulant. However, some difficulties can be experienced with certain laxatives. For example, bulking agents require a lot of fluid, and the amount required may be difficult to achieve in terminally ill patients. Moreover, motility is affected by opioids – with the result that bulking agents become less effective. High doses of lactulose, an osmotic laxative, can cause abdominal distension and flatulence, and make the patient feel dizzy; to be effective it has to be taken every 24–48 hours. It is not considered to be the best choice of laxative. Dantron colours the urine red which may cause skin irritation if left in prolonged contact with the skin. It is therefore unsuitable for patients troubled with urinary incontinence.

Diarrhoea

Before treating diarrhoea, it is important first to exclude the most common causes, namely, excessive use of laxatives, impaction with overflow, and diet. Profuse watery diarrhoea can leave the patient dehydrated and exhausted. A high intake of fluid is essential and the patient will need as much rest and assistance as required.

Dysphagia

Patients may have difficulty in swallowing because it is painful to do so (e.g. in oesophageal thrush) or because there is a partial obstruction (e.g. in oesophageal spasm or carcinoma), in which case food will be regurgitated. Mealtimes are no longer enjoyable, and yet the patient may still have a desire to eat. Weight may be lost quickly and the patient starts to feel weak.

Hiccup

Terminally ill patients sometimes develop persistent hiccup caused by gastric distension, which is exhausting. It interferes with eating, speaking and sleep, and may be a source of disturbance for others.

Mouth problems

Problems in or around the mouth are often a great source of discomfort to the dying patient. There may be problems in keeping the mouth clean and frequent attention is important. The mouth may be dry and make for difficulty in speaking and eating. Some drugs, notably morphine sulphate and antimuscarinics such as hyoscine, may make the mouth feel dry. Bacterial, viral or fungal infections of the mouth may cause severe pain and difficulty in swallowing. Halitosis may be a source of embarrassment to patients and/or their families (see also p. 435).

Respiratory symptoms

Dyspnoea

As with all other symptoms in terminal illness, any underlying cause should be treated if possible. For example, if there is evidence of airways reversibility, bronchodilators may be used. Otherwise, opioids are used to control dyspnoea.

If the patient is already receiving morphine, for example, the morphine dose should be increased. Nebulised drugs require little effort by the patient and are often helpful. There may be a place for using anxiolytics in some patients.

Positioning the patient in bed with the help of suitably placed pillows or nursing the patient comfortably in an upright chair instead of in bed creates a challenge for the nurse. Methods of promoting relaxation should be provided. Loose clothing, an open window or a fan may assist. Fluids and oral care may have to be increased to relieve dryness of the mouth caused by mouth breathing and oxygen therapy.

Intractable cough

Like hiccup, a persistent cough can be painful and distressing, leaving the patient exhausted and others disturbed. Simple linctuses may be tried as well as moist inhalations. Oral morphine hydrochloride solution may be needed and is given initially as 5 mg every 4 hours.

Skin symptoms

Pruritus

Itching of the skin is a troublesome feature of terminal illness and can be the source of irritability and disturbed sleep. Especially problematic is itching due to obstructive jaundice, which may be extremely persistent and difficult to manage in some patients and yet mysteriously vanish in others. A soap substitute should be used when bathing.

Sweating

Underlying causes such as anxiety, menopausal flushing, infection and thyrotoxicosis should be excluded. Hot drinks and hot baths should be avoided. The patient may be tepid sponged if unable to take a cool shower. Clothes and bedding should be made of cotton and changed as soon as they are damp. The patient may appreciate having the hair washed or at least dried. The use of a single room may allow the environmental temperature to be controlled without upsetting other patients. A bedside fan may offer some relief if carefully positioned. Care must be taken to prevent chilling the patient. Cold drinks and oral hygiene are important.

CNS symptoms

Insomnia

It is important to assess the situation fully and to establish what 'difficulty in sleeping' means to the individual patient. Any obvious causes should be treated. Patients should be discouraged from taking naps during the day and should stick to their normal bedtime. Various methods of relaxation may be utilised. Stimulant drugs should be used only in the early part of the day. A milky drink free from caffeine may help before going to bed. As well as a quiet, comfortable environment, peace of mind is essential.

Anxiety

Listening is of paramount importance. Patients will need reassurance about their worries and fears, and the meaning of their symptoms. Drug treatment takes second place to identifying and dealing with the underlying cause of the patient's anxiety.

Confusion

Where it can be identified, the underlying cause should be treated. There are many possible reasons why a patient may be confused including hypoxia, cerebral metastases, infection, hypercalcaemia, uraemia and constipation. Confusion may also be drug-induced or result from withdrawal from a drug.

A quiet, well-lit room should be provided and care delivered in a calm, reassuring manner. Staff should introduce themselves and explain any procedure before they begin. Relatives will also require understanding care.

Depression

It is important to recognise that the patient may become clinically depressed at this time. Emotional support and encouragement will be needed. Antidepressant therapy generally takes about 3 weeks to take effect.

Many patients respond to this type of treatment, although not all.

Ascites

The development of peritoneal metastases from primary tumours of the bronchus or breast results in the distressing accumulation of fluid in the peritoneal cavity known as ascites. A slow reduction in the ascites may be achieved with the administration of spironolactone 200–400 mg daily by mouth or furosemide (frusemide) 40–80 mg daily by mouth. For quicker effect, these drugs may be given in combination.

REFERENCES

O'Neill B, Fallon M 1997 Principles of palliative care and pain control. British Medical Journal 315:801–804

White I D, Hoskin P J, Hanks G W et al 1989 Morphine and dryness of the mouth. British Medical Journal 298:1222–1223

World Health Organization (WHO) 1990 Cancer pain relief and palliative care. WHO, Geneva

FURTHER READING

Doyle D (ed) 1986 International symposium on pain control. Royal Society of Medicine Services Limited, London

Kinghorn S, Gamlin R (eds) 2001 Palliative nursing: bringing comfort and hope. Baillière Tindall, Edinburgh, in conjunction with the Royal College of Nursing

Modern Medicine Postgraduate Partwork Series. Palliative care. February 1990. Caring for the dying patient at home. Modern Medicine, London

Montgomery F 2002 Pain management in palliative care. Pharmaceutical Journal 268:254–256

Regnard C F B, Tempest S 1992 A guide to symptom relief in advanced cancer, 3rd edn. Haigh and Hochland, Manchester

Russell K 1992 Pharmacology of pain. Surgical Nurse 5(6):18–22

Glossary and Appendices

SECTION CONTENTS

Glossary

Absorption. Process by which a drug reaches the general circulation and becomes biologically available.

ACE inhibitors. Drugs which act on the renin–angiotensin–aldosterone system, inhibiting the angiotensin-converting enzyme.

Active immunisation. Injection of an antigen in the form of live or attenuated organisms or their products to provide protection against certain infections.

Active transport. Cellular activity that transfers a drug from an area of low concentration to one of higher concentration.

Addiction. Inability to control craving for a drug.

Additive. Substance added to, for example, an existing solution.

Adjunctive therapy. An added substance, not essentially part of the treatment.

Adjuvant. Substance included in the formulation of a medicine to improve stability of the dosage form.

Adjuvant therapy. The simultaneous use of different forms of treatment, e.g. drugs with other types of drugs, drugs with radiotherapy and/or surgery.

Adsorption. The taking up of a liquid or vapour on the surface of a solid.

Adverse drug reaction. Any response to a drug which is noxious or unintended and occurs at doses used for prophylaxis, diagnosis or therapy (see also Side-effect).

Aerobe. An organism which can only live and grow in the presence of free oxygen.

Agonist. Drug with an affinity for a receptor resulting in stimulation of the receptor's functional properties.

Alkylating drugs. Cytotoxic agents that act by providing an unbreakable link between the strands of DNA, thus blocking cell replication.

Allergy. Hypersensitivity reaction to an intrinsically harmful substance varying from a mild form to severe life-threatening.

Ampoule. A sterile glass or plastic container that contains a single dose of a solution to be administered parenterally.

Anaerobe. An organism which can only live and grow in the absence of oxygen.

Analogue. A drug that resembles another in structure and constituents but has different effects.

Anaphylaxis. Life-threatening reaction to a foreign protein or other substance.

Antagonist. An agent that exerts an opposite action to an agonist.

Anticoagulant. Substance which delays or prevents clotting of the blood.

Anticholinergic drug. Substance which competes with the neurotransmitter acetylcholine for its receptor sites at synaptic junctions.

Antimuscarinic drug. Substance which inhibits the stimulation of postganglionic fibres.

Antimetabolites. Cytotoxic agents that mimic the respective partners for purines and pyrimidines and because of imperfect pairing arrest the development of new DNA.

Apoptosis. Programmed cell death.

Attenuated. Reduction of virulence of a microorganism with retention of antigenic properties.

Bactericidal. Destroying bacteria.

Bacteriostatic. Inhibiting growth or multiplication of bacteria.

Beta-blocker. Agent that inhibits the action of catecholamines at beta-adrenergic receptor sites.

Bioavailability. Amount and rate of appearance of a drug in the blood after administration of the dosage form.

Buccal. Between the gum and the cheek.

Chemotherapy. Treatment using drugs – generally used when referring to cytotoxic therapy.

Clinical pharmacy. Discipline concerned with application of pharmaceutical expertise to help maximise drug efficacy and minimise drug toxicity in individual patients and patient populations.

Colloid. Microscopic insoluble particles.

Compliance. The extent to which the patient's behaviour coincides with medical or health advice.

Concordance. Partnership between prescriber and patient where there are shared objectives aimed at achieving a therapeutic outcome.

Controlled drug. Drug of addiction subject to strict regulatory control.

Cycloplegic. An agent that causes paralysis of the ciliary muscle of the eye used prior to ophthalmic examination or surgery.

Crystalloid. Microscopic solute particle.

Cytotoxic. Capable of destroying cells.

Diuretic. A drug which increases the manufacture of urine by the kidneys.

Drug. Substance used to prevent, diagnose or treat disease.

Excipient. Substance mixed with a medicine to provide consistency, bulk or stability of a formulation.

Enteral. Via the intestine.

Enteric coating. An acid-resistant coating of tablets or compounds which prevents release of active ingredient(s) until the dosage form reaches the alkaline medium of the small intestine where release and absorption takes place.

Extemporaneous. One-off production of a preparation to meet an individual patient's requirement.

Extravasation. Escape of body fluid (usually blood) from a vessel into the surrounding tissues.

Femtolitre. A thousand-million-millionth of a litre (10^{-15}).

Fingertip unit. Amount of cream or ointment (steroid preparations) expressed from a tube with a standard 5-mm diameter nozzle, applied from the distal crease to the tip of the adult index finger.

First-pass effect. Effect, caused by metabolism of a drug mainly by the liver, resulting in only part of the drug reaching the systemic circulation.

Formulary. Approved list of pharmaceutical items for routine use together with information to assist in rational prescribing.

Formulation. Form in which a medicine is made up, e.g. tablet, capsule, solution, suspension, etc.

Gene therapy. Treatment of diseases by insertion into the body of genetic material.

Half-life. Time taken for a drug to lose 50% of its effect in a person's body.

Hickman catheter. Example of a device used to access a central vein for the infusion of large amounts of fluid and irritant substances, and for obtaining blood samples.

Hydrophilic. Associating freely with water and readily entering into aqueous solution.

Hygroscopic. Absorbing moisture from the air.

Hypercalcaemia. Abnormal increase of calcium in the blood.

Hyperglycaemia. Abnormal increase in blood glucose level.

Hyperkalaemia. Abnormal increase of potassium in the blood.

Hypernatraemia. Abnormal increase of sodium in the blood.

Hypersensitivity reaction. Exaggerated response to a drug.

Hypertonic. Of a solution, having a higher osmotic pressure than a specified solution.

Hypocalcaemia. Abnormal reduction in blood calcium level.

Hypoglycaemia. Abnormal reduction in blood glucose level.

Hypokalaemia. Abnormal reduction in blood potassium level.

Hyponatraemia. Abnormal reduction in blood sodium level.

Hypotonic. Of a solution, having a lower osmotic pressure than a specified solution.

Iatrogenic. Of a condition, caused by treatment.

Idiosyncracy. An individual's unique hypersensitivity to a particular drug.

Immunoglobulin. Humoral antibody produced by the blood.

Inotropic. Controlling muscular contraction especially in the heart.

Intrathecal. Within the subarachnoid space.

Loading dose. Initial dose of a drug which is twice the maintenance dose given, to allow the effective blood concentration to be reached promptly.

Medicine. Formulation of a drug into a suitable preparation for administration.

Microgram. One-thousandth of a milligram.

Milligram. One-thousandth of a gram.

Monoclonal. Pertaining to a group of cells derived from a single cell.

Mydriatic. A drug that dilates the pupil of the eye by contraction of the muscle of the iris.

Nanogram. One-thousandth of a microgram.

Nosocomial infection. Hospital-acquired infection.

Over-the-counter medicines. Medicines available without a prescription.

Palliative. Providing relief as opposed to a cure.

Parenteral. Other than the alimentary canal; by injection.

Passive immunisation. Injection of antibodies from immunised animals against the invading organism.

Pharmaceutical care. Direct pharmaceutical contribution to patient care.

Pharmacokinetics. Study of actions of drugs within the body.

Pharmacology. The science of drugs.

Pharmacy. Concerned with preparing, compounding, dispensing and safe use of medicines.

Picogram. A million-millionth of a gram.

Piggyback technique. Method of administering intermittent intravenous medication via a small secondary container attached by tubing to a primary infusion line.

Placebo. Inactive substance prescribed as if it were an effective medication dose, e.g. in clinical trials.

Polymer. One of a series of substances alike in composition but differing in molecular weight.

Polypharmacy. Use of many different drugs in treatment of disease.

Polysaccharide. A carbohydrate that hydrolyses into more than one molecule of simple sugars.

Potency. Of a drug, the relative amount of a drug required to produce the desired response.

Prophylaxis. Disease prevention.

Proprietary drug. Any pharmaceutical preparation protected from commercial competition by trademark.

Recreational drug. One that is used for its stimulating psychological or physical effects with no therapeutic intent.

Scheduled drugs. Drugs classified by legislation into categories known as schedules (of which there are five) according to their potential to cause harm if abused.

Shared-care protocol. Signed agreement between hospital specialist and general practitioner which clearly defines roles and responsibilities when a patient requires care from both hospital and primary care.

Side-effect. Undesirable, unwanted or unexpected effect of a drug administered within the therapeutic range (see also Adverse drug reaction).

Subcutaneous. Fatty layer beneath the dermis of the skin.

Sublingual. Under the tongue.

Sympathomimetic. Mimicking the sympathetic nervous system by producing similar effects.

Systemic. Pertaining to the whole body.

Tolerance. Ability to endure a substance without it causing physiological or psychological harm.

Topical. For local effect; often used to refer to a drug applied to the skin.

Vasoconstriction. Narrowing of the lumen of blood vessels.

Vial. Small glass rubber-capped container holding a drug either as a liquid or as a powder for reconstitution.

Xanthine. Nitrogenous by-product of metabolism of nucleoproteins, normally found in muscles, liver, spleen, pancreas and the urine.

Appendix 1

Abbreviations

ABVD	adriamycin, bleomycin, vinblastine, DTIC
ACAG	acute closed-angle glaucoma
ACBS	Advisory Committee on Borderline Substances
ACE	angiotensin-converting enzyme
ACTH	adrenocorticotrophic hormone
AIDS	acquired immune deficiency syndrome
APTT	activated partial thromboplastin time
ART	assisted reproduction therapy
AZT	zidovudine (azidothymidine)
BCG	bacille Calmette–Guérin
BEAM	BCNU, etoposide, cytarabine, melphalan
BEP	bleomycin, etoposide, cisplatin
BIPP	bismuth iodoform paraffin paste
BM-test	Boehringer–Mannheim reagent strips for blood glucose monitoring
BNF	British National Formulary
BP	British Pharmacopoeia
BPC	British Pharmaceutical Codex
CAPD	continuous ambulatory peritoneal dialysis
CAV	cyclophosphamide, adriamycin, vincristine
CCK-PZ	cholecystokinin-pancreozymin
CD	controlled drug
CFCs	chlorofluorocarbons
ChlVPP	chlorambucil, vinblastine, procarbazine, prednisolone
CHOP	cyclophosphamide, adriamycin, vincristine, prednisolone
CIVAS	central intravenous additive service
CMF	cyclophosphamide, methotrexate, fluorouracil
CMV	cytomegalovirus
COC	combined oral contraception
COSHH	control of substances hazardous to health
COX	cyclo-oxygenase
CSM	Committee on Safety of Medicines
CTZ	chemoreceptor trigger zone

CVP	cyclophosphamide, vincristine, prednisolone
D&TC	Drug and Therapeutics Committee
DdATP	dideoxyadenosine triphosphate
ddC	zalcitabine
DDC	zalcitabine
ddCTP	dideoxycytidine-5-triphosphate
ddI	didanosine
DDI	didanosine
dL	decilitre
DMARD	disease-modifying antirheumatic drug
DMSO	dimethylsulphoxide
DNA	deoxyribonucleic acid
DT	diphtheria/tetanus
DTP	diphtheria/tetanus/pertussis
DUMP	disposal of unwanted medicines and pills
e/c	enteric-coated
FBC	full blood count
fL	femtolitre
FTU	fingertip unit (adult)
g	gram
G6PD	glucose-6-phosphate dehydrogenase
GABA	gamma-aminobutyric acid
G-CSF	granulocyte-colony stimulating factor
GFR	glomerular filtration rate
GP10	General Practitioner prescription
GSL	General Sale List
HBP(A)	hospital-based prescribers' form (Scotland)
HDCV	human diploid cell vaccine
HDL	high-density lipoprotein
HFAs	hydrofluoroalkanes
Hib	*Haemophilus influenzae* type b
HIV	human immunodeficiency virus
HRT	hormone replacement therapy
HT	hydroxytryptamine
HTBS	Health Technology Board for Scotland
ID	intradermal
IDDM	insulin-dependent diabetes mellitus
IM	intramuscular
INHAL	inhalational
INR	international normalised ratio
IOP	intraocular pressure
IPV	inactivated poliomyelitis vaccine
ISA	intrinsic sympathomimetic activity
IV	intravenous
kg	kilogram
L	litre
LDL	low-density lipoprotein
LFTs	liver function tests
MAOI	monoamine-oxidase inhibitor
MBC	minimum bactericidal concentration
MCA	Medicines Control Agency
mg	milligram
MIC	minimum inhibitory concentration
MIMS	Monthly Index of Medical Specialities
mL	millilitre
MMR	mumps/measles/rubella
MOPP	chlormethine (mustine), vincristine, procarbazine, prednisolone
m/r	modified-release
MRSA	methicillin-resistant *Staphylococcus aureus*
MST	morphine sulphate tablets
NEFA	non-esterified fatty acid
ng	nanogram
NG	nasogastric
NHS	National Health Service
NICE	National Institute for Clinical Excellence
NIDDM	non-insulin-dependent diabetes mellitus
NMC	Nursing and Midwifery Council
NNRTIs	non-nucleoside reverse transcriptase inhibitors
NPF	Nurse Prescribers' Formulary
NSAID	non-steroidal anti-inflammatory drug
OGTT	oral glucose tolerance test
OPV	oral poliomyelitis vaccine
ORS	oral rehydration salts
ORT	oral rehydration therapy
OTC	over-the-counter
PCA	patient-controlled analgesia
PEFR	peak expiratory flow rate
PEG	percutaneous endoscopic gastrostomy
pg	picogram
PGD	patient group direction
POAG	primary open-angle glaucoma
PODs	patients' own drugs
PoM	prescription-only medicine
POP	progestogen-only pill
PPD	purified protein derivative
PPI	proton pump inhibitor
PR	per rectum
PTT	partial thromboplastin time
PUVA	psoralen + long-wave ultraviolet irradiation
PV	per vaginam
PVA	polyvinyl alcohol

RCV rubber-capped vial
RIMA reversible inhibitor of monoamine-oxidase A
rINN recommended International Non-proprietary Name
RNA ribonucleic acid
RT reverse transcriptase

s/c sugar-coated
SC subcutaneous
SI units Système International
SIGN Scottish Intercollegiate Guidelines Network
SL sublingual
SPF sun protection factor
SSRI selective serotonin reuptake inhibitor

Tab tablet
TENS transcutaneous electrical nerve stimulation
TIVA total intravenous anaesthetic
TPN total parenteral nutrition

U and Es urea and electrolytes
UVA ultraviolet radiation (long wavelength)
UVB ultraviolet radiation (medium wavelength)

WBC white blood count

CHAPTER CONTENTS

Appendix 2

Normal values

BIOCHEMICAL

Venous blood: approximate adult reference values

Acid phosphatase	
Total	up to 12 IU/L
Prostatic	up to 4 IU/L
Alkaline phosphatase	30–120 IU/L
Bicarbonate	22–30 mmol/L
Bilirubin	0–17 micromol/L
Calcium	2.26–2.60 mmol/L
Chloride	95–105 mmol/L
Cholesterol	
Male	2.5–7.9 mmol/L
Female	2.5–8.8 mmol/L
Copper	12–26 micromol/L
Creatinine	
Male	50–100 micromol/L
Female	50–80 micromol/L
Glucose (fasting)	2.9–6.4 mmol/L
Iron	
Male	14–32 mmol/L
Female	10–28 mmol/L
Iron-binding capacity	45–72 mmol/L
Lactate dehydrogenase (LDH)	100–300 IU/mL
Magnesium	0.70–1.20 mmol/L
pH	7.36–7.44
Phosphate	0.80–1.45 mmol/L
Potassium	3.4–5.2 mmol/L
Proteins	
Total	60–80 g/L
Albumin	35–58 g/L
Sodium	133–144 mmol/L
Urea	2.5–7.5 mmol/L

Uric acid	
Male	0.15–0.42 mmol/L
Female	0.10–0.36 mmol/L

HAEMATOLOGICAL

Venous blood: approximate adult reference values

Erythrocyte sedimentation rate (ESR)	0–6 mm in 1 hour
Fibrinogen	150–400 mg/dL
Folate	2.1–21 micrograms/L
Haemoglobin (Hb)	
Male	13–18 g/dL
Female	11.5–16.5 g/dL
Leucocytes: differential count	
Neutrophils	2.5–7.5 × 10^9/L
Lymphocytes	1.5–3.5 × 10^9/L
Monocytes	0.2–0.8 × 10^9/L
Eosinophils	0.015–0.1 × 10^9/L
Basophils	0.04–0.44 × 10^9/L
Mean cell haemoglobin (MCH)	27–32 pg (1.7–2.0 pg/cell)
Mean cell haemoglobin concentration (MCHC)	30–35 g/dL
Mean cell volume (MCV)	78–98 fL
Packed cell volume (PCV)	
Male	0.40–0.54
Female	0.35–0.47
Platelet count	150–400 × 10^9/L
Prothrombin time (PT)	10–14 seconds
Reticulocytes	0.2–2.0% of red blood cells
Vitamin B_{12}	120–600 micrograms/L

Arterial blood: approximate adult reference values

Carbon dioxide (P_aCO_2)	4.8–6.0 kPa (36–45 mmHg)
Oxygen (P_aO_2)	11–13 kPa (83–98 mmHg)

Index

A

B

C

D

E

F

I

M

N

O

Q

R

S

T

U

V

W

X

Y

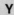

Z